Atlas of
Surgical Techniques for the Colon, Rectum, and Anus

Other Volumes in the Surgical Techniques Atlas Series

Atlas of **Endocrine Surgical Techniques**
Edited by Quan-Yang Duh, MD, Orlo H. Clark, MD, and Electron Kebebew, MD

Atlas of **Breast Surgical Techniques**
Edited by V. Suzanne Klimberg, MD

Atlas of **Surgical Techniques for the Upper Gastrointestinal Tract and Small Bowel**
Edited by Jeffrey R. Ponsky, MD, and Michael J. Rosen, MD

Atlas of **Thoracic Surgical Techniques**
Edited by Joseph B. Zwischenberger, MD

Atlas of **Cardiac Surgical Techniques**
Edited by Frank W. Sellke, MD, and Marc Ruel, MD

Atlas of **Minimally Invasive Surgical Techniques**
Edited by Ashley H. Vernon, MD, and Stanley W. Ashley, MD

Atlas of **Pediatric Surgical Techniques**
Edited by Dai H. Chung, MD, and Mike Kuang Sing Chen, MD

Atlas of Surgical Techniques for the Colon, Rectum, and Anus

A Volume in the Surgical Techniques Atlas Series

Editors

James W. Fleshman, Jr., MD
Professor of Surgery
Chief
Section of Colon and Rectal Surgery
Washington University School of Medicine
St. Louis, Missouri

Elisa H. Birnbaum, MD
Professor of Surgery
Section of Colon and Rectal Surgery
Washington University School of Medicine
St. Louis, Missouri

Steven R. Hunt, MD
Assistant Professor of Surgery
Section of Colon and Rectal Surgery
Washington University School of Medicine
St. Louis, Missouri

Matthew G. Mutch, MD
Associate Professor of Surgery
Section of Colon and Rectal Surgery
Washington University School of Medicine
St. Louis, Missouri

Ira J. Kodner, MD
Professor of Surgery
Section of Colon and Rectal Surgery
Washington University School of Medicine
St. Louis, Missouri

Bashar Safar, MD
Assistant Professor of Surgery
Section of Colon and Rectal Surgery
Washington University School of Medicine
St. Louis, Missouri

Series Editors

Courtney M. Townsend, Jr., MD
Professor and John Woods Harris Distinguished Chairman
Robertson-Poth Distinguished Chair in General Surgery
Department of Surgery
The University of Texas Medical Branch
Galveston, Texas

B. Mark Evers, MD
Professor and Vice-Chair for Research
Department of Surgery
Markey Cancer Foundation Endowed Chair
Director
Markey Cancer Center
University of Kentucky
Lexington, Kentucky

SAUNDERS
ELSEVIER

ELSEVIER
SAUNDERS

1600 John F. Kennedy Blvd.
Ste 1800
Philadelphia, PA 19103-2899

ATLAS OF SURGICAL TECHNIQUES FOR THE COLON, RECTUM, AND ANUS ISBN: 978-1-4160-5222-7

Library of Congress Cataloging-in-Publication Data

Atlas of surgical techniques for the colon, rectum, and anus / editors, James W. Fleshman ... [et al.].
p. ; cm.—(Surgical techniques atlas series)
Includes bibliographical references and index.
ISBN 978-1-4160-5222-7 (hardcover : alk. paper)
I. Fleshman, James. II. Series: Surgical techniques atlas series.
[DNLM: 1. Colon—surgery—Atlases. 2. Anal Canal—surgery—Atlases. 3. Rectum—surgery—Atlases. WI 17]
LC classification not assigned
617.5′547—dc23 2012017975

Executive Content Strategist: Michael Houston
Content Development Specialist: Rachel A. Miller
Publishing Services Manager: Patricia Tannian
Senior Project Manager: Linda Van Pelt
Design Direction: Steve Stave

Printed in China
Last digit is the print number: 9 8 7 6 5 4 3 2 1

Contributors

Elisa H. Birnbaum, MD
Professor of Surgery
Section of Colon and Rectal Surgery
Washington University School of Medicine
St. Louis, Missouri

James W. Fleshman, Jr., MD
Professor of Surgery
Chief
Section of Colon and Rectal Surgery
Washington University School of Medicine
St. Louis, Missouri

Steven R. Hunt, MD
Associate Professor of Surgery
Section of Colon and Rectal Surgery
Washington University School of Medicine
St. Louis, Missouri

Ira J. Kodner, MD
Professor of Surgery
Section of Colon and Rectal Surgery
Washington University School of Medicine
St. Louis, Missouri

Anne Y. Lin, MD
Assistant Professor
Colon and Rectal Surgery
David Geffen School of Medicine at UCLA
Los Angeles, California

Matthew G. Mutch, MD
Associate Professor of Surgery
Section of Colon and Rectal Surgery
Washington University School of Medicine
St. Louis, Missouri

Bashar Safar, MD
Assistant Professor of Surgery
Section of Colon and Rectal Surgery
Washington University School of Medicine
St. Louis, Missouri

FOREWORD

"A picture is worth a thousand words."

This atlas is for the practicing surgeon, surgical residents, and medical students for review of and preparation for surgical procedures. New procedures are developed and old ones are replaced as technologic and pharmacologic advances occur. The topics presented are contemporaneous surgical procedures with step-by-step illustrations, along with preoperative and postoperative considerations as well as pearls and pitfalls, taken from the personal experience and surgical practice of the authors. Their results have been validated in their surgical practices involving many patients. Operative surgery remains a manual art in which the knowledge, judgment, and technical skill of the surgeon come together for the benefit of the patient. A technically perfect operation is the key to this success. Speed in operation comes from having a plan and devoting sufficient time to completion of each step, in order, one time. The surgeon must be dedicated to spending the time to do it right the first time; if not, there will never be enough time to do it right at any other time. Use this atlas; study it for your patients.

"An amateur practices until he gets it right; a professional practices until she can't get it wrong."

Courtney M. Townsend, Jr., MD
B. Mark Evers, MD

Preface

The idea to develop an atlas of the common operative procedures performed by colon and rectal surgeons was stimulated by a need to have a clear, pictorial reference for residents-in-training in colon and rectal surgery. As time constraints increase for residency training and opportunities to gain experience become less available during general surgical residency, colon and rectal surgeons are faced with a limited time to cover all aspects of colon and rectal surgery with trainees. This text, an atlas, relies on actual photographs of critical steps and critical views to instruct trainees step by step in the common operations performed for colorectal diseases.

My colleagues in the Section of Colon and Rectal Surgery at Washington University have contributed their expertise, time, and love of teaching to this project. For that, I am very grateful, and I am very proud that we could develop a tool that may improve our ability to reach our residents-in-training.

The use of an atlas for common colorectal operations should not be limited to colorectal residents-in-training but should be available to general surgery residents, who are also under the same time constraints. These operations are performed in almost every tertiary care institution across the country, where many of the training programs are found for both general surgery and colon and rectal surgery. It is our hope that this book will be used by trainers, educators, and program directors to improve the preoperative preparation of our residents. This preoperative preparation can enhance the intraoperative experience of the trainee and is therefore paramount to improving efficiency of training for the future. In a future edition, we hope to add more procedures and to enhance the current photographic atlas with a video atlas.

I would like to acknowledge the efforts of Dr. Jonathan Chun (during his clinical research fellowship) and Mr. Oscar Wolff in obtaining and categorizing the numerous photographs for this project. I would also like to acknowledge the extraordinary efforts and time dedicated to this project by Liz Nordike, our administrative assistant and office manager at Washington University. As always, each of us owes a great debt of gratitude to our families, who have tolerated our tardiness, physical absence, and sometimes mental absence during the writing of this book. We hope the residents of future generations find this helpful. Finally, we would like to thank Drs. Townsend and Evers for the concept and for their ongoing support for the atlas.

James W. Fleshman, Jr., MD

Contents

Atlas of
Surgical Techniques for the Colon, Rectum, and Anus

CHAPTER 1

Open Right Colectomy

Steven R. Hunt

Step 1: Clinical Anatomy

The right colon lies on the patient's right side suspended laterally by peritoneal attachments to the right side of the abdominal wall, superiorly by attachments to the undersurface of the liver and posterior diaphragm, and medially by its mesentery. The ileocolic artery and vein and the right colic vessels, if they are present, run through this leaf of mesentery. The colon is adherent to the retroperitoneum on the right side of the abdomen and covers the right gonadal vessels and right ureter. The inferior vena cava is the next most medial structure on the right side. The hepatic flexure, the fold at the junction between the right colon and transverse colon, is adherent to the anterior surface of the kidney by avascular attachments to Gerota's fascia. The first and second portions of the duodenum are adherent to the undersurface of the mesentery of the right colon and proximal transverse colon. The gallbladder is sometimes adherent to the cephalad surface of the transverse colon at the hepatic flexure. The space behind the right colon is triangular shaped with the flat horizontal surface at the hepatic flexure running from the abdominal side wall toward the midline along the line of the greater curve of the stomach. The vertical axis follows the right lateral side wall of the abdomen. The hypotenuse runs from the fusion plane of the cecum at the pelvic brim over the top of the right iliac artery and vein at about the point where the ureter passes over the iliac vessels toward the midline over the aorta up to the base of the pancreas along the third portion of the duodenum. This triangular retroperitoneal area is a potential space with avascular attachments and allows the right colon to be lifted completely from the retroperitoneum during dissection. Release of all suspensory attachments allows the right colon to be made into a midline structure. The ileocolic artery and vein arise from the superior mesenteric artery (SMA) and superior mesenteric vein in the midportion of the SMA below the duodenum. The right colic artery is a variable structure and may be present as a separate structure or as part of the ileocolic trunk. The right branch of the middle colic artery exits through the pancreatic tissue from its origin on the SMA as a portion of the middle colic trunk at the base of the transverse mesocolon (Figure 1-1).

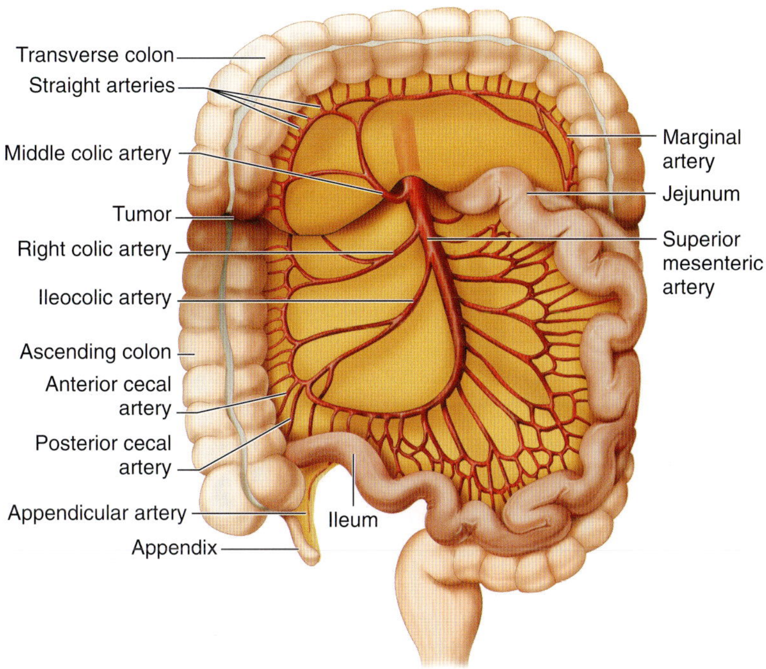
Transverse colon
Straight arteries
Middle colic artery
Tumor
Right colic artery
Ileocolic artery
Ascending colon
Anterior cecal artery
Posterior cecal artery
Appendicular artery
Appendix
Ileum
Marginal artery
Jejunum
Superior mesenteric artery

Figure 1-1

Step 2: Preoperative Considerations

Right colectomy is most commonly performed for neoplastic disease or inflammatory bowel disease, such as Crohn's disease. The patient requires very few preoperative preparations. Prophylactic antibiotics are appropriate for a colectomy to reduce the risk of wound infection. A mechanical bowel preparation is not necessary for a right colectomy. However, most patients seem to do better with clear liquids before an operation. Patients require routine deep vein thrombosis prophylaxis and instructions on postoperative care.

Step 3: Operative Steps

- The patient is placed in the supine position with sequential compression devices on the calves, Foley catheter in place, and the arms stretched to the side for access to the vessels and for blood pressure monitoring. General endotracheal anesthesia is required. An oral gastric tube helps decompress the stomach during the procedure.
- A vertical midline incision is made from the epigastrium to the mid low pelvis; a Bookwalter retractor (Codman, Raynham, Mass.) is placed for exposure with the abdominal incision stretched widely.
- The right colon is lifted from the pelvis, and a hand is placed from the medial aspect of the abdomen under the peritoneal attachments of the terminal ileum and right colon at the level of the pelvic brim and the white line of Toldt, or the peritoneal attachments along the right gutter are stretched over the index finger (Figure 1-2). The peritoneal attachments are incised with electrocautery to expose the duodenum at the base of the mesentery of the right colon. The right colon is lifted up and medially (Figure 1-3).
- The right colon is pulled toward the left leg, the space that has been generated over the top of the duodenum is developed bluntly up to the undersurface of the liver, and the suspensory peritoneal attachments along the base of the liver toward the gallbladder are incised with electrocautery (Figure 1-4).
- The attachments of the gastrocolic omentum are divided along the cephalad surface of the transverse colon outside the gastroepiploic arcade of the omentum between ties. The omentum is completely released, allowing the posterior aspect of the stomach and the entire lesser sac to be seen (Figure 1-5*A* and *B*).

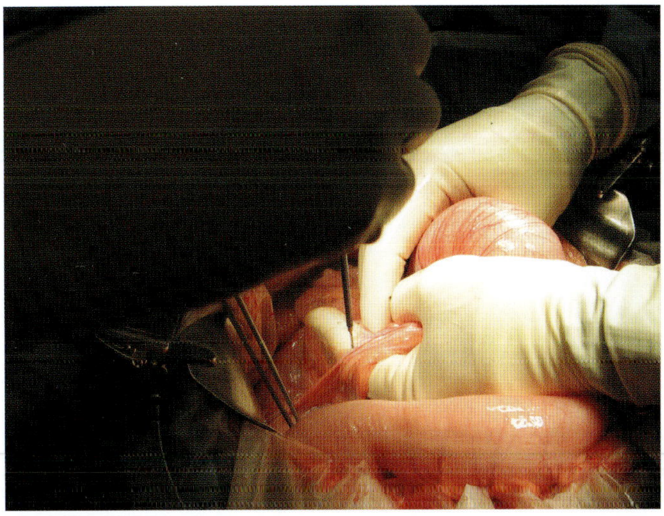

Figure 1-2

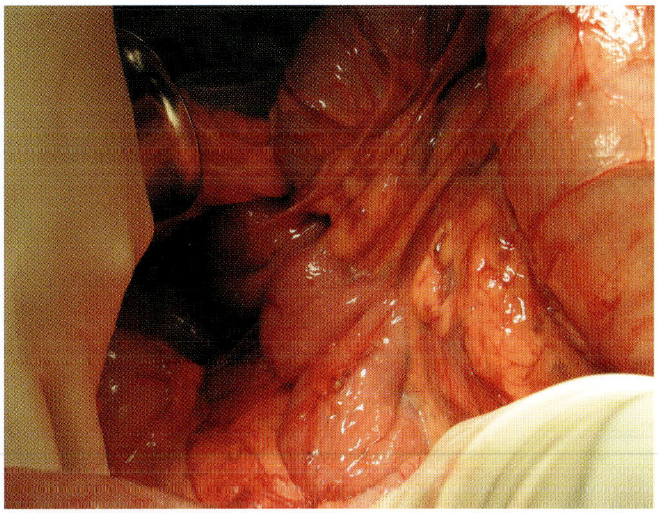

Figure 1-3

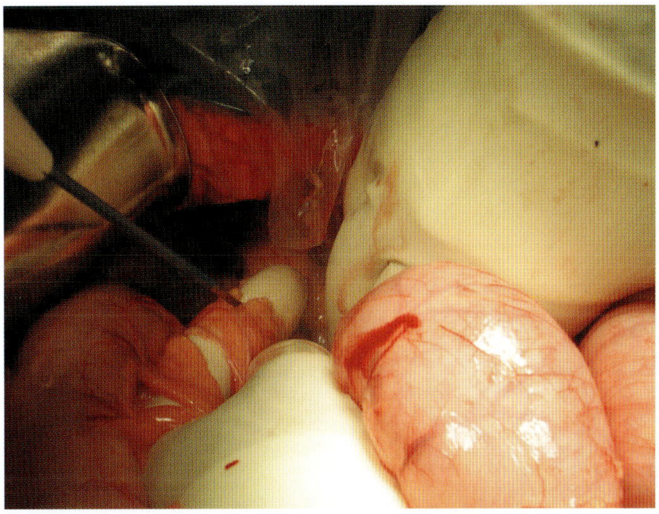

Figure 1-4

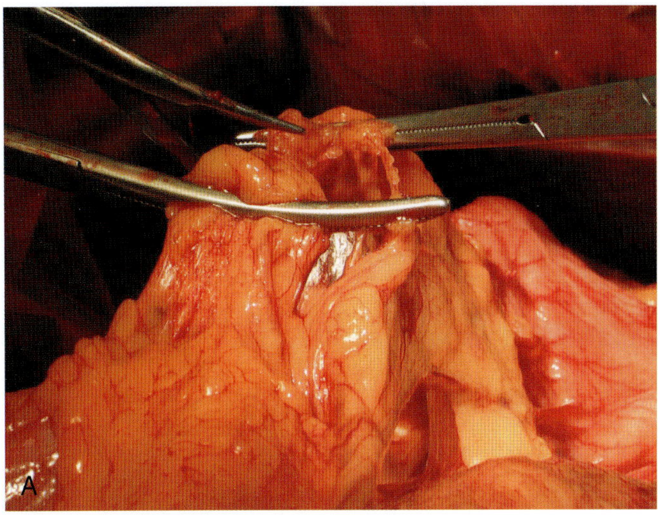

Figure 1-5A

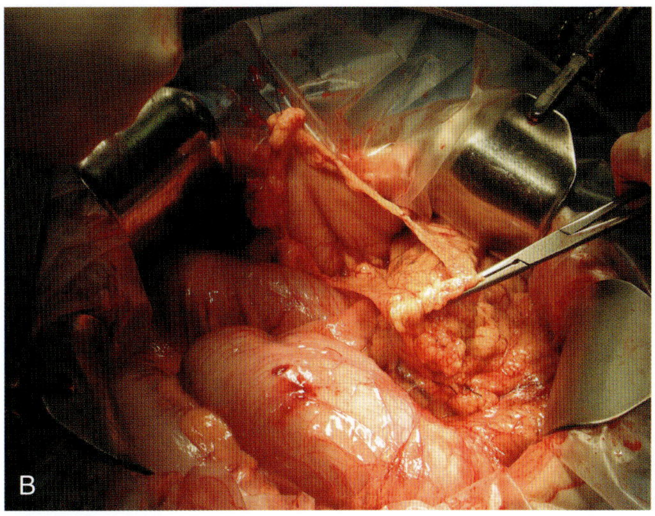

Figure 1-5B

- The colon is returned to its anatomic position with the right colon along the right gutter and the hepatic flexure up in the right upper quadrant. The SMA is identified in its tract to the terminal ileum; a window is seen in the base of the mesentery of the right colon proximal and distal to a large vascular trunk. This trunk is the ileocolic artery and vein arising from the SMA and superior mesenteric vein (Figure 1-6). An incision is made at the base of this window to expose and divide the ileocolic vessels at their origin (Figure 1-7).
- The vessels of the terminal ileal mesentery are divided; the terminal ileum is transected with a linear cutter stapler, and the transverse colon is divided in its proximal portion just distal to the hepatic flexure, also using a linear cutter stapler (Figures 1-8*A* and *B* and 1-9).

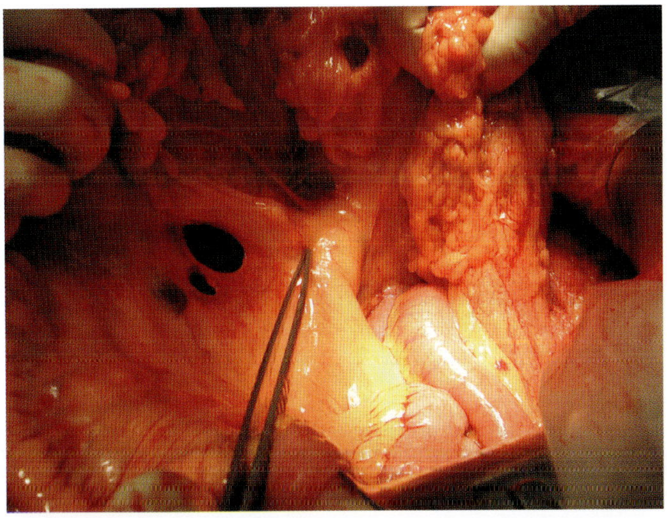

Figure 1-6

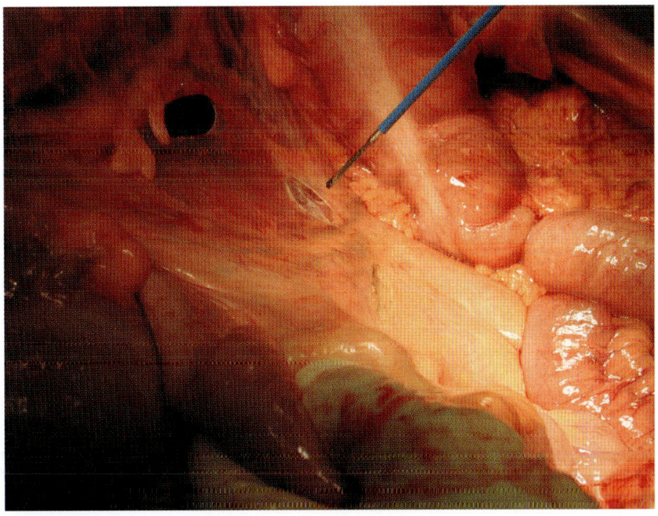

Figure 1-7

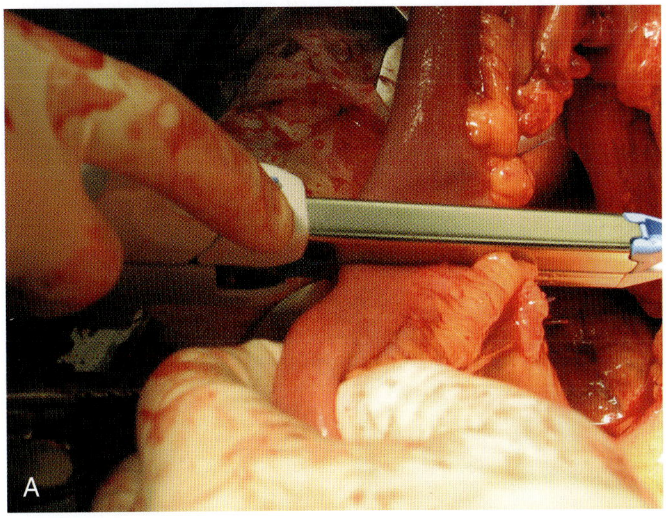

Figure 1-8A

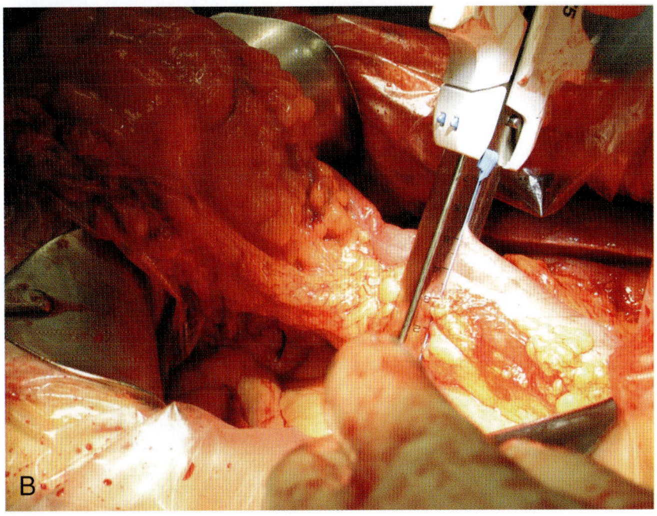

Figure 1-8B

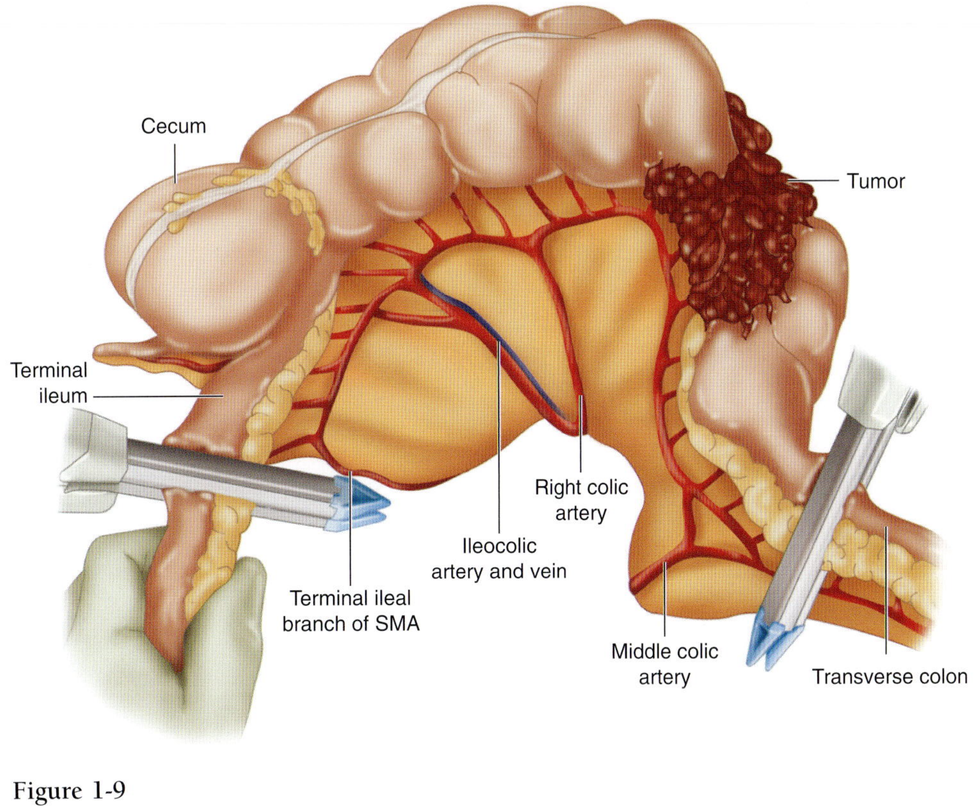

Figure 1-9

- Once the specimen has been passed off, the corners of the antimesenteric end of the transverse staple lines on the transverse colon and terminal ileum are removed, and the separated arms of the linear cutter stapler are passed into the lumen of the aligned loops of bowel. A side-to-side anastomosis is constructed between the terminal ileum and the transverse colon with the lumen aligned as a functional end-to-end anastomosis (Figures 1-10 and 1-11*A-F*). The internal staple line is distracted as widely as possible (Figure 1-11*E*, inset).

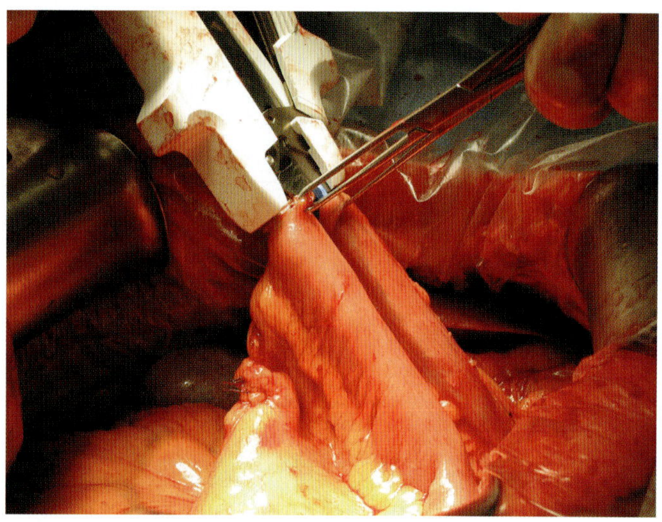

Figure 1-10

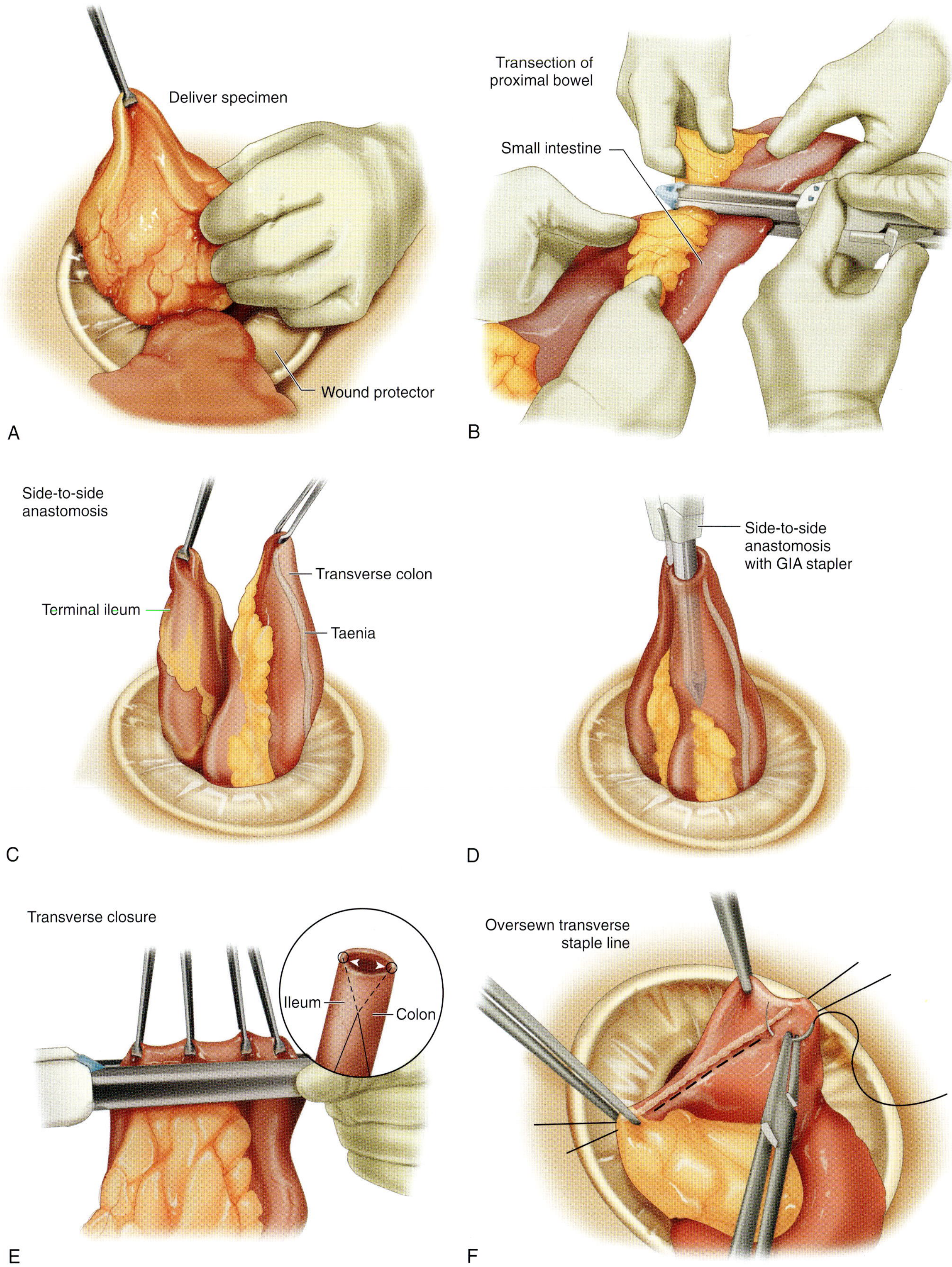

Figure 1-11A-F

- The transverse opening of the anastomosis is stretched to spread the "V" of the GIA staple line and increase the transverse opening as widely as possible before placing a second staple line across the transverse opening (Figure 1-12*A* and *B*). The mesenteric defect can be closed with a running suture to prevent torsion or internal hernia.

Step 4: Postoperative Care

The abdomen is generally closed with a running No. 1 looped absorbable suture and staples, and a sterile gauze is applied. Patients are ambulated early. Intravenous fluid replacement is given to maintain a urine output of greater than 30 mL/hr. Nasogastric decompression is not required unless the patient becomes nauseated. Most patients tolerate clear liquids within 24 to 48 hours, and the diet can be advanced as tolerated. Patients should be given prophylactic antibiotics for 24 hours, incentive spirometry, and deep vein thrombosis prophylaxis and encouraged to ambulate as much as possible during the early postoperative period. The usual hospital stay after an open right colectomy is 4 to 5 days; the hospital stay is shorter when the patient is placed on a fast-track postoperative regimen. Postoperative analgesia is usually managed with patient-controlled analgesia followed by a switch to oral analgesics.

Step 5: Pearls and Pitfalls

The most common and most feared complication after a right colectomy is anastomotic leak. These leaks can be prevented if the staple line at the apex of the GIA stapler is protected with a suture placed in a Lembert fashion with seromuscular depth to close the crotch between the two portions of bowel. The transverse staple line can be oversewn with a running 3-0 absorbable suture using Lembert suture placement (seromuscular rather than full-thickness oversewing). To prevent twisting at the anastomosis, the mesentery defect can be closed with a running absorbable suture when the anastomosis is complete; this also prevents herniation or volvulus at the anastomotic site. This closure is not required, but it is a safety procedure that has been shown to be effective. The anastomosis can be covered with a portion of the remaining omentum. Adhesion barriers can be used to prevent adhesions and to prevent the development of small bowel obstruction in the future. Powderless gloves and good surgical technique can also help avoid adhesions.

Selected Readings

West NP, Hohenberger W, Weber K, et al. Complete mesocolic excision with central vascular ligation produces an oncologically superior specimen compared with standard surgery for carcinoma of the colon. J Clin Oncol 2010;28:272–8.

West NP, Sutton KM, Ingeholm P, et al. Improving the quality of colon cancer surgery through a surgical education program. Dis Colon Rectum 2010;53:1594–603.

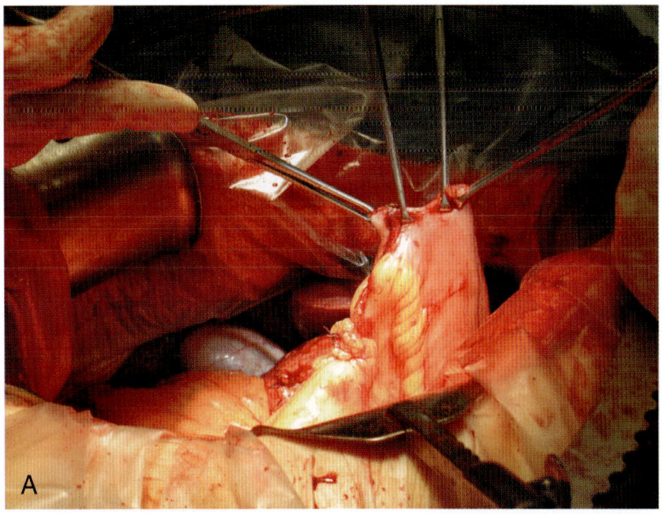

Figure 1-12A

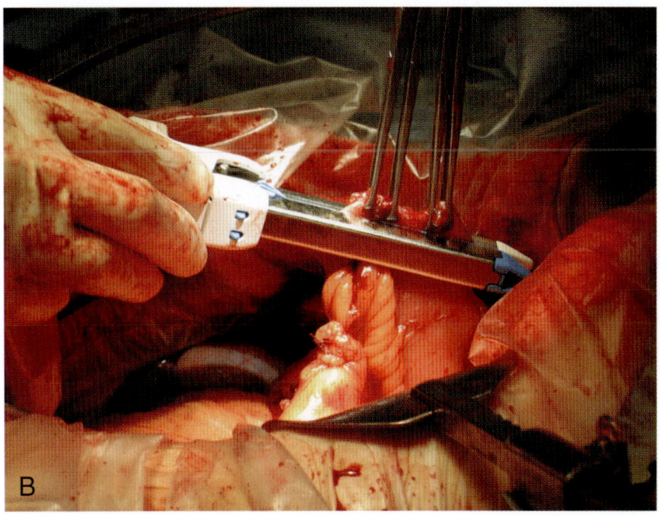

Figure 1-12B

CHAPTER 2

Laparoscopic Right Colectomy

Steven R. Hunt

Step 1: Clinical Anatomy

The right colon lies on the patient's right side suspended laterally by peritoneal attachments to the right side of the abdominal wall, superiorly by attachments to the undersurface of the liver and posterior diaphragm, and medially by its mesentery. The ileocolic artery and vein and the right colic vessels, if they are present, run through this leaf of mesentery. The colon is adherent to the retroperitoneum on the right side of the abdomen and covers the right gonadal vessels and right ureter. The inferior vena cava is the next most medial structure on the right side. The hepatic flexure, the fold at the junction between the right colon and transverse colon, is adherent to the anterior surface of the kidney by avascular attachments to Gerota's fascia. The first and second portions of the duodenum are adherent to the undersurface of the mesentery of the right colon and proximal transverse colon. The gallbladder is sometimes adherent to the cephalad surface of the transverse colon at the hepatic flexure. The space behind the right colon is triangular shaped with the flat horizontal surface at the hepatic flexure running from the abdominal side wall toward the midline along the line of the greater curve of the stomach. The vertical axis follows the right lateral side wall of the abdomen. The hypotenuse runs from the fusion plane of the cecum at the pelvic brim over the top of the right iliac artery and vein at about the point where the ureter passes over the iliac vessels toward the midline over the aorta up to the base of the pancreas along the third portion of the duodenum. This triangular retroperitoneal area is a potential space with avascular attachments and allows the right colon to be lifted completely from the retroperitoneum during dissection. Release of all suspensory attachments allows the right colon to be made into a midline structure. The ileocolic artery and vein arise from the superior mesenteric artery (SMA) and superior mesenteric vein in the midportion of the SMA below the duodenum. The right colic artery is a variable structure and may be present as a separate structure or as part of the ileocolic trunk. The right branch of the middle colic artery exits through the pancreatic tissue from its origin on the SMA as a portion of the middle colic trunk at the base of the transverse mesocolon (Figure 2-1).

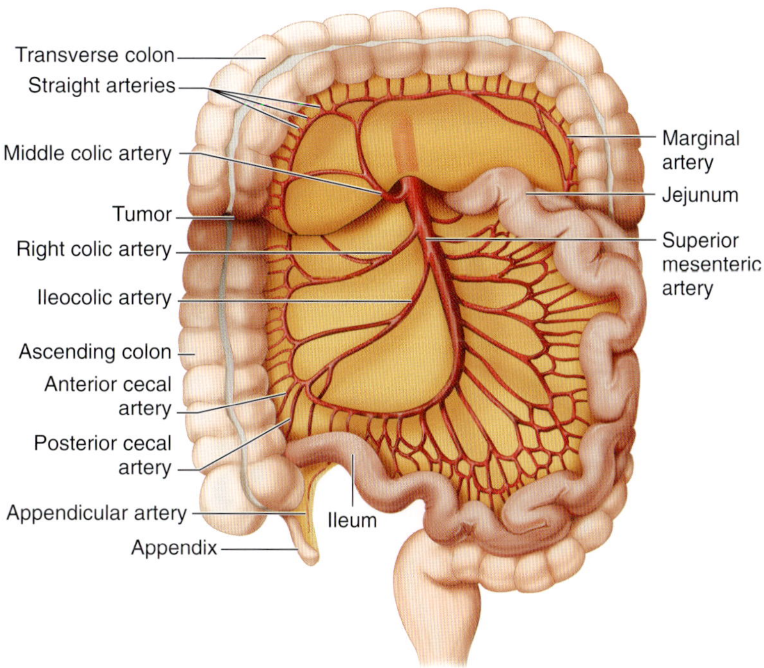
Transverse colon
Straight arteries
Middle colic artery
Tumor
Right colic artery
Ileocolic artery
Ascending colon
Anterior cecal artery
Posterior cecal artery
Appendicular artery
Appendix
Ileum
Marginal artery
Jejunum
Superior mesenteric artery

Figure 2-1

Step 2: Preoperative Considerations

The clinical anatomy for laparoscopic colectomy is the same as an open right colectomy. The indications for laparoscopic resection are also similar to indications for open right colectomy with the restriction that laparoscopy cannot be done as easily in the setting of large inflammatory masses or large advanced tumors. The amount of colon resected depends on the blood supply of the segment. The tumor determines the amount of bowel resected only if it is at the extremes of the right colon, either at the hepatic flexure or at the cecum near the ileocecal valve. In these circumstances, there should be an added proximal or distal margin to ensure adequate bowel and mesentery removal. A mid right colon tumor requires a right colectomy with removal of the entire right colon and anastomosis of the terminal ileum to the transverse colon. This procedure results in removal of the entire lymph node–draining area of the bowel segment.

As with open colectomy, there is no need for bowel preparation. The same type of antibiotic and deep vein thrombosis prophylaxis should be used. Laparoscopy adds the additional risk of decreased blood flow through the inferior vena cava under a pneumoperitoneum of 15 mm Hg, and sequential compression of the legs and proper positioning become critical. The laparoscopic procedure is performed in the modified lithotomy position using Allen's stirrups with the legs flexed no more than 5 degrees at the hips and the knees flexed at 90 degrees to keep the legs out of the field of the instruments as they traverse the lower quadrants during dissection. Figure 2-2 shows the positioning of the patient with leg flexion.

Step 3: Operative Steps

- The patient is positioned in the modified lithotomy position with the legs in Allen's stirrups with sequential compression boots in place. A beanbag, attached directly to the operating table with Velcro, is rolled around the patient and deflated to fix the patient in position. The beanbag keeps the arms at the patient's side and allows the table to be placed in steep Trendelenburg and airplaned (tilted) to the left during the operation. The trocar site placement is typically at the umbilicus and the suprapubic and left flank positions. The camera operator stands at the patient's left shoulder and operates the camera through the umbilical port. The operating surgeon stands at the patient's left hip or between the legs as needed and operates instruments through the left flank and suprapubic ports (Figure 2-3).

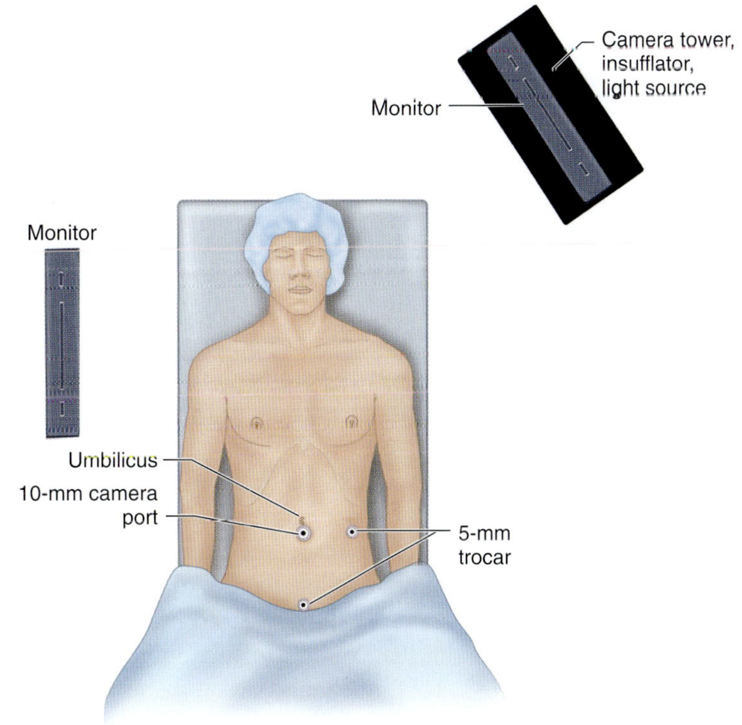

Figure 2-2

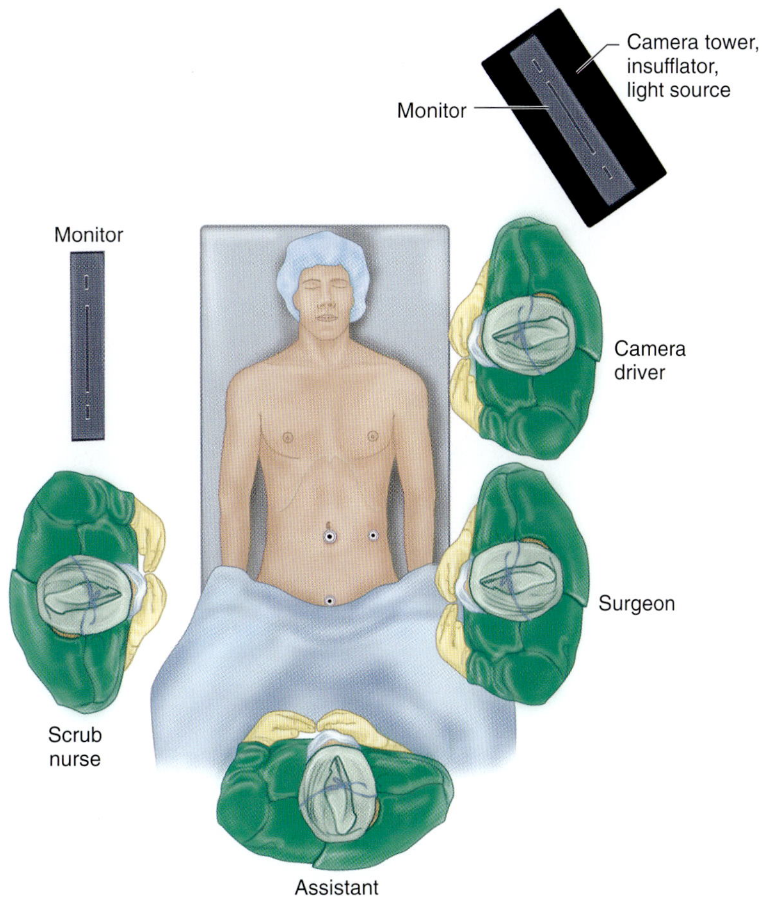

Figure 2-3

- The 15-mm Hg pneumoperitoneum is maintained with a pressure-controlled insufflator. The camera cord, light cord, and carbon dioxide cord are passed off of the table from the patient's left shoulder to the instrumentation tower. A monitor is placed opposite the operating surgeon and camera operator. If two monitors are available, one is at the right shoulder, and one is at the right hip (Figure 2-3). The operation is begun by abdominal exploration by using the laparoscope and instruments to move the abdominal contents before placing the table in steep Trendelenburg and airplane left. The liver should be evaluated. After the table is positioned, the omentum should be placed over the stomach to the left upper quadrant, and the small bowel should be retracted from the pelvis to lie in the left upper quadrant. The 5-mm wavy grasper is a good instrument to flip the small bowel up into the left upper quadrant with a reverse "C" motion; the principle should be to avoid grasping any individual piece of bowel on the bowel itself. Using mesenteric fat or epiploic fat to move portions of intestine is appropriate. The cecum is lifted to the anterior abdominal wall using the 5-mm grasper through the suprapubic port in the operator's left hand. An energy source, such as bipolar or monopolar cautery or Harmonic scalpel, can be used to incise along the base of the peritoneum from the pelvic brim over the iliac vessels toward the duodenum at the midline of the abdominal cavity (Figure 2-4*A*). This incision allows a plane to be developed in the retroperitoneum over the structures that are found posteriorly (Figure 2-5*A*). The right ureter is identified crossing the iliac vessels close to the bifurcation of the aorta; the gonadal vessels are further lateral and run parallel to the iliac vessels (Figure 2-4*B*). The psoas muscle lies posteriorly and should be a boundary of dissection. The avascular plane that is encountered is used as the dissection plane and can be bluntly dissected in a posterior sweeping direction to allow the mesentery and cecum to separate anteriorly from the posterior structures.

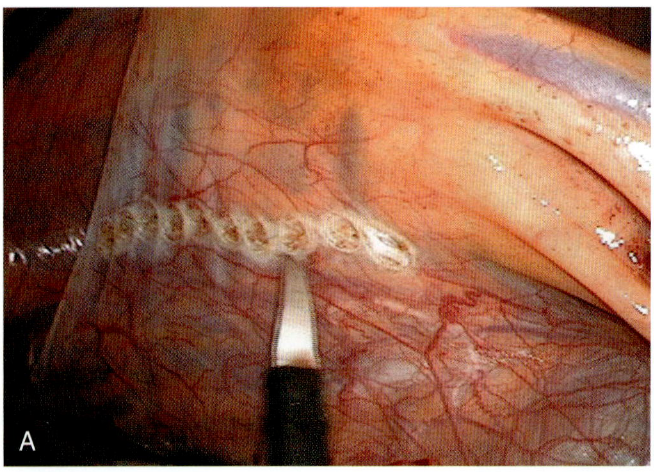

Figure 2-4A

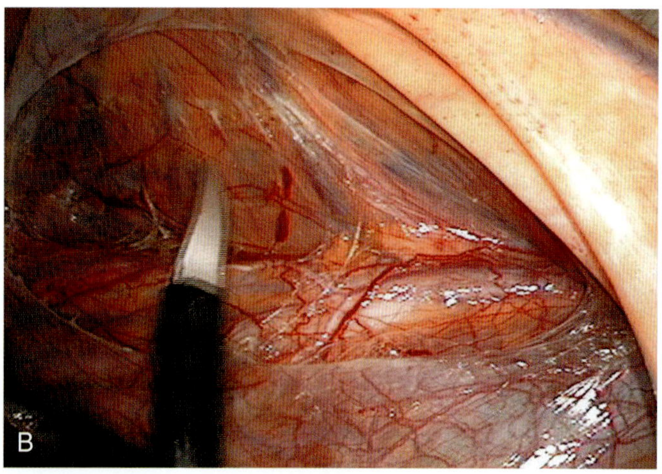

Figure 2-4B

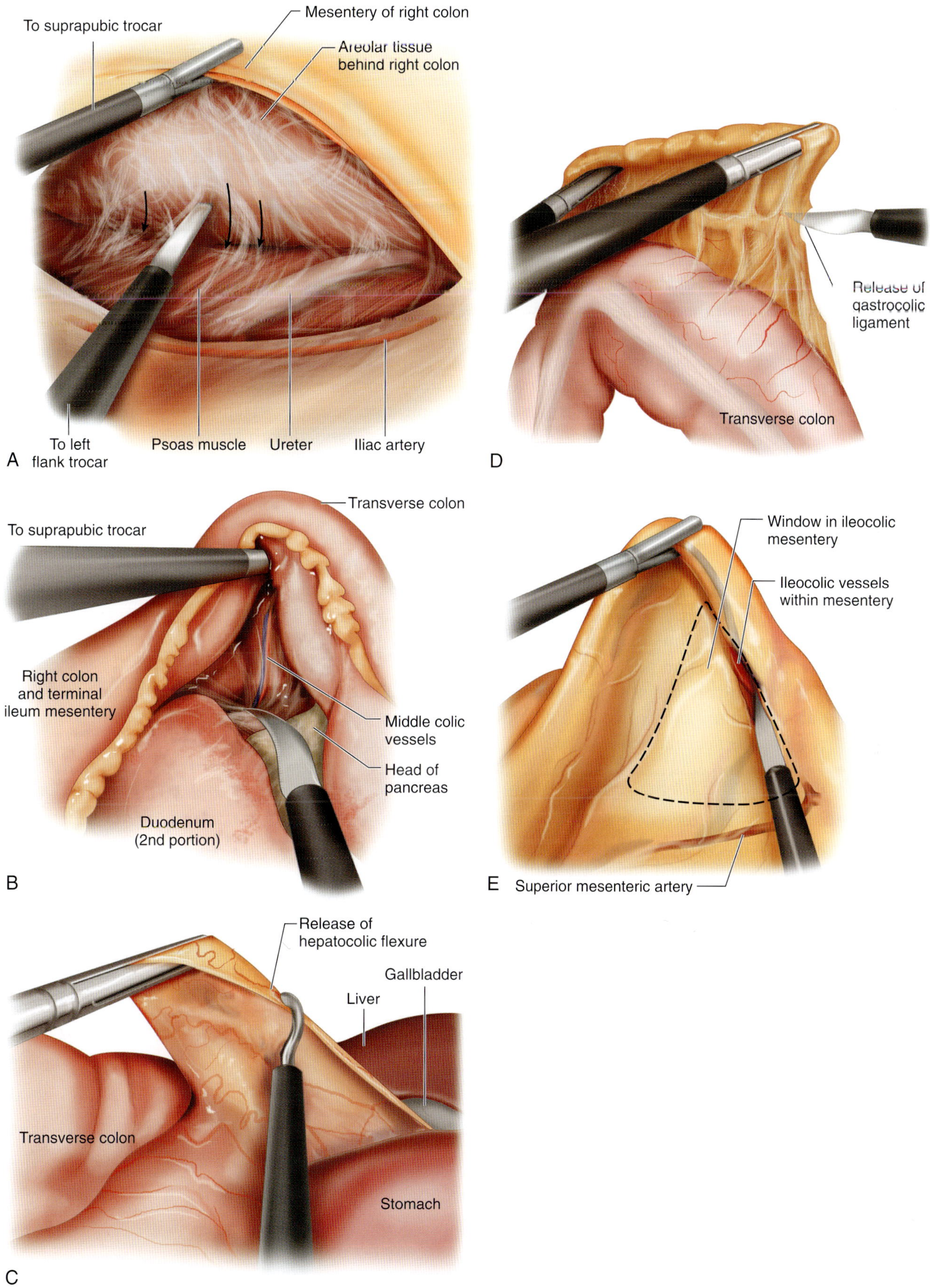
To suprapubic trocar
Mesentery of right colon
Areolar tissue behind right colon
To left flank trocar
Psoas muscle
Ureter
Iliac artery
A
Release of gastrocolic ligament
Transverse colon
D
Transverse colon
To suprapubic trocar
Right colon and terminal ileum mesentery
Middle colic vessels
Head of pancreas
Duodenum (2nd portion)
B
Window in ileocolic mesentery
Ileocolic vessels within mesentery
E
Superior mesenteric artery
Release of hepatocolic flexure
Gallbladder
Liver
Transverse colon
Stomach
C

Figure 2-5A-E

- The cecum should be completely mobilized from the retroperitoneum all the way out to the side wall of the abdomen using the left-hand grasper for retraction upward and the right-hand instrument to develop the plane. The dissection is carried in this posterior plane up to and around and on top of the surface of the duodenum (Figure 2-6). The duodenum should be separated from the overlying mesentery of the right colon using the left hand for anterior retraction. The dissection is continued up to the hepatic flexure peritoneal attachments, exposing the entire sweep of the duodenum, a portion of the head of the pancreas, and the lateral aspect of the middle colic vessels (Figure 2-5*B*). The anterior portion of the kidney is exposed with this same maneuver with upward traction and downward countertraction. The mesentery and right colon are lifted toward the anterior abdominal wall while pulling the avascular tissue posteriorly using the instrument in the operator's right hand. Most of the retraction is accomplished with the left hand on the grasper through the suprapubic port.
- The patient is placed in *reverse* Trendelenburg position, and the attachments of the hepatic flexure to the retroperitoneum are lifted anteriorly and divided with an energy source along the line between the liver and the transverse colon (Figure 2-5*C*). This maneuver allows entry in the previously dissected plane of the right colon posteriorly and is seen in Figure 2-7*A* as a purple hue in the posterior peritoneum.
- Figure 2-7*B* illustrates the separation of the omentum attached to the transverse colon so that the lesser sac can be entered and the transverse colon released from the lesser sac, head of the pancreas, and undersurface of the antrum of the stomach all the way out to the right side wall of the abdomen (Figure 2-5*D*).
- The hepatic flexure is completely mobilized from the undersurface of the liver, and the posterior dissection is connected to the right upper quadrant dissection.
- The patient is returned to Trendelenburg position, and the cecum is grasped at the ileocecal valve and lifted anteriorly to the abdominal wall. This maneuver provides the tension needed to allow the ileocolic vessel to be easily seen in the mesentery of the right colon (Figure 2-7*C*).
- Dissection on either side of the ileocolic vessel provides windows to allow transection of the ileocolic vessels at their origin along the SMA, as seen in Figures 2-5*E* and 2-7*D*.
- The final laparoscopic maneuver of the right colon dissection is the release of the lateral attachments of the colon from the right side wall of the abdomen (Figure 2-8). The cecum is grasped and lifted anteriorly with the left hand on a grasper through the suprapubic site, and the energy source through the left lower quadrant can divide the lateral attachments. Alternatively, the left hand could also run the energy source through the suprapubic trocar, and the right hand on a grasper through the left flank site could retract the cecum toward the midline to facilitate the division of the lateral attachments. This maneuver allows the right colon to become a midline structure from the middle of the transverse colon all the way to the terminal ileum.

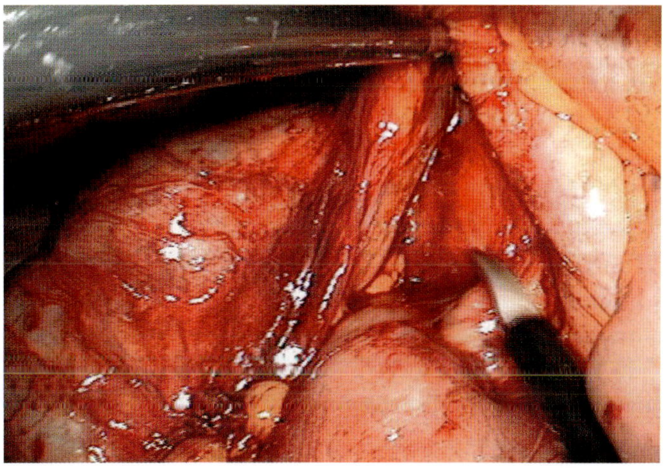

Figure 2-6

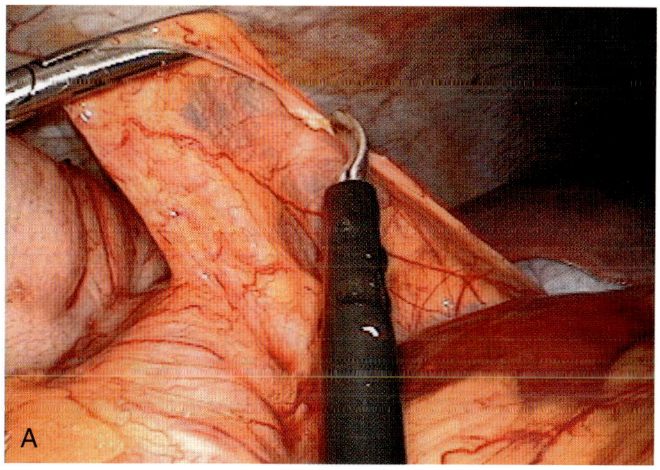

Figure 2-7A

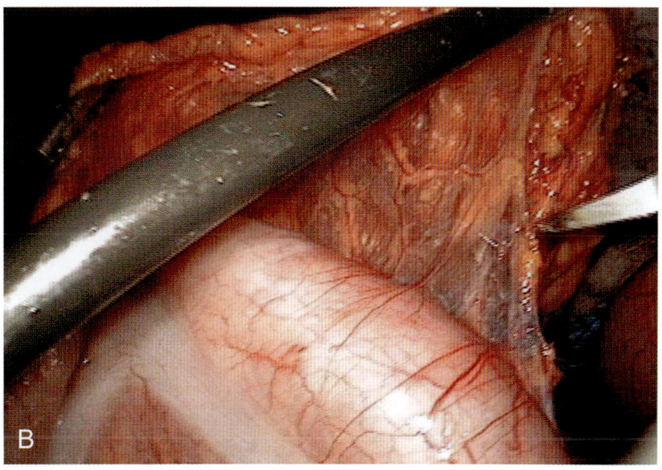

Figure 2-7B

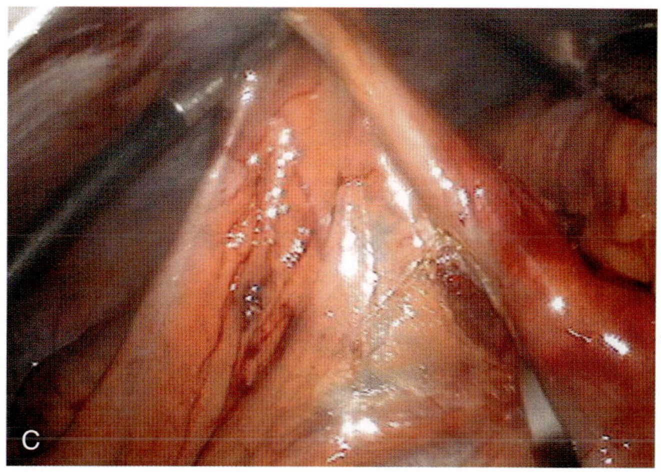

Figure 2-7C

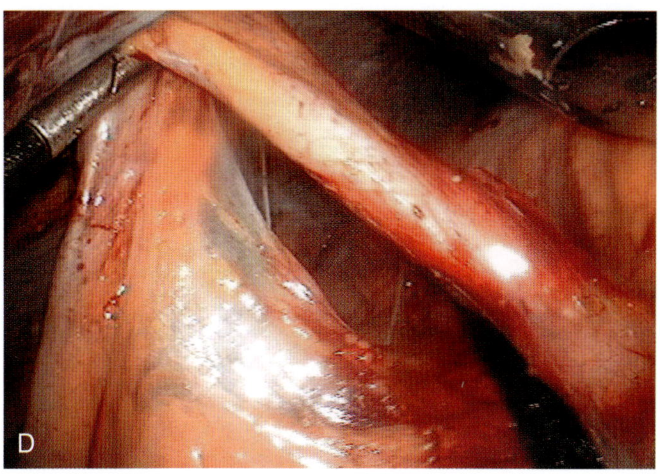

Figure 2-7D

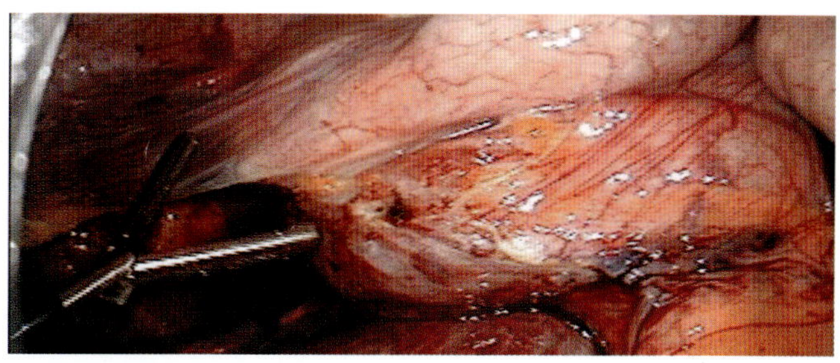

Figure 2-8

- The umbilical trocar site is enlarged to 5 cm, and a wound protector is placed through the incision to allow the specimen to be delivered through the 5-cm incision at the umbilicus. The specimen is delivered through the anterior abdominal wall in its anatomic position, as seen in Figure 2-9, and the transverse colon is transected with a 75-mm linear cutter stapler at the level of the abdominal wall. The terminal ileum is delivered through the abdominal wall adjacent to the transverse colon and transected at a point appropriate to the disease process, usually 10 cm proximal to the ileal cecal valve with a 75-mm linear cutter stapler (Figures 2-10 and 2-11*A* and *B*).

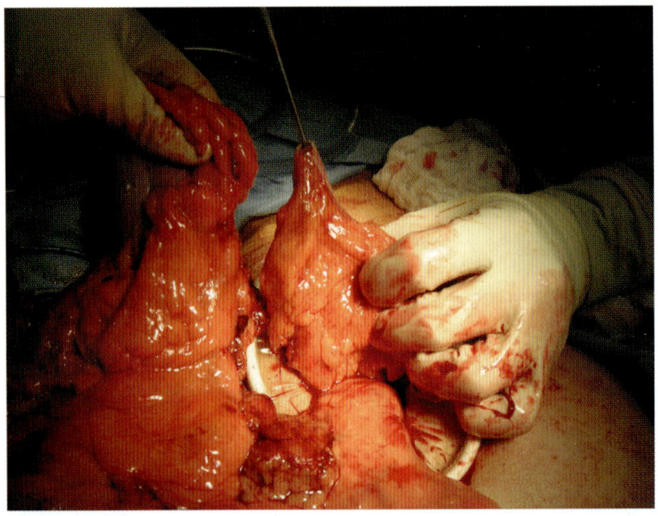

Figure 2-9

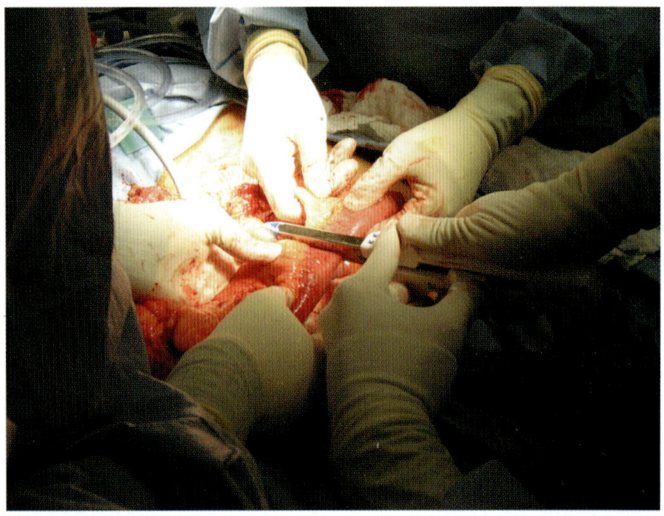

Figure 2-10

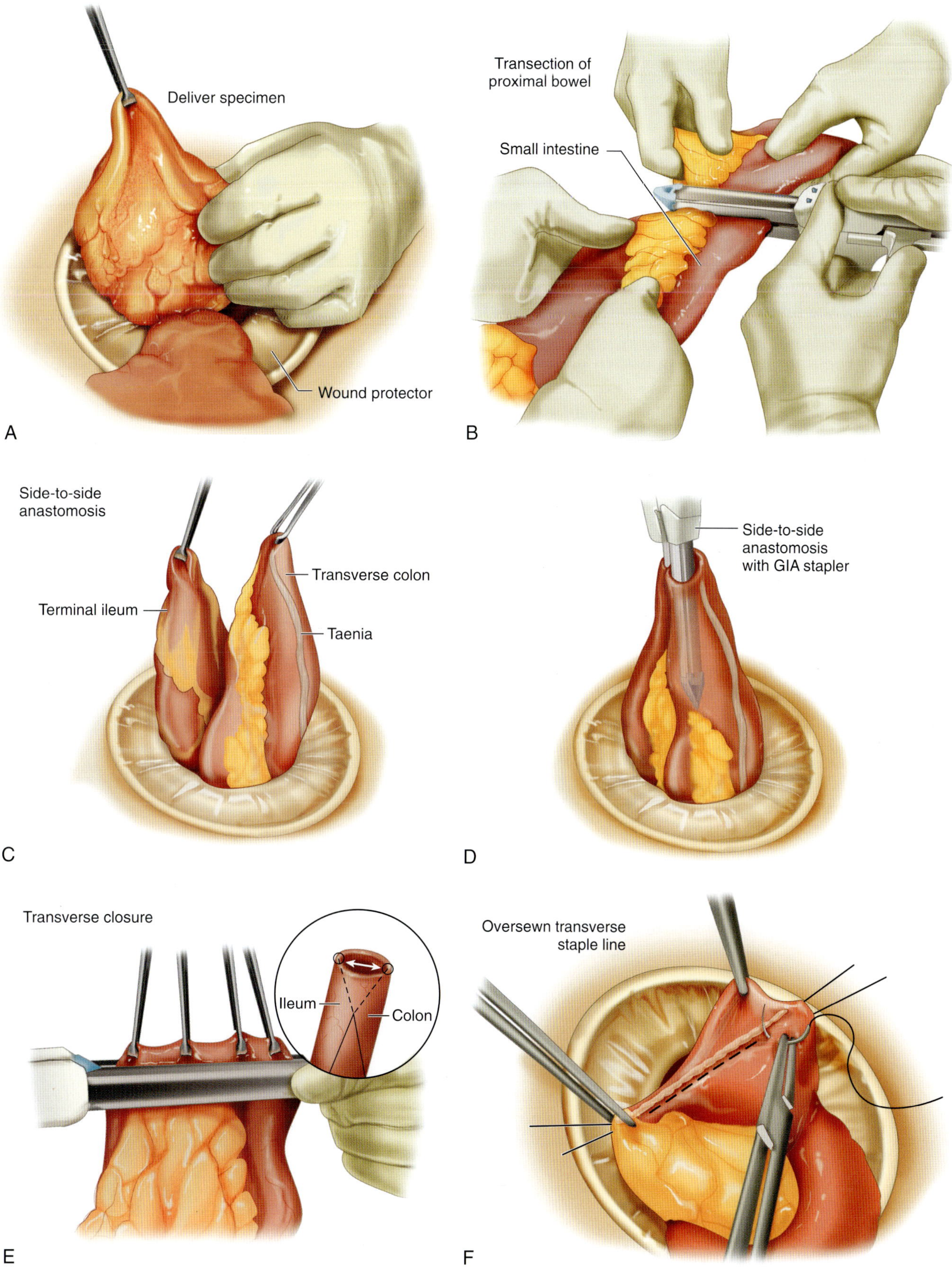

Figure 2-11A-F

- The two cut ends of the bowel, which include the transverse colon and the terminal ileum, are lifted through the abdominal opening and aligned for stapled anastomosis (Figures 2-11*C* and 2-12).
- A functional end-to-end, side-to-side anastomosis is accomplished by placing the two sides of the linear cutter stapler through the antimesenteric corners of the transverse staple line to attach the terminal ileum to the transverse colon (Figures 2-11*D* and 2-13).
- The transverse opening is then closed with Allis clamps, and a 75-mm linear cutter stapler is placed across the transverse opening with the staple lines of the linear cutter stapler distracted as far as possible to create a triangular anastomosis (Figures 2-11*E* and 2-14). The transverse staple line is oversewn with an inverting Lembert absorbable suture to invert the transverse staple line (Figures 2-11*F* and 2-15).
- The mesenteric defect between the transverse colon and the terminal ileum can be closed with a running 3-0 absorbable suture to help ensure that there are no twists in the bowel and prevent herniation through the opening in the mesenteric defect. A 3-0 absorbable suture is usually also placed at the apex of the ileocolic GIA anastomosis to protect the crotch of the GIA staple line (Figure 2-16).
- The wound protector is removed, and the abdominal incision is closed with a running No. 1 looped absorbable suture. The skin can be closed with skin staples or subcuticular suture to result in a 5-cm incision (Figure 2-17).
- The amount of bowel resected and the positioning of the bowel on the abdominal wall can facilitate maintaining the bowel without twists and verifying that the appropriate specimen has been removed (Figure 2-9).

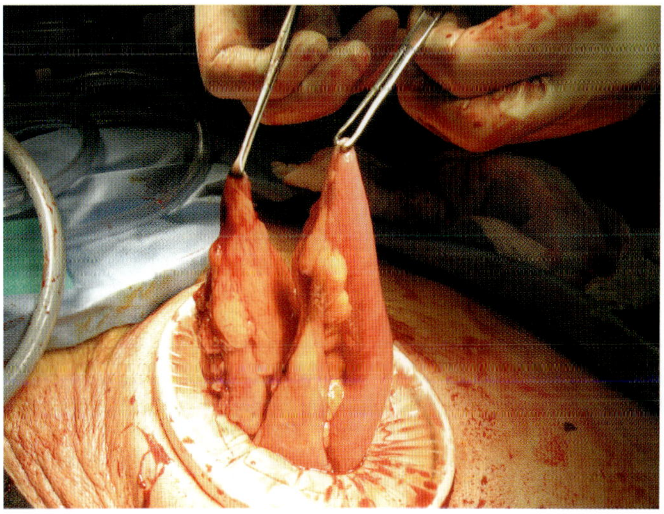
Figure 2-12

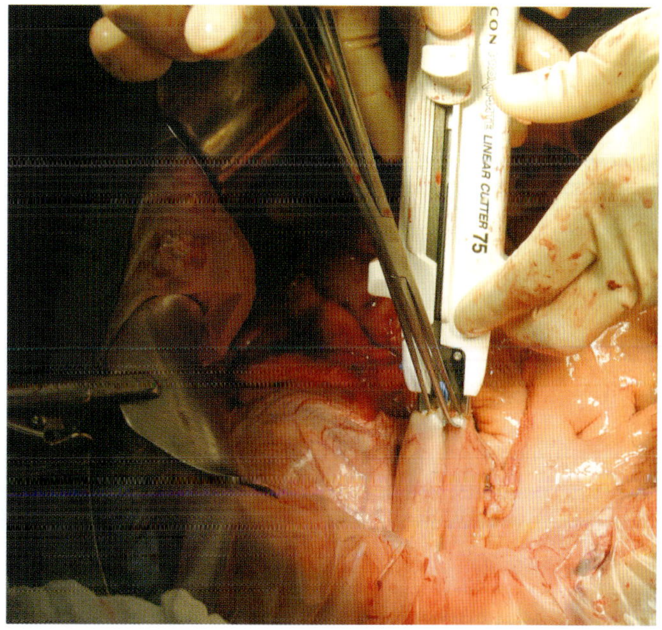

Figure 2-13

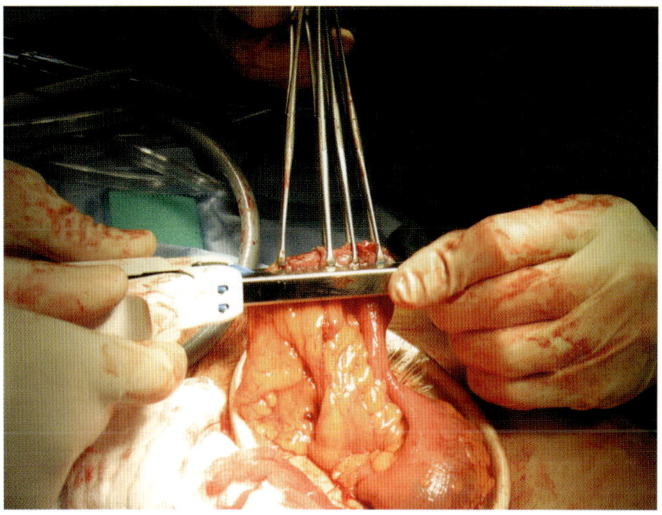
Figure 2-14

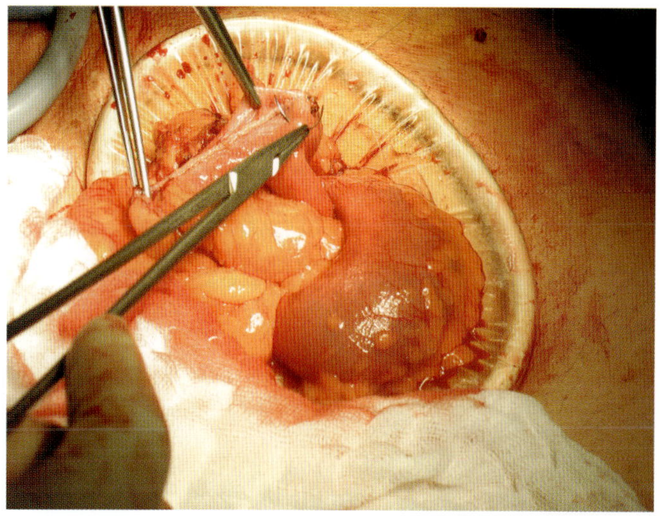
Figure 2-15

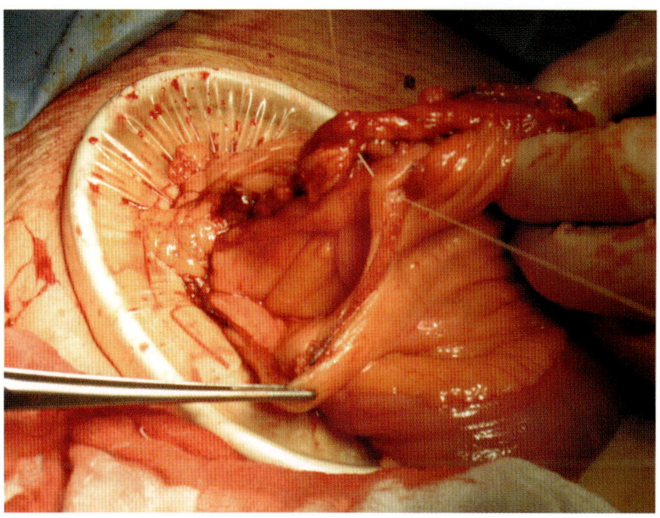
Figure 2-16

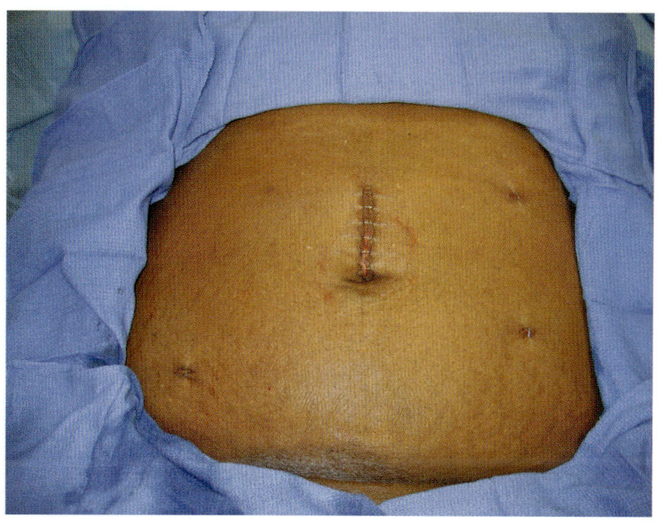
Figure 2-17

Step 4: Postoperative Care

Patients are maintained on intravenous fluids until they can tolerate an oral diet. They are offered liquids on the first postoperative day, and the diet is advanced as tolerated. Patients are discharged only when they have demonstrated bowel function and tolerated a regular diet, usually after 4 days or less. Prophylactic antibiotics for 24 hours and sequential compression deep vein thrombosis prophylaxis are appropriate for all patients. Supplemental subcutaneous heparin is appropriate for patients with neoplastic disease. Ambulation should be started on the first postoperative day and continued aggressively. A urinary catheter is needed for only 1 or 2 days until the patient is fully ambulatory and able to get to the bathroom alone. Incentive spirometry is provided and encouraged. Analgesics are started with patient-controlled analgesia and switched to oral analgesics fairly rapidly.

Step 5: Pearls and Pitfalls

Twisting of the anastomosis can be a problem. It is helpful to maintain the bowel in its anatomic position at all times when it comes through the extraction wound. Adequate mobilization of the transverse colon away from the stomach and division of the right branch of the middle colic artery and vein may be necessary to allow the transverse colon to reach the anterior abdominal wall in obese patients; this avoids excessive tension during the anastomosis. As mentioned, closing the mesenteric defect prevents twisting, but this may not always be possible in obese patients. Closing the defect through the extraction site is almost always possible. A retractor is placed from the right upper quadrant, lifting the abdominal wall away from the bowel. The mesenteric edges from the anastomosis down to the apex of the defect in the mesentery are closed with a running stitch. Anastomotic leak is the most feared complication; oversewing the transverse staple line and protecting the GIA staple line can usually prevent this from happening. The omentum can be placed over the anastomosis to give some protection.

Selected Readings

Baker RP, Titu LV, Hartley JE, et al. A case-control study of laparoscopic right hemicolectomy vs. open right hemicolectomy. Dis Colon Rectum 2004;47:1675–9.

Kim J, Edwards E, Bowne W, et al. Medial-to-lateral laparoscopic colon resection: a view beyond the learning curve. Surg Endosc 2007;21:1503–7.

CHAPTER 3

Extended Right Colectomy with Ileosigmoid Anastomosis

Steven R. Hunt

Step 1: Clinical Anatomy

The right colon lies on the patient's right side suspended laterally by peritoneal attachments to the right side of the abdominal wall, superiorly by attachments to the undersurface of the liver and posterior diaphragm, and medially by its mesentery. The ileocolic artery and vein and the right colic vessels, if they are present, run through this leaf of mesentery. The colon is adherent to the retroperitoneum on the right side of the abdomen and covers the right gonadal vessels and right ureter. The inferior vena cava is the next most medial structure on the right side. The hepatic flexure, the fold at the junction between the right colon and transverse colon, is adherent to the anterior surface of the kidney by avascular attachments to Gerota's fascia. The first and second portions of the duodenum are adherent to the undersurface of the mesentery of the right colon and proximal transverse colon. The gallbladder is sometimes adherent to the cephalad surface of the transverse colon at the hepatic flexure. The space behind the right colon is triangular shaped with the flat horizontal surface at the hepatic flexure running from the abdominal side wall toward the midline along the line of the greater curve of the stomach. The vertical axis follows the right lateral side wall of the abdomen. The hypotenuse runs from the fusion plane of the cecum at the pelvic brim over the top of the right iliac artery and vein at about the point where the ureter passes over the iliac vessels toward the midline over the aorta up to the base of the pancreas along the third portion of the duodenum. This triangular retroperitoneal area is a potential space with avascular attachments and allows the right colon to be lifted completely from the retroperitoneum during dissection. Release of all suspensory attachments allows the right colon to be made into a midline structure. The ileocolic artery and vein arise from the superior mesenteric artery (SMA) and superior mesenteric vein in the midportion of the SMA below the duodenum. The right colic artery is a variable structure and may be present as a separate structure or as part of the ileocolic trunk. The right branch of the middle colic artery exits through the pancreatic tissue from its origin on the SMA as a portion of the middle colic trunk at the base of the transverse mesocolon (Figure 3-1).

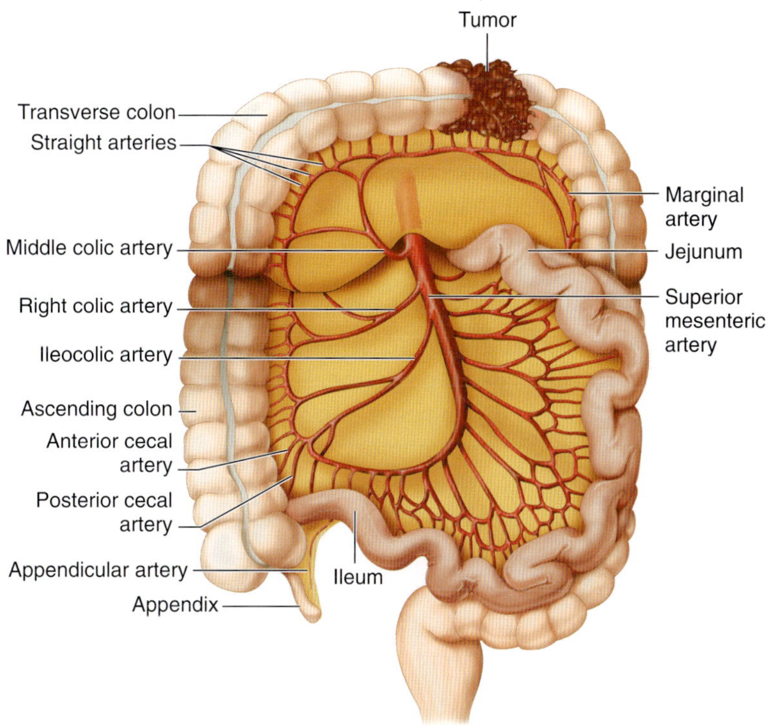
Tumor
Transverse colon
Straight arteries
Middle colic artery
Right colic artery
Ileocolic artery
Ascending colon
Anterior cecal artery
Posterior cecal artery
Appendicular artery
Appendix
Ileum
Marginal artery
Jejunum
Superior mesenteric artery

Figure 3-1

The left branches of the middle colic artery and vein exit adjacent to the right branch of the middle colic and are found at the third portion of the duodenum over the pancreas. The inferior mesenteric vein (IMV) travels along the window of the base of the mesentery of the colon and enters the portal vein adjacent to the ligament of Treitz at the base of the splenic flexure mesentery (Figure 3-2). This area of the vasculature to the colon is extremely complex and should be studied carefully before mobilization of the transverse colon. The mesentery of the transverse colon itself is sometimes attached to filmy attachments of the posterior aspect of the stomach. The omentum falls from the gastroepiploic artery along the greater curve of the stomach over the transverse colon, where it attaches tangentially to the antimesenteric surface of the transverse colon and continues to the lower aspect of the abdomen, free-floating over the surface of the small bowel.

The splenic flexure of the colon sits in the left upper quadrant with a surface adherent to the undersurface of the tip of the spleen, the anterior surface of the left kidney, and the anterior surface of the tail of the pancreas. A portion of the base of the mesentery of the transverse colon is attached to the undersurface of the tail of the pancreas starting at the level of the IMV and extending laterally toward the left side of the abdomen. These attachments can be released by developing avascular planes given knowledge of the peritoneal windows, areolar tissue planes, and structural relationships. The left colon itself is adherent to the retroperitoneum in the left gutter via an avascular filmy tissue plane that attaches the mesentery and left colon to the posterior abdominal wall, where the ureter and gonadal vessels are found. The peritoneal attachments along the left gutter of the abdomen suspend the left colon from the left side of the abdomen from the pelvic brim all the way up to the splenic flexure. The splenic flexure is a fold of the colon with its apex attached to the tip of the spleen by omental congenital adhesions.

The splenic flexure is usually covered by the omentum as it falls over the top of the transverse colon along the left gutter, and numerous embryologic attachments can occur between the antimesenteric surface of the proximal left colon and the omentum at the splenic flexure. The left colon descends along the left gutter to the level of the pelvic brim, where the colon becomes free from the pelvic side wall and falls into a sigmoid-appearing structure known as the sigmoid colon. The sigmoid colon lies free in the pelvis, attached posteriorly only to its vascular attachments at the midline over the sacral promontory.

The inferior mesenteric artery (IMA) arises from the anterior surface of the aorta proximal to the origin of the common iliac vessels. The IMA branches to give the superior hemorrhoidal artery descending into the posterior mesorectal vessel and the ascending left colic vessel, which sweeps up toward the splenic flexure. The IMV runs across the base of the mesentery of the left colon, crossing the superior hemorrhoidal and left colic vessels on its way to the duodenum. There is a clear peritoneal window between the aorta and the IMV, which can be used to enter the avascular plane behind the left colon mesentery and the retroperitoneum.

Step 2: Preoperative Considerations

Extended right colectomy is most commonly performed for mid to distal transverse colon cancers or splenic flexure cancers. The patient requires very few preoperative preparations. Prophylactic antibiotics are appropriate for a colectomy to reduce the risk of wound infection. A mechanical bowel preparation is not necessary for a right colectomy. However, most patients seem to do better with clear liquids and several enemas before an operation. Patients require routine deep vein thrombosis prophylaxis and instructions on postoperative care. The decision to perform an extended right colectomy is influenced by the need to remove at least two major lymphatic drainage fields (tumor at a flexure) or anticipated difficulty in stretching the proximal resection line to the distal colonic resection line without compromising vascular supply or bowel lumen patency. A wedge resection of the transverse colon with right colon–to–left colon anastomosis yields a stretched anastomosis over the pancreas and a large window between the respective mesenteries with opportunity for internal hernia.

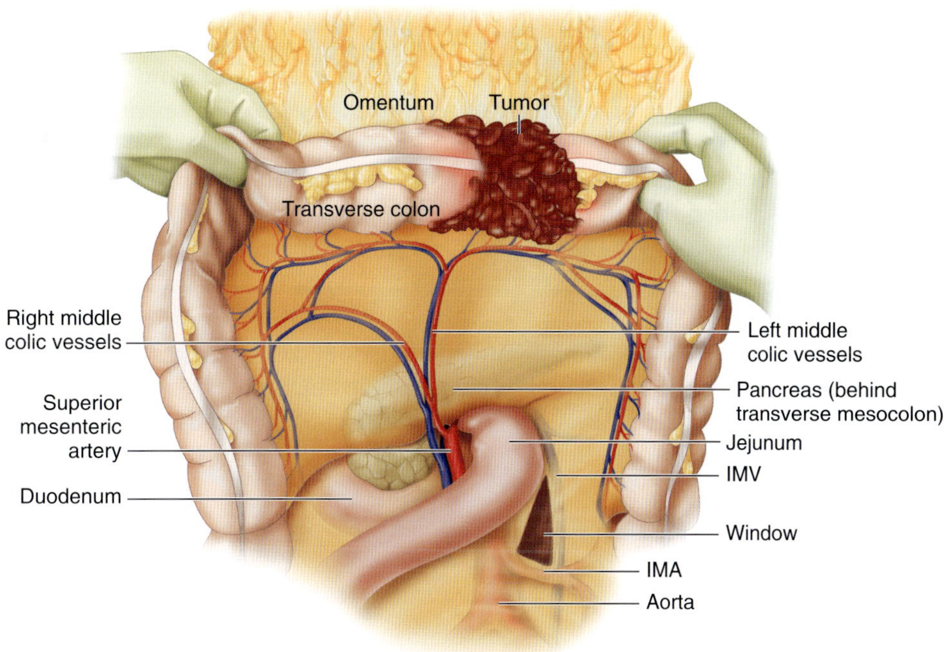
Omentum
Tumor
Transverse colon
Right middle colic vessels
Superior mesenteric artery
Duodenum
Left middle colic vessels
Pancreas (behind transverse mesocolon)
Jejunum
IMV
Window
IMA
Aorta

Figure 3-2

Step 3: Operative Steps

- The patient is placed in the supine position with sequential compression devices on the calves, Foley catheter in place, and the arms stretched to the side for access to the vessels and for blood pressure monitoring. General endotracheal anesthesia is required. An oral gastric tube helps decompress the stomach during the procedure.
- A vertical midline incision is made from the epigastrium to the mid low pelvis, and a Bookwalter retractor (Codman, Raynham, Mass.) is placed for exposure with the abdominal incision stretched widely.
- The right colon is lifted from the pelvis, and a hand is placed from the medial aspect of the abdomen under the peritoneal attachments of the terminal ileum and right colon at the level of the pelvic brim and the white line of Toldt, or the peritoneal attachments along the right gutter are stretched over the index finger as seen in Figure 3-3. The peritoneal attachments are incised with electrocautery to expose the duodenum at the base of the mesentery of the right colon. As seen in Figure 3-4, the right colon is lifted up and medially.
- The right colon is pulled toward the left leg. The space that has been generated over the top of the duodenum is developed bluntly up to the undersurface of the liver. The suspensory peritoneal attachments along the base of the liver toward the gallbladder are incised with electrocautery (Figure 3-5).
- The attachments of the gastrocolic omentum are divided along the cephalad surface of the transverse colon outside the gastroepiploic arcade of the omentum between ties. The omentum is completely released, which allows the posterior aspect of the stomach and the entire lesser sac to be seen (Figure 3-6*A* and *B*).

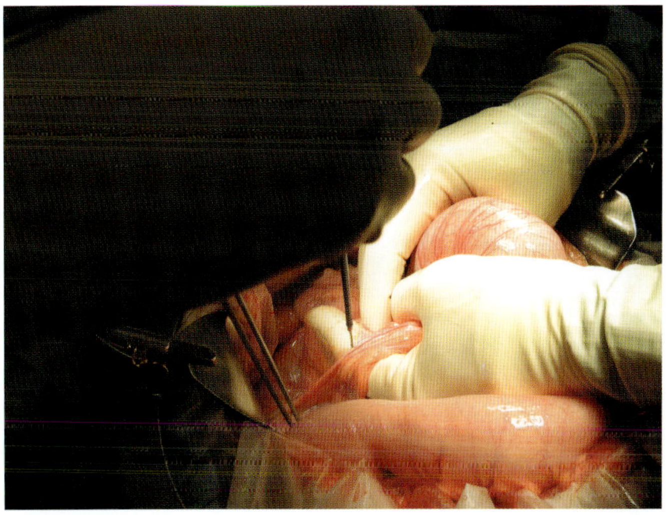

Figure 3-3

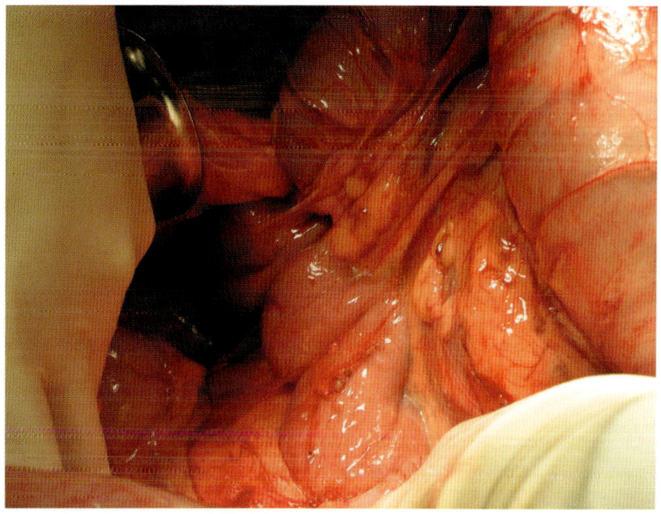

Figure 3-4

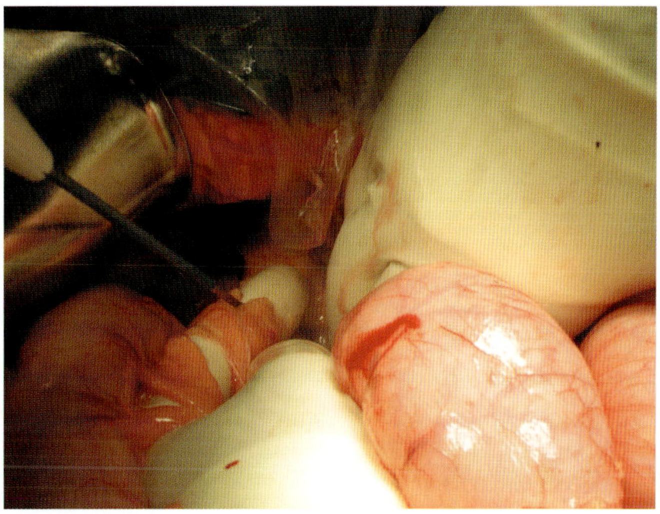

Figure 3-5

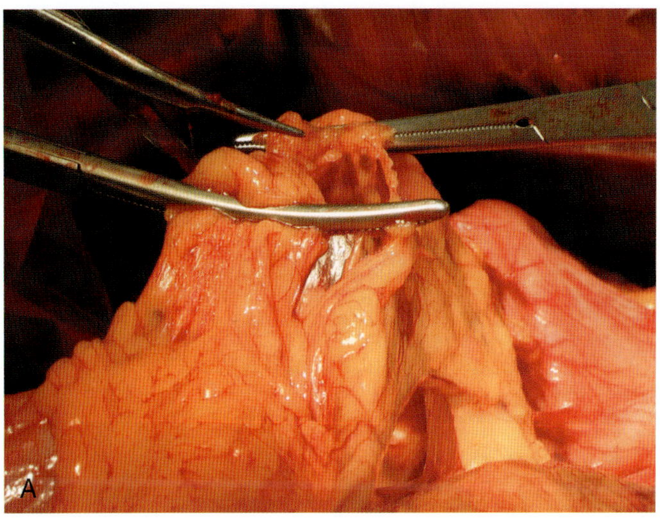

Figure 3-6A

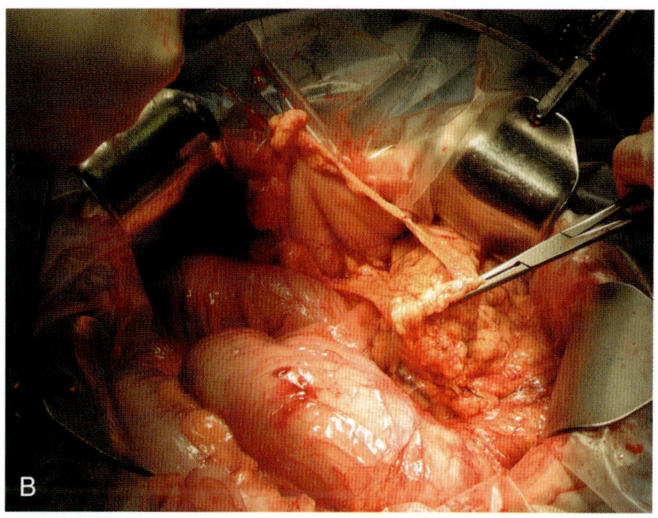

Figure 3-6B

- The colon is returned to its anatomic position with the right colon along the right gutter and the hepatic flexure up in the right upper quadrant. The SMA is identified in its tract to the terminal ileum, and a window is seen in the base of the mesentery of the right colon proximal and distal to a large vascular trunk. This trunk is the ileocolic artery and vein arising from the SMA and superior mesenteric vein (Figure 3-7). An incision is made at the base of this window to expose and divide the ileocolic vessels at their origin (Figure 3-8).

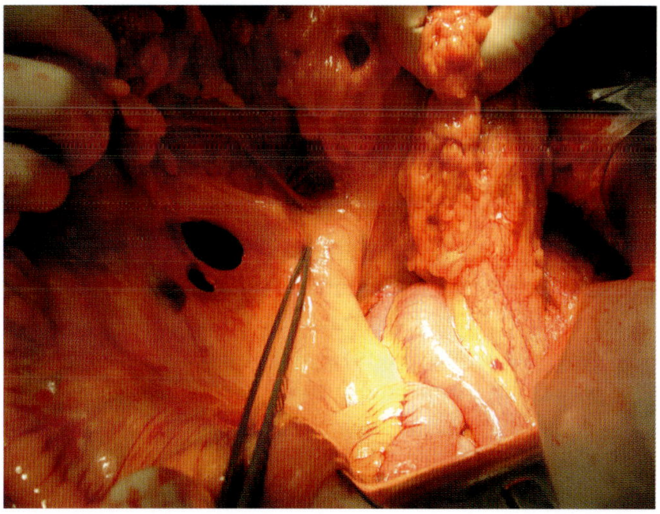

Figure 3-7

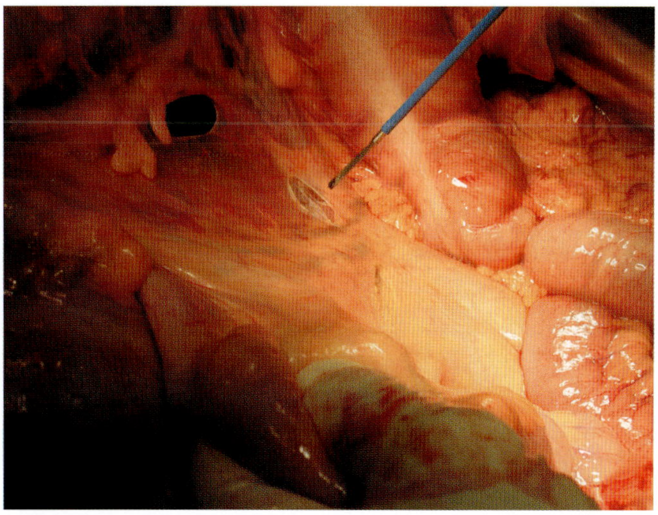

Figure 3-8

- The terminal ileal vessels are divided, and the terminal ileum is transected with a linear cutter stapler proximal to the ileocecal valve (Figure 3-9).
- The sigmoid colon and left colon are retracted to the midline to expose the left gutter and the lateral aspect of the left colon (Figures 3-10*A* and 3-11). The peritoneal surface of the left gutter is incised along the congenital fusion plane at the base of the left colon mesentery

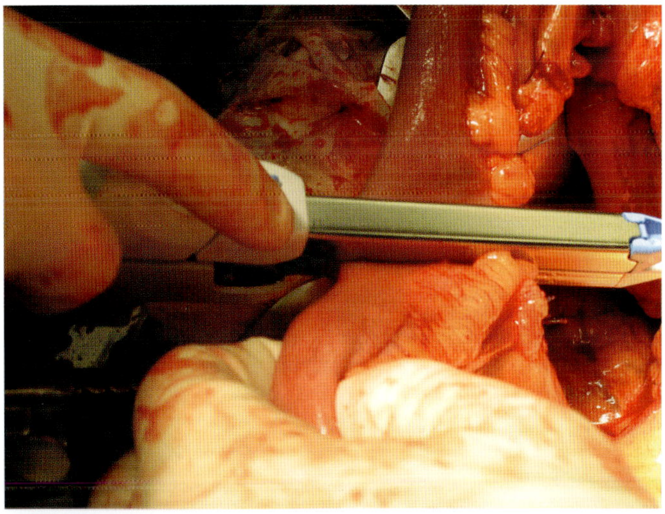

Figure 3-9

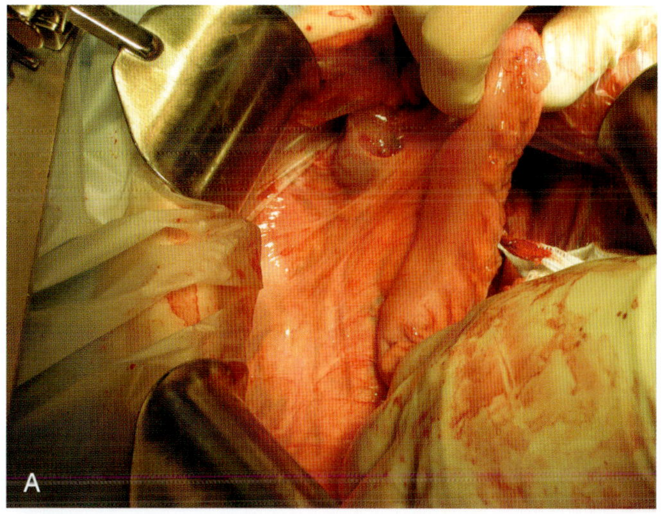

Figure 3-10A

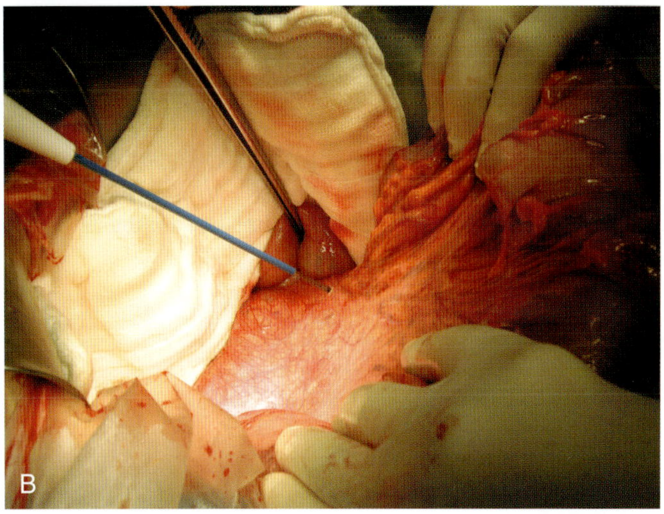

Figure 3-10B

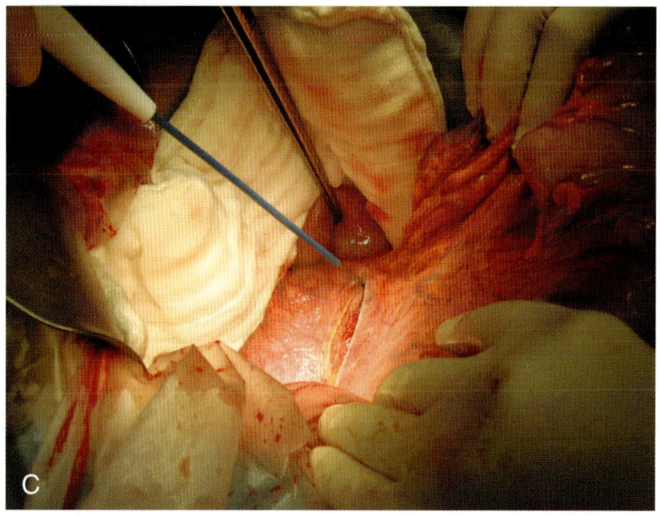

Figure 3-10C

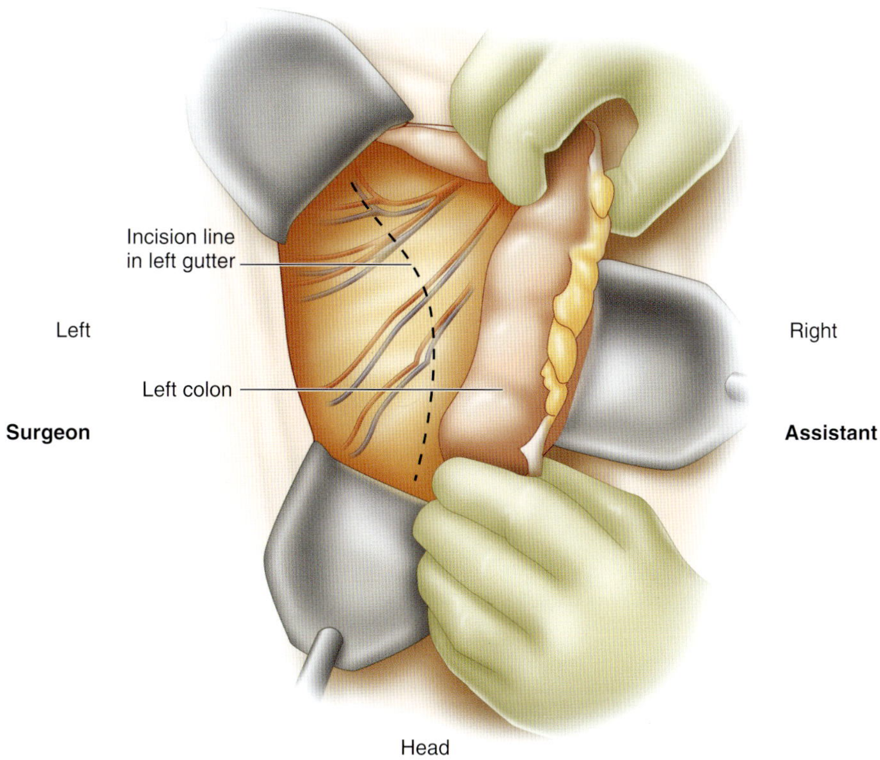

Figure 3-11

to enter an avascular plane from the pelvic brim all the way up to the splenic flexure (Figures 3-10*B* and 3-12). The areolar tissue plane is developed toward the midline to release the mesentery and colon from the retroperitoneal structures, exposing the left ureter and gonadal vessels (Figure 3-10*C*). As the left colon is pushed toward the midline bluntly, the left ureter, gonadal vessels, and areolar tissue plane are dropped posteriorly all the way down to the pelvic brim at the sacral promontory and up to the splenic flexure and all the way to the midline at the aorta (Figure 3-13*A* and *B*).

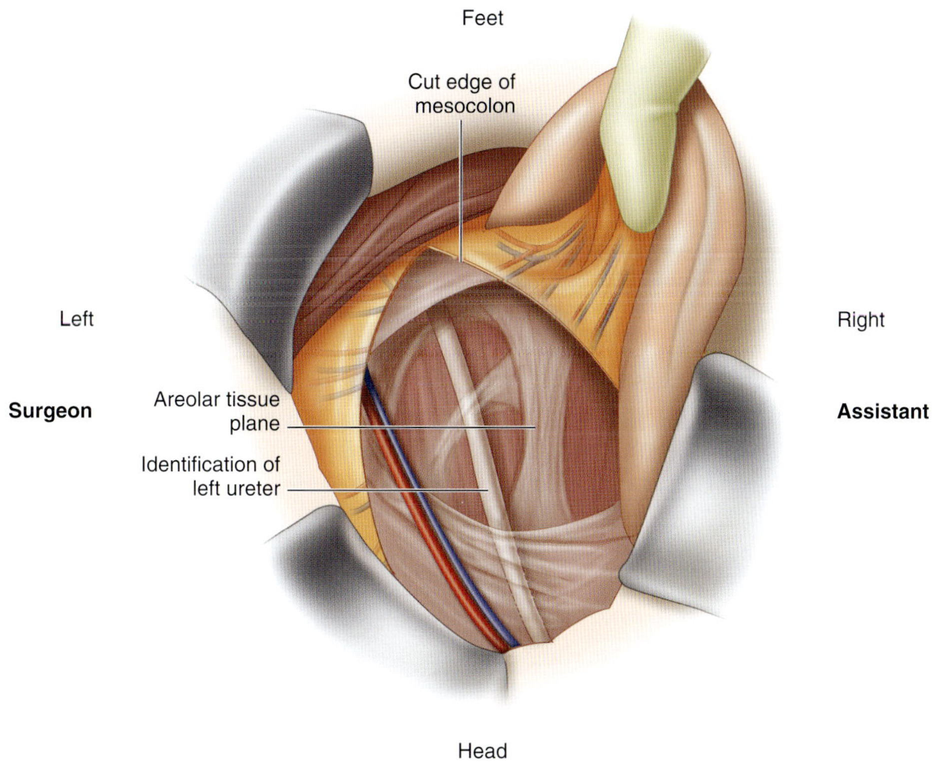

Figure 3-12

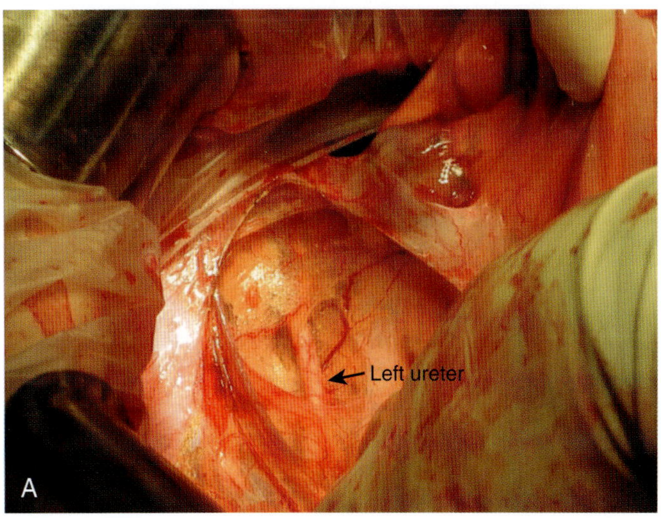

Figure 3-13A

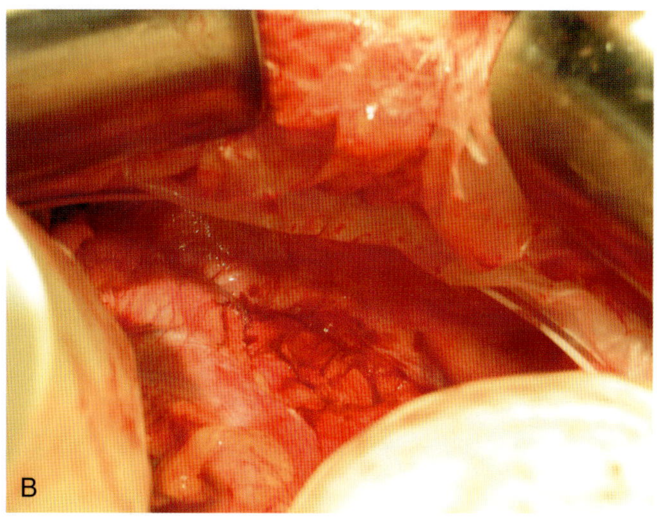

Figure 3-13B

- The splenic flexure is released from the left upper quadrant by incising the lateral peritoneal attachments with a finger placed in the avascular tissue plane posteriorly and extended up toward the tip of the spleen. The peritoneum is incised over the finger using the finger as a guide (Figure 3-14*A*). As the splenic flexure is released medially, the dissection turns toward the pancreas, and the attachments of the splenic flexure to the undersurface of the tail of the pancreas are incised using electrocautery over the finger as a guide (Figure 3-14*B*). The splenic flexure attachments are occasionally very dense and attached to the spleen; these adhesions are freed from the tip of the spleen and the vascular pedicle of the spleen to allow the splenic flexure to move toward the midline (Figure 3-14*C*). The omental attachments along the anterior surface of the splenic flexure and transverse colon are incised with electrocautery to preserve the omentum and release the colon from the undersurface of the omentum toward the previously dissected right colon (Figure 3-14*D*).

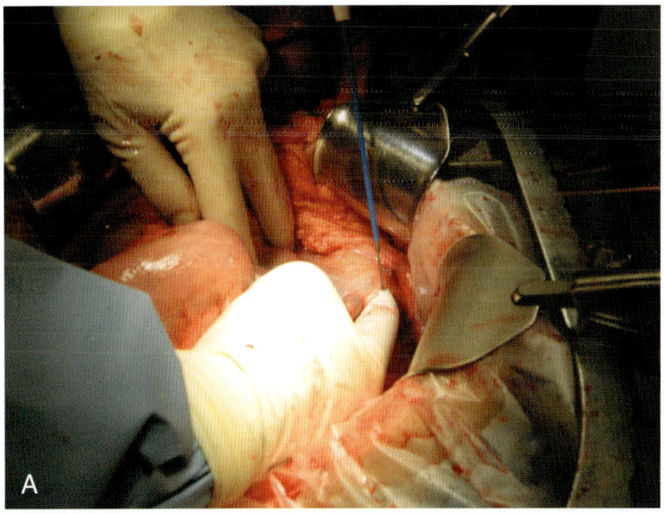

Figure 3-14A

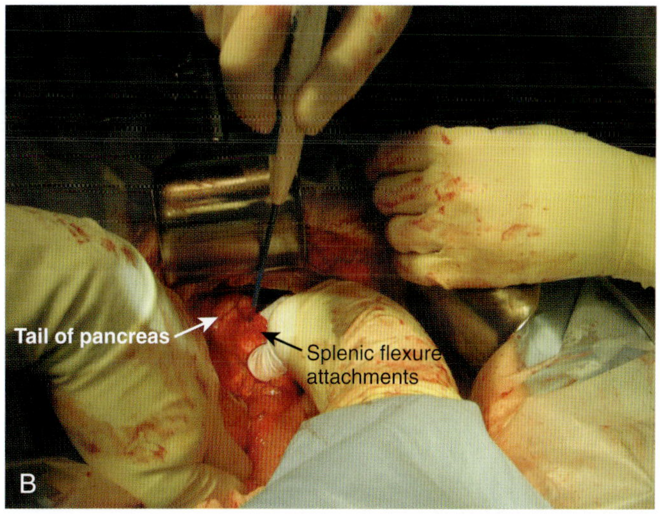

Figure 3-14B

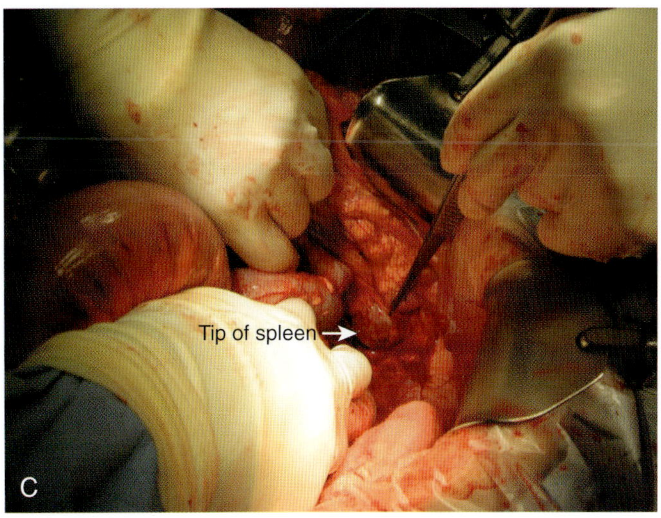

Figure 3-14C

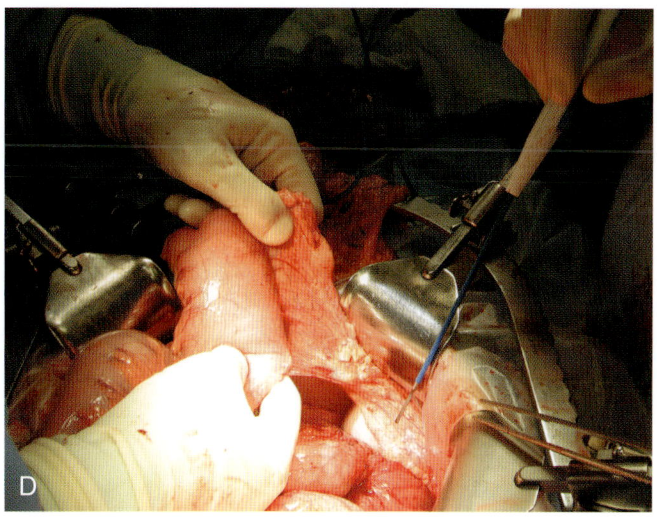

Figure 3-14D

- When the left colon has been mobilized, the sigmoid colon can be transected at a point appropriate for the disease process anywhere along its surface from the rectum to descending colon. The sigmoid colon is transected in a mesenteric-to-antimesenteric direction with a linear cutter stapler at the sacral promontory to provide the distal end of the anastomosis (Figures 3-15 and 3-16).
- The IMA pedicle or the left colic vessels can be divided at their origin or along the vessel pedicle at a point appropriate for the disease process as the left colon is now mobilized from the retroperitoneal structures (Figure 3-17). The IMV can be ligated at its origin adjacent to the third portion of the duodenum with the left colon retracted anteriorly and the small bowel and right colon retracted to the patient's right (Figure 3-18).

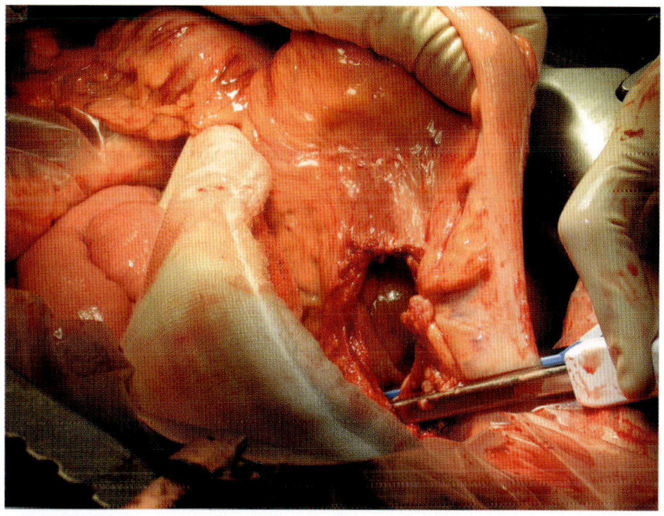

Figure 3-15

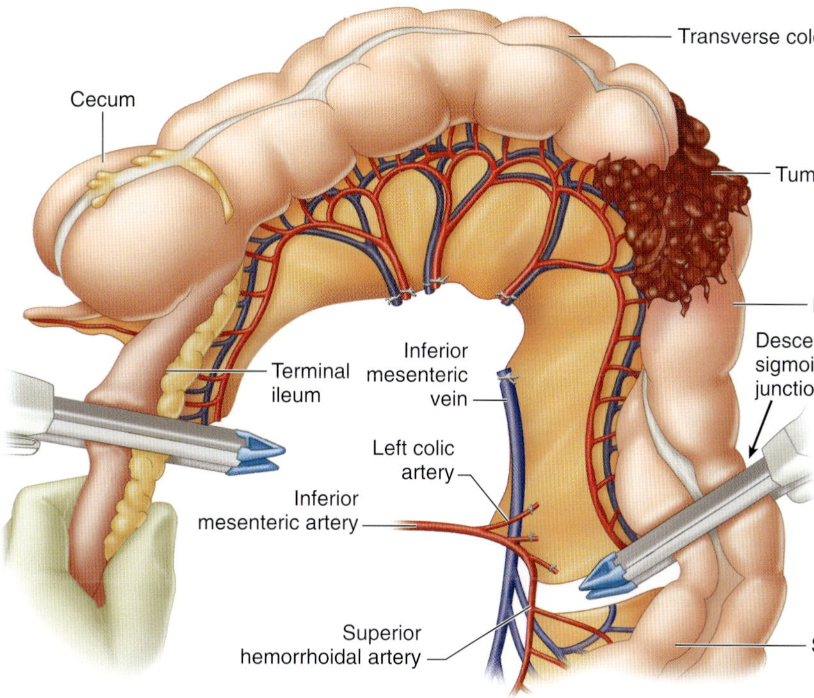

Figure 3-16

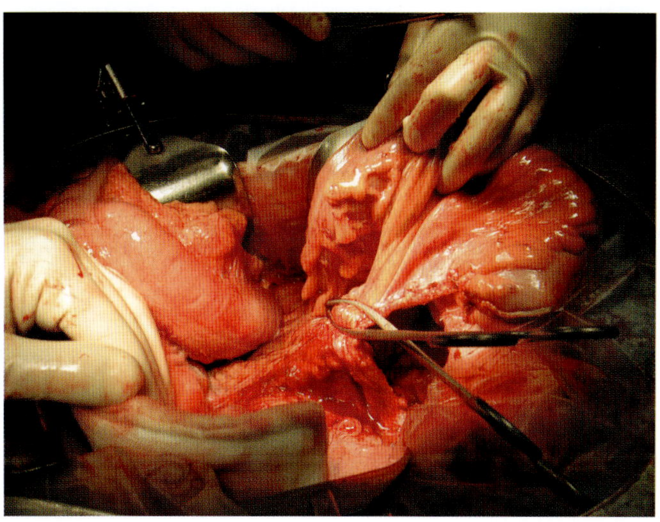

Figure 3-17

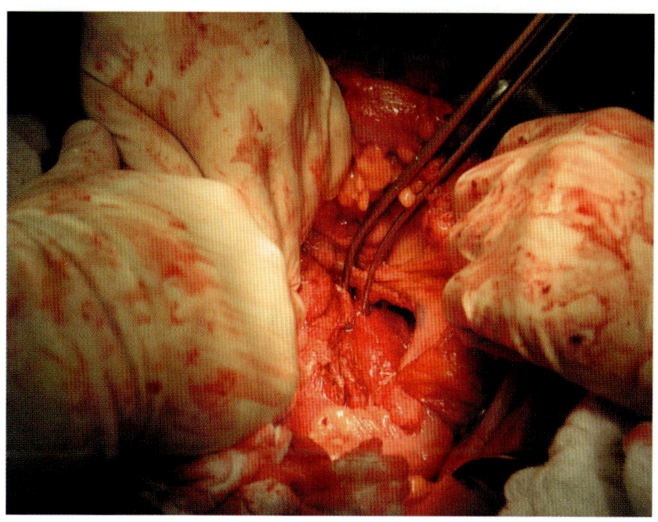

Figure 3-18

- The final step is to divide the transverse colon mesentery and vessels at the middle colic vessel origin over the anterior surface of the pancreas. The base of the right colon mesentery is pulled to the patient's right, and an incision is made across the base of the mesentery of the left colon on the patient's left. The transverse colon can be lifted anteriorly to reveal the final attachments of the colon at the third portion of the duodenum. The base of the mesentery of the transverse colon, as the transverse colon is lifted anteriorly, reveals the middle colic vessels as they form a "V." These vessels are divided outside the pancreatic tissue to protect the anterior surface of the pancreas (Figure 3-19).
- The anastomosis is accomplished by opening the antimesenteric corner of the transverse staple line on the sigmoid colon and the ileum. The small bowel is positioned to the left side of the abdomen with the cut edge of the mesentery placed toward the midline (Figure 3-20). The terminal ileum is allowed to fall to the left side of the pelvis, and the small bowel is brought up along the edge of the left side of the sigmoid colon. The sigmoid is positioned along the right side of the pelvis, and the linear cutter stapler is placed down the open corners of the transverse staple lines to create a side-to-side anastomosis (Figures 3-21 and 3-22).

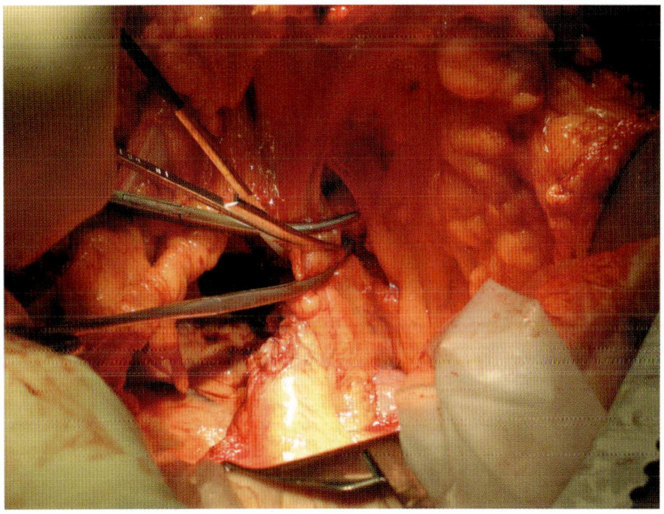

Figure 3-19

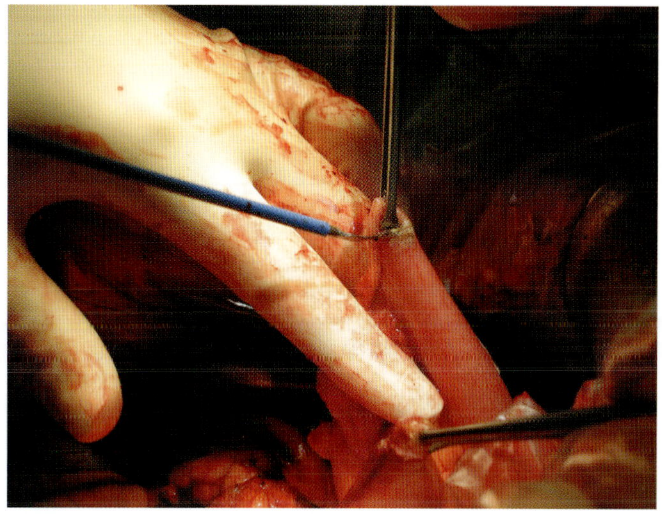

Figure 3-20

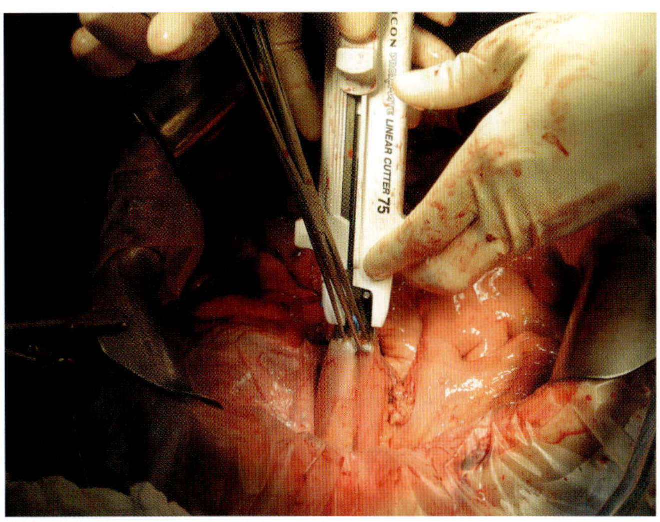

Figure 3-21

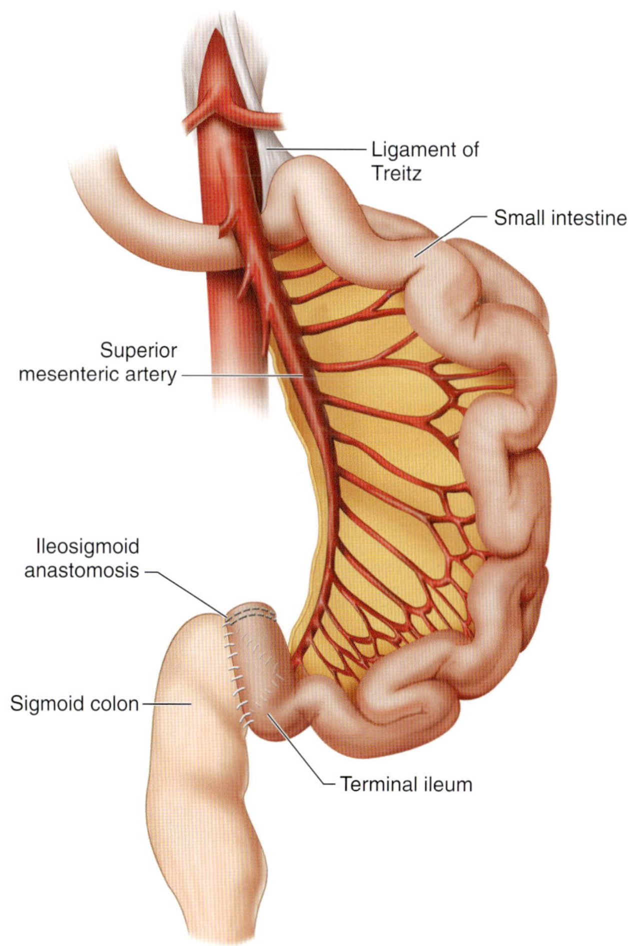

Figure 3-22

- The transverse opening of the anastomosis is opened widely, the GIA staple lines are distracted as far as possible, and the opening is brought together with Allis clamps. The transverse opening is closed with a second firing of the 75-mm linear cutter stapler (Figure 3-23). The mesenteric defect is closed by placing a running suture from the pelvic brim down the mesentery of the sigmoid colon along the mesentery of the small bowel all the way to the base of the duodenum to prevent herniation and twisting (Figure 3-24). The transverse staple line of the ileosigmoid anastomosis is oversewn with a running Lembert suture line of 3-0 absorbable suture to invert and protect the transverse staple line (Figure 3-25). An adhesive barrier can be applied, and the abdomen is closed with a running No. 1 loop absorbable suture.

Step 4: Postoperative Care

Patients are ambulated early. They are given intravenous fluid replacement to maintain a urine output of greater than 30 mL/hr. Nasogastric decompression is not required unless the patient becomes nauseated. Most patients tolerate clear liquids within 24 to 48 hours, and the diet can be advanced as tolerated. Patients should be given prophylactic antibiotics for 24 hours, incentive spirometry, and deep vein thrombosis prophylaxis and encouraged to ambulate as much as possible during the early postoperative period. Usual hospital stay after an open right colectomy is 4 to 5 days; the hospital stay is shorter when the patient is placed on a fast-track postoperative regimen. Postoperative analgesia is usually managed with patient-controlled analgesia followed by a switch to oral analgesics.

Step 5: Pearls and Pitfalls

The most commonly feared complication after an extended right colectomy and ileosigmoid anastomosis is anastomotic leak. Anastomotic leak can be prevented by oversewing the transverse staple line and careful construction of the anastomosis without risk of twist, tension, or ischemia. Closure of the mesenteric defect also prevents herniation and torsion. Occasionally, patients develop a syndrome known as "ileosigmoid" or "ileorectal" syndrome, in which the patient develops an ileus after the initial early return of bowel function. The small bowel becomes distended, bowel function ceases, and the patient becomes nauseated with emesis. A nasogastric tube is required as well as support with intravenous fluids and parenteral nutrition. Decompression of the rectal or sigmoid stump with a 34-F mushroom catheter can sometimes be helpful. This syndrome typically resolves over 4 to 5 days of bowel rest to allow slow resumption of enteral feedings. Most patients have 6 to 10 bowel movements a day at first; this can be modified with the addition of fiber and antidiarrheals over time.

Selected Readings

Parry S, Win AK, Parry B, et al. Metachronous colorectal cancer risk for mismatch repair gene mutation carriers: the advantage of more extensive colon surgery. Gut 2011;60:950-7.

You YN, Chua HK, Nelson H, et al. Segmental vs. extended colectomy: measurable differences in morbidity, function, and quality of life. Dis Colon Rectum 2008;51:1036-43.

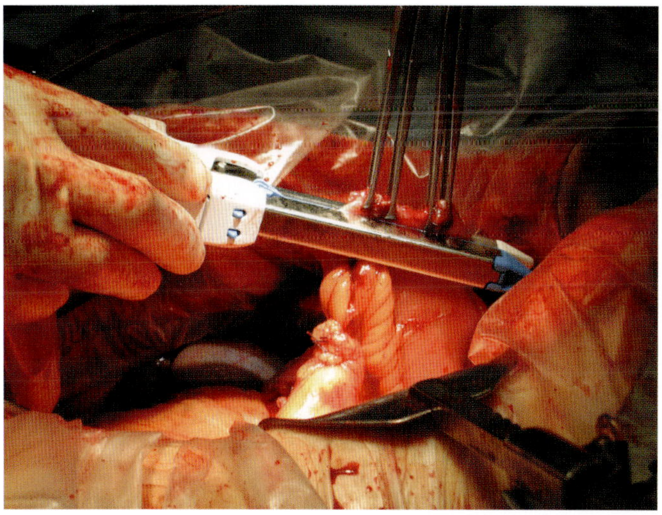

Figure 3-23

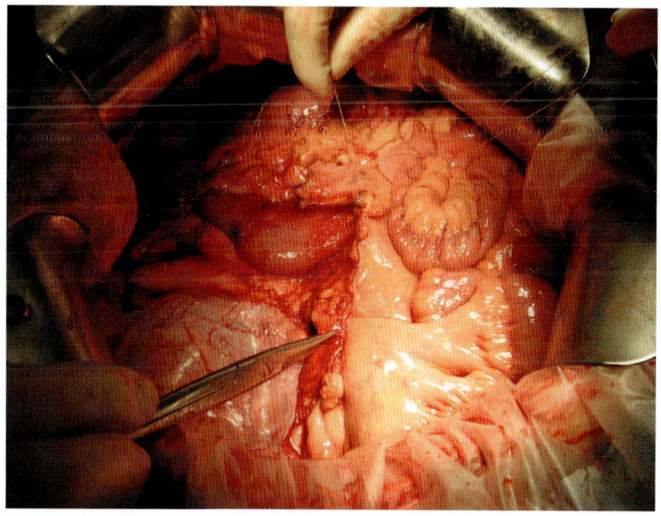

Figure 3-24

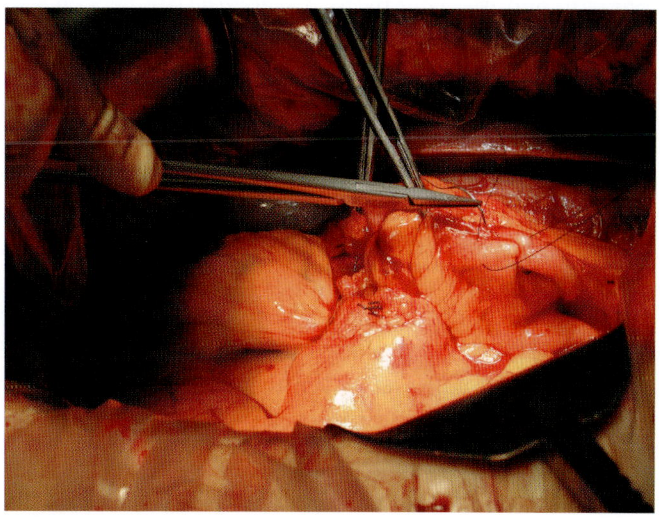

Figure 3-25

CHAPTER 4

Extended Left Colectomy with Right Colon–to–Rectal Anastomosis

Steven R. Hunt

Step 1: Clinical Anatomy

The right colon lies on the patient's right side suspended laterally by peritoneal attachments to the right side of the abdominal wall, superiorly by attachments to the undersurface of the liver and posterior diaphragm, and medially by its mesentery. The ileocolic artery and vein and the right colic vessels, if they are present, run through this leaf of mesentery. The colon is adherent to the retroperitoneum on the right side of the abdomen and covers the right gonadal vessels and right ureter. The inferior vena cava is the next most medial structure on the right side. The hepatic flexure, the fold at the junction between the right colon and transverse colon, is adherent to the anterior surface of the kidney by avascular attachments to Gerota's fascia. The first and second portions of the duodenum are adherent to the undersurface of the mesentery of the right colon and proximal transverse colon. The gallbladder is sometimes adherent to the cephalad surface of the transverse colon at the hepatic flexure. The space behind the right colon is triangular shaped with the flat horizontal surface at the hepatic flexure running from the abdominal side wall toward the midline along the line of the greater curve of the stomach. The vertical axis follows the right lateral side wall of the abdomen. The hypotenuse runs from the fusion plane of the cecum at the pelvic brim over the top of the right iliac artery and vein at about the point where the ureter passes over the iliac vessels toward the midline over the aorta up to the base of the pancreas along the third portion of the duodenum. This triangular retroperitoneal area is a potential space with avascular attachments and allows the right colon to be lifted completely from the retroperitoneum during dissection. Release of all suspensory attachments allows the right colon to be made into a midline structure. The ileocolic artery and vein arise from the superior mesenteric artery (SMA) and superior mesenteric vein in the midportion of the SMA below the duodenum. The right colic artery is a variable structure and may be present as a separate structure or as part of the ileocolic trunk. The right branch of the middle colic artery exits through the pancreatic tissue from its origin on the SMA as a portion of the middle colic trunk at the base of the transverse mesocolon (Figure 4-1*A* and *B*).

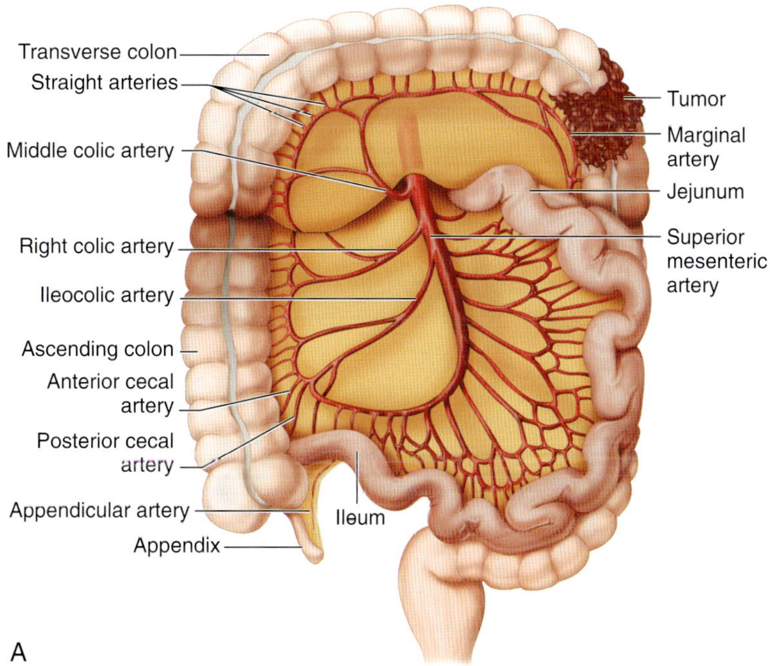

Figure 4-1A

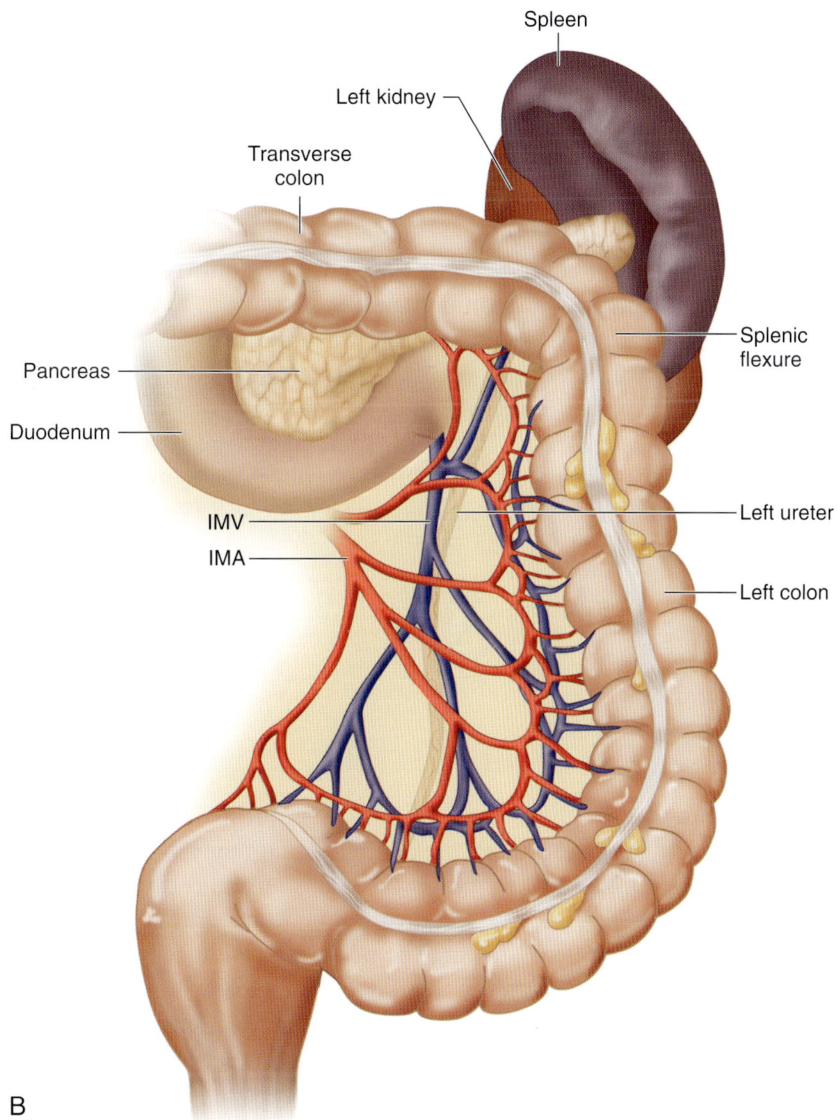

Figure 4-1B

The left branches of the middle colic artery and vein exit adjacent to the right branch of the middle colic and are found at the third portion of the duodenum over the pancreas. The inferior mesenteric vein (IMV) travels along the window of the base of the mesentery of the colon and enters the portal vein adjacent to the ligament of Treitz at the base of the splenic flexure mesentery (Figure 4-2). This area of the vasculature to the colon is extremely complex and should be studied carefully before mobilization of the transverse colon. The mesentery of the transverse colon itself is sometimes attached to filmy attachments of the posterior aspect of the stomach. The omentum falls from the gastroepiploic artery along the greater curve of the stomach over the transverse colon where it attaches tangentially to the antimesenteric surface of the transverse colon and continues to the lower aspect of the abdomen free-floating over the surface of the small bowel.

The splenic flexure of the colon sits in the left upper quadrant with a surface adherent to the undersurface of the tip of the spleen, the anterior surface of the left kidney, and the anterior surface of the tail of the pancreas. A portion of the base of the mesentery of the transverse colon is attached to the undersurface of the tail of the pancreas starting at the level of the IMV and extending laterally toward the left side of the abdomen. These attachments can be released by developing avascular planes given knowledge of the peritoneal windows, areolar tissue planes, and structural relationships. The left colon itself is adherent to the retroperitoneum in the left gutter via an avascular filmy tissue plane, which attaches the mesentery and left colon to the posterior abdominal wall where the ureter and gonadal vessels are found. The peritoneal attachments along the left gutter of the abdomen suspend the left colon from the left side of the abdomen from the pelvic brim all the way up to the splenic flexure. The splenic flexure is a fold of the colon with its apex attached to the tip of the spleen by omental congenital adhesions.

The splenic flexure is usually covered by the omentum as it falls over the top of the transverse colon along the left gutter, and numerous embryologic attachments can occur between the antimesenteric surface of the proximal left colon and the omentum at the splenic flexure. The left colon descends along the left gutter to the level of the pelvic brim, where the colon becomes free from the pelvic side wall and falls into a sigmoid-appearing structure known as the sigmoid colon. The sigmoid colon lies free in the pelvis, attached posteriorly only to its vascular attachments at the midline over the sacral promontory.

The inferior mesenteric artery (IMA) arises from the anterior surface of the aorta proximal to the origin of the common iliac vessels. The IMA branches to give the superior hemorrhoidal artery descending into the posterior mesorectal vessel and the ascending left colic vessel, which sweeps up toward the splenic flexure. The IMV runs across the base of the mesentery of the left colon, crossing the superior hemorrhoidal and left colic vessels on its way to the duodenum. There is a clear peritoneal window between the aorta and the IMV, which can be used to enter the avascular plane behind the left colon mesentery and the retroperitoneum.

Step 2: Preoperative Considerations

Extended left colectomy with right colon–to–rectal anastomosis is indicated for patients with a splenic flexure cancer or multiple cancers involving the sigmoid, the left colon, and the transverse colon. Occasionally, inflammatory bowel disease is an indication for this complex operation. The patient requires very few preoperative preparations and should be informed of the possibility that a diverting loop ileostomy may be performed should the need arise. Prophylactic antibiotics are appropriate for a colectomy to reduce the risk of wound infection. A mechanical bowel preparation is not necessary for an extended left colectomy, but clear liquids may be given the day before the procedure to reduce the volume of stool in the right colon. It is helpful to use two Fleet enemas the night before as well. Patients require routine deep vein thrombosis prophylaxis and instructions on postoperative care.

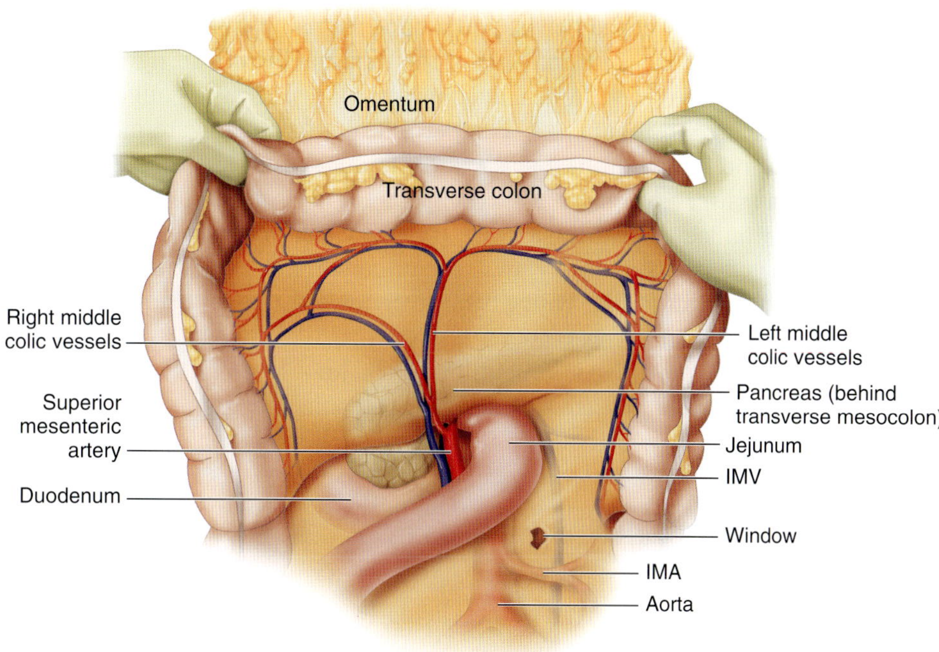
Omentum
Transverse colon
Right middle colic vessels
Superior mesenteric artery
Duodenum
Left middle colic vessels
Pancreas (behind transverse mesocolon)
Jejunum
IMV
Window
IMA
Aorta

Figure 4-2

Step 3: Operative Steps

- The patient is placed in the supine position with sequential compression devices on the calves, urinary bladder catheter in place, and arms stretched to the side for access to the vessels and for blood pressure monitoring. General endotracheal anesthesia is required. An oral gastric tube helps decompress the stomach during the procedure.
- A vertical midline incision is made from the epigastrium to the mid low pelvis, and a Bookwalter retractor (Codman, Raynham, Mass.) is placed for exposure with the abdominal incision stretched widely.
- The right colon is lifted from the pelvis, and a hand is placed from the medial aspect of the abdomen under the peritoneal attachments of the terminal ileum and right colon at the level of the pelvic brim. The lateral peritoneal attachments along the right gutter are stretched over the index finger as seen in Figure 4-3. The peritoneal attachments are incised with electrocautery to expose the retroperitoneal space and the duodenum at the base of the mesentery of the right colon, as seen in Figure 4-4. The right colon is lifted upward and medially.
- The right colon is pulled toward the left leg, the space that has been generated over the top of the duodenum is developed bluntly up to the undersurface of the liver, and the suspensory peritoneal attachments along the base of the liver toward the gallbladder are incised with electrocautery (Figure 4-5).
- The attachments of the gastrocolic omentum are divided between ties along the cephalad surface (antimesenteric) of the transverse colon outside the gastroepiploic arcade of the omentum. The omentum is completely released, which allows the posterior aspect of the stomach and the entire lesser sac to be seen (Figure 4-6).
- The colon is returned to its anatomic position with the right colon along the right gutter and the hepatic flexure in the right upper quadrant. The SMA is identified along its course running caudally to the terminal ileum; a window is seen in the base of the mesentery of the right colon proximal and distal to a large perpendicularly directed vascular trunk. This trunk is the ileocolic artery and vein arising from the SMA and superior mesenteric vein (Figure 4-7). The ileocolic trunk is preserved. The hepatic flexure is transected in a well-vascularized area with the 75-mm linear cutter stapler (Figure 4-8).

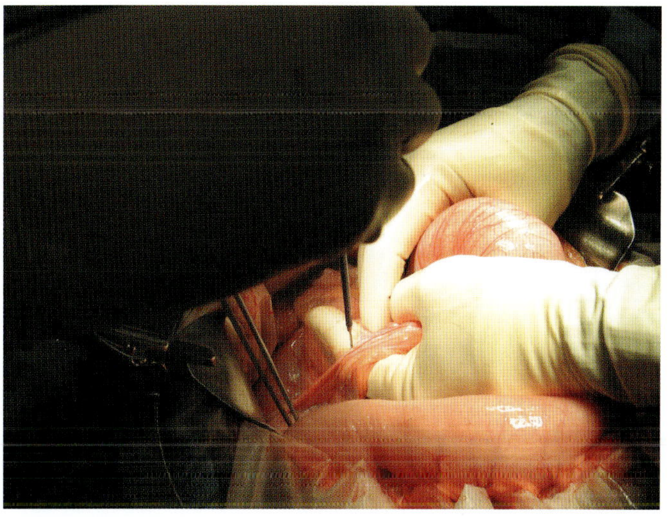

Figure 4-3

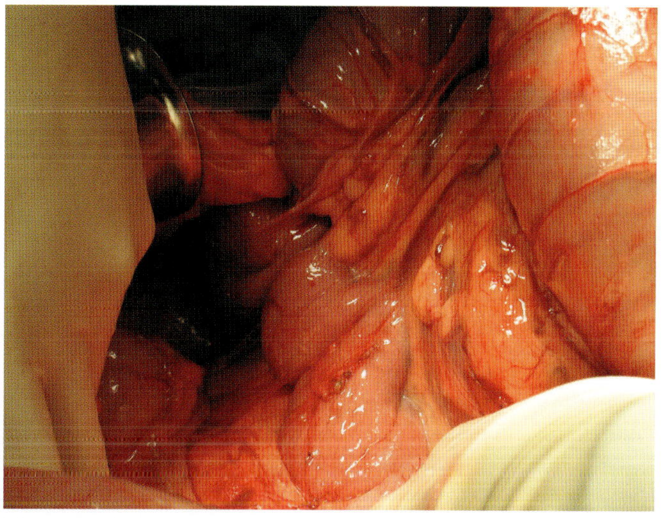

Figure 4-4

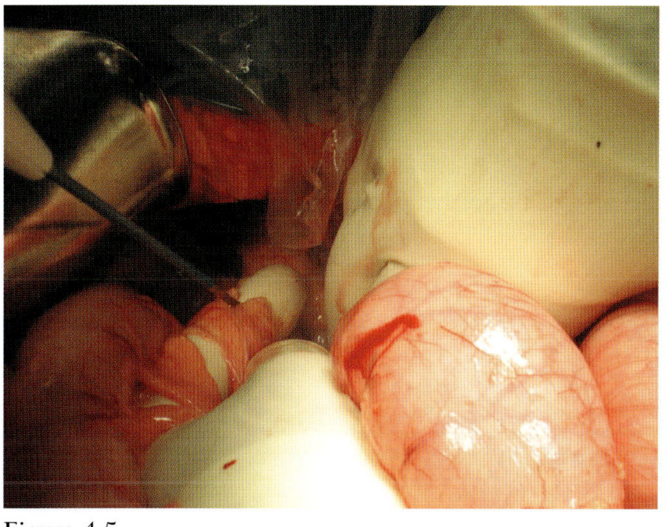

Figure 4-5

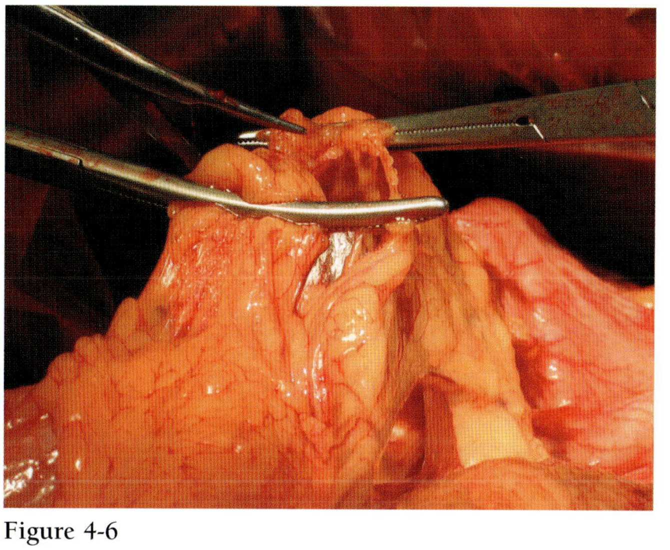

Figure 4-6

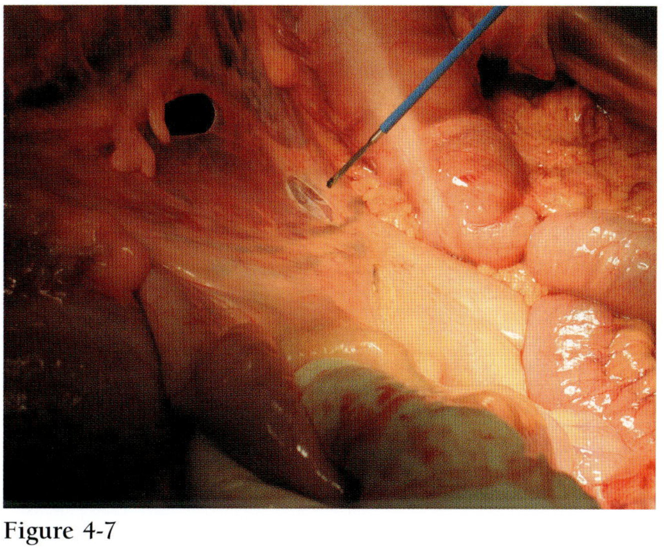

Figure 4-7

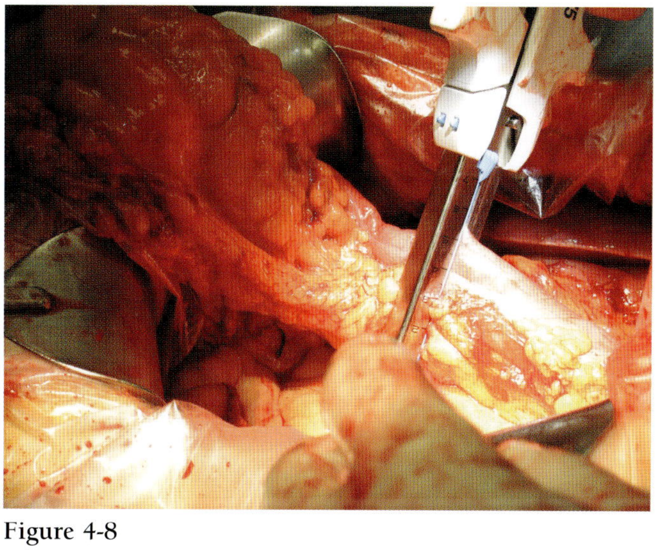

Figure 4-8

- The sigmoid colon and left colon are retracted to the midline to expose the left gutter and the line of incision along the mesentery of the left colon (Figure 4-9*A*). The peritoneal surface of the left gutter is incised along the congenital fusion plane at the base of the left colon mesentery to enter an avascular plane from the pelvic brim all the way up to the splenic flexure (Figure 4-9*B*). The areolar tissue plane is developed toward the midline to release the mesentery and colon from the retroperitoneal structures, exposing the left ureter and gonadal vessels (Figure 4-10). The left colon is pushed toward the midline bluntly as the left ureter, gonadal vessels, and areolar tissue plane are dropped posteriorly to the level of the pelvic brim and sacral promontory. The process is carried out up to the splenic flexure and all the way to the midline at the aorta (Figure 4-11).

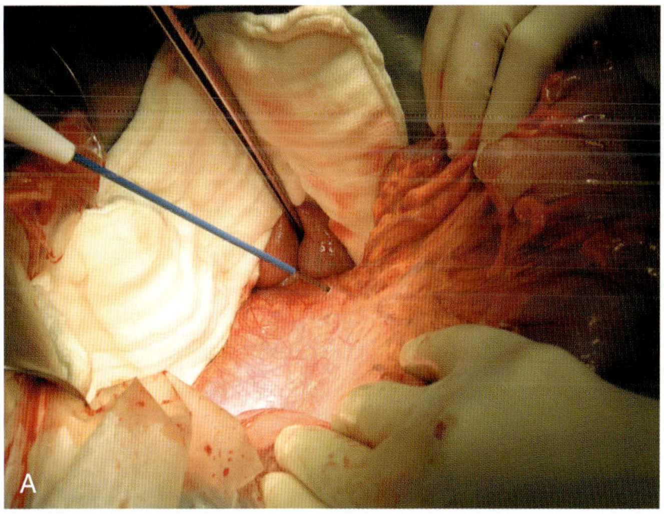

Figure 4-9A

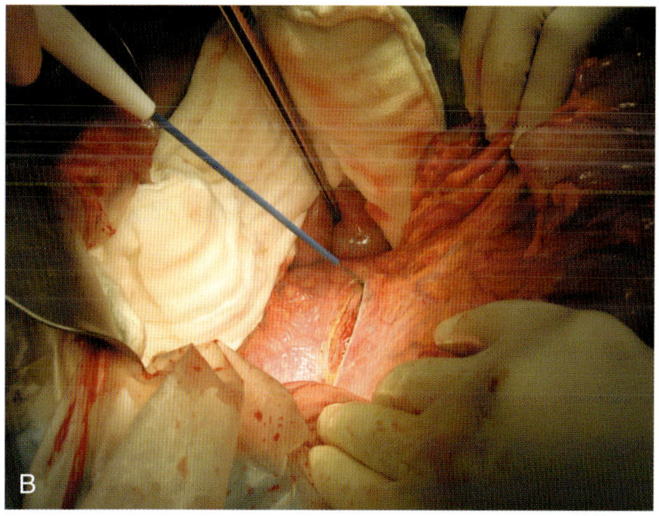

Figure 4-9B

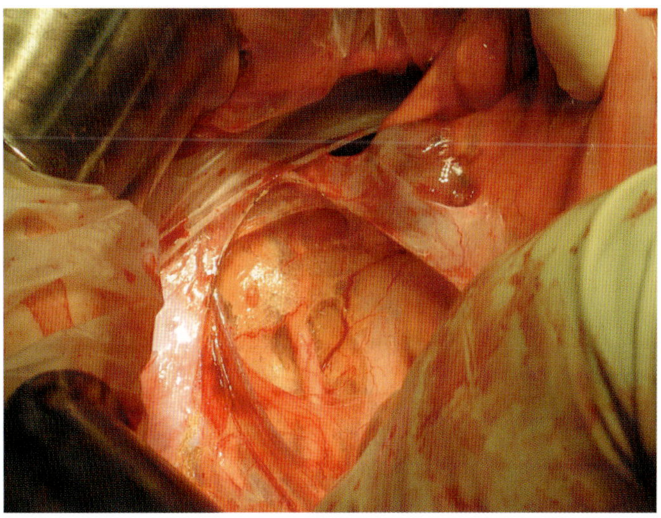

Figure 4-10

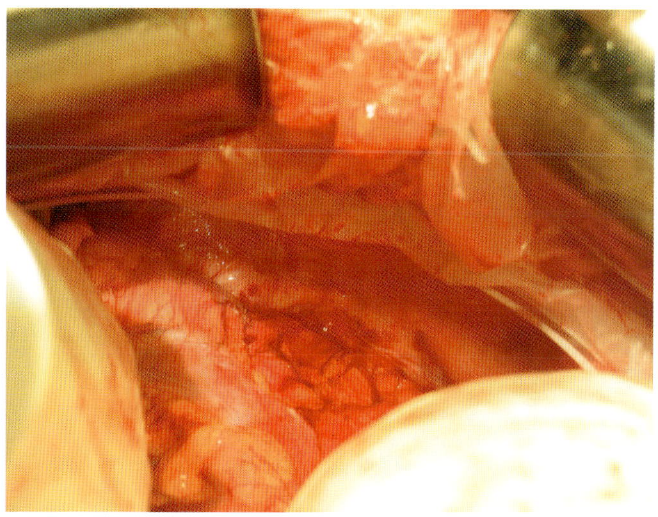

Figure 4-11

- The splenic flexure is released from the left upper quadrant by incising the lateral peritoneal attachments over a finger placed in the avascular tissue plane posteriorly and extended up toward the tip of the spleen. The peritoneum is incised over the finger as a guide (Figure 4-12*A*). As the splenic flexure is released medially, the dissection turns toward the pancreas, and the attachments of the splenic flexure to the undersurface of the tail of the pancreas are incised over the finger with electrocautery, using the finger as a guide (Figure 4-12*B*). The splenic flexure attachments, which are occasionally very dense and attached to the spleen, are freed from the tip of the spleen and the vascular pedicle of the spleen to allow the splenic flexure to move toward the midline (Figure 4-12*C*). The omental attachments along the anterior surface of the splenic flexure and transverse colon are incised with electrocautery to preserve the omentum and release the colon from the undersurface of the omentum toward the transected hepatic flexure (Figure 4-12*D*).
- The rectosigmoid colon is transected in an antimesenteric direction with a linear cutter stapler at the sacral promontory to provide the distal end of the anastomosis (Figure 4-13).

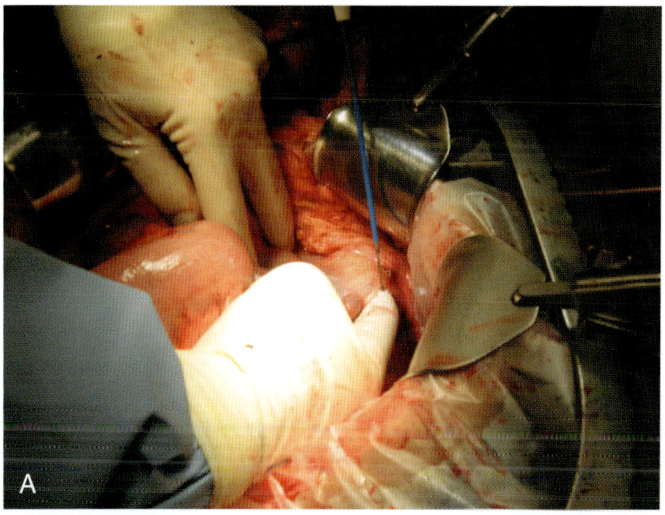
Figure 4-12A

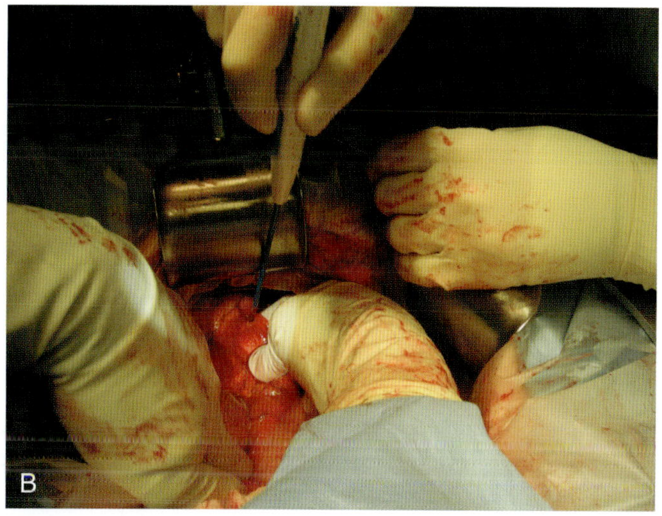
Figure 4-12B

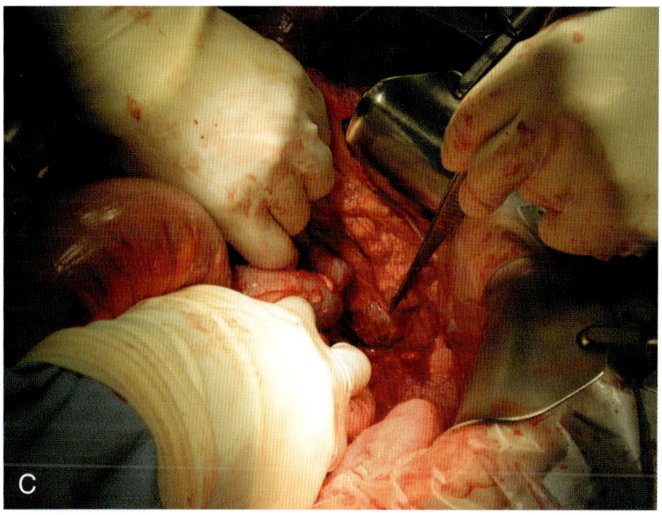
Figure 4-12C

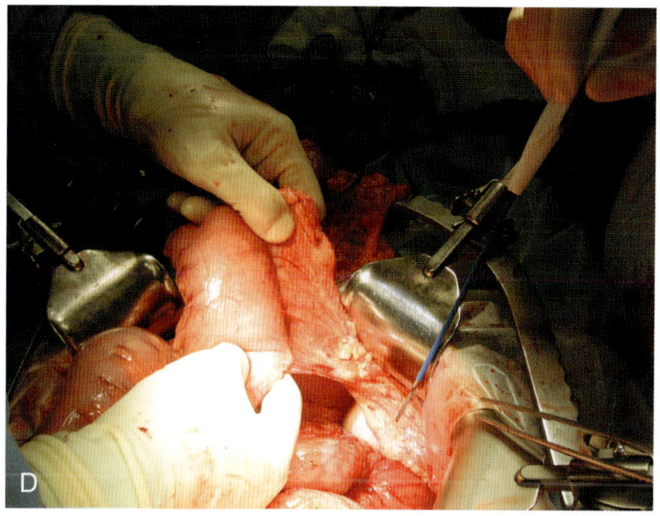
Figure 4-12D

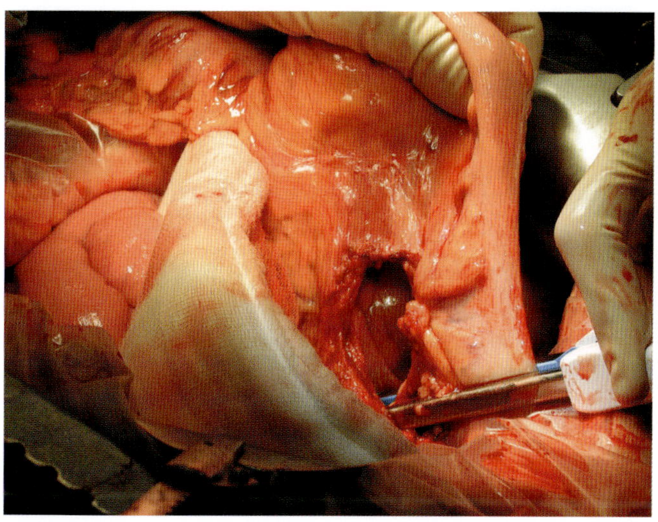
Figure 4-13

- The IMA pedicle is divided at its origin on the aorta (Figure 4-14). The IMV is ligated at its origin adjacent to the third portion of the duodenum with the left colon retracted anteriorly and the small bowel and right colon retracted to the patient's right (Figure 4-15).
- The final step of the bowel resection is to transect the middle colic vessels at their origin over the anterior surface of the pancreas. The base of the right colon mesentery and the base of the mesentery of the left colon are lifted anteriorly, exposing the final attachments of the colon cephalad to the third portion of the duodenum at the base of the mesentery of the transverse colon. With the transverse colon retracted cephalad, these vessels form a "V" and can be easily identified and divided outside the pancreatic tissue protecting the anterior surface of the pancreas (Figure 4-16).
- After removing the transverse, left, and sigmoid colon as a specimen, the hepatic flexure is rotated 180 degrees counterclockwise to place the right colon and terminal ileum in the midline of the abdomen with a straight, untwisted edge of cut mesentery extending from the duodenum to the pelvic brim (Figure 4-17*A*). The hepatic flexure and right colon fall to the pelvis (with the cecum at the pelvic brim) to lie to the left of the midline rectal stump. The staple line of the hepatic flexure is pulled up to lie adjacent to the cut end of the rectum. A functional end-to-end, side-to-side anastomosis is accomplished with a firing of the 75-mm linear cutter stapler through the open antimesenteric corners of the transverse staple lines through the right colon and the rectum (Figure 4-17*B*). The resulting opening is closed using a transversely placed staple line of the 75-mm linear cutter stapler, with the GIA staple lines distracted as far as possible. The transverse staple line is inverted with a continuous 3-0 absorbable suture with Lembert sutures. The apex of the GIA staple line at the crotch between

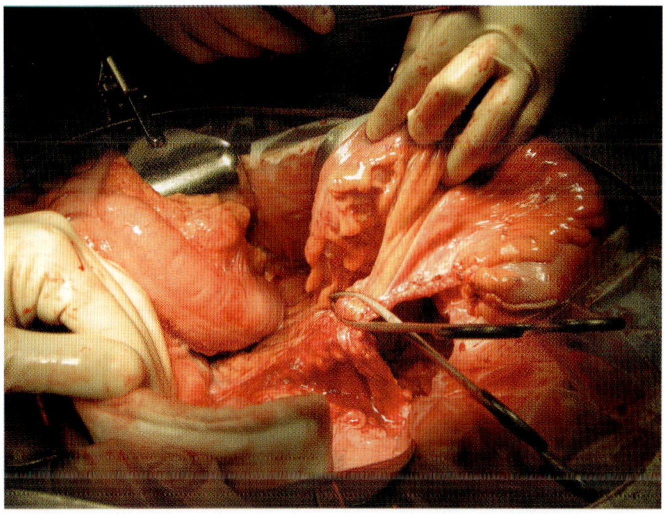

Figure 4-14

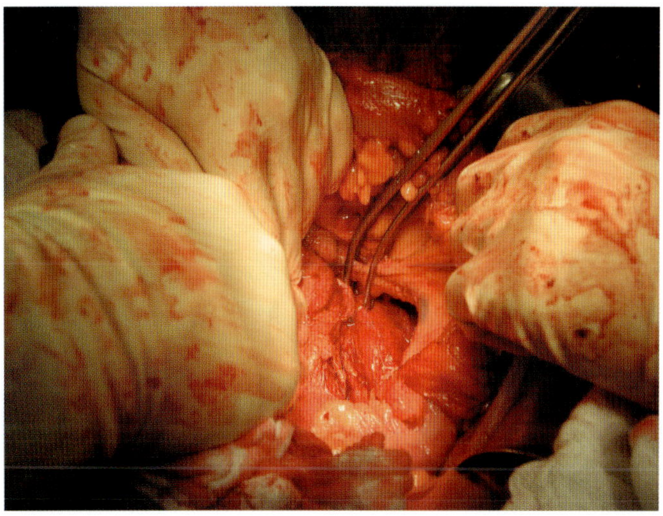

Figure 4-15

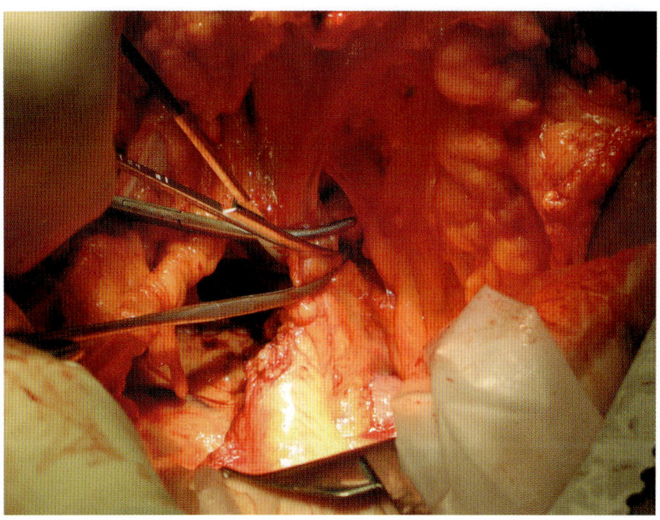

Figure 4-16

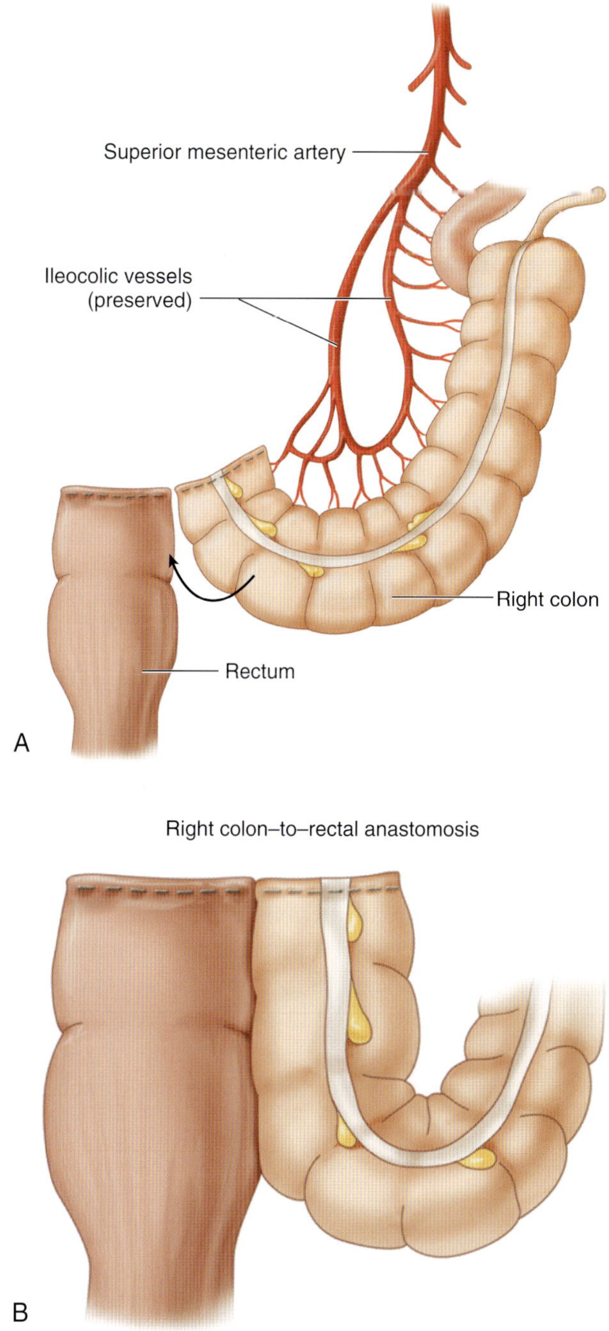

Figure 4-17A-B

the right colon and the rectum is protected with a 3-0 absorbable suture between the portions of bowel. The mesenteric defect is closed with a continuous absorbable suture from the duodenum along the mesenteric edge of the terminal ileum and right colon down to the level of the sacral promontory and the rectal stump; this may prevent volvulus and internal herniation (Figure 4-18).

Step 4: Postoperative Care

The abdomen is closed with a running No. 1 loop absorbable suture and staples, and sterile gauze is applied. Patients are ambulated early. Intravenous fluid replacement is given to maintain a urine output of greater than 30 mL/hr. Nasogastric decompression is not required unless the patient becomes nauseated. Most patients tolerate clear liquids within 24 to 48 hours, and the diet can be advanced as tolerated. Patients should be given prophylactic antibiotics for 24 hours, incentive spirometry, and deep venous thrombosis prophylaxis and encouraged to ambulate as much as possible during the early postoperative period. Usual hospital stay after an open extended left colectomy is 4 to 5 days; the hospital stay is shorter when the patient is placed on a fast-track postoperative regimen. Postoperative analgesia is usually managed with patient-controlled analgesia followed by a switch to oral analgesics.

Step 5: Pearls and Pitfalls

The most commonly feared complication after an extended left colectomy and right colon-to-rectal anastomosis is anastomotic leak. These leaks can be prevented with oversewing of the transverse staple line and careful construction without risk of twist, tension, or ischemia. The closure of the mesenteric defect also prevents herniation and torsion. An incidental appendectomy may be prudent to prevent difficulty with diagnosis of acute appendicitis and its related complications because the appendix may now reside in the left lower quadrant. Most patients have 6 to 10 bowel movements a day at first; this can be modified with the addition of fiber and antidiarrheals over time. Preservation of the water-absorptive surface of the right colon should yield improved bowel function over time.

Selected Readings

Adriano T, Gianluca M, Vittorio F. A technique for colorectal anastomosis after extended left colectomy. Eur J Surg 1998;164:627-8.
Le TH, Gathright JB Jr. Reconstitution of intestinal continuity after extended left colectomy. Dis Colon Rectum 1993;36:197-8.

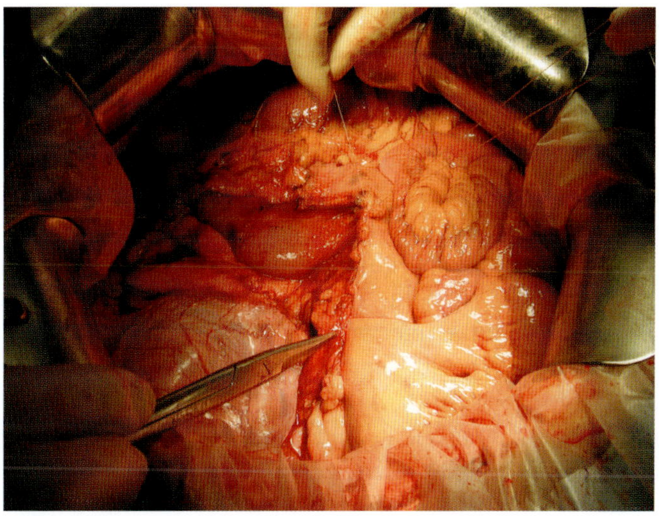

Figure 4-18

CHAPTER 5

Open Left and Sigmoid Colectomy

Matthew G. Mutch

Step 1: Clinical Anatomy

The left colon lies along the left side of the abdomen suspended from the splenic flexure to the pelvic brim by lateral peritoneal attachments. The mesentery of the left colon arises from the midline of the abdomen along the aorta. The sigmoid colon has no lateral peritoneal attachments other than some congenital adhesions, which fix the apex of the sigmoid to the pelvic brim and the iliac fossa. Otherwise, the sigmoid colon is attached to the retroperitoneum through a midline mesentery arising from the inferior mesenteric artery (IMA) and extending down into the pelvis to the mesorectum. The splenic flexure is attached to the undersurface of the tip of the spleen, the lower edge of the tail of the pancreas, and the anterior surface of the left kidney by various levels of suspensory ligaments and peritoneal extensions. The blood supply to the left colon is based on the IMA, which arises from the anterior surface of the aorta just above the bifurcation of the common iliac arteries. The IMA extends anteriorly and bifurcates to produce the superior rectal artery feeding the sigmoid colon and the rectum. The left colic artery extends cephalad to provide the left colon and distal splenic flexure with blood supply through the arcade at the mesenteric edge known as the marginal artery of Drummond. The retroperitoneum behind the left colon contains the left ureter and the gonadal vessels lying over the psoas muscle. The ureter crosses the iliac vessels at the bifurcation of the iliac vessels into the external and internal iliac branches (Figure 5-1).

Step 2: Preoperative Considerations

A mechanical bowel preparation may be beneficial because it eliminates formed stool in the distal colon and improves handling and anastomosis formation. However, it is not required, and enemas may suffice. Antibiotic prophylaxis begun preoperatively and continuing for 24 hours postoperatively is recommended. Deep vein thrombosis prophylaxis by means of sequential compression devices is required and may be supplemented with subcutaneous heparin. Preoperative tattooing of a neoplastic lesion is very helpful to identify a small lesion intraoperatively.

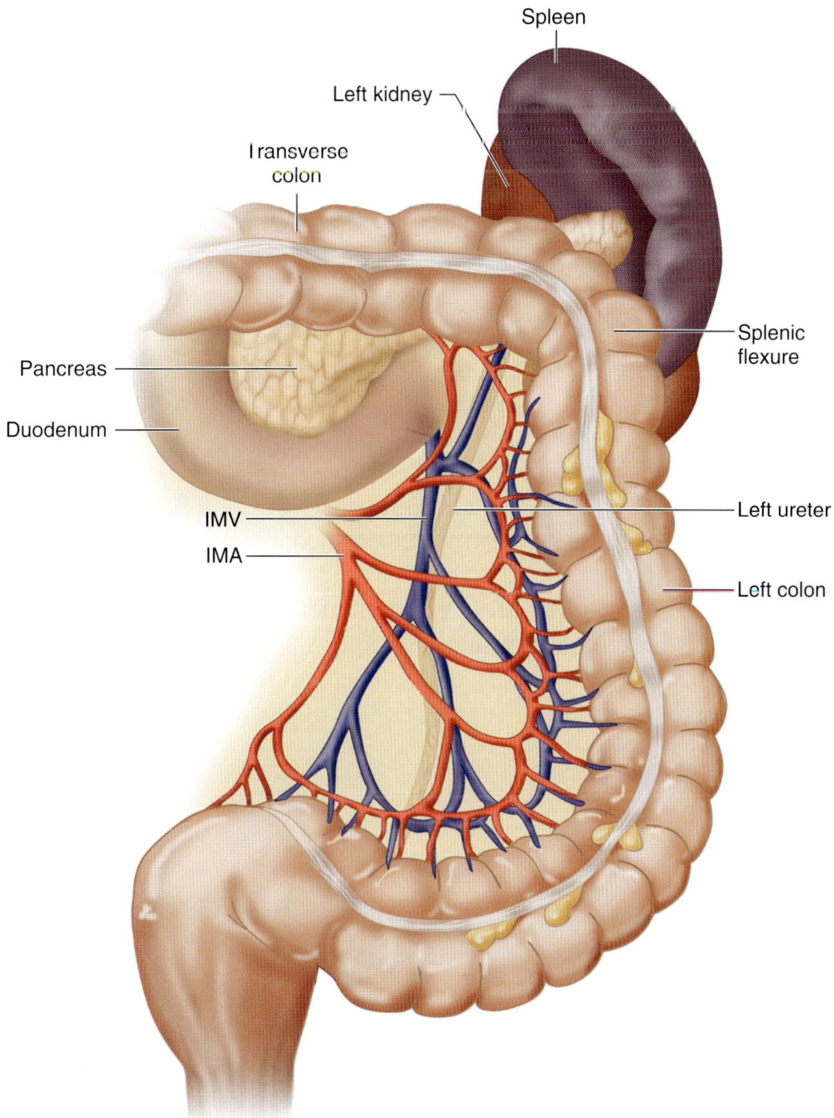
Spleen
Left kidney
Transverse colon
Splenic flexure
Pancreas
Duodenum
Left ureter
IMV
IMA
Left colon

Figure 5-1

Step 3: Operative Steps

- The patient is placed in lithotomy position using Allen's stirrups with sequential compression devices and bladder catheter in place. The rectum is irrigated to clear the rectum of any solid stool. The patient's arms are placed with the left arm extended and the right arm tucked to allow an overhead Mayo stand placed for draping. The abdomen is entered through a vertical midline incision from xiphoid to pubis, and the Bookwalter retractor (Codman, Raynham, Mass.) is placed for exposure and opened widely. The small bowel is retracted to the right upper quadrant and upper midline.
- An incision is made at the base of the lateral aspect of the left colon mesentery along the white line of Toldt with the left colon retracted medially and anteriorly (Figure 5-2). The incision is extended from the pelvis to the left upper quadrant. The exposed areolar tissue plane allows dissection anterior to the retroperitoneum (Figure 5-3). Blunt dissection frees the left colon from the retroperitoneum and exposes the ureter and gonadal vessels within the retroperitoneum (Figure 5-4). The blunt dissection is carried medially to the base of the aorta and cephalad to the splenic flexure level, freeing the left colon from the anterior surface of the kidney (Figure 5-5).

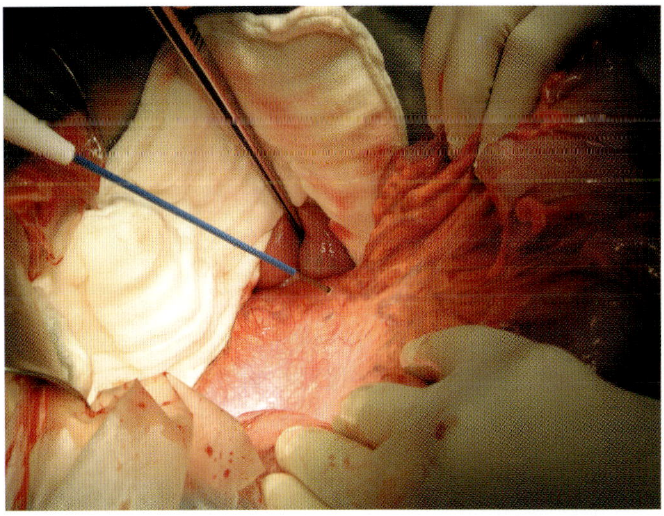
Figure 5-2

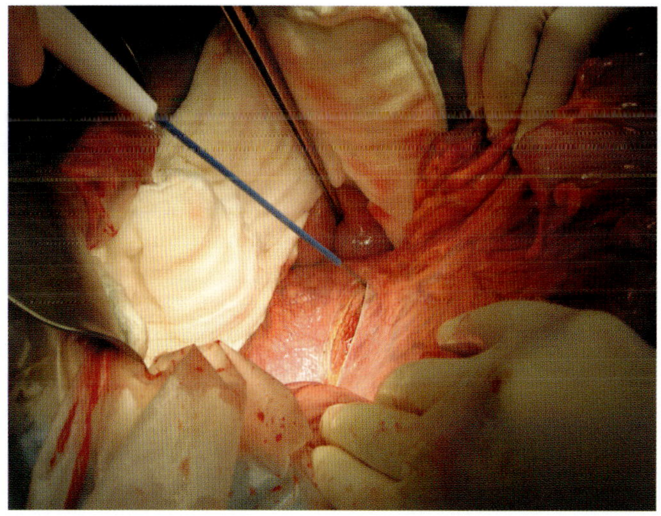
Figure 5-3

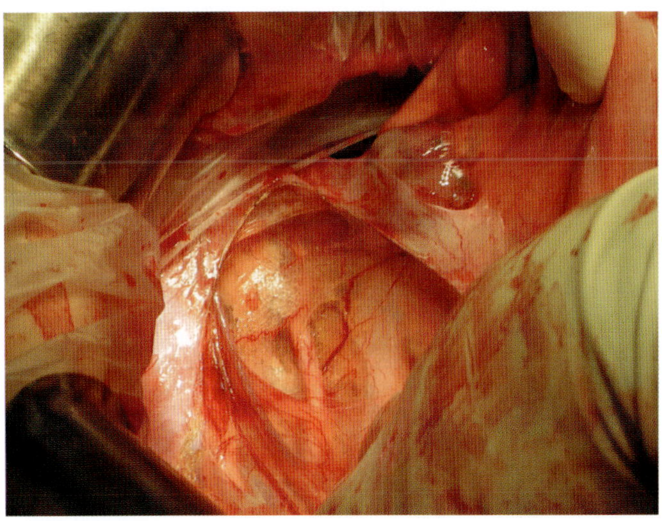
Figure 5-4

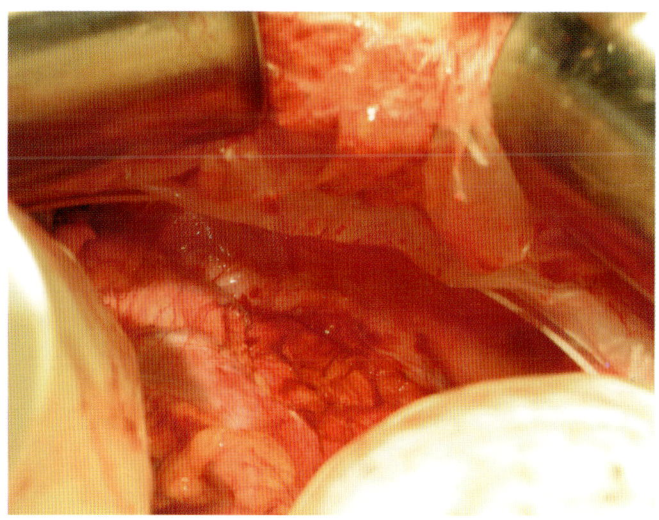
Figure 5-5

- An incision is made on the peritoneal attachments of the splenic flexure using the finger as a guide, incising lateral to medial to release the splenic flexure from the undersurface of the tip of the spleen, the lateral aspect of the abdominal cavity, and the anterior surface of the kidney (Figure 5-6). The tip of the spleen is freed from the splenic flexure, releasing the multiple congenital adhesions and incising the omental attachment to release the splenic flexure toward the midline (Figure 5-7). The attachments of the splenic flexure to the undersurface of the tail of the pancreas and the retroperitoneum are incised all the way to the midline toward the duodenum at the ligament of Treitz (Figure 5-8).
- The omental attachments to the anterior surface of the transverse colon are incised, releasing the splenic flexure from the left upper quadrant. The omental attachments to the transverse colon are incised all the way to the middle of the transverse colon or to the right colon itself (Figure 5-9).

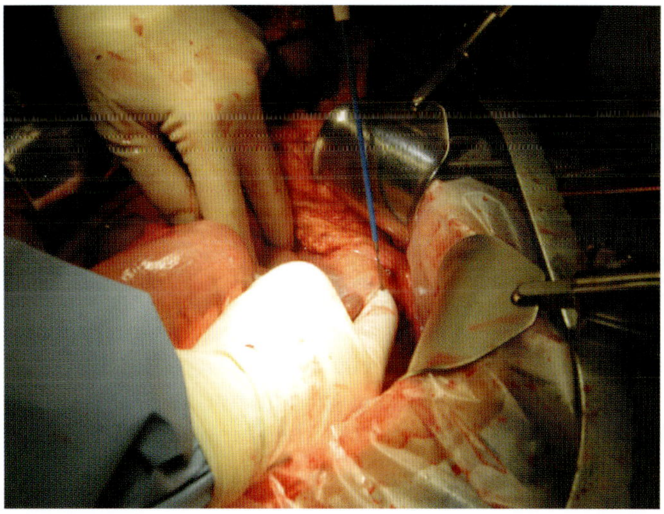

Figure 5-6

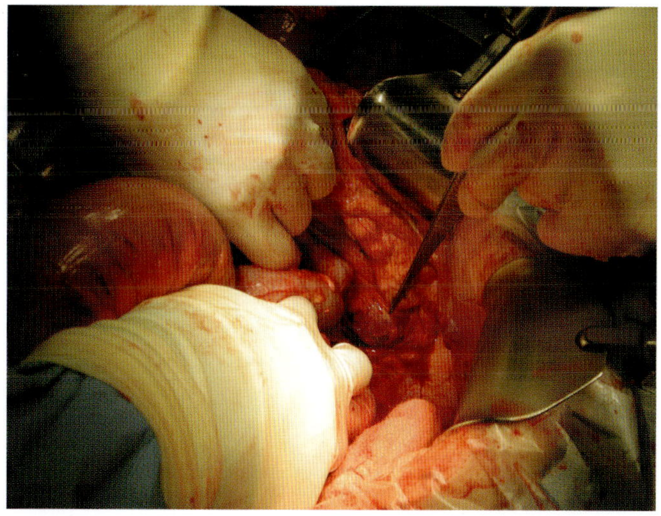

Figure 5-7

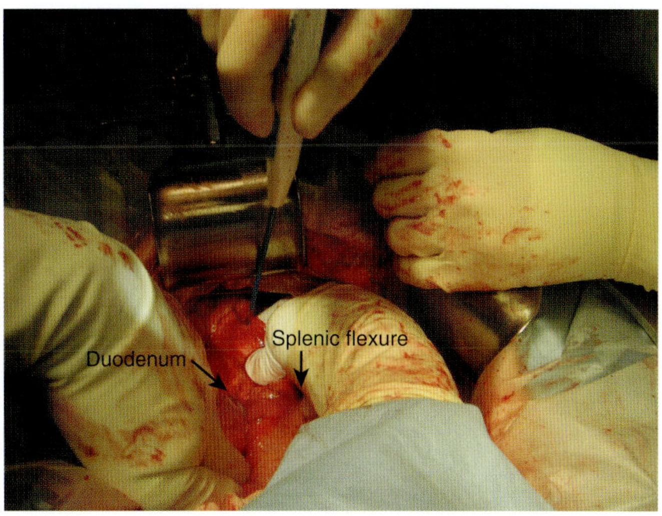

Figure 5-8

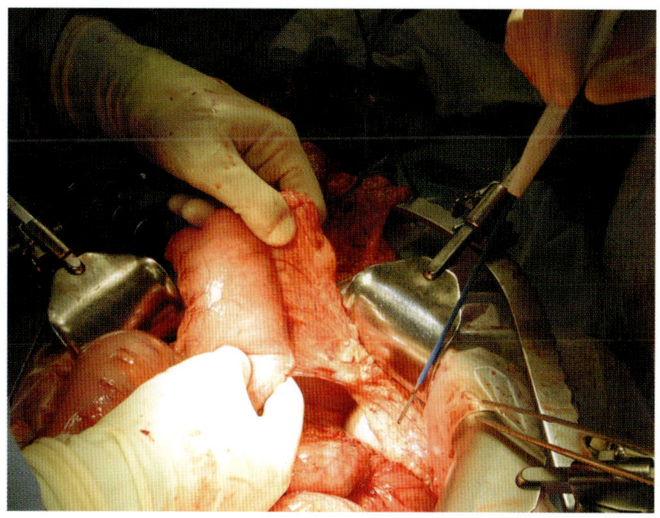

Figure 5-9

- The left colon is lifted from the abdomen and is pulled to the patient's left, exposing the medial aspect of the left colon mesentery over the aorta. The IMA is encountered at the level of the aorta just above the bifurcation of the common iliac artery and vein. The inferior mesenteric vein (IMV) is identified at the level of the ligament of Treitz at the base of the mesentery of the left colon above a window of clear peritoneum along the anterior surface of the aorta (Figures 5-10 and 5-11). The IMA and IMV are isolated at their origins and divided between ties (Figures 5-12 and 5-13).

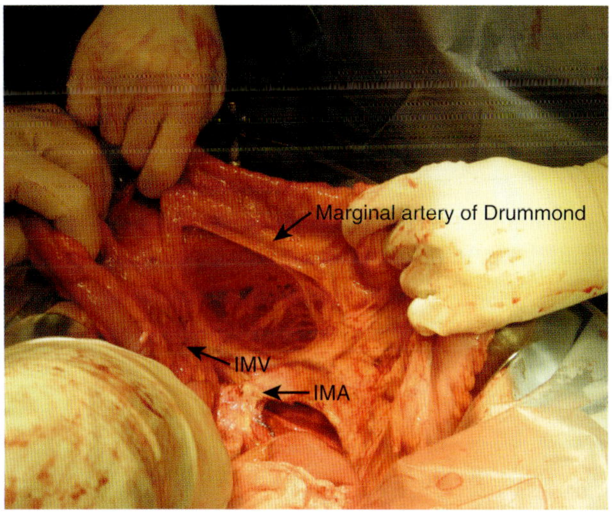

Figure 5-10

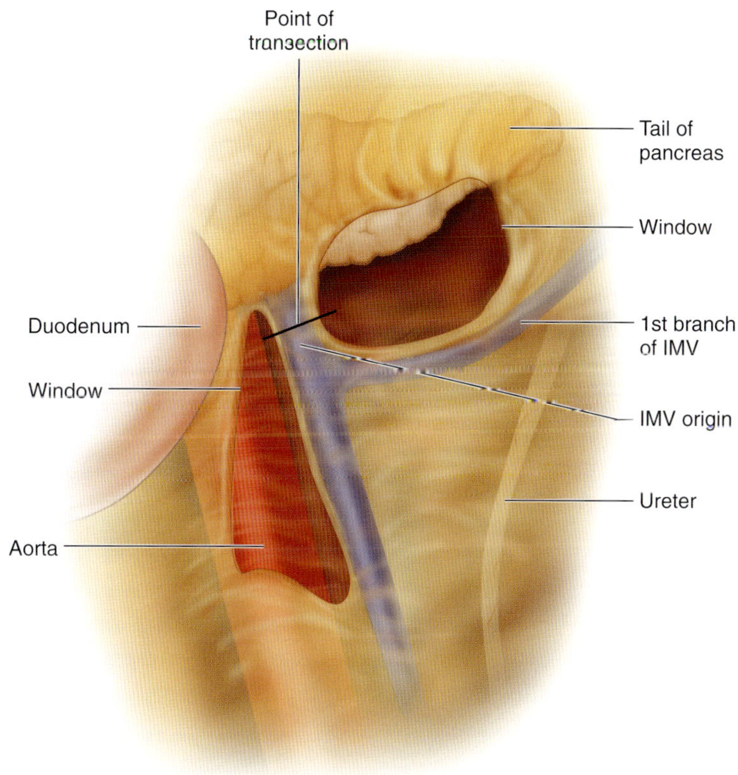

Figure 5-11

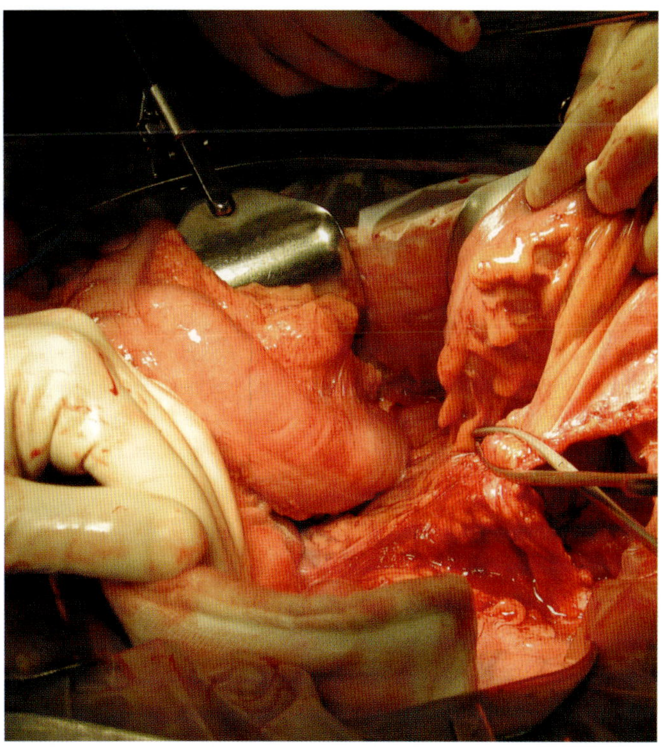

Figure 5-12

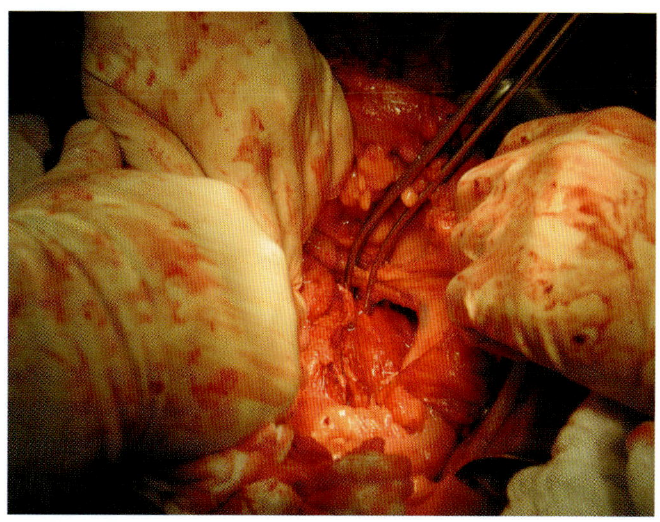

Figure 5-13

- The left colon is stretched all the way to the pelvis, bringing the splenic flexure to near the pelvic brim; this allows the left colon to be evaluated for point of transection, removing adequate proximal and distal margins for the lesion (Figure 5-14). A purse-string instrument is used to place a purse-string suture, or a hand-sewn purse-string suture is placed at the site of transection after dividing the mesenteric vessels. The purse-string suture is placed so that adequate blood supply is available and there is no tension or twisting (Figures 5-15 and 5-16*A* and *B*).

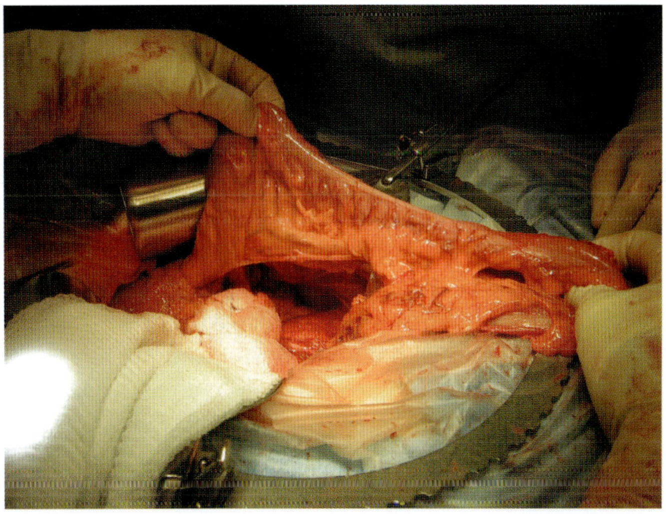

Figure 5-14

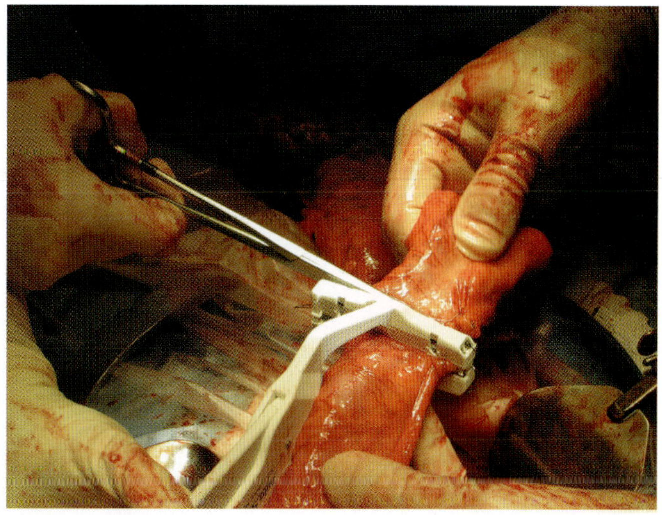

Figure 5-15

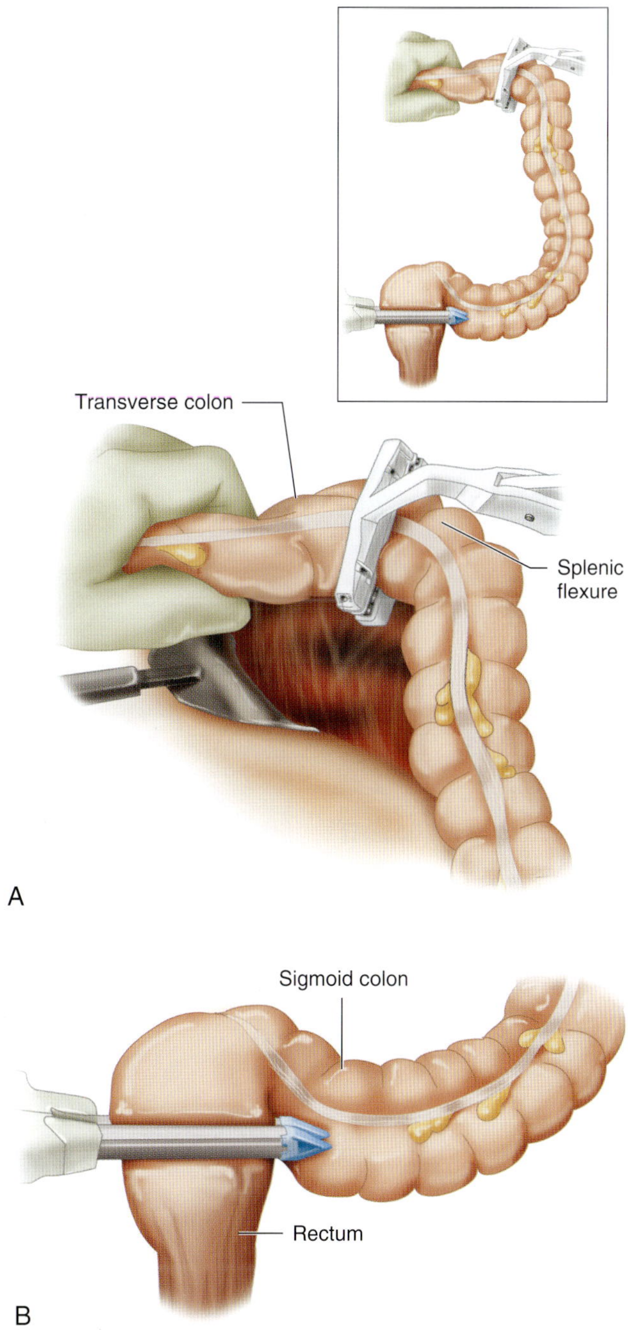

Figure 5-16A-B

- For a stapled circular anastomosis, the circular stapler anvil and shaft are secured in the proximal purse-string suture and reinforced with ties as needed to complete the doughnut around the base of the shaft of the stapling instrument head (Figure 5-17). The sigmoid or rectum is transected at the level of the sacral promontory using either a linear cutter stapler or a transverse linear stapler to create the transverse staple line (Figure 5-18). The circular stapler itself is introduced through the anal canal to the level of the transverse staple line, and the post is inserted and extended through the midportion of the rectal stump at the midportion of the transverse staple line. The left colon is brought into the pelvis without twisting (Figure 5-19*A*). The stapler is reconnected and closed under direct vision, maintaining good orientation with the mesentery of the left colon directed posteriorly (Figures 5-19*B* and 5-20*A-D*).
- The anastomosis can be checked by insufflating air through a rigid proctoscope, with the bowel proximal to the stapled anastomosis occluded and the pelvis filled with saline, to create an underwater test. Any bubbles seen would indicate a leak at the staple line, and this should be oversewn with Lembert sutures of 3-0 absorbable suture.
- The abdomen is closed after irrigation, and the small bowel is returned in gentle S-shaped curves and is covered with adhesion barrier.

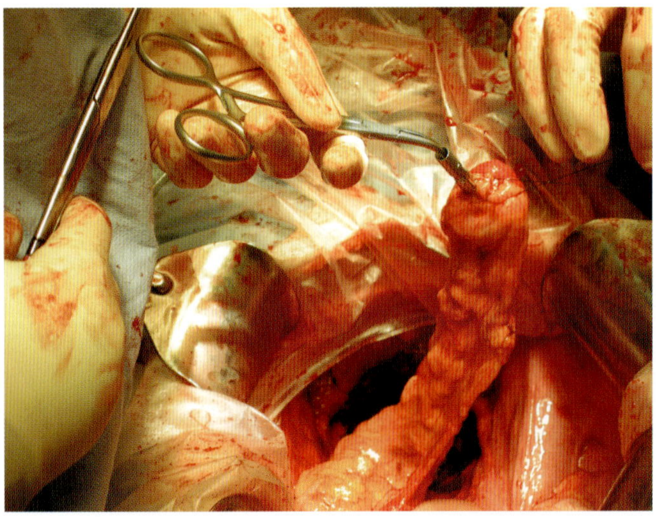

Figure 5-17

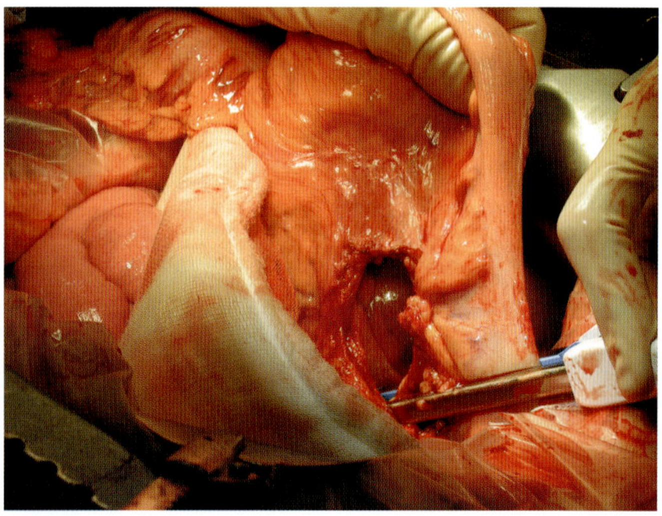

Figure 5-18

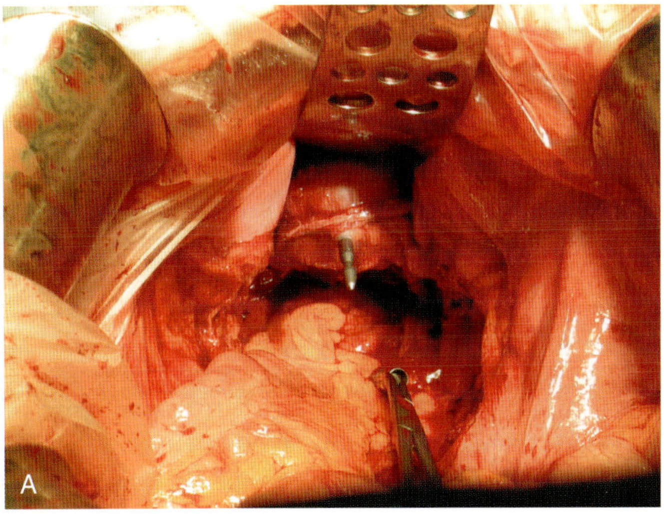

Figure 5-19A

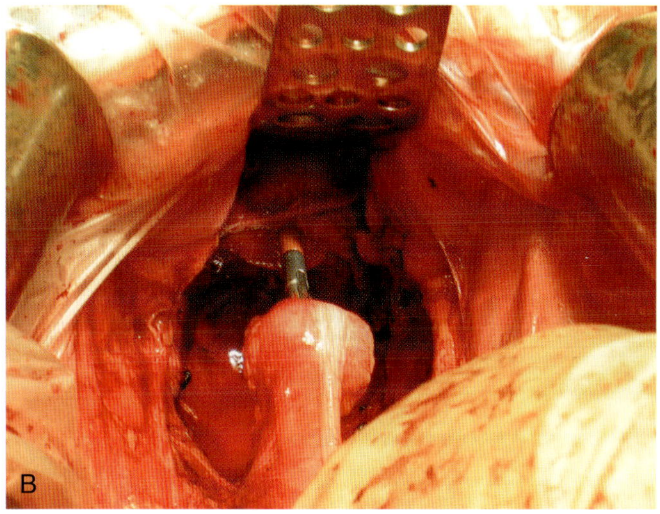

Figure 5-19B

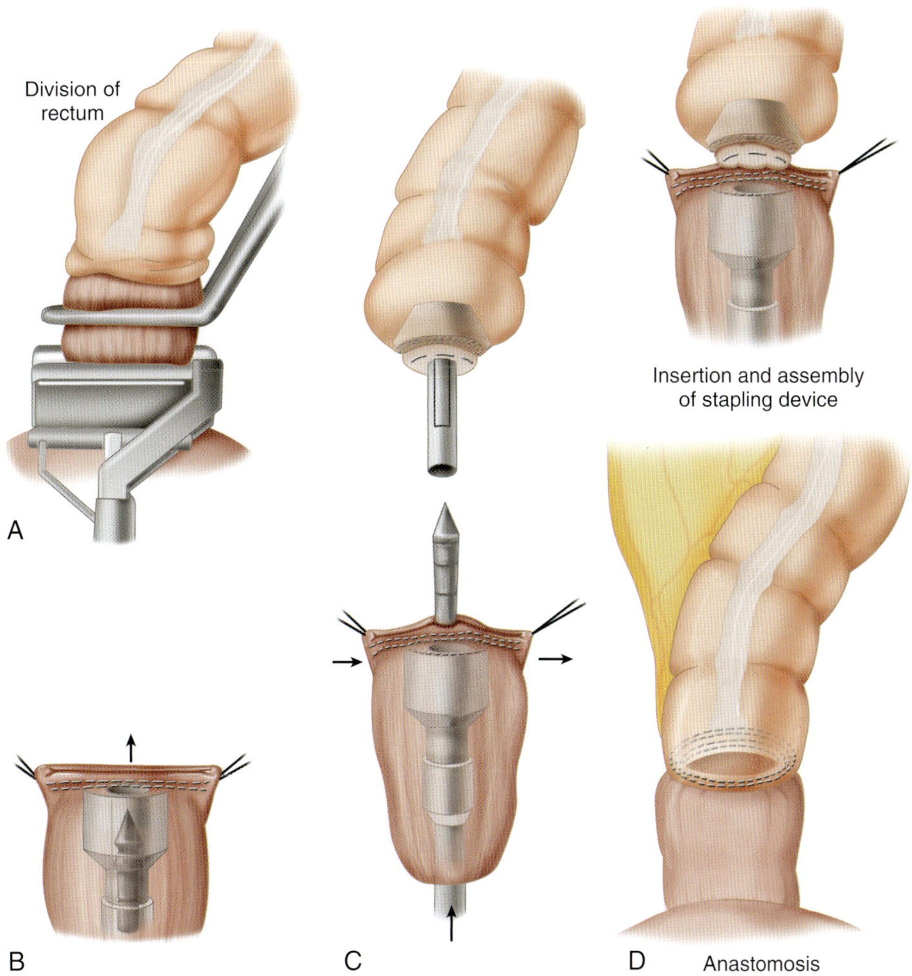

Figure 5-20A-D

Step 4: Postoperative Care

The abdomen is generally closed with a running No. 1 loop absorbable suture and staples. Patients are ambulated early. Intravenous fluid replacement is given to maintain a urine output of greater than 30 mL/hr. Nasogastric decompression is not required unless the patient becomes nauseated. Most patients tolerate clear liquids within 24 to 48 hours, and the diet can be advanced as tolerated. Patients should be given prophylactic antibiotics for 24 hours, incentive spirometry, and deep vein thrombosis prophylaxis and encouraged to ambulate as much as possible during the early postoperative period. Usual hospital stay after an open left colectomy is 4 to 5 days; the hospital stay is shorter when the patient is placed on a fast-track postoperative regimen. Postoperative analgesia is usually managed with patient-controlled analgesia followed by a switch to oral analgesics.

Step 5: Pearls and Pitfalls

The most critical aspect of left colectomy is ensuring an airtight anastomosis with no tension with good blood supply and no twisting; this can be accomplished with routine attention to detail. The patient may be best served by placement of a pelvic drain if the dissection is carried into the pelvis and there is enough oozing from surfaces to justify continued drainage. A pelvic drain does not eliminate the possibility of a leak, but drainage may be an early indicator of breach of anastomotic integrity. The patient can be fed on a fast-track basis (early recovery process). It is important to ensure that the patient can evacuate either gas or stool before discharge to avoid undetected anastomotic leak.

Adequate length for the left colon is guaranteed only if the splenic flexure is mobilized. Some surgeons hesitate to add this complexity to the case, but, if done routinely, it becomes a straightforward procedure on every patient. Ligation of the IMV and IMA at their origin also adds an extra dimension of length to the left colon specimen, while adding a degree of radicality. This maneuver is actually a simplification of the procedure because only two vessels are required for ligation. The decision regarding vessel division in the proximal left colon mesentery becomes much simpler because of the easy mobility of the colon and the possibility for using the splenic flexure itself as the proximal anastomotic segment.

Selected Readings

Adachi Y, Sato K, Kakisako K, et al. Quality of life after laparoscopic or open colonic resection for cancer. Hepatogastroenterology 2003;50:1348–51.

Seitz G, Seitz EM, Kasparek MS, et al. Long-term quality-of-life after open and laparoscopic sigmoid colectomy. Surg Laparosc Endosc Percutan Tech 2008;18:162–7.

CHAPTER 6

Laparoscopic Left Colectomy

Matthew G. Mutch

Step 1: Clinical Anatomy

The left colon lies along the left side of the abdomen suspended from the splenic flexure to the pelvic brim by lateral peritoneal attachments. The mesentery of the left colon arises from the midline of the abdomen along the aorta. The sigmoid colon has no lateral peritoneal attachments other than some congenital adhesions, which fix the apex of the sigmoid to the pelvic brim and the iliac fossa. Otherwise, the sigmoid colon is attached to the retroperitoneum through a midline mesentery arising from the inferior mesenteric artery (IMA) and extending down into the pelvis to the mesorectum. The splenic flexure is attached to the undersurface of the tip of the spleen, the lower edge of the tail of the pancreas, and the anterior surface of the left kidney by various levels of suspensory ligaments and peritoneal extensions. The blood supply to the left colon is based on the IMA, which arises from the anterior surface of the aorta just above the bifurcation of the common iliac arteries. The IMA extends anteriorly and bifurcates to produce the superior rectal artery feeding the sigmoid colon and the rectum. The left colic artery extends cephalad to provide the left colon and distal splenic flexure with blood supply through the arcade at the mesenteric edge known as the marginal artery of Drummond. The retroperitoneum behind the left colon contains the left ureter and the gonadal vessels lying over the psoas muscle. The ureter crosses the iliac vessels at the bifurcation of the iliac vessels into the external and internal iliac branches (Figure 6-1).

Step 2: Preoperative Considerations

The indications for laparoscopic left colectomy include colon cancer, diverticulitis, and isolated inflammatory bowel disease such as Crohn's disease. The preparation for a left colectomy usually includes a mechanical bowel preparation. The patient receives preoperative antibiotic prophylaxis and deep vein thrombosis prophylaxis with sequential compression devices and anticoagulation for malignancy. The preferred anastomotic technique for a left colectomy involves a circular stapled end-to-end anastomosis, which may be made anywhere along the rectum or sigmoid colon depending on blood supply, indication, and disease limitations.

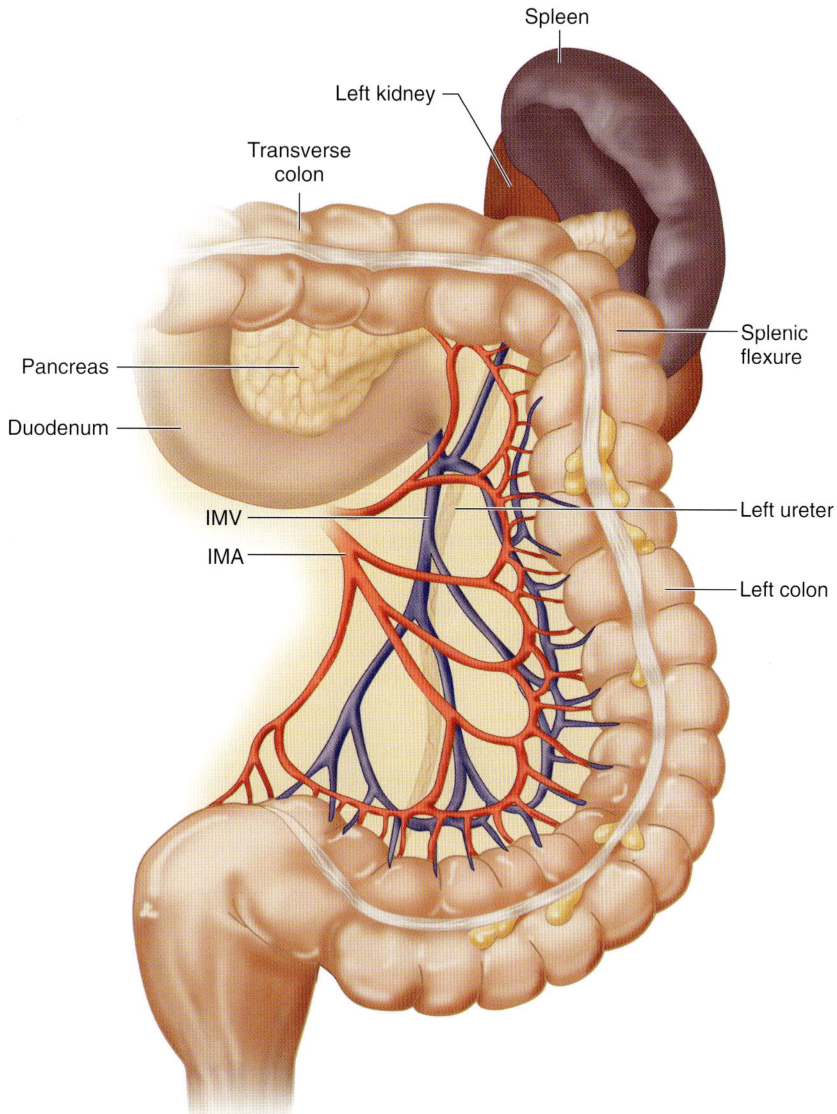
Spleen
Left kidney
Transverse colon
Splenic flexure
Pancreas
Duodenum
IMV
IMA
Left ureter
Left colon

Figure 6-1

Step 3: Operative Steps

- The patient is positioned in a lithotomy position, with Allen's stirrups, lower extremity sequential compression devices, and bladder catheter in place. A beanbag attached directly to the table is deflated, to allow steep Trendelenburg and airplane to the patient's right for maximum gravity benefit from positioning. Two monitors are required, one at the left shoulder and one at the left hip (Figure 6-2). The camera operator and surgeon stand on the patient's right side, working toward the monitor across the table from the diseased area. If a hand-assisted approach is used, the hand assistant stands between the legs with a hand through a suprapubic port.
- The abdomen is prepared, and a 1-cm incision is made above the umbilicus in the midline to establish a pneumoperitoneum of carbon dioxide to a pressure of 15 mm Hg. A 12-mm trocar is placed at the umbilical incision, to allow insertion of a flexible tip, 10-mm or 5-mm scope. A 5-mm trocar is placed in the left lower quadrant in the anterior axillary line at the level of the umbilicus and right upper quadrant and right lower quadrant in the anterior axillary line 4 cm below the costal margin and above the anterior superior iliac spine. A 10-mm trocar is placed at the suprapubic vertical midline, or a hand port incision is made at the site of the suprapubic midline. The small bowel is swept from the pelvis into the right upper quadrant with grasping instruments, and the base of the mesentery of the left colon is exposed (Figure 6-3). The IMA is identified at its origin on the aorta proximal to the sacral promontory. The space posterior to the superior hemorrhoidal artery and anterior to the sacral promontory is exposed. Anterior traction is exerted on the superior hemorrhoidal artery with a clamp through the suprapubic port. An energy source is introduced through the right lower quadrant trocar site, and a 5-mm bowel grasper is introduced through the right upper quadrant trocar site. The presacral window is easily seen with this retraction plan (Figure 6-4). For hand-assisted cases, the hand assistant places the left hand through the suprapubic site and provides traction to expose the base of the left colon mesentery.

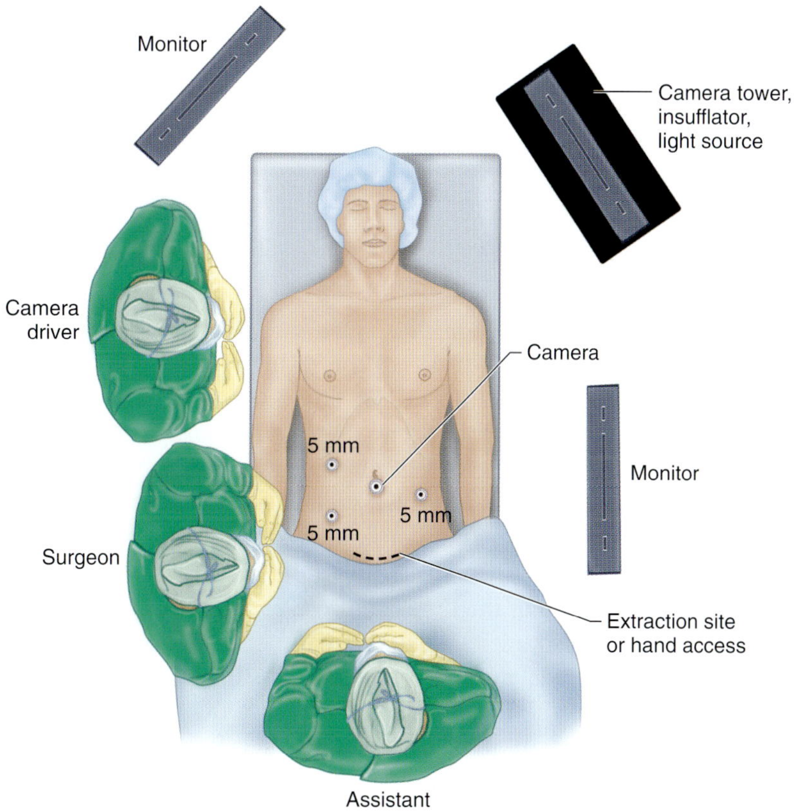

Figure 6-2

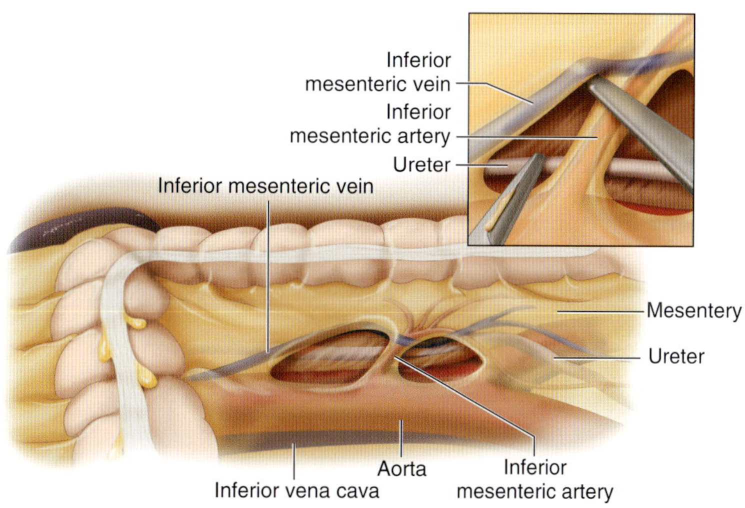

Figure 6-3

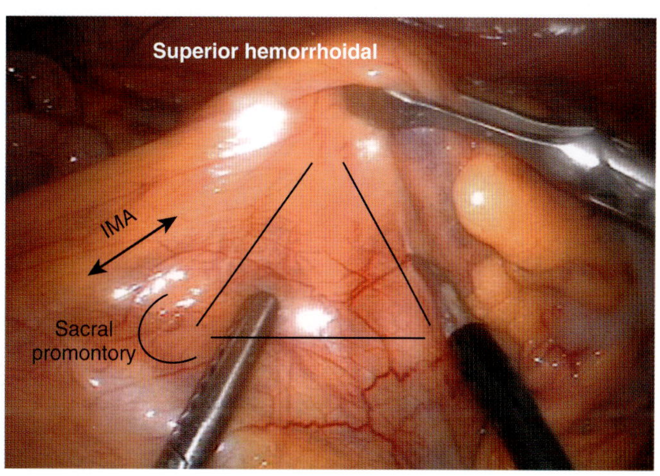

Figure 6-4

- The peritoneum is incised along the base of the triangle to expose the areolar tissue plane behind the superior hemorrhoidal artery but anterior to the retroperitoneum, where the gonadal vessels and the ureter are found crossing the left iliac artery and vein (Figure 6-5). This avascular plane is bluntly developed all the way out to the left abdominal side wall behind the mesentery of the sigmoid and left colon.
- The medial to lateral dissection is carried around the IMA to the peritoneal window beneath the inferior mesenteric vein (IMV) and anterior to the aorta. The window is incised, and the opening is developed cephalad to the IMA (Figure 6-6). The IMA is skeletonized and divided at its origin with an energy source. The artery may be divided at the bifurcation of the left colic and superior hemorrhoidal arteries if the disease is benign to prevent all risk of injuring nerves of sexual function in the preaortic plexus (Figure 6-7).
- Medial to lateral blunt dissection of the avascular plane is carried from the pelvic brim to the tail of the pancreas and laterally to the side wall of the abdomen beneath the left colon and its mesentery. The right upper quadrant trocar site provides access for the retracting blunt instrument, and the right lower quadrant trocar site provides access for the energy source or dissecting instrument. The suprapubic site allows the second retracting grasper to lift the edge of the mesentery anteriorly to provide a tenting effect, while the camera (in the umbilical port) looks beneath and laterally (Figure 6-8). The hand provides the retraction in a case with hand assistance.
- The IMV is exposed at its origin at the level of the ligament of Treitz, proximal to the first branch of the IMV, which travels to the splenic flexure. The vein is transected with an energy source or stapling instrument to release the base of the mesentery of the left colon (Figure 6-9). The left colon is released from the lateral side wall of the abdomen from the pelvic brim to the splenic flexure, exposing the previously dissected retroperitoneum with the protected structures posteriorly (Figure 6-10).

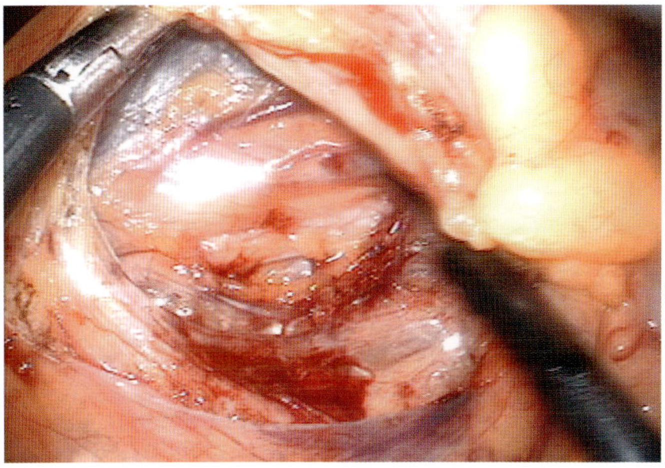

Figure 6-5

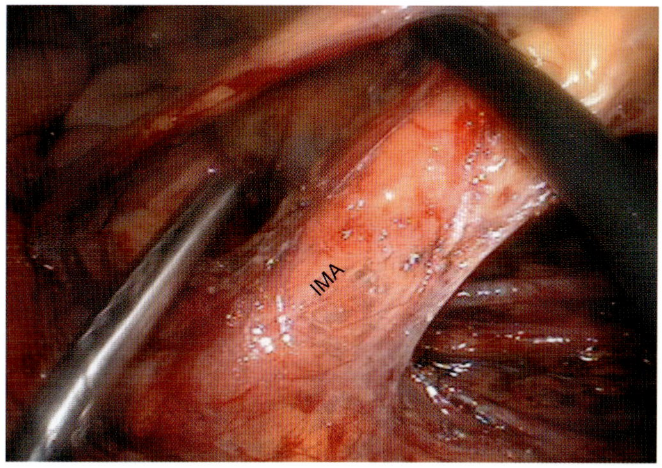

Figure 6-6

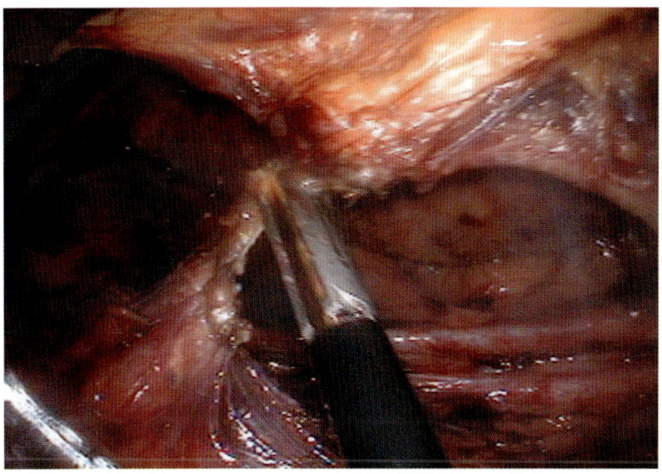

Figure 6-7

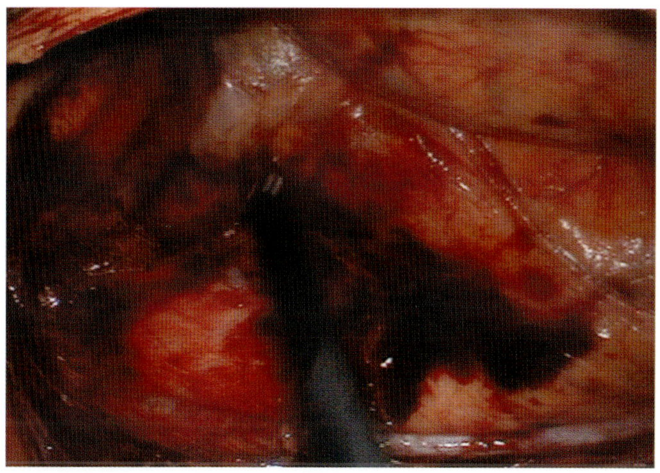

Figure 6-8

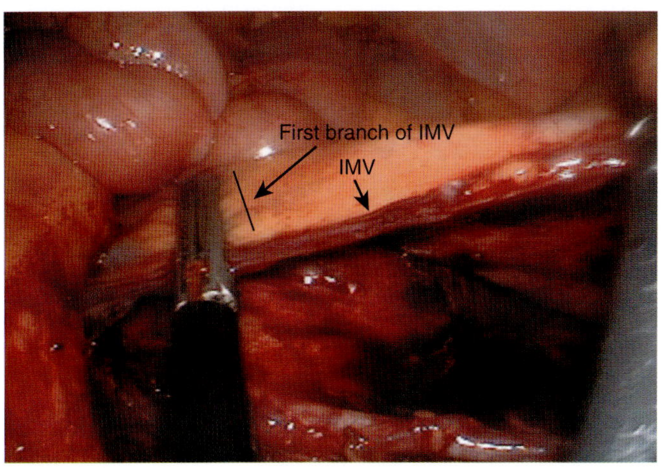

Figure 6-9

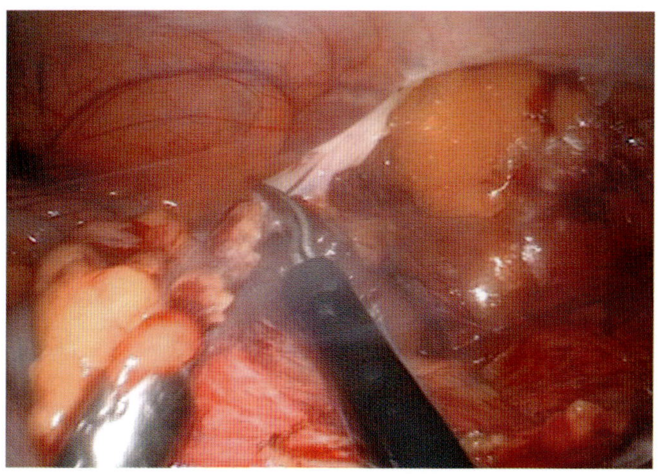

Figure 6-10

- The patient is placed in reverse Trendelenburg, still airplaned to the right, and the splenic flexure attachments are incised along the left side wall of the pelvis up to the level of the spleen (Figures 6-11*A* and 6-12*A*). The tip of the spleen and the anterior surface of the kidney are exposed as the suspensory ligaments are divided and the splenic flexure is mobilized medially. The right upper quadrant trocar provides access for the assistant to place a 5-mm grasper and pull the splenic flexure toward the midline. The operating surgeon stands between the patient's legs and uses the 10-mm grasper (or left hand) through the suprapubic midline. The 5-mm port in the left lower quadrant is used to place the energy source to allow the instrument to reach closer to the splenic flexure. The tail of the pancreas and tip of the spleen and anterior surface of the kidney are exposed (Figures 6-11*B* and 6-12*B*).
- The omentum is released from the antimesenteric surface of the splenic flexure and transverse colon to enter the lesser sac around the corner of the splenic flexure. The right upper quadrant trocar site provides retracting access to lift the omentum anteriorly and cephalad, and the suprapubic trocar site provides access for retracting (with 10-mm Babcock endoscopic instrument or hand) the splenic flexure toward the feet and the left lower quadrant. The left flank trocar provides access for the energy source to divide the attachments of the omentum to the colon (Figure 6-11*C*). The pancreas is exposed in the base of the lesser sac, and its lower edge is freed from the attachments of the splenic flexure all the way to the stump of the IMV at the ligament of Treitz. The posterior wall of the stomach, the anterior surface of the pancreas, the tip of the spleen, and the anterior surface of the kidney are clearly visualized with this technique (Figure 6-11*D*).

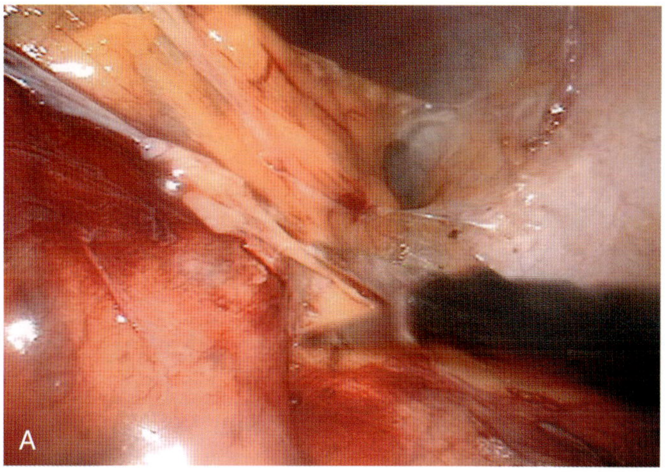

Figure 6-11A

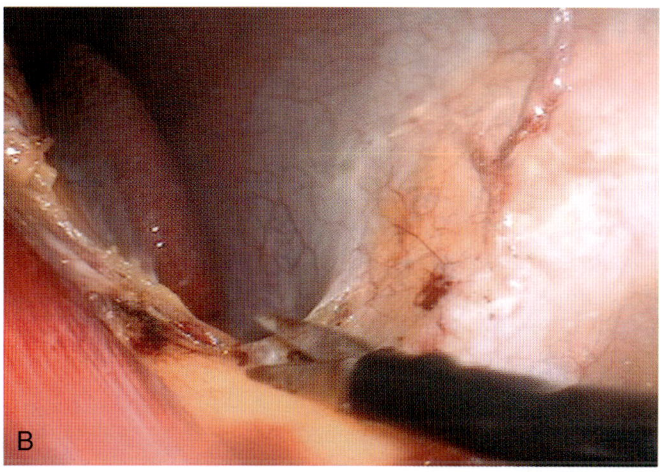

Figure 6-11B

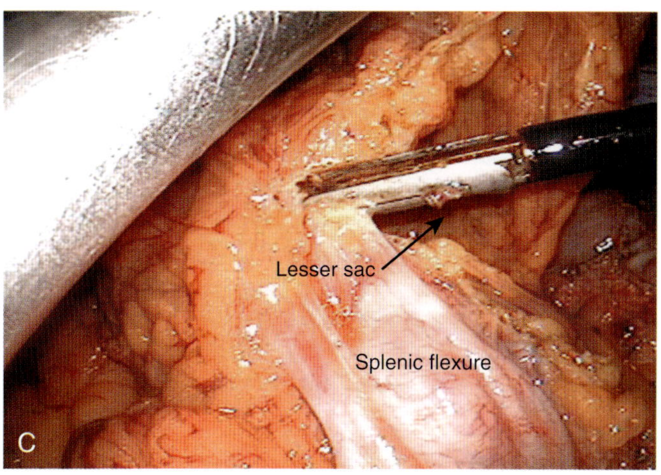

Figure 6-11C

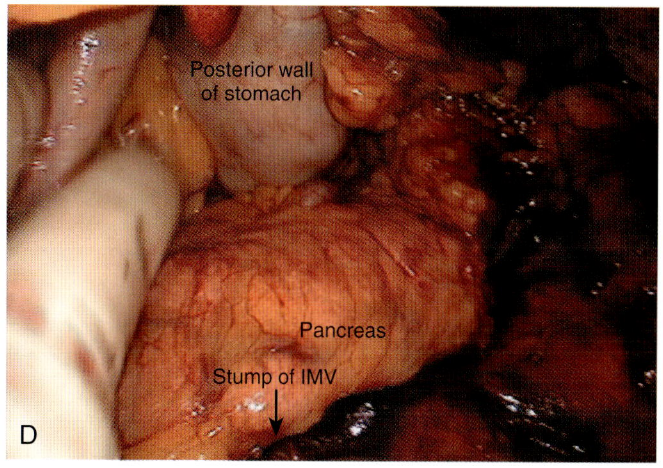

Figure 6-11D

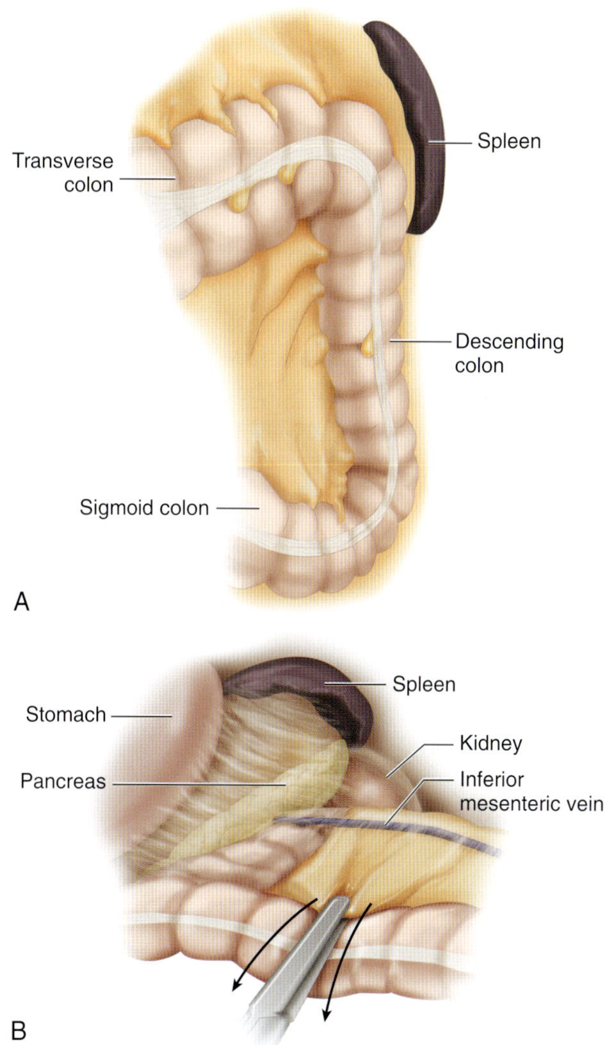

Figure 6-12A-B

- When the left colon is completely mobilized to the midline and freed from the attachments to the omentum to allow the splenic flexure to reach to the pelvic brim, an incision is made in the suprapubic area, either vertical midline or Pfannenstiel, and a wound protector is placed. Alternatively, if this were a hand-assisted case, the top of the hand access port would be removed, and the hand port would be used as an extraction site. The left colon is transected at a point appropriate for the disease using a purse-string instrument or noncrushing clamps. The mesenteric vessels at that level are transected between ties (Figure 6-13*A*). The rectosigmoid is transected through the access site at the level of the sacral promontory (Figure 6-13*B*).
- The end-to-end anastomosis is accomplished by using a purse-string instrument to place the proximal purse-string suture (Figure 6-14*A*) and secure the anvil and shaft of a 29-mm circular stapler in the proximal transection line of the colon (Figure 6-14*B*). The circular stapling instrument is inserted through the rectum to the level of the transverse staple line (Figure 6-15) and reconnected to the proximal handle and shaft (Figure 6-16). The anastomosis is checked by insufflating air through the rigid proctoscope with the proximal bowel occluded and the pelvis filled with saline to look for air leaks as the bowel is inflated. Any leaking can be repaired through the extraction site by reinforcing the staple line with sutures.
- The inner aspect of the supraumbilical trocar site is closed with a figure-eight suture of 0 absorbable suture, and the suprapubic incision is closed with a running No. 1 looped absorbable suture. The subcutaneous tissue is irrigated, and the skin is closed with a skin stapler or subcuticular closure. Adhesive bandages and gauze dressings are applied.

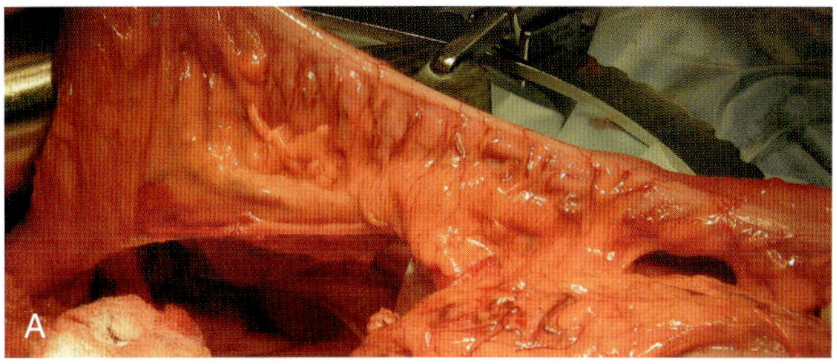

Figure 6-13A

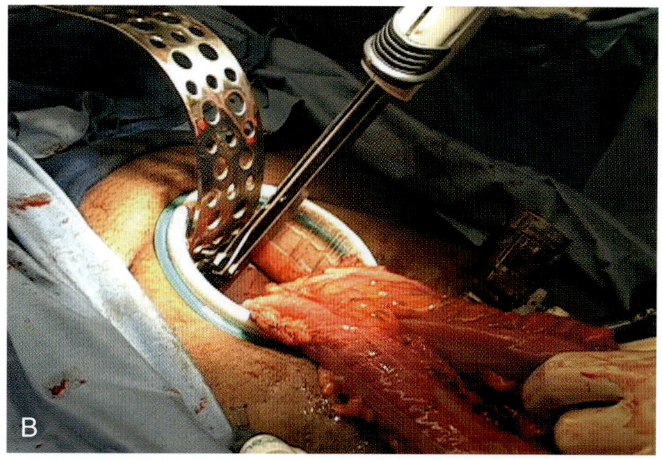

Figure 6-13B

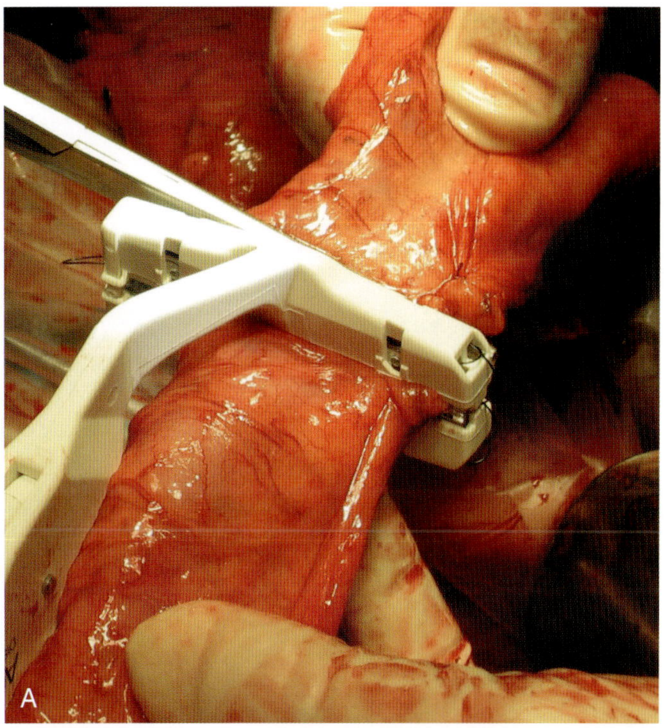

Figure 6-14A

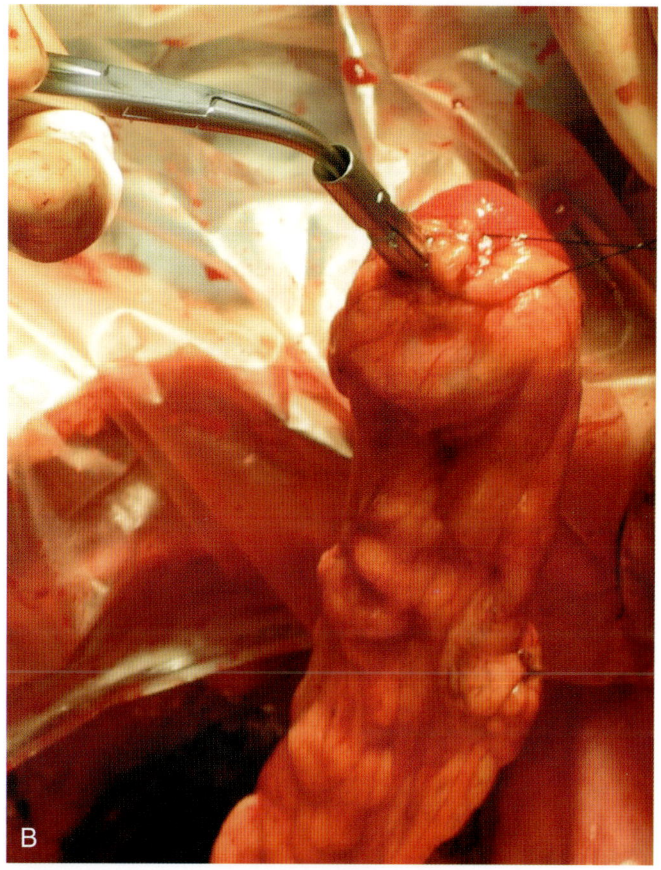

Figure 6-14B

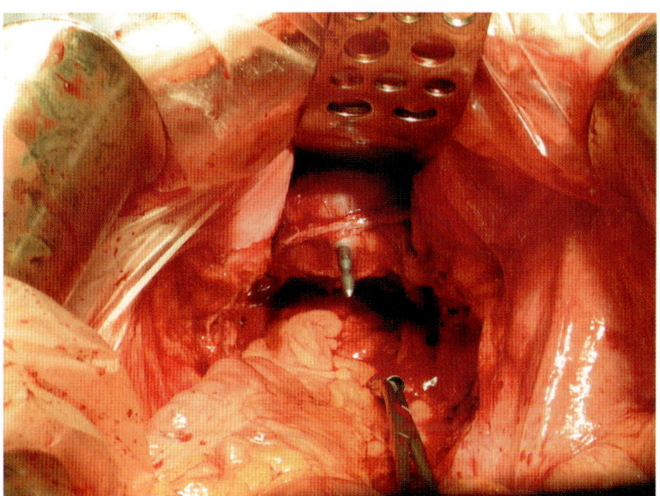

Figure 6-15

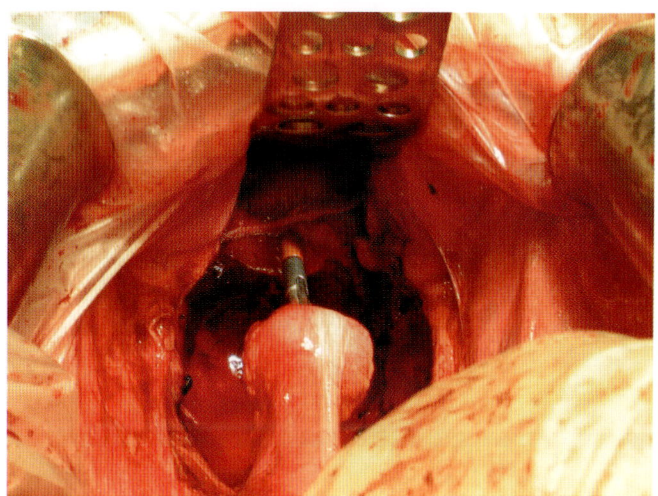

Figure 6-16

Step 4: Postoperative Care

Patient-controlled analgesia is appropriate for pain management supplemented with epidural morphine or anti-inflammatory agents as needed. The patient is fed an oral diet when nausea abates, and diet is advanced as tolerated. The patient is discharged within 4 to 5 days only after having had a bowel movement. A Jackson-Pratt drain is used only if indicated by continued blood or serum accumulation in the pelvis. The bladder catheter is left in place until the patient is able to ambulate and reach the bathroom independently.

Step 5: Pearls and Pitfalls

As with open left colectomy, the major risk consideration is anastomotic leak. A tension-free, nontwisted, well-vascularized anastomosis has the greatest chance of healing. The patient should be monitored for signs of sepsis with a low threshold for computed tomographic scanning to look for a perianastomotic collection. An interventional radiologist is able to place a percutaneous drain in most cases to prevent anastomotic breakdown and to control a small leak if present. Care is needed during stretching the left colon to the pelvis to avoid twisting the colon. The taenia of the colon can be followed to check for twisting before final firing of the circular stapler.

The patient should be informed that three to four bowel movements per day is typical after this operation. Bowel movements are more urgent than before the operation. The patient can be managed with antidiarrheals and bulking agents to normalize the bowel pattern. The patient should be told that this change slowly resolves over 6 months.

If during the operation any suspected complications arise, if the blood supply is questionable, or if anastomotic leaks are identified and repaired, consideration should be given to a diverting loop ileostomy for several months until the anastomosis can be guaranteed healed. A diverting loop ileostomy does not prevent anastomotic leaks, but it decreases the impact of the leak itself and allows the anastomosis to heal over time with minimal intervention such as percutaneous drainage.

Selected Readings

Fleshman J, Sargent DJ, Green E, et al. Laparoscopic colectomy for cancer is not inferior to open surgery based on 5-year data from the COST Study Group trial. Ann Surg 2007;246:655–62.

Marcello PW, Fleshman JW, Milsom JW, et al. Hand-assisted laparoscopic vs. laparoscopic colorectal surgery: a multicenter, prospective, randomized trial. Dis Colon Rectum 2008;51:818–26.

CHAPTER 7

Open Total Abdominal Colectomy with Ileorectal Anastomosis

Matthew G. Mutch

Step 1: Clinical Anatomy

The right colon lies on the patient's right side suspended laterally by peritoneal attachments to the right side of the abdominal wall, superiorly by attachments to the undersurface of the liver and posterior diaphragm, and medially by its mesentery. The ileocolic artery and vein and the right colic vessels, if they are present, run through this leaf of mesentery. The colon is adherent to the retroperitoneum on the right side of the abdomen and covers the right gonadal vessels and right ureter. The inferior vena cava is the next most medial structure on the right side. The hepatic flexure, the fold at the junction between the right colon and transverse colon, is adherent to the anterior surface of the kidney by avascular attachments to Gerota's fascia. The first and second portions of the duodenum are adherent to the undersurface of the mesentery of the right colon and proximal transverse colon. The gallbladder is sometimes adherent to the cephalad surface of the transverse colon at the hepatic flexure. The space behind the right colon is triangular shaped with the flat horizontal surface at the hepatic flexure running from the abdominal side wall toward the midline along the line of the greater curve of the stomach. The vertical axis follows the right lateral side wall of the abdomen. The hypotenuse runs from the fusion plane of the cecum at the pelvic brim over the top of the right iliac artery and vein at about the point where the ureter passes over the iliac vessels toward the midline over the aorta up to the base of the pancreas along the third portion of the duodenum. This triangular retroperitoneal area is a potential space with avascular attachments and allows the right colon to be lifted completely from the retroperitoneum during dissection. Release of all suspensory attachments allows the right colon to be made into a midline structure. The ileocolic artery and vein arise from the superior mesenteric artery (SMA) and superior mesenteric vein in the midportion of the SMA below the duodenum. The right colic artery is a variable structure and may be present as a separate structure or as part of the ileocolic trunk. The right branch of the middle colic artery exits through the pancreatic tissue from its origin on the SMA as a portion of the middle colic trunk at the base of the transverse mesocolon (Figure 7-1).

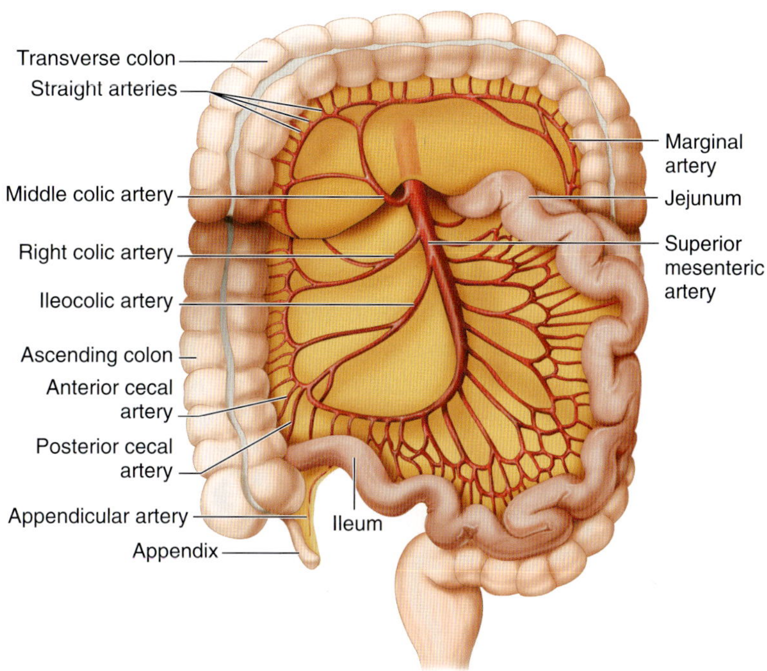
Transverse colon
Straight arteries
Middle colic artery
Right colic artery
Ileocolic artery
Ascending colon
Anterior cecal artery
Posterior cecal artery
Appendicular artery
Appendix
Ileum
Marginal artery
Jejunum
Superior mesenteric artery

Figure 7-1

The left branches of the middle colic artery and vein exit adjacent to the right branch of the middle colic and are found at the third portion of the duodenum over the pancreas. The inferior mesenteric vein (IMV) travels along the window of the base of the mesentery of the colon and enters the portal vein adjacent to the ligament of Treitz at the base of the splenic flexure mesentery (Figure 7-2). This area of the vasculature to the colon is extremely complex and should be studied carefully before mobilization of the transverse colon. The mesentery of the transverse colon itself is sometimes attached to filmy attachments of the posterior aspect of the stomach. The omentum falls from the gastroepiploic artery along the greater curve of the stomach over the transverse colon where it attaches tangentially to the antimesenteric surface of the transverse colon and then continues to the lower aspect of the abdomen free-floating over the surface of the small bowel.

The splenic flexure of the colon sits in the left upper quadrant with a surface adherent to the undersurface of the tip of the spleen, the anterior surface of the left kidney, and the anterior surface of the tail of the pancreas. A portion of the base of the mesentery of the transverse colon is attached to the undersurface of the tail of the pancreas starting at the level of the IMV and extending laterally toward the left side of the abdomen. These attachments can be released by developing avascular planes given knowledge of the peritoneal windows, areolar tissue planes, and structural relationships. The left colon itself is adherent to the retroperitoneum in the left gutter via an avascular filmy tissue plane that attaches the mesentery and left colon to the posterior abdominal wall where the ureter and gonadal vessels are found. The peritoneal attachments along the left gutter of the abdomen suspend the left colon from the left side of the abdomen from the pelvic brim all the way up to the splenic flexure. The splenic flexure is a fold of the colon with its apex attached to the tip of the spleen by omental congenital adhesions.

The splenic flexure is usually covered by the omentum as it falls over the top of the transverse colon along the left gutter, and numerous embryologic attachments can occur between the antimesenteric surface of the proximal left colon and the omentum at the splenic flexure. The left colon descends along the left gutter to the level of the pelvic brim where the colon becomes free from the pelvic side wall and falls into a sigmoid-appearing structure known as the sigmoid colon. The sigmoid colon lies free in the pelvis, attached only posteriorly to its vascular attachments at the midline over the sacral promontory.

The inferior mesenteric artery (IMA) arises from the anterior surface of the aorta proximal to the origin of the common iliac vessels. The IMA branches to give the superior hemorrhoidal artery descending into the posterior mesorectal vessel and the ascending left colic vessel, which sweeps up toward the splenic flexure. The IMV runs across the base of the mesentery of the left colon, crossing the superior hemorrhoidal and left colic vessels on its way to the duodenum. There is a clear peritoneal window between the aorta and the IMV, which can be used to enter the avascular plane behind the left colon mesentery and the retroperitoneum.

Step 2: Preoperative Considerations

Common indications for a total abdominal colectomy with ileorectal anastomosis include synchronous colon cancers, familial cancer syndromes (hereditary nonpolyposis colorectal cancer, familial adenomatous polyposis with rectal sparing, and cancer in patients <40 years old), colonic inertia, Crohn's colitis with rectal sparing, and gastrointestinal bleeding. The preparation of the patient is dictated by the specific indication, and the appropriate evaluations should be undertaken. A mechanical bowel preparation with oral agents is not necessary but is frequently performed. The left side of the colon can be adequately cleansed with several enemas before surgery. Patients require routine deep vein thrombosis prophylaxis and instructions on postoperative care. Patients should receive education on the expected functional outcome of an ileorectal anastomosis. They can expect to have four to five semisolid, pasty bowel movements a day with good bowel control.

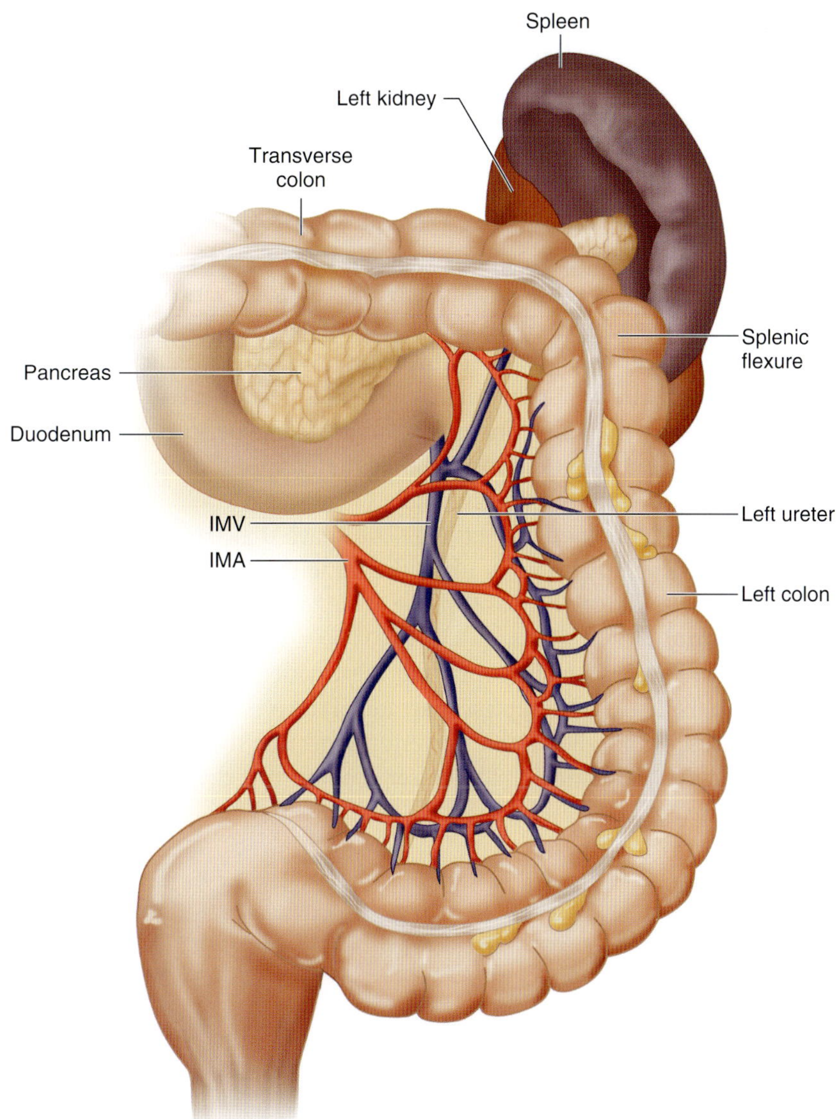
Spleen
Left kidney
Transverse colon
Splenic flexure
Pancreas
Duodenum
Left ureter
IMV
IMA
Left colon

Figure 7-2

Step 3: Operative Steps

- The patient is placed on the operating table in the lithotomy position. One of the arms is tucked to the patient's side so that the Mayo stand and scrub nurse can be at the head of the patient.
- A vertical midline incision is made from the epigastrium to the mid low pelvis. A Bookwalter retractor (Codman, Raynham, Mass.) is placed for exposure with the abdominal incision stretched widely.
- The right colon can be mobilized from a lateral, inferior, or posterior approach. Regardless of the approach, the cecum, ascending colon, and right colon mesentery are mobilized off the retroperitoneum, and the duodenum is reflected safely into the retroperitoneum. The right colon is lifted from the pelvis, and a hand is placed from the medial aspect of the abdomen under the peritoneal attachments of the terminal ileum and right colon at the level of the pelvic brim and the white line of Toldt, or the peritoneal attachments along the right gutter are stretched over the index finger (Figure 7-3). The peritoneal attachments are incised with electrocautery to expose the duodenum at the base of the mesentery of the right colon when the right colon is lifted up and medially (Figure 7-4).
- The right colon is pulled toward the left leg. The space that has been generated over the top of the duodenum is developed bluntly up to the undersurface of the liver, and the suspensory peritoneal attachments along the base of the liver toward the gallbladder are incised with electrocautery (Figure 7-5).
- The attachments of the gastrocolic omentum are divided along the cephalad surface of the transverse colon outside the gastroepiploic arcade of the omentum between ties. The omentum is completely released and allows the posterior aspect of the stomach and the entire lesser sac to be seen (Figure 7-6*A* and *B*). The lesser omentum is divided as far toward the splenic flexure as possible.

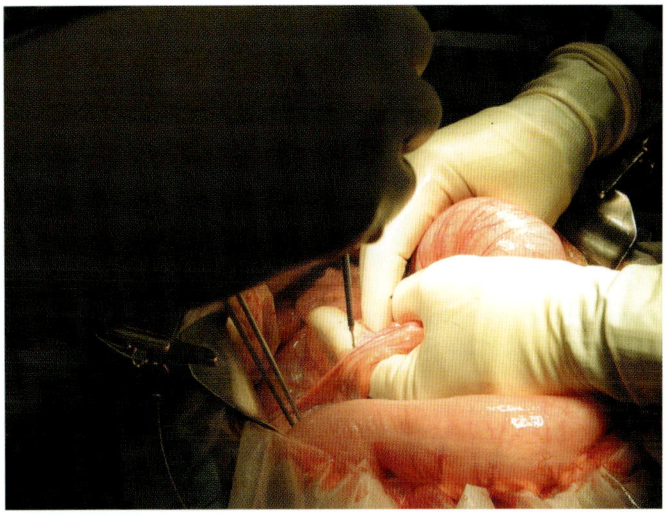

Figure 7-3

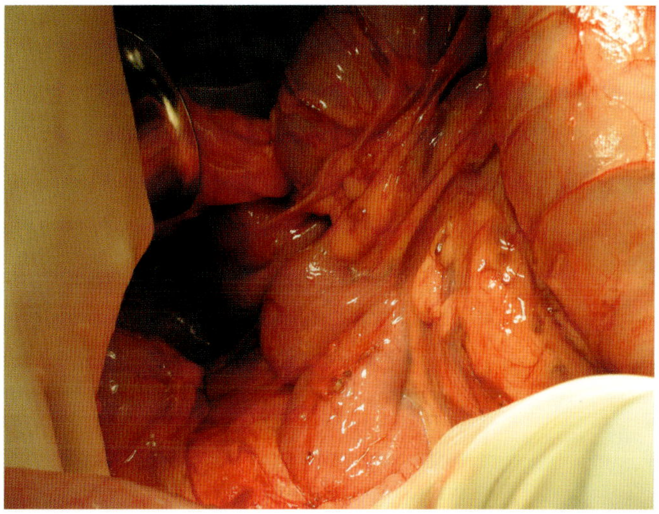

Figure 7-4

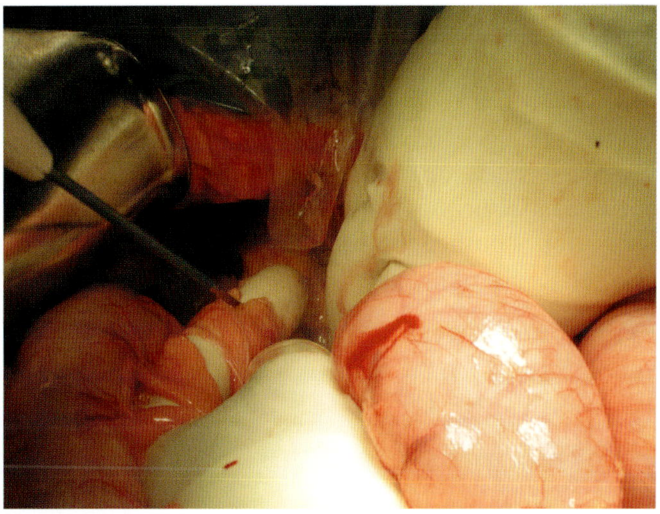

Figure 7-5

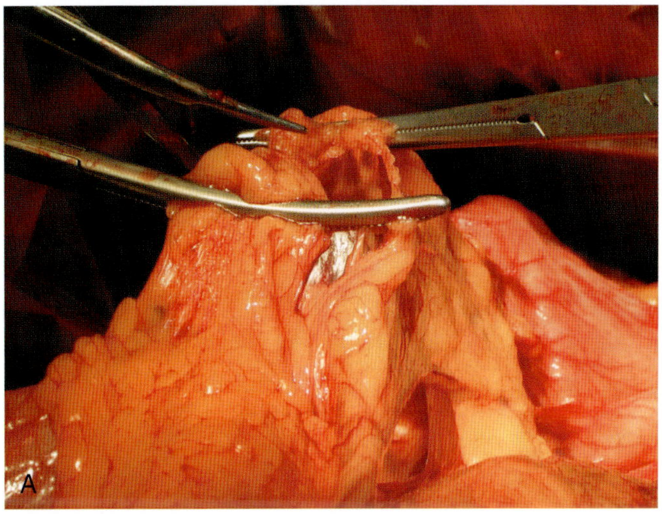

Figure 7-6A

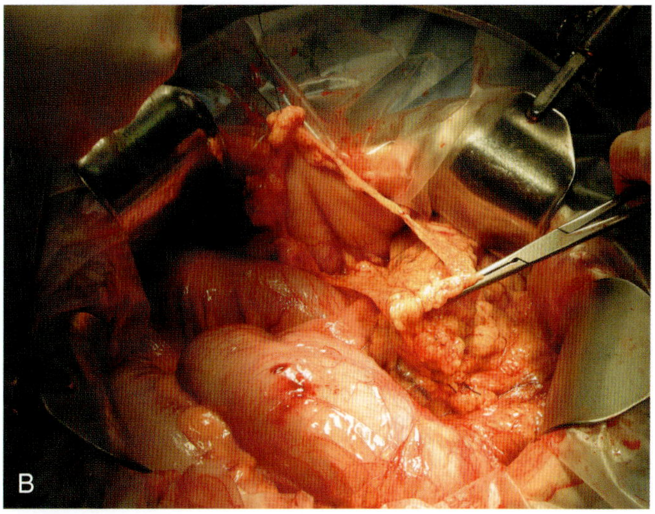

Figure 7-6B

- The colon is returned to its anatomic position with the right colon along the right gutter and the hepatic flexure up in the right upper quadrant. The SMA is identified in its track to the terminal ileum, and a window is seen in the base of the mesentery of the right colon proximal and distal to a large vascular trunk. This trunk is the ileocolic artery and vein arising from the SMA and superior mesenteric vein (Figure 7-7). An incision is made at the base of this window to expose and divide the ileocolic vessels at their origin (Figure 7-8).
- The terminal ileal mesentery is divided up to the level of the bowel. The type of anastomosis performed dictates this step. Options include an end-to-end, side-to-end, or side-to-side anastomosis. A side-to-side anastomosis is described here. The terminal ileum is divided with a linear cutter stapler (Figure 7-9).
- The sigmoid colon and left colon are retracted to the midline to expose the left gutter and the lateral aspect of the left colon (Figure 7-10*A*). The peritoneal surface of the left gutter is incised along the congenital fusion plane at the base of the left colon mesentery to enter an avascular plane from the pelvic brim all the way up to the splenic flexure (Figure 7-10*B*). The areolar tissue plane is developed toward the midline to release the mesentery and colon from the retroperitoneal structures exposing the left ureter and gonadal vessels (Figure 7-10*C*). As the left colon is pushed toward the midline bluntly, the left ureter gonadal vessels

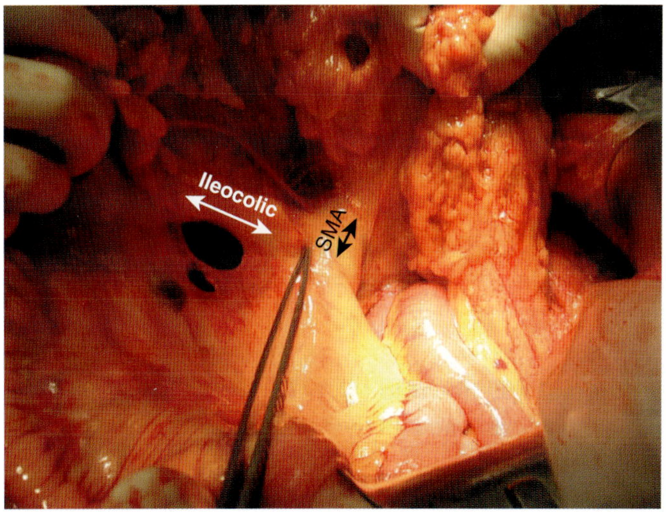

Figure 7-7

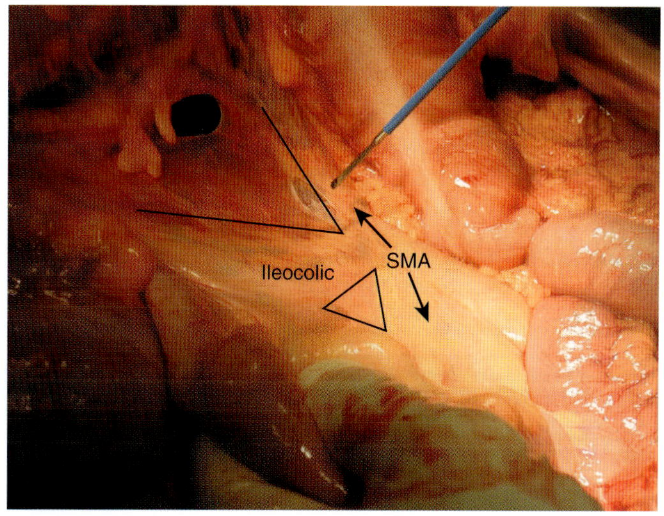

Figure 7-8

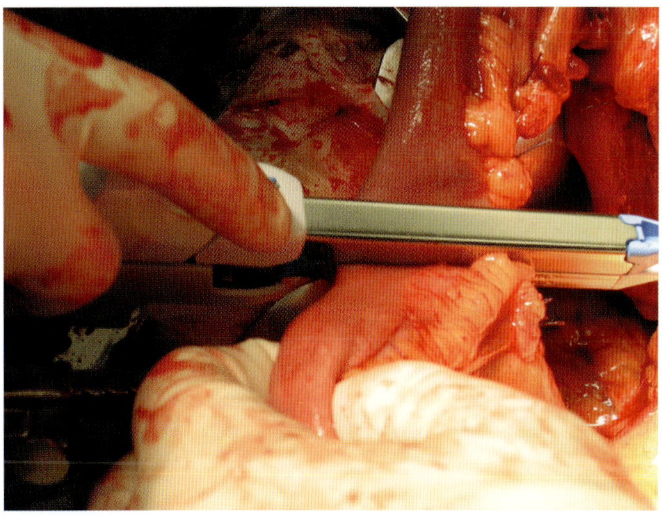

Figure 7-9

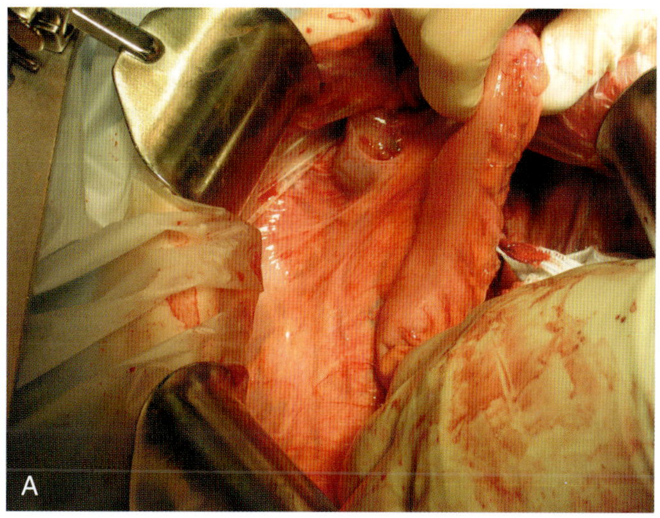

Figure 7-10A

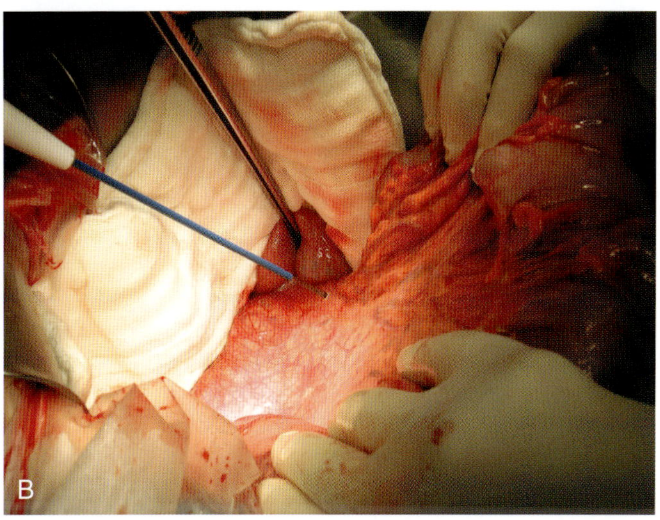

Figure 7-10B

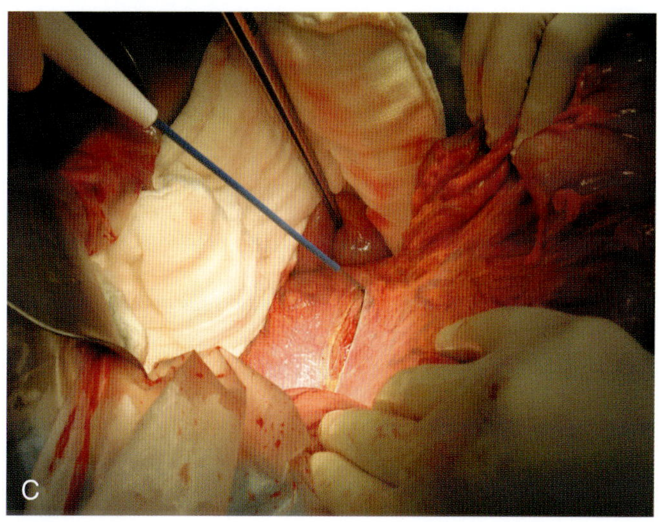

Figure 7-10C

and areolar tissue plane are dropped posteriorly all the way down to the pelvic brim at the sacral promontory (Figure 7-11*A*) and up to the splenic flexure and all the way to the midline at the aorta (Figure 7-11*B*).

- The splenic flexure is released from the left upper quadrant by incising the lateral peritoneal attachments with a finger placed in the avascular tissue plane posteriorly and extended up toward the tip of the spleen. The peritoneum is incised over the finger using the finger as a guide (Figure 7-12*A*). As the splenic flexure is released medially, the dissection turns toward the pancreas, and the attachments of the splenic flexure to the undersurface of the tail of the pancreas are incised with electrocautery over the finger as a guide (Figure 7-12*B*). The splenic flexure attachments, which are occasionally very dense and attached to the spleen, are freed from the tip of the spleen and the vascular pedicle of the spleen to allow the splenic flexure to move toward the midline (Figure 7-12*C*). The omental attachments along the anterior surface of the splenic flexure and transverse colon are incised with electrocautery to preserve the omentum and release the colon from the undersurface of the omentum toward the previously dissected right colon (Figure 7-12*D*).

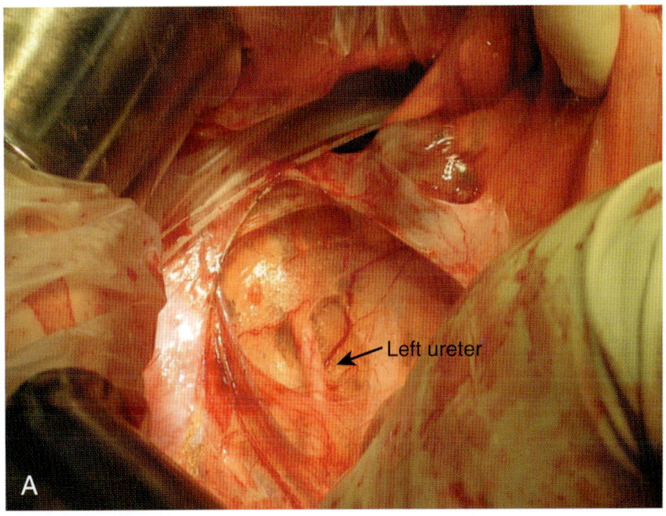

Figure 7-11A

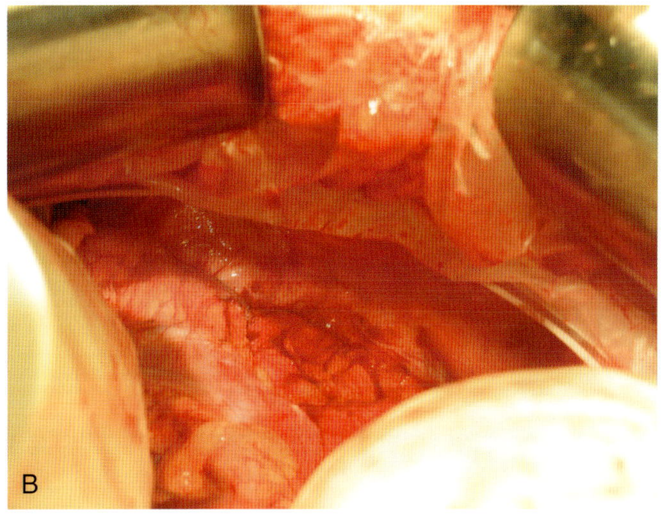

Figure 7-11B

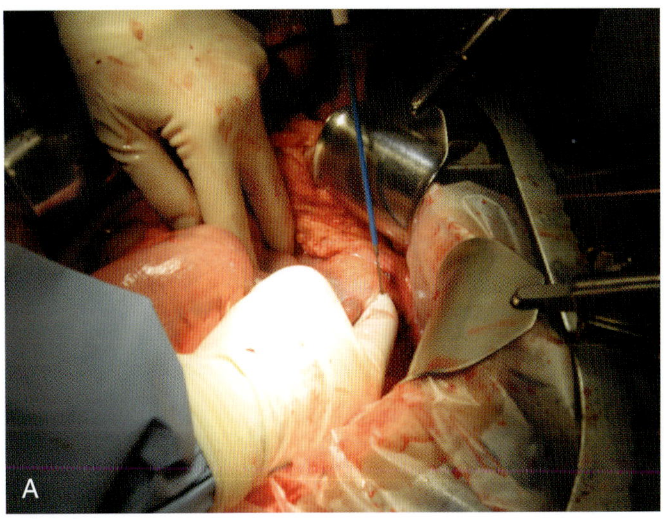

Figure 7-12A

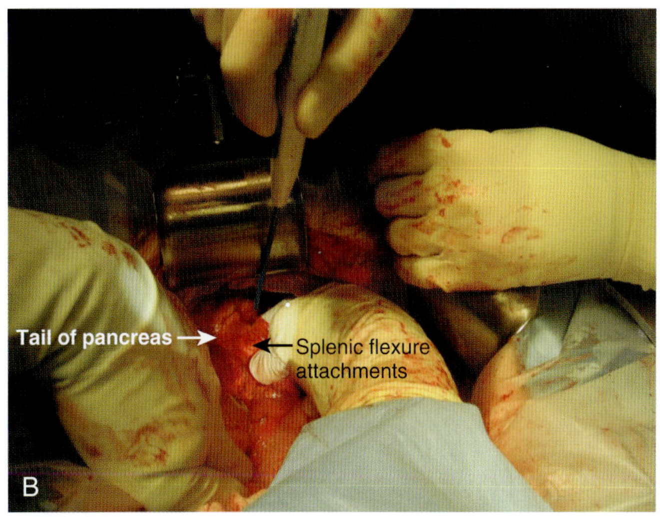

Figure 7-12B

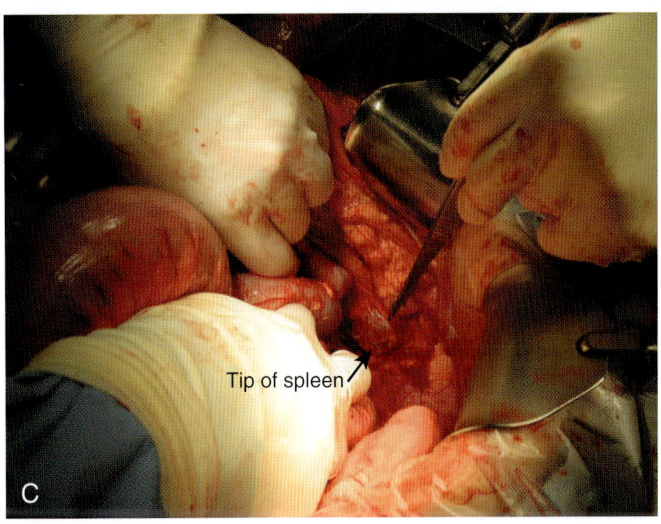

Figure 7-12C

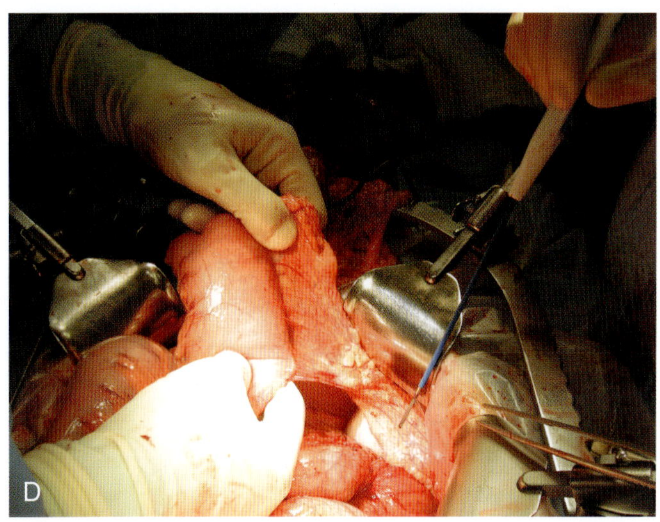

Figure 7-12D

- After the left colon has been mobilized, the sigmoid colon can be transected anywhere along its surface from rectum to descending colon that is appropriate for the disease process. The rectosigmoid colon is transected in a mesenteric-to-antimesenteric direction with a linear cutter stapler at the sacral promontory to provide the distal end of the anastomosis (Figure 7-13).
- The IMA pedicle or the left colic vessels can be divided at their origin or along the vessel pedicle at a point appropriate for the disease process as the left colon is mobilized from the retroperitoneal structures (Figure 7-14). The IMV can be ligated at its origin adjacent to the third portion of the duodenum with the left colon retracted anteriorly and the small bowel and right colon retracted to the patient's right (Figure 7-15).
- The transverse colon is pulled inferiorly. The surgeon's left hand is passed through the defect of the ileocolic vessels and encircles the middle colic vessels. These vessels form a "V" and can be easily identified and divided outside the pancreatic tissue to protect the anterior surface of the pancreas (Figure 7-16).

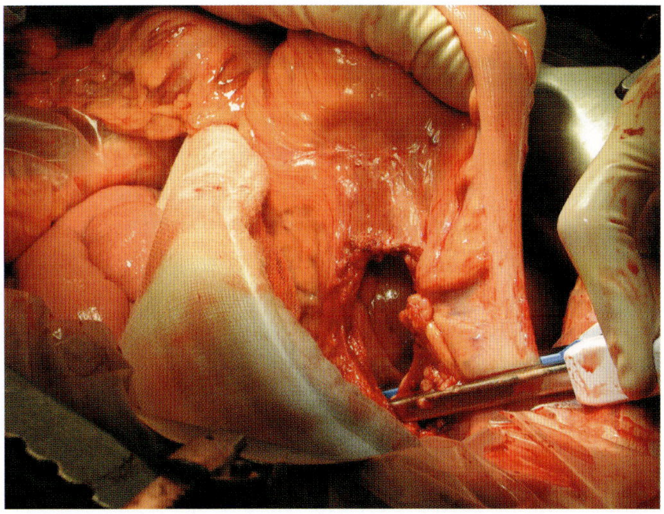

Figure 7-13

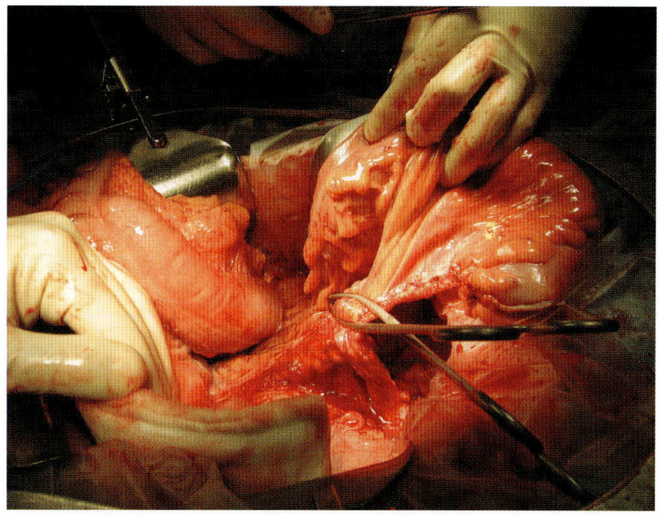

Figure 7-14

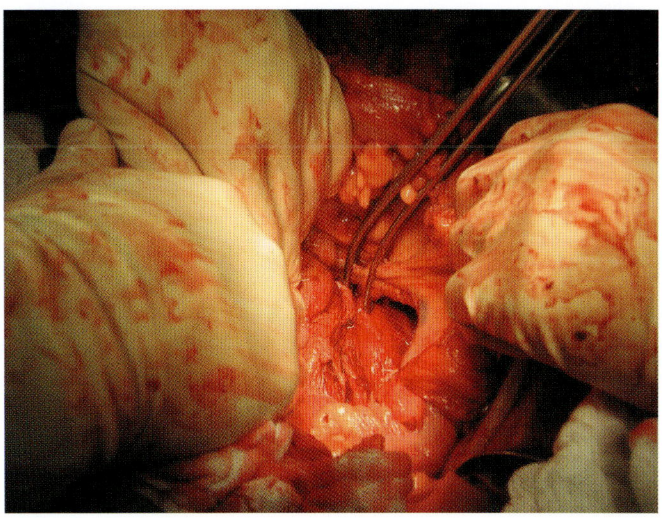

Figure 7-15

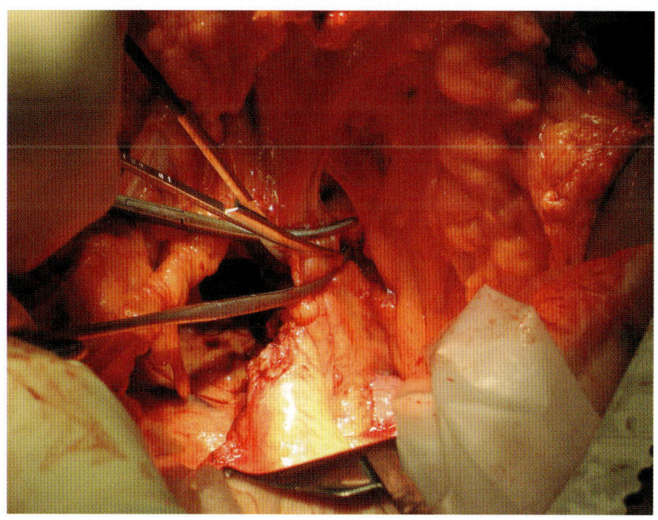

Figure 7-16

- The anastomosis is accomplished by opening the antimesenteric corner of the transverse staple line on the sigmoid colon and the ileum. The small bowel is positioned to the left side of the abdomen with the cut edge of the mesentery placed toward the midline. The terminal ileum is allowed to fall to the left side of the pelvis, and the small bowel is brought up along the edge of the left side of the rectum (Figure 7-17*A*). The sigmoid is positioned along the right side of the pelvis, and the linear cutter stapler is placed down the open corners of the transverse staple lines to create a side-to-side anastomosis (Figures 7-17*B* and 7-18).
- The transverse opening of the anastomosis is opened widely, the longitudinal staple lines are distracted as far as possible, and the opening is brought together with Allis clamps. The transverse opening is closed with a second firing of the linear cutter stapler (Figure 7-19). The mesenteric defect is closed by placing a running suture from the pelvic brim down the mesentery of the sigmoid colon along the mesentery of the small bowel all the way up to the base of the duodenum to prevent herniation and twisting (Figure 7-20). The transverse staple line of the ileosigmoid anastomosis is oversewn with a running Lembert suture line of 3-0 absorbable suture to invert and protect the transverse staple line (Figure 7-21).
- An adhesive barrier can be applied, and the abdomen is closed with a running No. 1 loop absorbable suture.

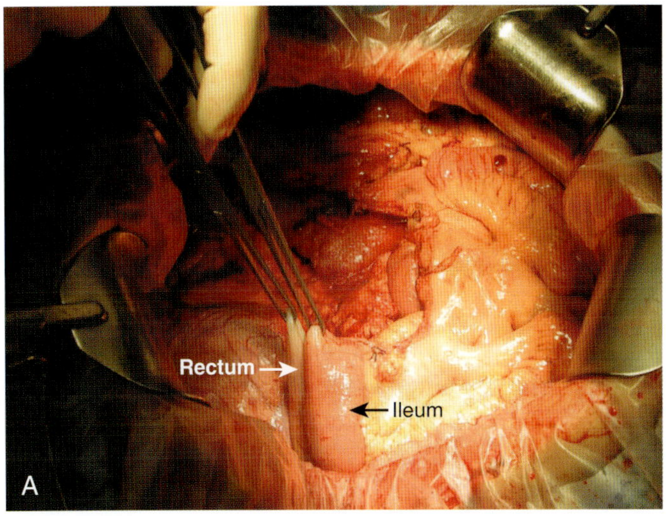

Figure 7-17A

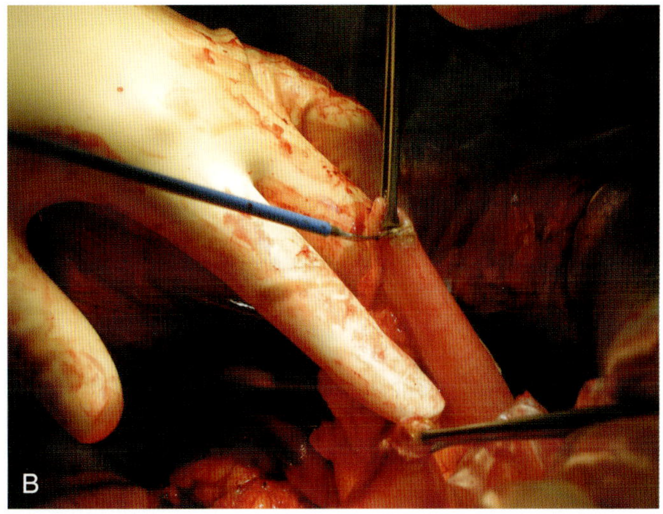

Figure 7-17B

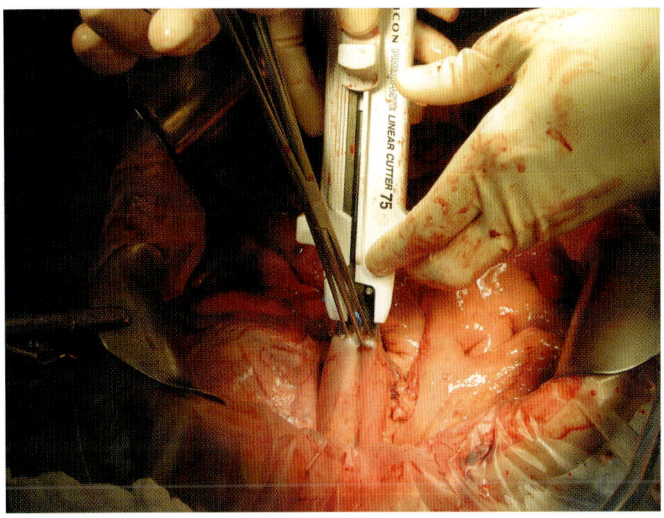

Figure 7-18

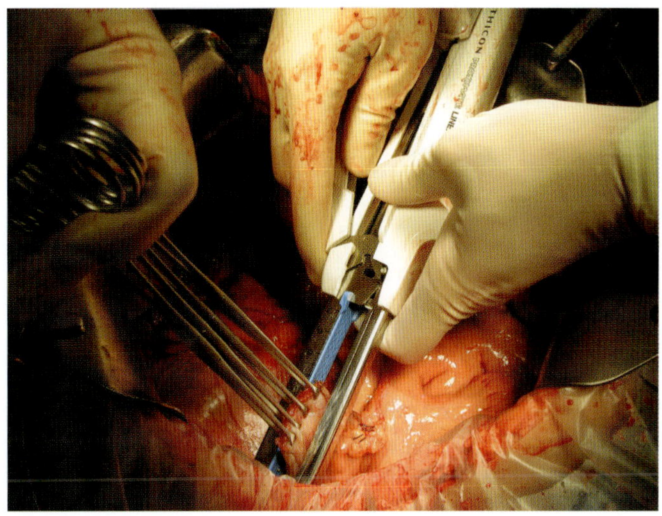

Figure 7-19

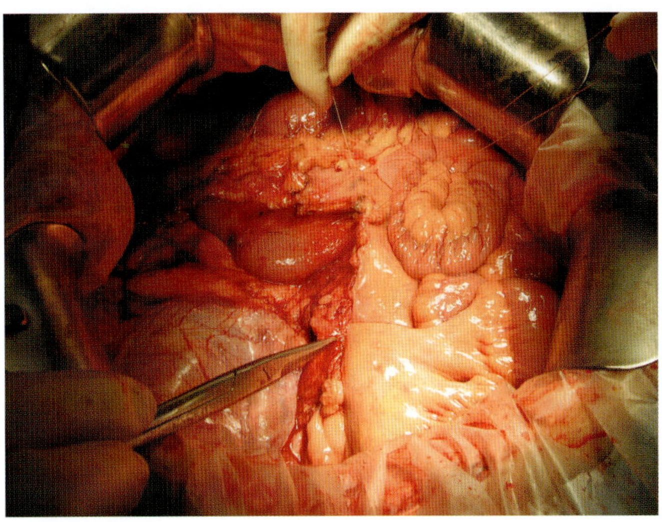

Figure 7-20

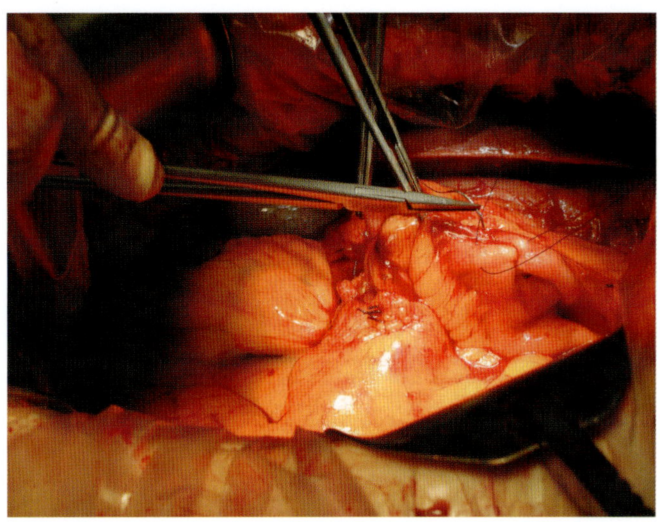

Figure 7-21

Step 4: Postoperative Care

Patients are ambulated early. Intravenous fluid replacement is given to maintain a urine output of greater than 30 mL/hr. Nasogastric decompression is not required unless the patient becomes nauseated. Most patients tolerate clear liquids within 24 to 48 hours, and the diet can be advanced as tolerated. Patients should be given prophylactic antibiotics for 24 hours, incentive spirometry, and deep vein thrombosis prophylaxis and encouraged to ambulate as much as possible during the early postoperative period. Usual hospital stay after an open right colectomy is 4 to 5 days; the hospital stay is shorter when the patient is placed on a fast-track postoperative regimen. Postoperative analgesia is usually managed with patient-controlled analgesia followed by a switch to oral analgesics.

Step 5: Pearls and Pitfalls

The ileorectal anastomosis sometimes begins functioning rapidly and suddenly stops causing nausea, vomiting, and general malaise. This "ileorectal syndrome" may be due to the small intestine being exposed to a higher pressure created by the rectal vault. Placement of a 34-F mushroom catheter in the rectum during the first week of recovery may alleviate this problem or prevent it from occurring. The bowel slowly recovers over 7 to 10 days. An anastomotic leak must be ruled out. Parenteral nutrition allows the patient time to recover normal bowel function. When feeding resumes, a liquid diet is usually best until function normalizes.

The rectum varies in length in individuals. The usual length of 12 to 15 cm is adequate to provide a meaningful reservoir. Occasionally, the blood supply provided by the middle hemorrhoidal vessels via the internal iliac artery through the anterior lateral ligaments is inadequate. If this inadequacy can be determined preoperatively or suspected intraoperatively, the superior hemorrhoidal artery can be saved during sigmoid mesenteric dissection and good blood supply guaranteed. If the IMA has been sacrificed, and blood supply fails to the upper rectum, the only option is to resect more rectum to find well-vascularized tissue. Continued uncertainty regarding blood supply should lead to a decision to perform an end ileostomy and leave a Hartmann's stump at the level of reasonable blood supply.

The length of the rectal stump is also mandated by the need to perform long-term surveillance for malignancy. Patients with familial adenomatous polyposis, hereditary nonpolyposis colorectal cancer, or Crohn's disease require endoscopic surveillance. A short (12-cm) stump is easy to follow in the office setting.

Selected Readings

Church J, Burke C, McGannon E, et al. Risk of rectal cancer in patients after colectomy and ileorectal anastomosis for familial adenomatous polyposis: a function of available surgical options. Dis Colon Rectum 2003;46:1175–81.

Kalady MF, McGannon E, Vogel JD, et al. Risk of colorectal adenoma and carcinoma after colectomy for colorectal cancer in patients meeting Amsterdam criteria. Ann Surg 2010;252:507–11.

CHAPTER 8

Laparoscopic Total Abdominal Colectomy and Ileorectal Anastomosis

James W. Fleshman, Jr.

Step 1: Clinical Anatomy

The right colon lies on the patient's right side suspended laterally by peritoneal attachments to the right side of the abdominal wall, superiorly by attachments to the undersurface of the liver and posterior diaphragm, and medially by its mesentery. The ileocolic artery and vein and the right colic artery, if it is present, run through this leaf of mesentery. The colon is adherent to the retroperitoneum on the right side of the abdomen and covers the right gonadal vessels and right ureter. The inferior vena cava is the next most medial structure on the right side. The hepatic flexure, the fold at the junction between the right colon and transverse colon, is adherent to the anterior surface of the kidney by avascular attachments to Gerota's fascia. The first and second portions of the duodenum are adherent to the undersurface of the mesentery of the right colon and proximal transverse colon. The gallbladder is sometimes adherent to the cephalad surface of the transverse colon at the hepatic flexure.

The space behind the right colon is triangular shaped with the flat horizontal surface at the hepatic flexure running from the abdominal side wall toward the midline along the line of the greater curve of the stomach. The vertical axis follows the right lateral side wall of the abdomen. The hypotenuse runs from the fusion plane of the cecum at the pelvic brim over the top of the right iliac artery and vein at about the point where the ureter passes over the iliac vessels toward the midline over the aorta up to the base of the pancreas along the third portion of the duodenum. This triangular retroperitoneal area is a potential space with avascular attachments and allows the right colon to be lifted completely from the retroperitoneum during dissection. Release of all suspensory attachments allows the right colon to be made into a midline structure. The ileocolic artery and vein arise from the superior mesenteric artery (SMA) and superior mesenteric vein in the midportion of the SMA below the duodenum. The right colic artery is a variable structure and may be present as a separate structure or as part of the ileocolic trunk. The right branch of the middle colic artery exits through the pancreatic tissue from its origin on the SMA as a portion of the middle colic trunk at the base of the transverse mesocolon (Figure 8-1).

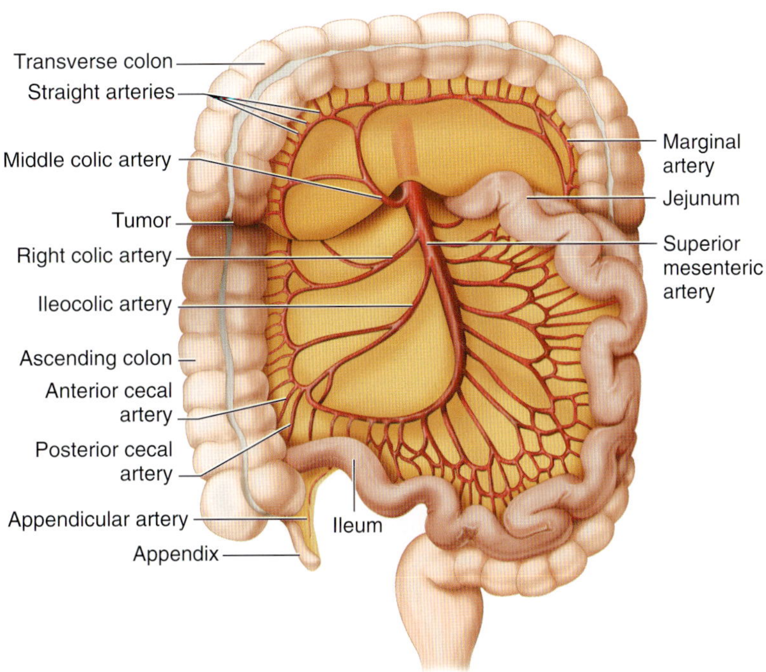
Transverse colon
Straight arteries
Middle colic artery
Tumor
Right colic artery
Ileocolic artery
Ascending colon
Anterior cecal artery
Posterior cecal artery
Appendicular artery
Appendix
Ileum
Marginal artery
Jejunum
Superior mesenteric artery

Figure 8-1

The left branches of the middle colic artery and vein exit adjacent to the right branch of the middle colic and are found at the third portion of the duodenum over the pancreas. The inferior mesenteric vein (IMV) travels along the window of the base of the mesentery of the colon and enters the portal vein adjacent to the ligament of Treitz at the base of the splenic flexure mesentery. This area of the vasculature to the colon is extremely complex and should be studied carefully before mobilization of the transverse colon. The mesentery of the transverse colon itself is sometimes attached to filmy attachments of the posterior aspect of the stomach. The omentum falls from the gastroepiploic artery along the greater curve of the stomach over the transverse colon where it attaches tangentially to the antimesenteric surface of the transverse colon and then continues to the lower aspect of the abdomen free-floating over the surface of the small bowel.

The splenic flexure of the colon sits in the left upper quadrant with a surface adherent to the undersurface of the tip of the spleen, the anterior surface of the left kidney, and the anterior surface of the tail of the pancreas. A portion of the base of the mesentery of the transverse colon is attached to the undersurface of the tail of the pancreas starting at the level of the IMV and extending laterally toward the left side of the abdomen (Figure 8-2). These attachments can be released by developing avascular planes given knowledge of the peritoneal windows, areolar tissue planes, and structural relationships. The left colon itself is adherent to the retroperitoneum in the left gutter via an avascular filmy tissue plane that attaches the mesentery and left colon to the posterior abdominal wall where the ureter and gonadal vessels are found. The peritoneal attachments along the left gutter of the abdomen suspend the left colon from the left side of the abdomen from the pelvic brim all the way up to the splenic flexure. The splenic flexure is a fold of the colon with its apex attached to the tip of the spleen by omental congenital adhesions.

The splenic flexure is usually covered by the omentum as it falls over the top of the transverse colon along the left gutter, and numerous embryologic attachments can occur between the antimesenteric surface of the proximal left colon and the omentum at the splenic flexure. The left colon descends along the left gutter to the level of the pelvic brim where the colon becomes free from the pelvic side wall and falls into a sigmoid-appearing structure known as the sigmoid colon. The sigmoid colon lies free in the pelvis, attached only posteriorly to its vascular attachments at the midline over the sacral promontory.

The inferior mesenteric artery (IMA) arises from the anterior surface of the aorta proximal to the origin of the common iliac vessels. The IMA branches to give the superior hemorrhoidal artery descending into the posterior mesorectal vessel and the ascending left colic vessel, which sweeps up toward the splenic flexure. The IMV runs across the base of the mesentery of the left colon, crossing the superior hemorrhoidal and left colic vessels on its way to the duodenum. There is a clear peritoneal window between the aorta and the IMV, which can be used to enter the avascular plane behind the left colon mesentery and the retroperitoneum.

Step 2: Preoperative Considerations

Common indications for a laparoscopic total abdominal colectomy with ileorectal anastomosis are the same as for an open procedure and include synchronous colon cancers, familial cancer syndromes (hereditary nonpolyposis colorectal cancer, familial adenomatous polyposis with rectal sparing, and cancer in patients <40 years old), colonic inertia, Crohn's colitis with rectal sparing, and gastrointestinal bleeding. The preparation of the patient is dictated by the specific indication, and the appropriate evaluations should be undertaken. A mechanical bowel preparation with oral agents is not necessary but is frequently performed to reduce stool in the colon. If the patient has a history of constipation, the colon can be too heavy with retained stool to allow a safe laparoscopic approach. The left side of the colon can be adequately cleansed with several enemas before surgery. Routine deep vein thrombosis prophylaxis, prophylactic antibiotics, and instructions on postoperative care are required. Patients should receive education on

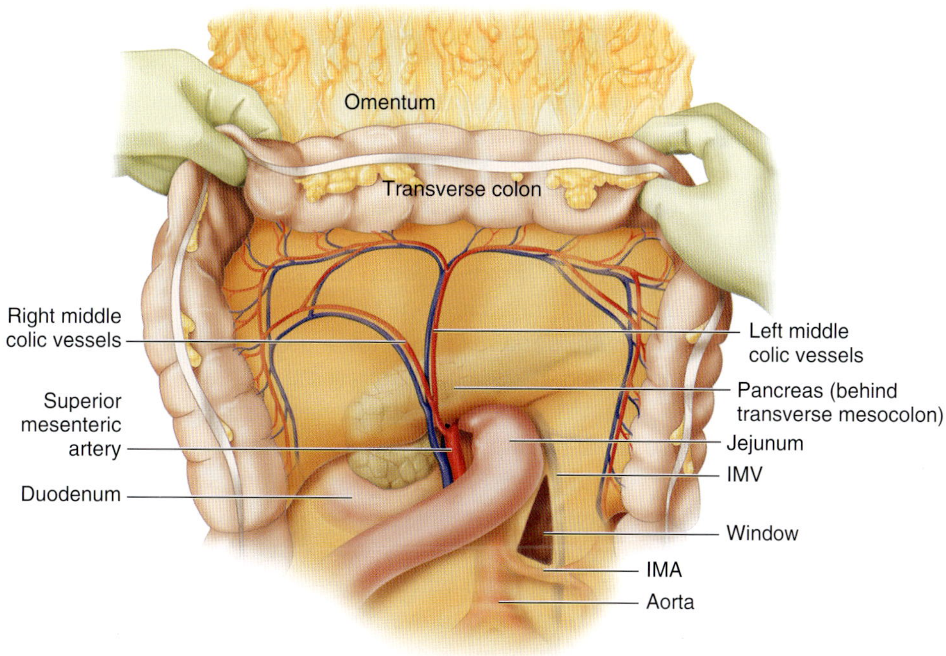
Omentum
Transverse colon
Right middle
colic vessels
Superior
mesenteric
artery
Duodenum
Left middle
colic vessels
Pancreas (behind
transverse mesocolon)
Jejunum
IMV
Window
IMA
Aorta

Figure 8-2

the expected functional outcome of an ileorectal anastomosis. They can expect to have four to five semisolid, pasty bowel movements a day with good bowel control after a period of accommodation (usually 6 months).

Step 3: Operative Steps

Right Colon

- The patient is positioned in the modified lithotomy position with the legs in Allen's stirrups and sequential compression leggings in place. A beanbag, attached directly to the operating table with Velcro, is folded around the patient, including the shoulders, and deflated to fix the patient in position. This beanbag keeps the arms at the patient's side and allows the table to be placed in steep Trendelenburg and airplaned to the left and right during the operation. The trocar site placement is typically at the umbilicus, right upper anterior axillary line, right lower anterior axillary line, suprapubic, and left flank positions. The camera operator stands to the patient's left shoulder and operates the camera through the umbilical port. The operating surgeon stands at the patient's left hip or between the legs as needed and operates instruments through the left flank and suprapubic ports (Figure 8-3).
- A 15-mm Hg pneumoperitoneum is maintained with a pressure-controlled insufflator. The camera cord, light cord, and carbon dioxide cord are passed off of the table from the patient's left shoulder to the instrumentation tower. A monitor is placed opposite the operating surgeon and camera operator. If two monitors are available, one is at the right shoulder, and one is at the right hip. The liver should be evaluated, the omentum should be placed over the stomach to the left upper quadrant, and the small bowel should be retracted from the pelvis to lie in the left upper quadrant. The 5-mm wavy grasper is a good instrument to flip the small bowel up into the left upper quadrant with a reverse "C" motion; the principle should be to avoid grasping any individual piece of bowel on the bowel itself. Using mesenteric fat or epiploic fat to move portions of intestine is appropriate.
- The cecum is lifted to the anterior abdominal wall using the 5-mm grasper through the suprapubic port in the operator's left hand. An instrument with a surgeon-controlled energy source can be used to incise along the base of the peritoneum from the pelvic brim over the iliac vessels toward the duodenum at the midline of the abdominal cavity (Figure 8-4*A*). This incision allows a plane to be developed in the retroperitoneum over the structures that are found posteriorly (Figure 8-5). The right ureter is identified crossing the iliac vessels close to the bifurcation of the aorta; the gonadal vessels are further lateral and run parallel to the iliac vessels (Figure 8-4*B*). The psoas muscle lies posteriorly and should be a boundary of dissection. The avascular plane that is encountered is used as the dissection plane and can be bluntly dissected in a posterior sweeping direction to allow the mesentery and cecum to separate anteriorly from the posterior structures.

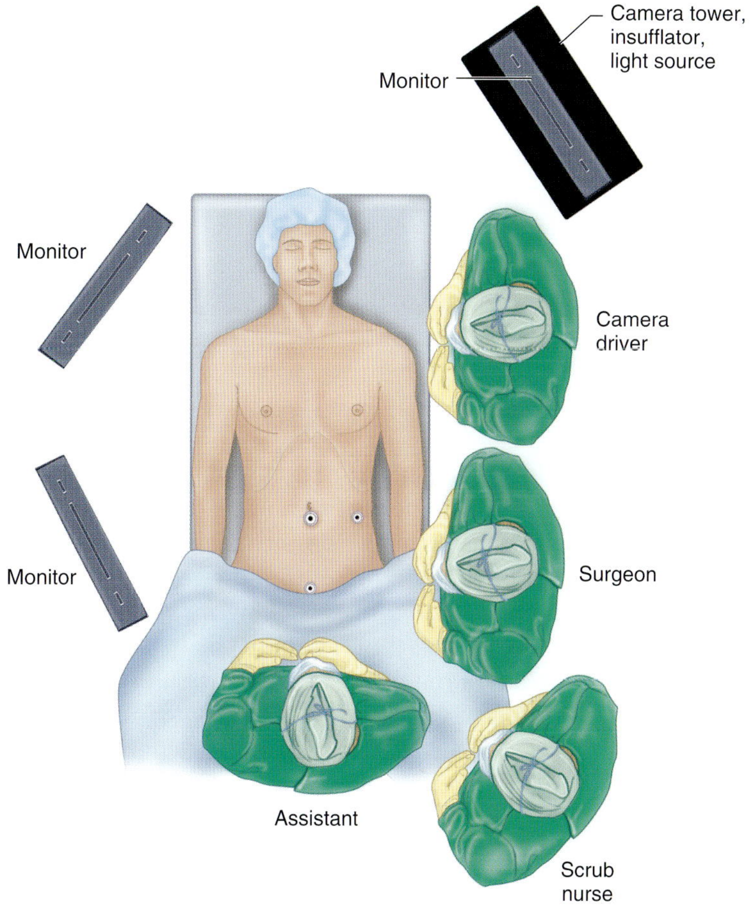

Figure 8-3

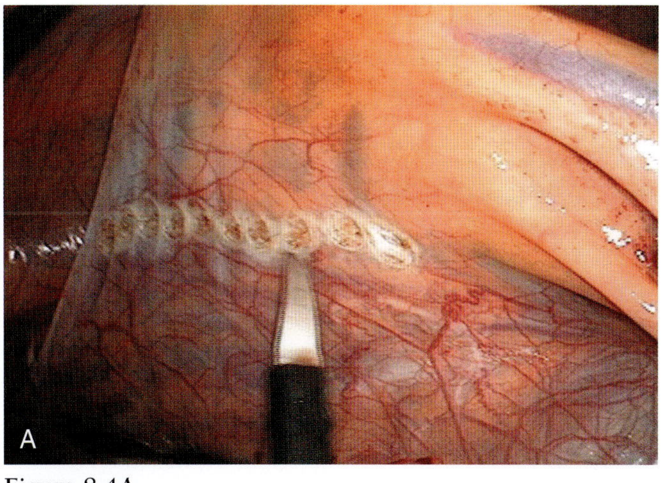

Figure 8-4A

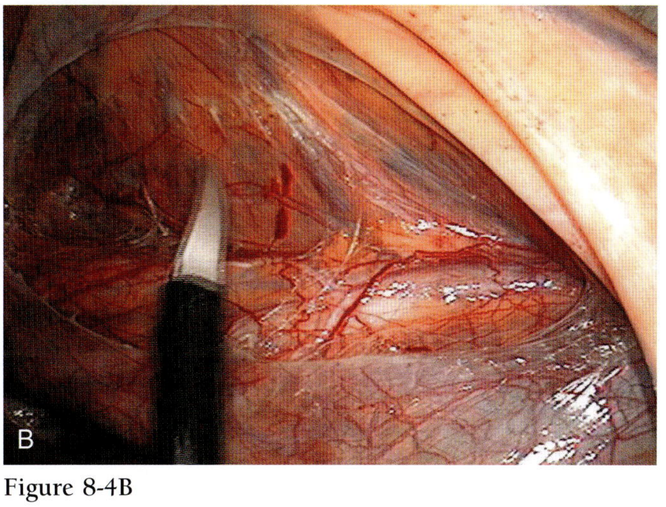

Figure 8-4B

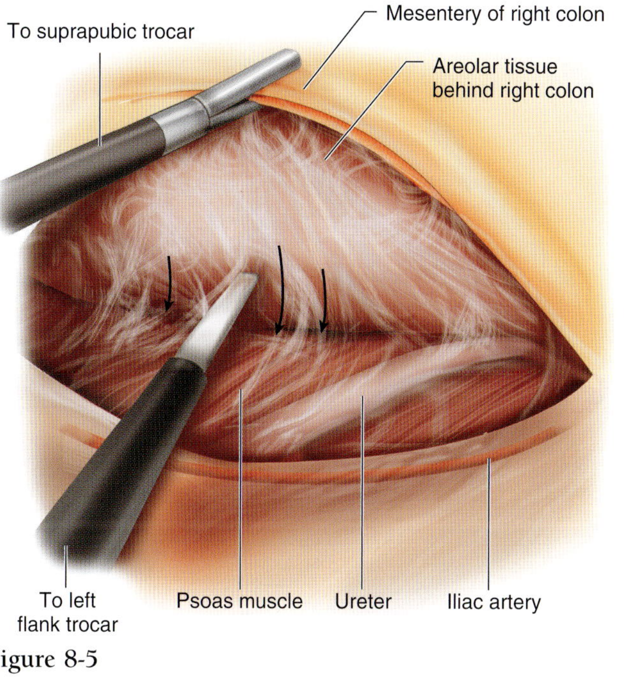

Figure 8-5

- The cecum should be completely mobilized from the retroperitoneum all the way out to the side wall of the abdomen using the left-hand grasper for retraction upward and the right-hand instrument to develop the plane. The dissection is carried in this posterior plane up to and around and on top of the surface of the duodenum (Figure 8-6). The duodenum should be separated from the overlying mesentery of the right colon using the left hand for anterior retraction all the way up to the hepatic flexure peritoneal attachments, exposing the entire sweep of the duodenum, a portion of the head of the pancreas, and the lateral aspect of the middle colic vessels (Figure 8-7). The anterior portion of the kidney is exposed with this same maneuver with upward traction and downward countertraction. The mesentery and right colon are lifted toward the anterior abdominal wall, while pulling the avascular tissue posteriorly with the blunt dissection using the instrument in the operator's right hand. Most of the retraction is accomplished with the left hand on the grasper through the suprapubic port.
- The patient is placed in reverse Trendelenburg position. The attachments of the hepatic flexure to the retroperitoneum are lifted anteriorly and divided with an energy source along the line between the liver and the transverse colon (Figure 8-8); this allows entry in the previously dissected plane of the right colon posteriorly in the area of purple hue in the posterior peritoneum (Figure 8-9*A*).

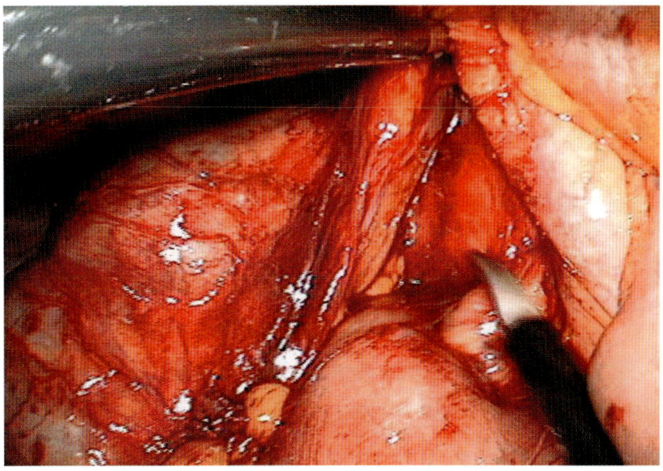
Figure 8-6

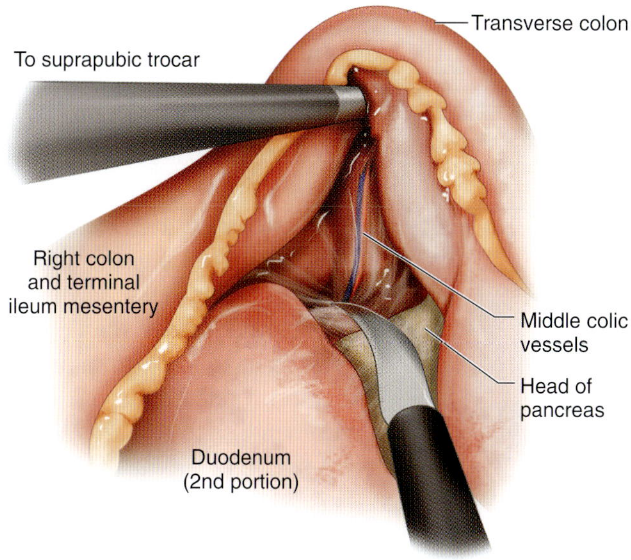

Figure 8-7

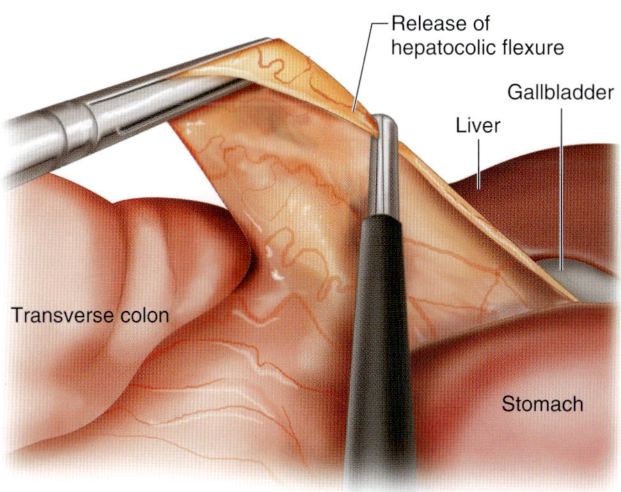

Figure 8-8

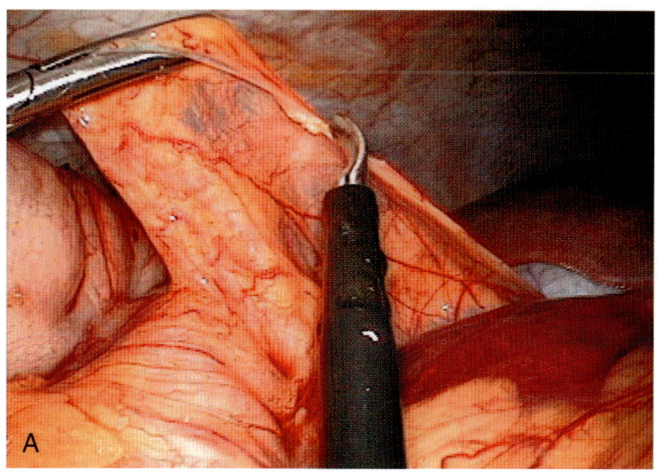

Figure 8-9A

- The omentum attached to the transverse colon is detached to enter the lesser sac (Figure 8-9*B*). The transverse colon is released from the lesser sac, head of the pancreas, and undersurface of the antrum of the stomach all the way out to the right side wall of the abdomen (Figure 8-10). The hepatic flexure is completely mobilized from the undersurface of the liver, and the posterior dissection is connected to the right upper quadrant dissection.
- The patient is returned to Trendelenburg position, and the cecum is grasped at the ileocecal valve and lifted anteriorly to the abdominal wall. This maneuver provides the tension needed to expose the ileocolic vessel in the mesentery of the right colon (Figure 8-9*C*).
- Dissection on either side of the ileocolic vessel provides windows to allow transection of the ileocolic vessels at their origin along the SMA (Figures 8-9*D* and 8-11).
- The right colon is released from the lateral attachments of the colon from the right side wall of the abdomen (Figure 8-12). The cecum is grasped and lifted anteriorly. The cecum is retracted toward the midline to facilitate the division of the lateral attachments with the energy source. This maneuver allows the right colon to become a midline structure from the middle of the transverse colon all the way to the terminal ileum.

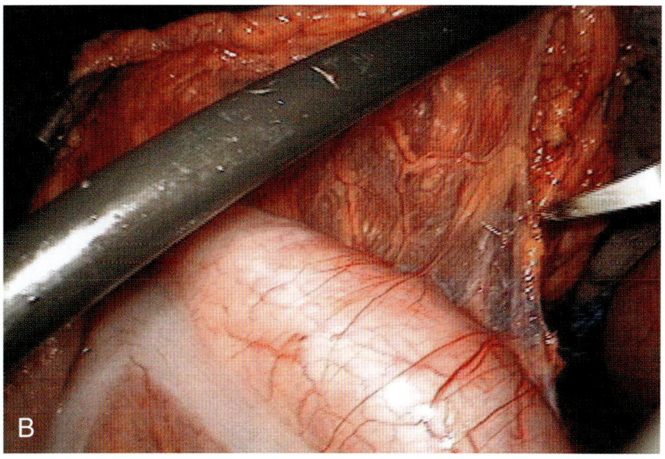

Figure 8-9B

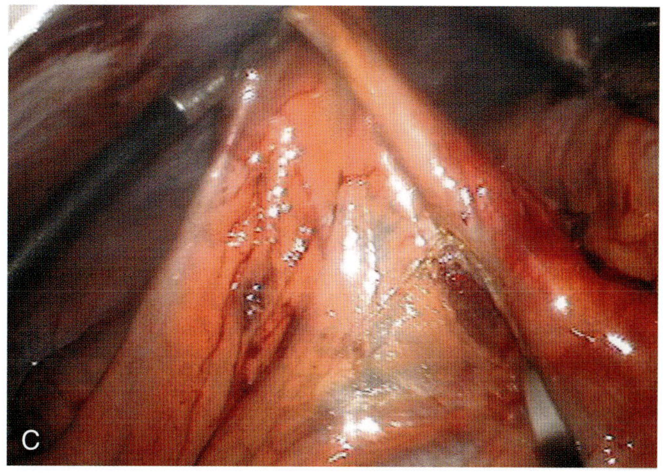

Figure 8-9C

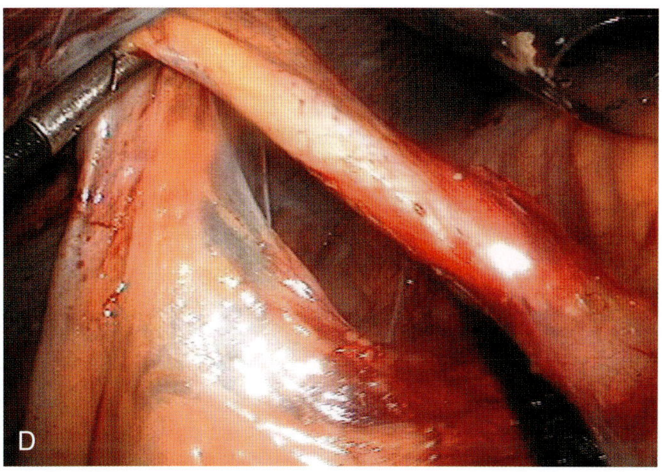

Figure 8-9D

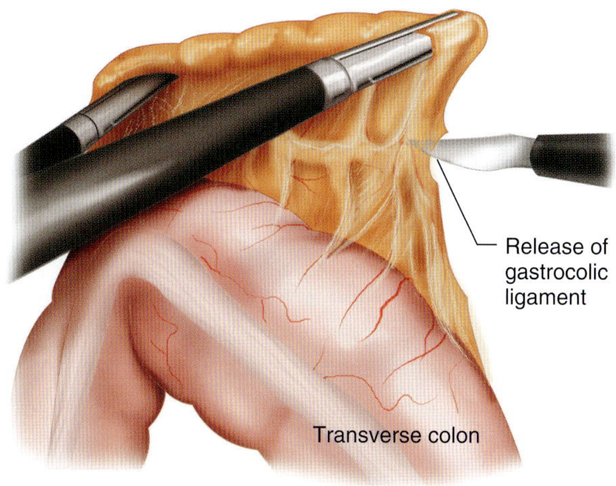

Figure 8-10

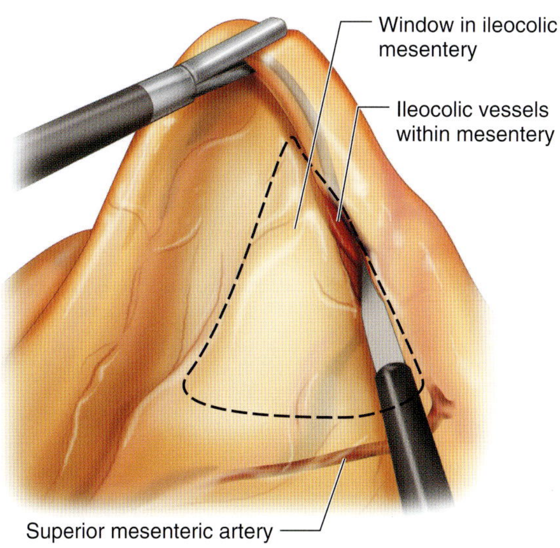

Figure 8-11

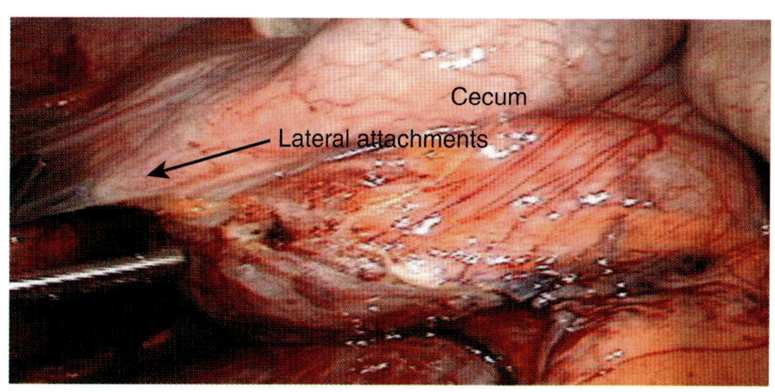

Figure 8-12

Left Colon

- The patient is placed in steep Trendelenburg and airplaned to the right. The surgeon stands to the right of the patient. The small bowel is swept from the pelvis into the right upper quadrant with grasping instruments, and the base of the mesentery of the left colon is exposed. The IMA is identified at its origin on the aorta proximal to the sacral promontory (Figure 8-13). The space posterior to the superior hemorrhoidal artery and anterior to the sacral promontory is exposed. Anterior traction is exerted on the superior hemorrhoidal artery with a clamp through the suprapubic port. An energy source is introduced through the right lower quadrant trocar site, and a 5-mm bowel grasper is introduced through the right upper quadrant trocar site. The presacral window is easily seen with this retraction plan (Figure 8-14).
- The peritoneum is incised along the base of the triangle to expose the areolar tissue plane behind the superior hemorrhoidal artery but anterior to the retroperitoneum where the gonadal vessels and the ureter are found along the left iliac artery and vein (Figure 8-15). This avascular plane is bluntly developed all the way out to the left abdominal side wall behind the mesentery of the sigmoid and left colon.

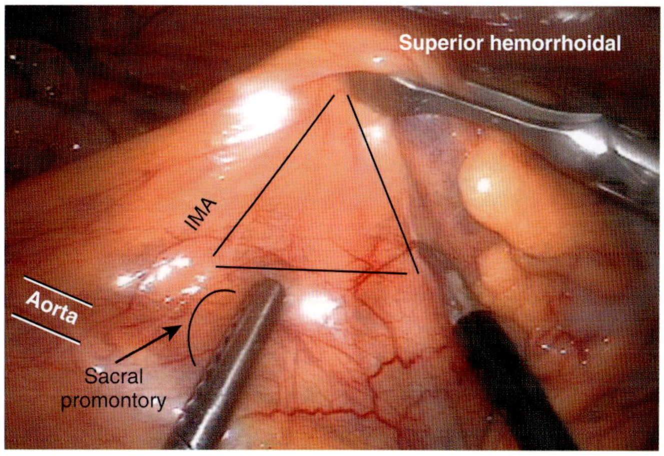

Figure 8-13

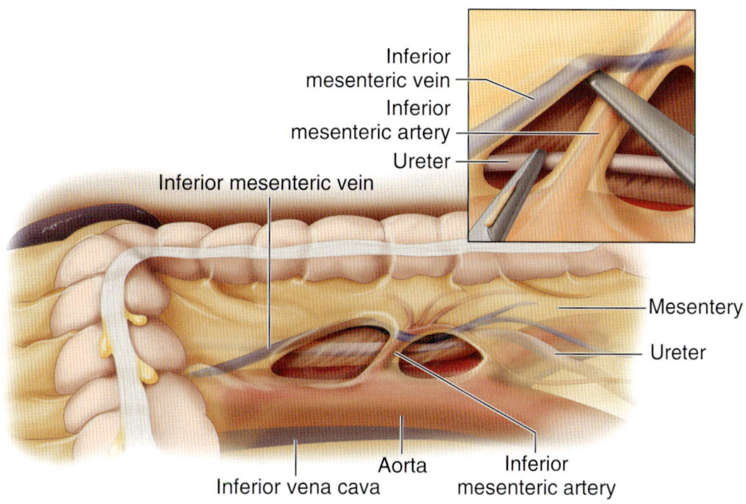

Figure 8-14

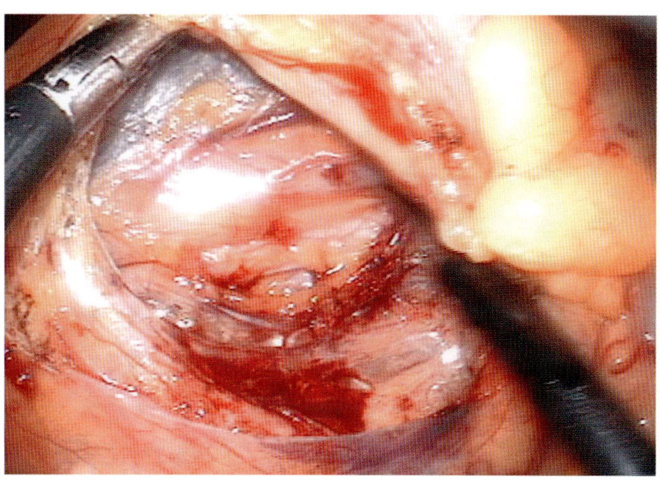
Figure 8-15

- The dissection is carried around the IMA to the peritoneal window beneath the IMV and anterior to the aorta. The window is incised, and the opening is developed cephalad to the IMA (Figure 8-16). The IMA is skeletonized and divided at its origin with an energy source (Figure 8-17). The artery may be divided at the bifurcation of the left colic and superior hemorrhoidal artery if the disease is benign to prevent all risk of injuring nerves of sexual function in the preaortic plexus.
- Blunt dissection of the avascular plane is carried from the pelvic brim to the tail of the pancreas and laterally to the side wall of the abdomen beneath the left colon and its mesentery (Figure 8-18). The right upper quadrant trocar site provides access for the retracting blunt instrument, and the right lower quadrant trocar site provides access for the energy source or dissecting instrument. The suprapubic site allows the second retracting grasper to lift the edge of the mesentery anteriorly to provide a tenting effect, while the camera (in the umbilical port) looks beneath and laterally.
- The IMV is exposed at its origin at the level of the ligament of Treitz, proximal to the first branch of the IMV, which travels to the splenic flexure. The vein is transected with an energy source or stapling instrument to release the base of the mesentery of the left colon (Figure 8-19). The left colon is released from the lateral side wall of the abdomen from the pelvic brim to the splenic flexure, exposing the previously dissected retroperitoneum with the protected structures posteriorly (Figure 8-20).

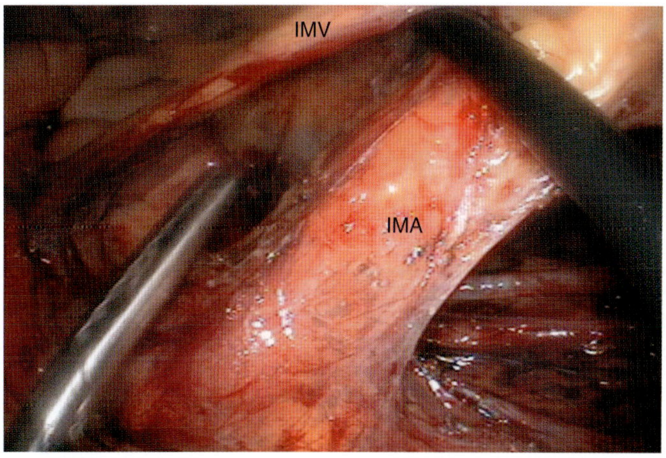

Figure 8-16

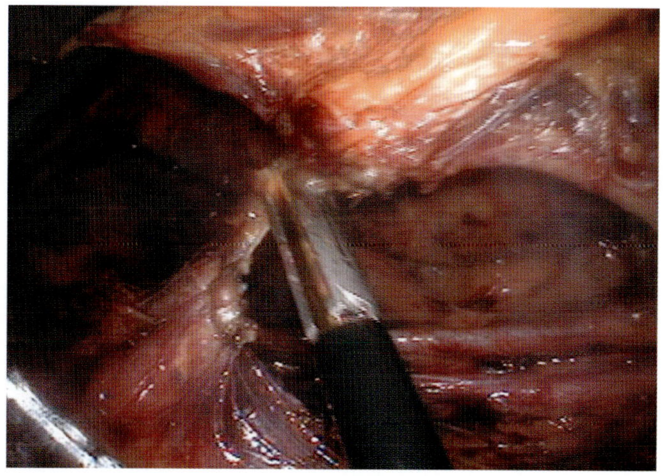
Figure 8-17

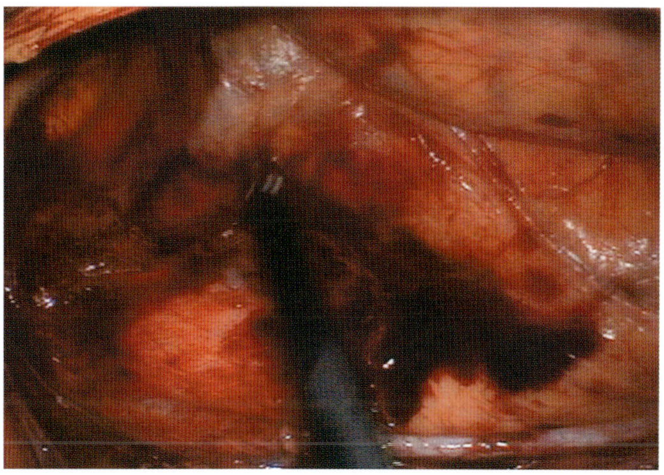
Figure 8-18

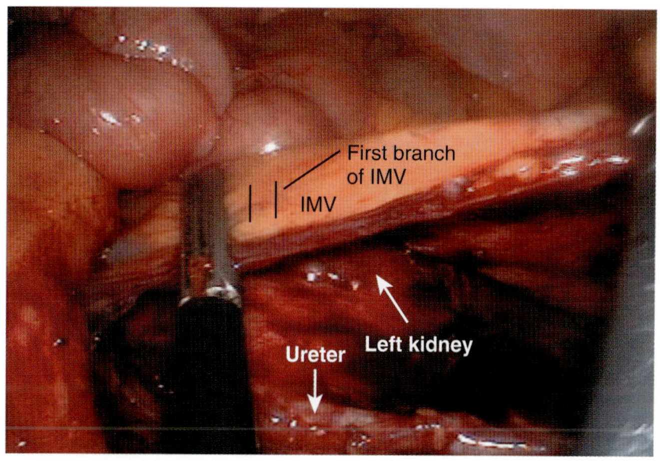

Figure 8-19

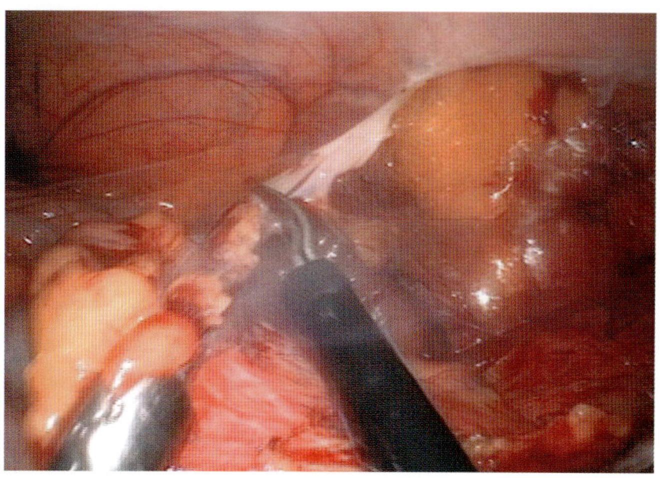
Figure 8-20

- The patient is placed in reverse Trendelenburg, still airplaned to the right, and the splenic flexure attachments are incised along the left side wall of the pelvis up to the level of the spleen (Figures 8-21 and 8-22). The tip of the spleen and the anterior surface of the kidney are exposed as the suspensory ligaments are divided, and the splenic flexure is mobilized medially (Figure 8-23). The right upper quadrant trocar provides access for the assistant to place a 5-mm grasper and pull the splenic flexure toward the midline. The operating surgeon stands between the legs and uses the 10-mm grasper through the suprapubic midline and the 5-mm port in the left lower quadrant to place the energy source to allow the instrument to reach closer to the splenic flexure. The tail of the pancreas and tip of the spleen and anterior surface of the kidney are exposed (Figure 8-24).
- Finally, the omentum is released from the antimesenteric surface of the splenic flexure and transverse colon to enter the lesser sac around the corner of the splenic flexure (Figure 8-25). The right upper quadrant trocar site provides retracting access to lift the omentum anteriorly and cephalad, while the suprapubic trocar site provides access for retracting the splenic flexure toward the feet, and the left lower quadrant trocar site provides access for the energy source to divide the attachments of the omentum to the colon. The pancreas is exposed in the base of the lesser sac, and its lower edge is freed from the attachments of the splenic flexure all the way to the stump of the IMV at the ligament of Treitz. The posterior wall of the stomach, the anterior surface of the pancreas, the tip of the spleen, and the anterior surface of the kidney are clearly visualized with this technique (Figure 8-26).

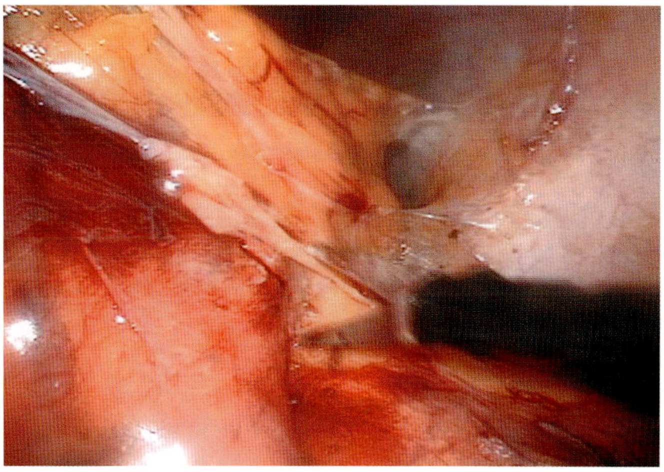

Figure 8-21

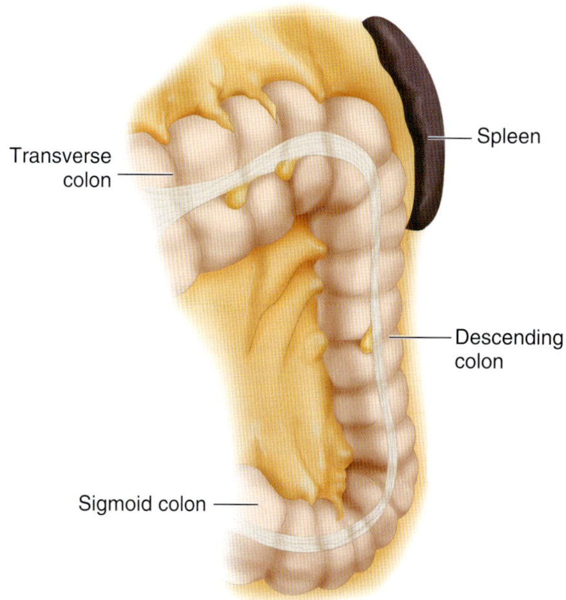

Figure 8-22

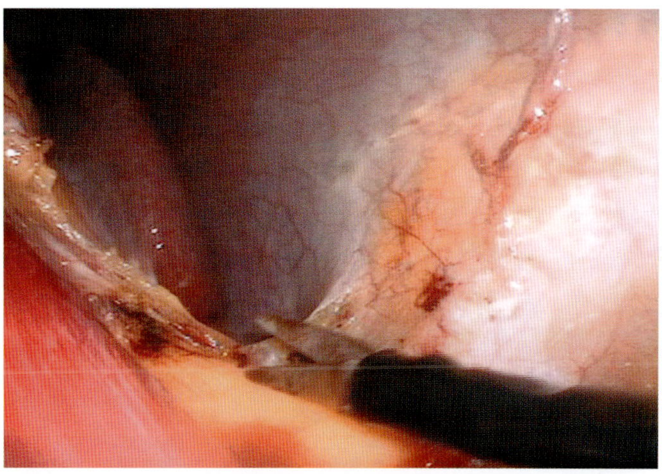

Figure 8-23

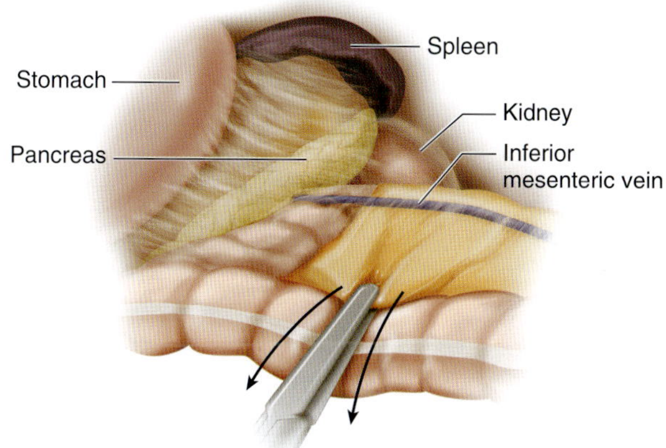

Figure 8-24

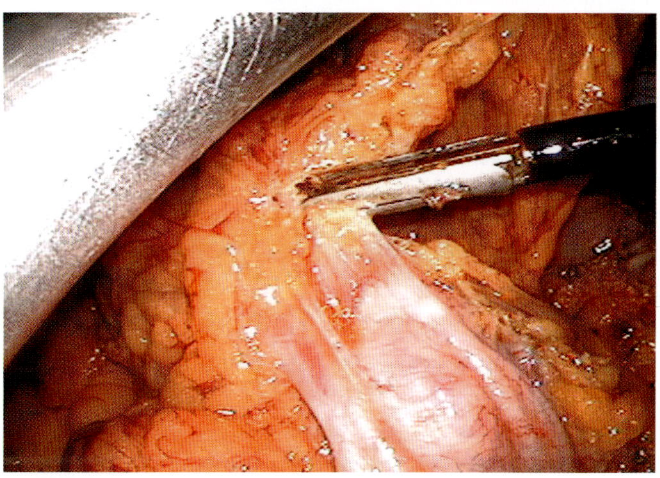

Figure 8-25

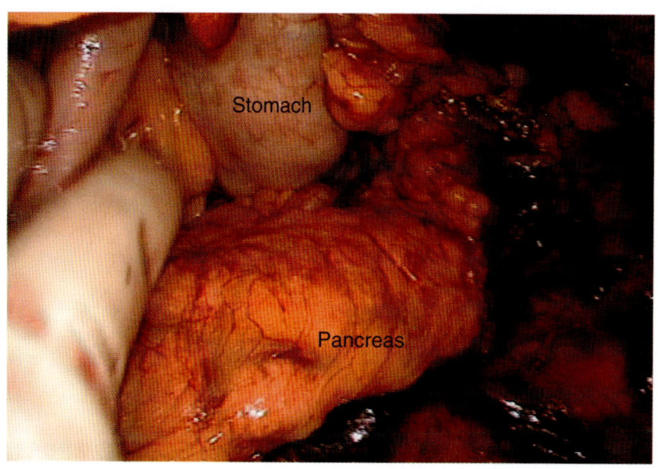

Figure 8-26

Isolation of Middle Colic Vessels

- After the left and right colon have been completely mobilized and the transverse colon completely freed from the gastrocolic ligament, the pedicle of the middle colic vessels can be identified at the inferior margin of the pancreas and the anterior surface of the third portion of the duodenum. In a hand-assisted approach, this pedicle is most easily identified by placing the left hand through the hand-access port with the operator standing between the legs. The operator identifies the windows of the mesentery on both sides of the vessels on either side of the midline (Figures 8-27*A* and *B* and 8-28); this allows the middle colic vessels to be lifted anteriorly, and the SMA and SMV are protected (Figure 8-27*A*). The flexible tip camera is turned to the right upper quadrant and flexed to the right to give a transverse view of the vessels as they are stretched and lifted. An endoscopic linear cutter stapler can be inserted through a 10-mm trocar placed in the right upper quadrant (Figure 8-29), or the bipolar sealing instrument can be used through the right upper quadrant to divide the base of the middle colic vessels carefully. Time should be taken to ensure adequate hemostasis because these vessels bear the pressure of aortic flow.

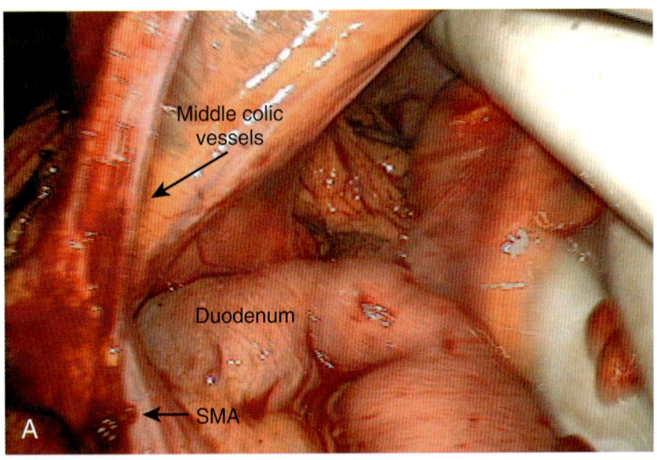

Figure 8-27A

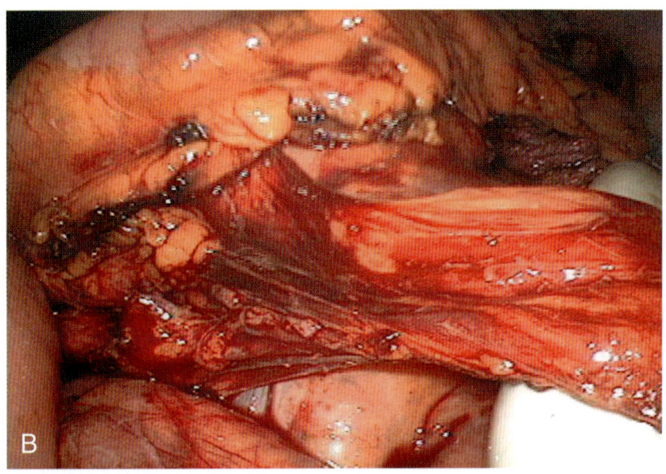

Figure 8-27B

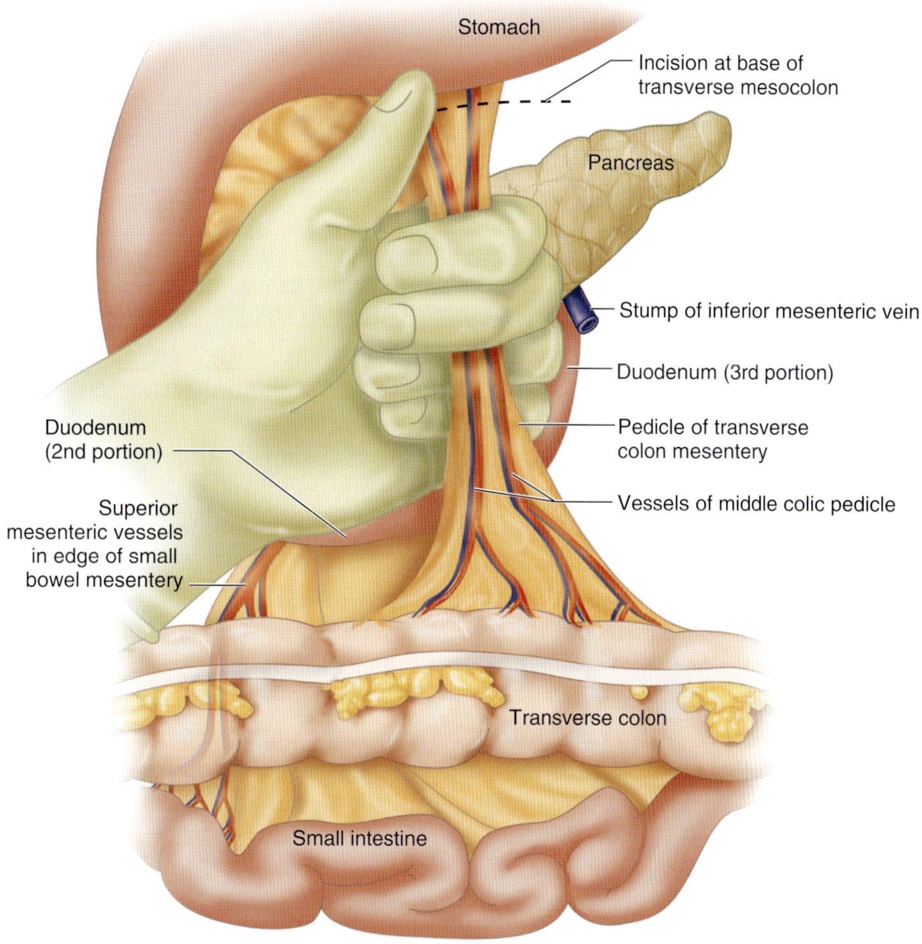

Figure 8-28

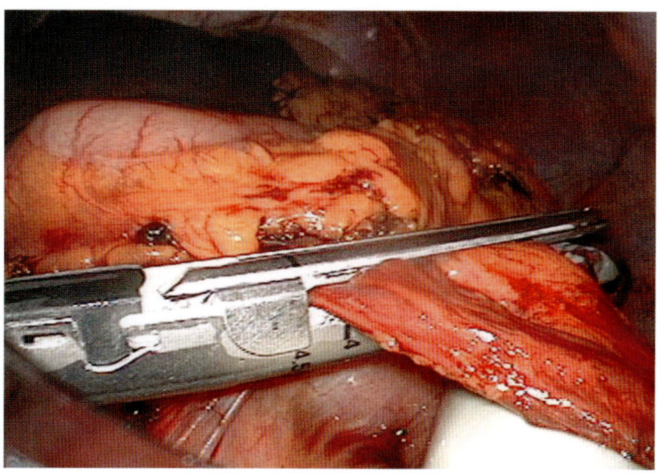

Figure 8-29

- The suprapubic incision is extended, and a wound protector is placed, or in a hand-assisted case, the cap of the gel port is removed, and the carbon dioxide is deflated. The colon and terminal ileum are extracted (Figure 8-30*A*). The mesentery of the sigmoid colon is identified, and the mesentery is divided at the level of the sacral promontory using either a clamp and tie technique or radiofrequency sealing with an appropriate device. The rectum can be divided at the level of the sacral promontory with a transverse stapler, endoscopic stapler, or linear cutter stapler through the suprapubic incision (Figure 8-30*B*).
- The terminal ileum is divided at the ileocecal valve using another firing of a GIA stapler (Covidien, Mansfield, Mass.). The colon and its mesentery from the right colon all the way to the top of the rectum are passed off as specimen.
- The terminal ileum is returned to the abdomen. The small bowel is allowed to fall to the patient's left, and the rectum is pulled to the right side of the pelvis. The ileum is allowed to loop down into the pelvis along the left side of the rectum and then curve back up along the antimesenteric border of the rectum to the level of the staple line (Figure 8-31). The two transverse staple lines are aligned; the corners of the staple lines are opened, and a linear cutter stapler is placed between the rectum and the terminal ileum to create a side-to-side anastomosis when fired (Figure 8-32).

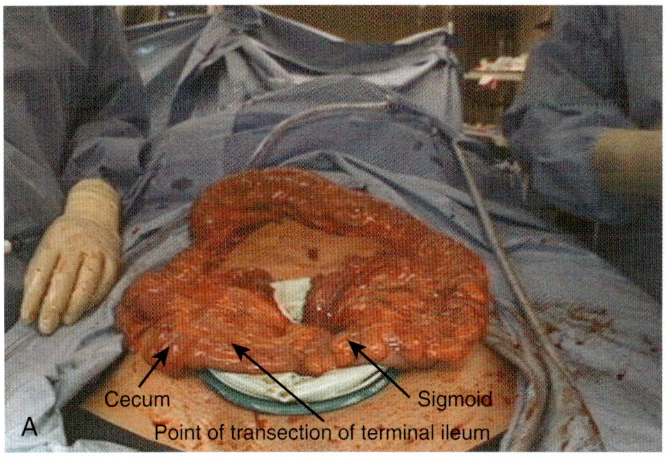

Figure 8-30A

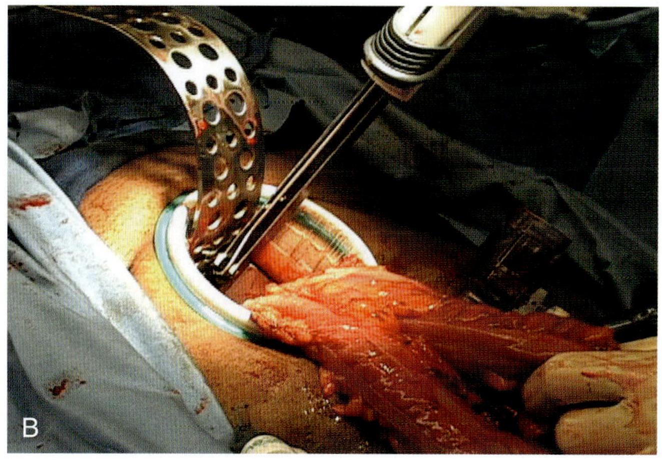

Figure 8-30B

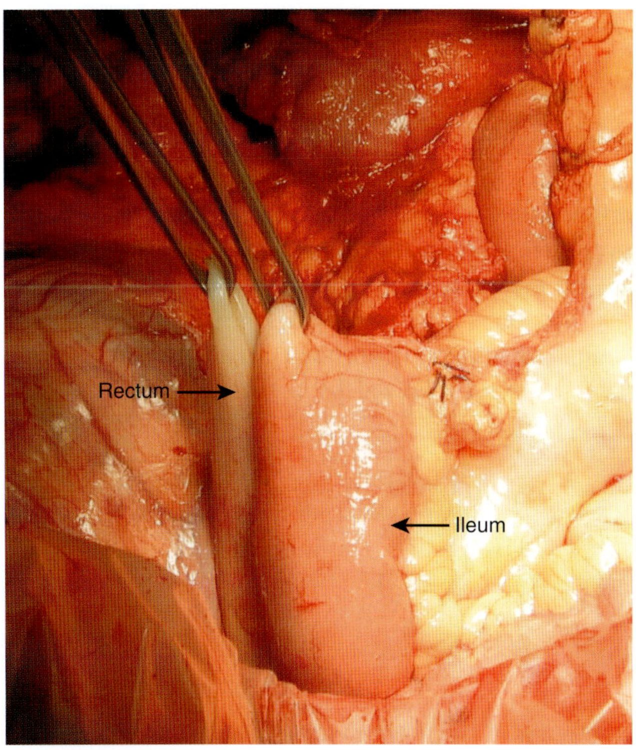

Figure 8-31

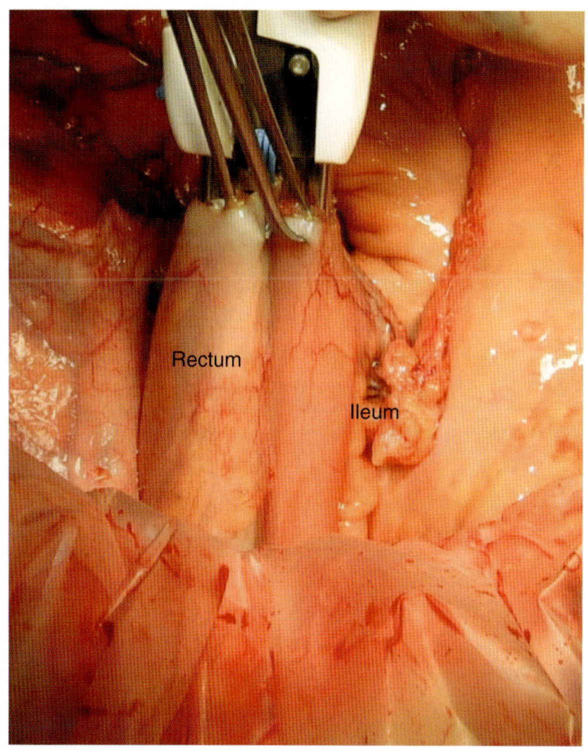

Figure 8-32

- The transverse opening is closed with another firing of the GIA stapler (Figure 8-33). The transverse staple line is inverted with a running monofilament absorbable suture. The apex of the GIA staple line is protected with an interrupted absorbable suture. The cut edge of the mesentery in the small bowel can usually be secured to the retroperitoneum along the side of the aorta on either side of the aorta using a running absorbable suture; this has the benefit of preventing internal herniation and guarantees that the small bowel is lying in an unrotated or twisted manner.
- The inner aspect of the umbilical trocar is closed with a figure-eight suture of 0 absorbable suture. The Pfannenstiel incision is closed with a running monofilament absorbable suture in the fascia. Subcutaneous tissue is irrigated with antibiotic solution at all sites. The skin is closed with skin staples, and adhesive bandages are applied.

Step 4: Postoperative Care

Patients are ambulated early. Intravenous fluid replacement is given to maintain a urine output of greater than 30 mL/hr. Nasogastric decompression is not required unless the patient becomes nauseated. Most patients tolerate clear liquids within 24 to 48 hours, and the diet can be advanced as tolerated. Patients should be given prophylactic antibiotics for 24 hours, incentive spirometry, and deep vein thrombosis prophylaxis and encouraged to ambulate as much as possible during the early postoperative period. Usual hospital stay is 4 to 5 days; the hospital stay is shorter when the patient is placed on a fast-track postoperative regimen. Postoperative analgesia is usually managed with patient-controlled analgesia followed by a switch to oral analgesics.

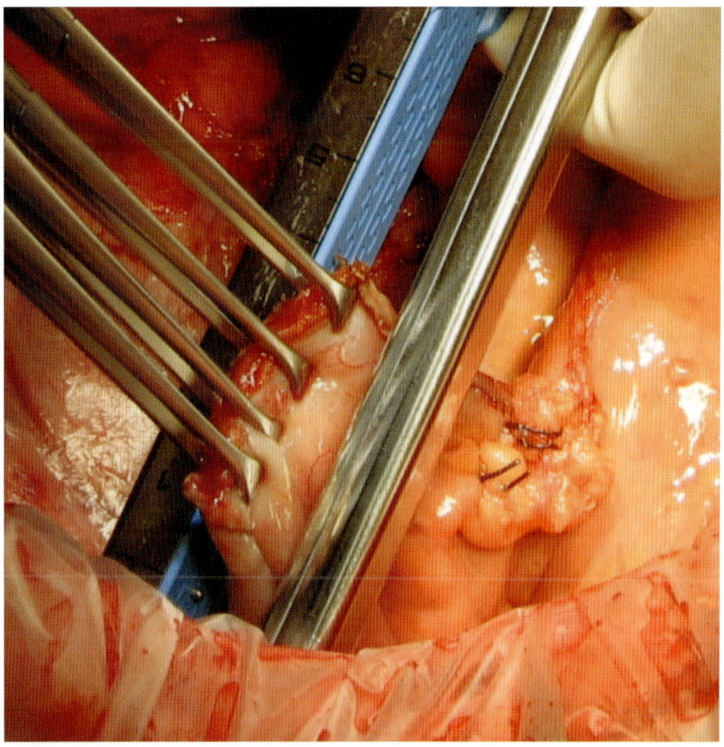

Figure 8-33

Step 5: Pearls and Pitfalls

Patients have a fairly rapid return of bowel function because of the laparoscopic approach. A large fluid shift is likely to occur because of the raw surfaces created. Adequate fluid replacement can avoid acute renal failure, dehydration, and an ileus.

As we have performed more ileorectal anastomoses for familial adenomatous polyposis and Crohn's disease, the frequent development of a delayed ileus has led us to describe a syndrome known as "ileorectal syndrome." This syndrome is possibly caused by the terminal ileum facing new high pressure intraluminally because of its attachment to the rectum with an intact sphincter only 12 cm away. The ileum interprets this high pressure as small bowel obstruction, and a high volume of intraluminal fluid is created that causes diarrhea, a bloating sensation, and nausea and vomiting. Treatment is best accomplished with a nasogastric tube, bowel rest, and total parenteral nutrition. This syndrome develops even when a 34-F mushroom catheter is left in the rectum in the early postoperative period to decompress and equalize the pressures in the rectum. The terminal ileum responds as if it were a blocked ileostomy with high outpouring of fluid; distention; and a syndrome of nausea, vomiting, and diarrhea. The patient should be reassured and supported, and the possibility of an anastomotic leak should be ruled out with a computed tomography (CT) scan.

The patient should be warned before surgery that 6 to 10 bowel movements a day is common. The early administration of loperamide (Imodium) can cause problems with a partial blockage-type syndrome as mentioned in the previous paragraph. The patient should be allowed to stabilize at 6 to 10 bowel movements a day in the first 2 weeks, and then Imodium or diphenoxylate (Lomotil) can be added to reduce bowel movements to 3 to 4 a day in the early months after surgery. The patient can expect continued decrease in frequency over time as the small bowel accommodates to its new position at the top of the rectum.

If the patient develops a postoperative obstructive clinical picture, it is important to rule out an internal herniation, especially if the mesentery has not been secured to the retroperitoneum. The internal herniation and volvulus around the SMA can result in disaster because infarction of a significant portion of the small bowel can occur resulting in short bowel syndrome and loss of the possibility for intestinal continuity. Rapid recognition and treatment by exploration and detorsion are essential in this situation.

Selected Readings

Boushey RP, Marcello PW, Martel G, et al. Laparoscopic total colectomy: an evolutionary experience. Dis Colon Rectum 2007;50:1512–9.

Chung TP, Fleshman JW, Birnbaum EH, et al. Laparoscopic vs. open total abdominal colectomy for severe colitis: impact on recovery and subsequent completion restorative proctectomy. Dis Colon Rectum 2009;52:4–10.

Marcello PW, Fleshman JW, Milsom JW, et al. Hand-assisted laparoscopic vs. laparoscopic colorectal surgery: a multicenter, prospective, randomized trial. Dis Colon Rectum 2008;51:818–26.

CHAPTER 9

Open Total Proctocolectomy and Ileal Pouch

James W. Fleshman, Jr.

Step 1: Clinical Anatomy

The right colon lies on the patient's right side suspended by peritoneal attachments to the right side of the abdominal wall, the undersurface of the liver and posterior diaphragm, and its mesentery from the medial aspect through which the ileocolic artery and vein and the right colic artery, if it is present, run. The colon is adherent to the retroperitoneum on the right side of the abdomen and covers the right gonadal vessels and right ureter. The inferior vena cava is the next most medial structure on the right side. The hepatic flexure, the fold at the junction between the right colon and transverse colon, is adherent to the anterior surface of the kidney by avascular attachments over the outside of Gerota's fascia. The first and second portions of the duodenum are adherent to the undersurface of the mesentery of the right colon and the proximal aspect of the transverse colon. The gallbladder is sometimes adherent to the cephalad surface of the transverse colon at the hepatic flexure.

The space behind the right colon is shaped like a triangle with the flat horizontal surface at the hepatic flexure running from the abdominal side wall toward the midline along the line of the greater curve of the stomach. The vertical axis is found along the right gutter at the peritoneal attachment to the lateral side wall of the abdomen, and the hypotenuse runs from the fusion plane of the cecum at the pelvic brim over the top of the right iliac artery and vein at about the point where the ureter passes over the iliac vessels toward the midline over the aorta up to the base of the pancreas along the third portion of the duodenum. This triangular retroperitoneal area is an avascular space and allows the right colon to be lifted completely from the retroperitoneum during dissection; this allows the right colon to be made into a midline structure. The ileocolic artery and vein arise from the superior mesenteric artery (SMA) and superior mesenteric vein in the midportion of the SMA below the point of exit above the duodenum. The right colic artery is a variable structure and may not exist or exist only as part of the ileocolic trunk. The right branch of the middle colic artery exits through the pancreatic tissue from its origin on the SMA as a portion of the middle colic trunk at the base of the transverse mesocolon (Figure 9-1).

The left branches of the middle colic artery and vein arise adjacent to the right branch of the middle colic and are found at the third portion of the duodenum over the pancreas. The inferior mesenteric vein (IMV) travels along the window of the base of the mesentery of the left colon

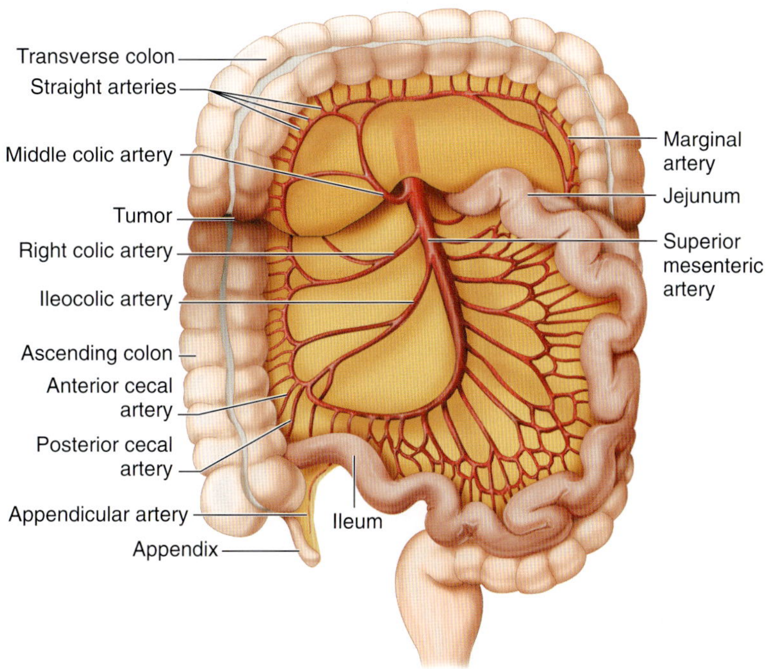
Transverse colon
Straight arteries
Middle colic artery
Tumor
Right colic artery
Ileocolic artery
Ascending colon
Anterior cecal artery
Posterior cecal artery
Appendicular artery
Appendix
Ileum
Marginal artery
Jejunum
Superior mesenteric artery

Figure 9-1

and joins the splenic vein adjacent to the ligament of Treitz at the base of the splenic flexure mesentery. This area of the vasculature to the colon is extremely complex and should be studied carefully before mobilization of the transverse colon. The mesentery of the transverse colon itself is sometimes attached to filmy attachments of the posterior aspect of the stomach. The omentum falls from the gastroepiploic artery along the greater curve of the stomach over the transverse colon where it attaches tangentially to the antimesenteric surface of the transverse colon and continues to the lower aspect of the abdomen free-floating over the surface of the small bowel.

The splenic flexure of the colon sits in the left upper quadrant with a surface adherent to the undersurface of the tip of the spleen, the anterior surface of the left kidney, and the anterior surface of the tail of the pancreas. A portion of the base of the mesentery of the transverse colon is attached to the undersurface of the tail of the pancreas starting at the level of the IMV and extending laterally toward the left side of the abdomen. These attachments can be released by developing avascular planes given knowledge of the peritoneal windows, areolar tissue planes, and structural relationships. The left colon itself is adherent to the retroperitoneum in the left gutter via an avascular filmy tissue plane that attaches the mesentery and left colon to the posterior abdominal wall where the ureter and gonadal vessels are found. The peritoneal attachments along the left gutter of the abdomen suspend the left colon from the left side of the abdomen from the pelvic brim all the way up to the splenic flexure. The splenic flexure is a fold of the colon with its apex attached to the tip of the spleen by omental congenital adhesions.

The splenic flexure is usually covered by the omentum as it falls over the top of the transverse colon along the left gutter, and numerous embryologic attachments can occur between the antimesenteric surface of the proximal left colon and the omentum at the splenic flexure. The left colon descends along the left gutter to the level of the pelvic brim where the colon becomes free from the pelvic side wall and falls into a sigmoid-shaped structure known as the sigmoid colon. The sigmoid colon lies free in the pelvis, attached only posteriorly to its vascular attachments at the midline over the sacral promontory.

The inferior mesenteric artery (IMA) arises from the anterior surface of the aorta, proximal to the bifurcation at the common iliac vessels (Figure 9-2). The IMA branches to give the superior hemorrhoidal artery, which becomes the posterior mesorectal vessels, and the ascending left colic vessel, which sweeps up toward the splenic flexure. The IMV runs across the base of the mesentery of the left colon, crossing the superior hemorrhoidal and left colic vessels on its way to the duodenum. There is a clear peritoneal window between the aorta and the IMV, which can be used to enter the avascular plane behind the left colon mesentery and the retroperitoneum.

Pelvic Anatomy

The pelvic anatomy is complex and has interrelationships between the rectum, vagina, uterus, ovaries, bladder, and prostate. The anatomy is important for pelvic dissection because of the various structures that are at risk, such as the splanchnic nerves innervating the bladder, the ureters, and the organs themselves.

The common iliac artery and vein on each side of the sacral promontory course along the posterior aspect of the pelvic brim. The hypogastric plexus of parasympathetic and sympathetic nerves is found between the bifurcation of the aorta and common iliacs. This plexus coalesces to the right and left to become the splanchnic pelvic nerves, which run along the inner aspect of the pelvic side wall to the level of the obturator fossa and the anterolateral ligaments carrying the middle hemorrhoidal vessels. Nerve fibers course from the splanchnic nerve to the rectum through the anterolateral ligaments along the middle hemorrhoidal vessels. Extension of these nerves continues to either the vagina or the prostate as the nervi erigentes. A clear understanding of this nerve anatomy is crucial because it is easily damaged during dissection and results in both sexual dysfunction and urinary bladder dysfunction.

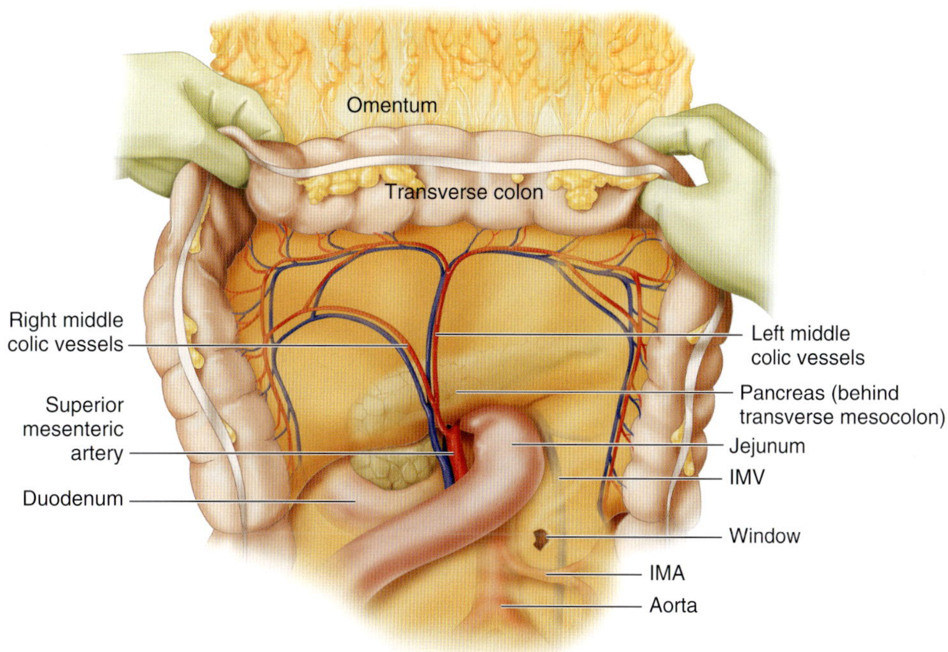
Omentum
Transverse colon
Right middle colic vessels
Superior mesenteric artery
Duodenum
Left middle colic vessels
Pancreas (behind transverse mesocolon)
Jejunum
IMV
Window
IMA
Aorta

Figure 9-2

At the level of the sacral promontory, an areolar tissue plane begins behind the superior hemorrhoidal artery (Figure 9-3*A* and *B*). The superior hemorrhoidal artery descends from the bifurcation of the IMA and splits at approximately S1-2 to give two major trunks down the posterior aspect of the rectum. The mesorectal "envelope" encases the fat, lymphatic, and vascular structures to the rectum. The areolar tissue plane outside the mesorectal envelope is known as the "holy plane" and guides the dissection in the pelvis. A cross-sectional diagram of the pelvis shows the visceral peritoneum encasing the mesorectum with the areolar tissue plane between the visceral peritoneum and the parietal peritoneum posteriorly (Figure 9-3*B*). The parietal peritoneum covers a nerve and venous plexus over the sacrum and the musculature of the side wall of the pelvis. Maintaining dissection within the areolar tissue plane between the parietal and the visceral peritoneal layers protects all of the crucial structures in the pelvis.

The rectum descends through the middle of the pelvis following the curve of the sacrum and at the level of the coccyx makes a right angle to exit through the pelvic floor via the anal canal. The levator ani muscles on either side of the pelvic floor form the support diaphragm of the pelvis and extend up onto the side wall of the pelvis to insert in the ischiospinous ligament attachments covering the nerves and vessels of the deep pelvic floor. The tip of the coccyx attaches to the pubococcygeal ligament, which supports the puborectalis muscle as a semicircular sling from the pubis around the back of the rectum. This muscle closes the top of the anal canal anterior to posterior.

The anterior pelvic structures, including the bladder, prostate, and vagina, are separated from the rectum by the rectoprostatic or rectovaginal septum. A visceral peritoneal layer known as Denonvilliers' fascia is the posterior boundary of the anterior structures. This fascia protects the seminal vesicles and prostate during dissection. The areolar tissue plane surrounding the fat mesorectum continues around the entire rectum to the anterior surface of the rectum below the cul-de-sac of the pelvis. The plane is found behind or posterior to Denonvilliers' fascia. The anterolateral ligaments of the rectum carry the middle hemorrhoidal vessels (terminal branches of the internal iliac artery and vein) into the mesorectal envelope through the visceral fascia from an anterolateral direction. Dissection and transection of these middle hemorrhoidal vessels reveals the anterior areolar tissue plane behind Denonvilliers' fascia, which can be followed all the way down to the anal canal.

The ureters, which have been described as running into the pelvic area over the pelvic brim crossing the common iliac artery and vein on either side of the pelvis, continue into the pelvis along the side wall of the pelvis toward the posterior aspect of the bladder. In the nonoperated, pristine pelvis, the ureters are higher up along the side wall of the pelvis aiming toward the posterior aspect of the trigone of the bladder. In females, the ureters run between the arterial blood supply of the uterus along the anterior lateral side wall of the pelvis. In males, ureters are not exposed during the distal pelvic dissection. The ureters may be drawn posteriorly after a previous operation but are normally fairly well protected anteriorly and laterally. In a previously operated pelvis, it is always wise to place ureteral stents at the beginning of the procedure to aid in identification of the aberrantly placed ureters.

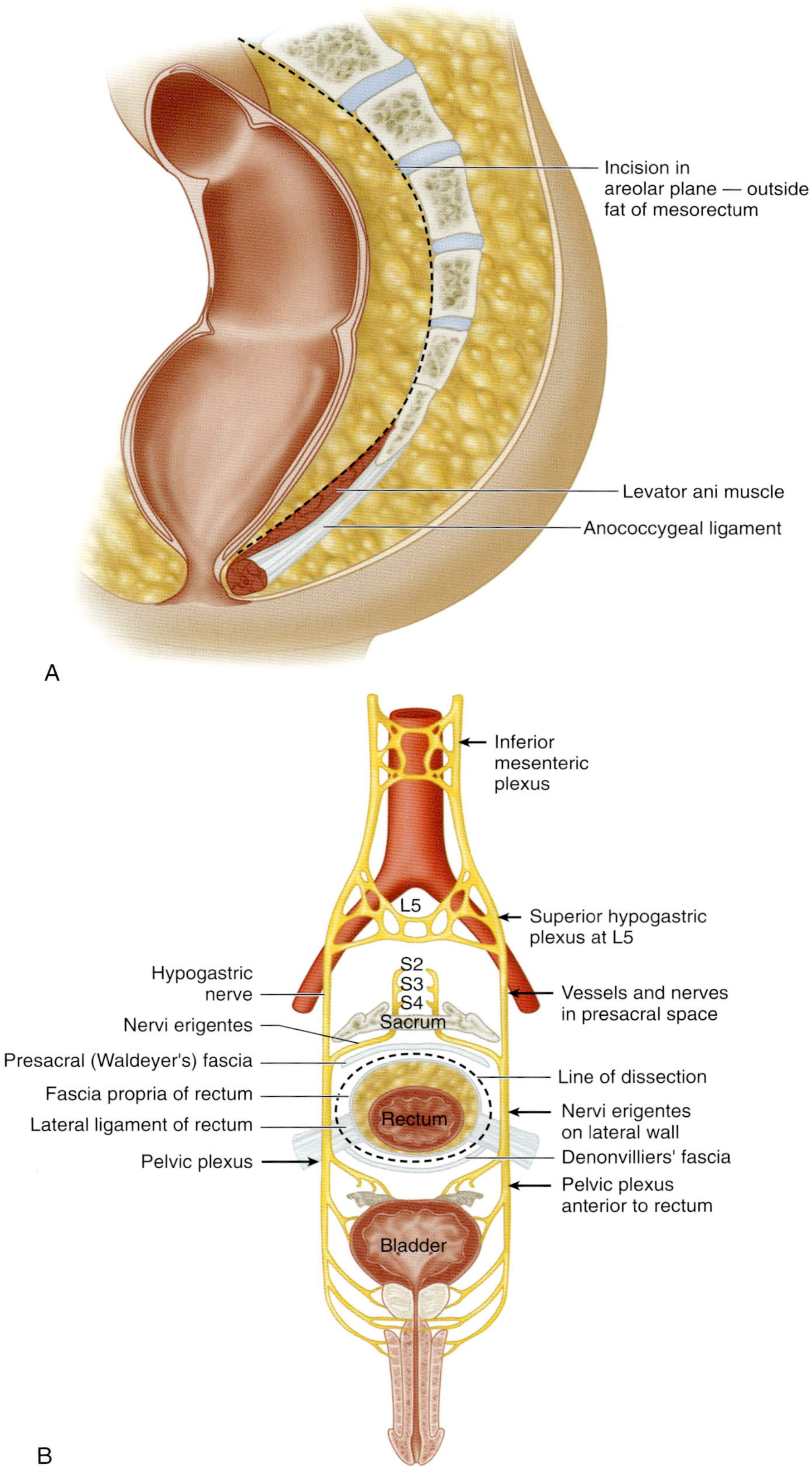
Incision in
areolar plane — outside
fat of mesorectum
Levator ani muscle
Anococcygeal ligament
A
Inferior
mesenteric
plexus
L5
Superior hypogastric
plexus at L5
Hypogastric
nerve
S2
S3
S4
Sacrum
Vessels and nerves
in presacral space
Nervi erigentes
Presacral (Waldeyer's) fascia
Line of dissection
Fascia propria of rectum
Rectum
Nervi erigentes
on lateral wall
Lateral ligament of rectum
Pelvic plexus
Denonvilliers' fascia
Pelvic plexus
anterior to rectum
Bladder
B

Figure 9-3A-B

Anal Anatomy

The upper anal canal begins at the puborectalis sling or the anorectal ring, which sits at the level of the pelvic floor and can be palpated through the anal canal as a bulge posteriorly (Figure 9-4). The longitudinal muscles of the rectum continue into the anus as the intersphincteric plane demarcating the line between autonomic internal sphincter and somatic external sphincter fibers all the way down to the level of the anal canal skin where the intersphincteric groove is palpable. Outside the circular fibers of the external sphincter that encircle the rectum, the ischiorectal fossa fat is found. The pudendal nerve and vessels traverse the ischiorectal fat from each ischial spine through Alcock's canal to the posterior lateral aspect of the anal canal. During the perineal portion of a procedure, the pudendal nerves and vessels must be controlled.

The rectovaginal and rectoprostatic septum descends all the way to the level of the perineum anteriorly. The transverse perinei muscle separates the anterior and posterior perineum. The terminal fibers of the longitudinal muscle of the rectum insert into the skin of the anal canal just outside the anal verge as the corrugator cutanei ani and cause the ridges that are noticed around the anal canal. The internal sphincter is the hypertrophied circular muscle of the wall of the rectum. The lowest portion of the internal sphincter can be palpated as a groove where the longitudinal fibers insert on the skin.

Within the anal canal, the dentate line is the junction between cuboidal epithelium of the anal transition zone, which is the terminal mucosal layer of the rectum, and the squamous epidermal cells of the anal canal skin. The anatomic anal canal extends from the dentate line to the hair-bearing skin of the inner buttocks. Gland openings (or crypts) are found in the dentate line at the base of the columns of Morgagni, which are interdigitating lines of squamous epithelium into the cuboidal and columnar epithelium of the distal rectum. The anal transition zone is the most highly innervated section of the rectum and anal canal and contains nerve fibers sensing temperature, vibration, electrical stimulation, pressure, liquid, solid, and gas. The dentate line lies approximately halfway along the "surgical anal canal." The surgical anal canal extends from the palpable anal verge all the way up to the anorectal ring palpated at the puborectalis sling posteriorly. The anoderm within the anal canal, cephalad to the anal verge, has no hair follicles.

Step 2: Preoperative Considerations

Total proctocolectomy and ileal pouch construction is recommended for patients with disease that is curable after complete extirpation of the colon and rectum, including patients with ulcerative colitis, familial polyposis, and multiple colon and rectal cancers. The ileal pouch reconstruction provides a restoration of continuity of the small bowel to the anal canal with fewer bowel movements than a straight ileoanal anastomosis. However, the 6 to 10 bowel movements a day that occur after ileal pouch reconstruction fall short of "normal" function for the average person. Patients with ulcerative colitis who are accustomed to 20 bowel movements a day because of inflammatory bowel disease find 6 to 10 bowel movements easily tolerable and an improvement in quality of life. Patients with familial polyposis who had one bowel movement a day or less may find this increased number of bowel movements to be a severe deterioration in quality of life. Emphasis must be placed on the actual function of the pouch after the operation to make patients fully aware of their expected bowel function and the effects on their quality of life.

In most circumstances, the total proctocolectomy and ileal pouch procedure is accompanied by a loop ileostomy for diversion to protect the pouch and the ileoanal anastomosis during the healing period. The ileostomy is a loop ileostomy and is best fashioned in the right lower quadrant with an underlying supporting rod if the patient is obese. The loop ileostomy need only be in place for 2 months to allow adequate healing. The patient must be educated and aware

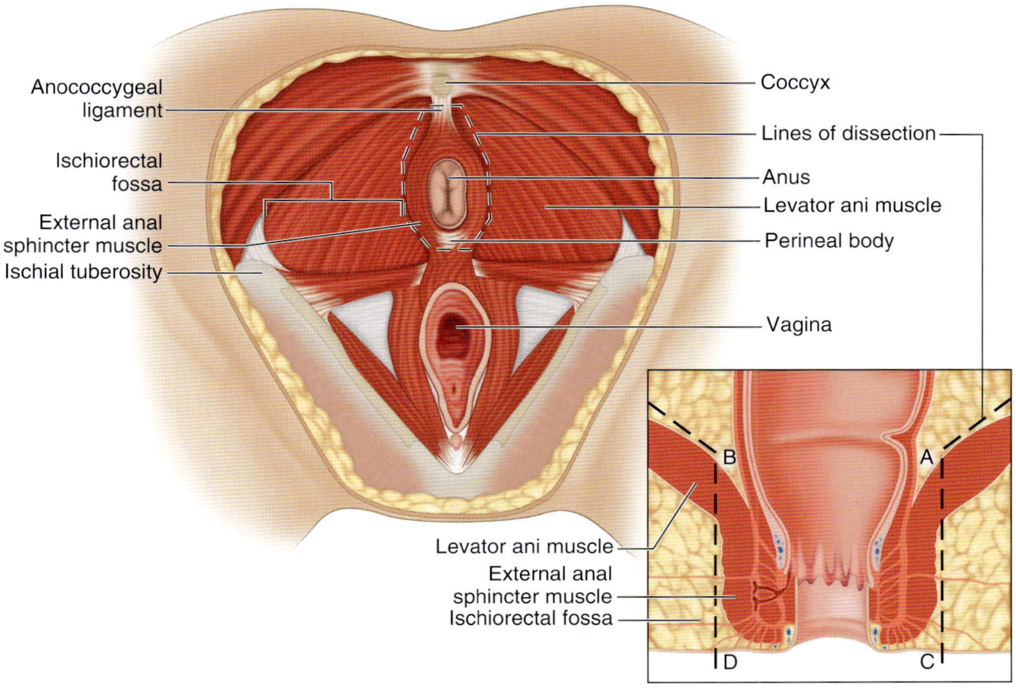
Anococcygeal ligament
Ischiorectal fossa
External anal sphincter muscle
Ischial tuberosity
Coccyx
Lines of dissection
Anus
Levator ani muscle
Perineal body
Vagina
B
A
Levator ani muscle
External anal sphincter muscle
Ischiorectal fossa
D
C

Figure 9-4

of potential complications of the ileostomy itself and the difficulties in managing the ileostomy.

When used as a diverting stoma and placed greater than 20 cm proximal to the terminal ileum, the ileostomy may have a high output. The selection of the portion of bowel should be as close to the J pouch inlet as possible to provide adequate absorption. The patient should be informed that antidiarrheals may be necessary to reduce the volume of output through the stoma to avoid dehydration and renal failure.

A patient with a loop ileostomy requires a second procedure to close the ileostomy. The patient should be informed that the recovery period is shorter for this second procedure. There is less pain, but it is still a significant operation and has inherent risks at the time of closure.

Diagnoses of ulcerative colitis, familial polyposis, and multiple cancers as indications for restorative proctocolectomy have been accepted by the surgical community. Long-standing Crohn's colitis with no evidence of anal disease or small bowel disease is a controversial indication. It has been suggested that a few of these patients with stable, isolated colitis are candidates for a total proctocolectomy and ileal pouch–anal anastomosis. The major indication for this operation in these patients would be the presence of high-grade dysplasia or cancer that would require removal of the entire "at-risk" colonic mucosa.

The most critical preoperative evaluation for patients being considered for ileal pouch–anal anastomosis is the status of the anal sphincter. In patients who have compromise of the sphincter mechanism, the ileal pouch–anal anastomosis would produce overwhelming, uncontrollable diarrhea. An intact, well-functioning sphincter that is capable of holding back liquid stool is an essential component of a successful ileal pouch–anal anastomosis procedure. Patients with suboptimal function should be strongly considered for a permanent end ileostomy as opposed to risking complete lack of control. Even patients with the strongest of sphincters report intermittent incontinence under special circumstances, such as heavy alcohol intake and the use of sedatives or sleeping aids. Nighttime incontinence remains a factor in quality-of-life determination for these patients.

Male and female patients risk compromise to their fertility after this operation. Women have more difficulty becoming pregnant because of trapping of the ovary in the pelvis and inadequate communication between fallopian tube and ovary given a moderate amount of adhesion formation in the pelvis. Laparoscopic techniques and the use of adhesion barriers may reduce this problem, but normal fecundity is not guaranteed.

Men are at risk for damage to the nerves controlling both ejaculation and erection based on the operative technique. Ejaculatory nerves are found at the base of the IMA around the anterior surface of the aorta. In patients with cancer, if the IMA must be removed at its origin for lymph node clearance, the risk of retrograde ejaculation is extremely high. In the deep pelvis, the nervi erigentes, which control erectile function, run behind the prostate and around the seminal vesicles. The lateral splanchnic pelvic nerves carry fibers controlling erectile function tissue; when these fibers are damaged, either by errant incision or by transmitted heat, complete or partial erectile dysfunction results. Nerve damage is resistant to pharmacologic agents that treat erectile dysfunction. Mechanical implants or injected substances that stimulate erection are the only alternative for these individuals. Fertility may also be decreased based on decreased production of semen. The risk of damage to fertility or sexual function in the setting of benign disease in a patient without inflammation is approximately 1%.

Bowel preparation is unnecessary for these patients, but most surgeons prefer to limit the amount of potential contamination during low dissection of the rectum. Reconstruction is easier in an empty low rectal cavity. The use of Fleet enemas to empty the rectum completely before the procedure is helpful. Irrigation of the rectum with antiseptic solution may reduce some of the contamination that occurs when transecting the rectum or when mucosal dissection is performed. Preoperative marking of the stoma site and preoperative education are essential for good outcome for a patient who is a new ostomate.

The type of anastomosis needed for ileoanal anastomosis depends on the disease state. A double-stapled circular anastomosis is appropriate in patients with no active neoplastic disease at the level of the dentate line; this includes patients with familial polyposis who do not have obvious polyps and patients with ulcerative colitis who have no high-grade dysplasia in the rectum or in the low rectum. A mucosal dissection with a hand-sewn ileoanal anastomosis between the ileal pouch at the level of the dentate line is appropriate in patients who have obvious close malignancy or a field of high-risk mucosa present in that area. In properly selected patients, the incidence of rectal cancer occurring during long-term follow-up after a double-stapled anastomosis 1 to 2 cm above the dentate line is the same as in patients undergoing mucosal dissection and hand-sewn ileoanal anastomosis at the dentate line.

Step 3: Operative Steps

- The patient is placed on the operating table in the lithotomy position. One of the arms is tucked to the patient's side so that the Mayo stand and scrub nurse can be over the head of the patient.
- A vertical midline incision is made from the epigastrium to the mid low pelvis, and a Bookwalter retractor is placed for exposure with the abdominal incision stretched widely.
- The right colon can be mobilized from a lateral, inferior, or posterior approach. Regardless of the approach, the cecum, ascending colon, and right colon mesentery are mobilized off the retroperitoneum, and the duodenum is reflected safely into the retroperitoneum. The right colon is lifted from the pelvis, and a hand is placed from the medial aspect of the abdomen under the peritoneal attachments of the terminal ileum and right colon at the level of the pelvic brim and the white line of Toldt, or the peritoneal attachments along the right gutter are stretched over the index finger (Figure 9-5). The peritoneal attachments are incised with electrocautery to expose the duodenum at the base of the mesentery of the right colon (Figure 9-6).
- The right colon is pulled toward the left leg, the space that has been generated over the top of the duodenum is developed bluntly up to the undersurface of the liver, and the suspensory peritoneal attachments along the base of the liver toward the gallbladder are incised with electrocautery (Figure 9-7).
- The attachments of the gastrocolic omentum are divided along the cephalad surface of the transverse colon outside the gastroepiploic arcade of the omentum between ties (Figure 9-8). The omentum is completely released, which allows the posterior aspect of the stomach and the entire lesser sac to be seen (Figure 9-9). The omentum is divided as far toward the splenic flexure as possible.

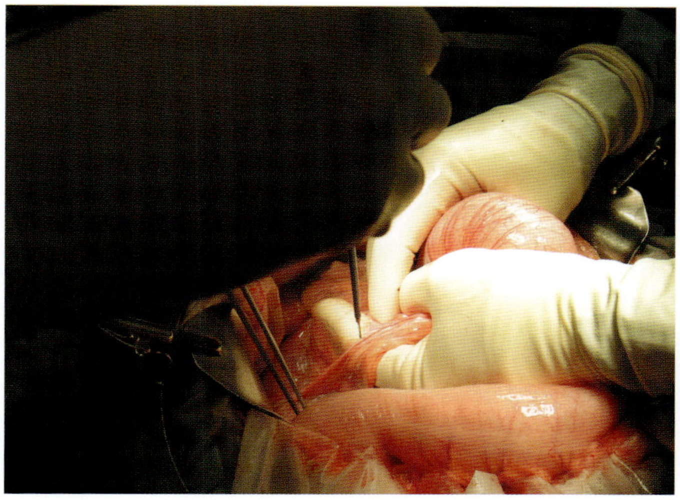

Figure 9-5

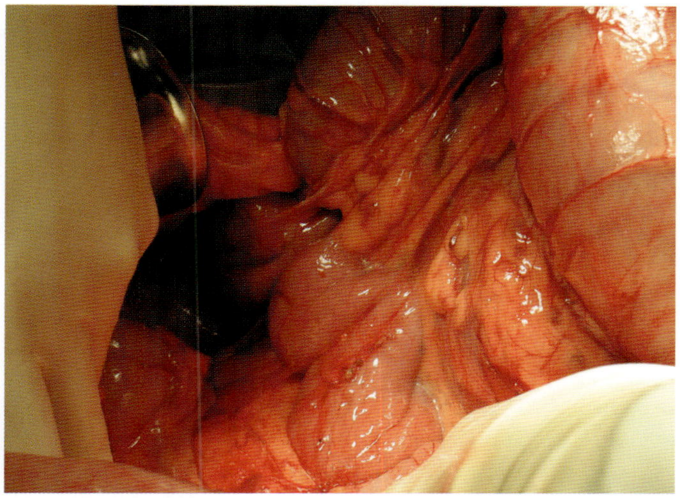

Figure 9-6

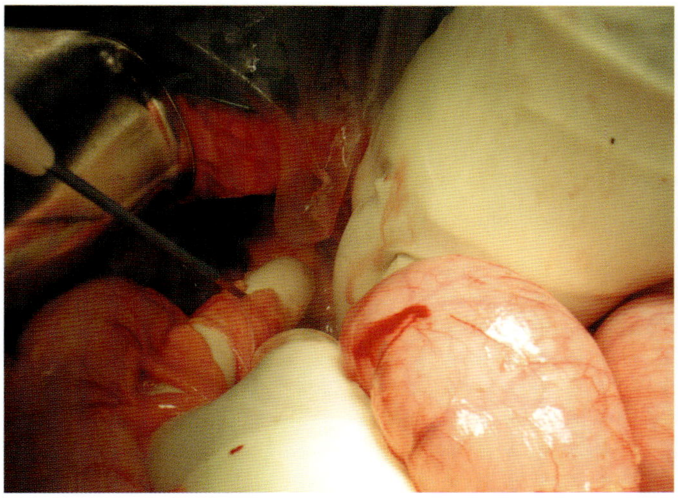

Figure 9-7

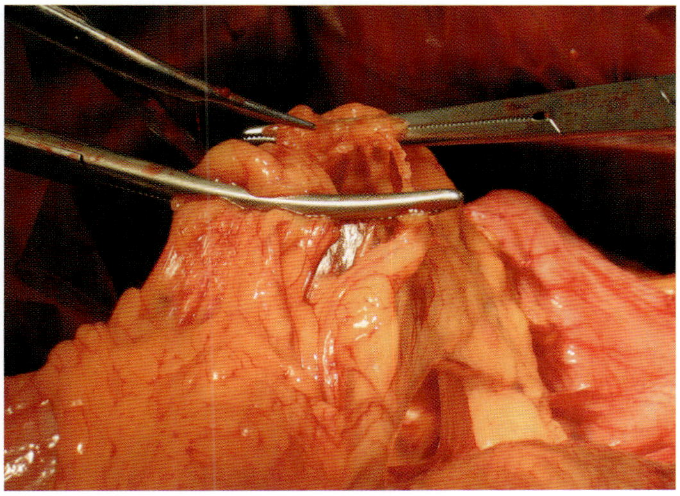

Figure 9-8

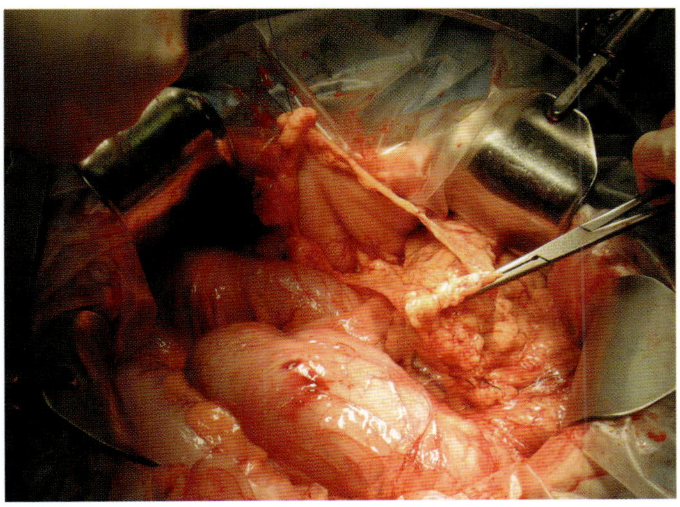

Figure 9-9

- The colon is returned to its anatomic position with the right colon along the right gutter and the hepatic flexure up in the right upper quadrant. The SMA is identified in its tract to the terminal ileum, and a window is seen in the base of the mesentery of the right colon proximal and distal to a large vascular trunk (Figure 9-10). This trunk is the ileocolic artery and vein arising from the SMA and vein. An incision is made at the base of this window to expose and divide the ileocolic vessels at their origin (Figure 9-11).
- The terminal ileal mesentery is divided up to the level of the bowel. The terminal ileum is divided with a linear cutter stapler (Figure 9-12).
- The transverse colon is pulled inferiorly. The surgeon's left hand is passed through the defect of the ileocolic vessels and encircles the middle colic vessels. These vessels form a "V" and can be easily identified and divided outside the pancreatic tissue to protect the anterior surface of the pancreas (Figure 9-13).

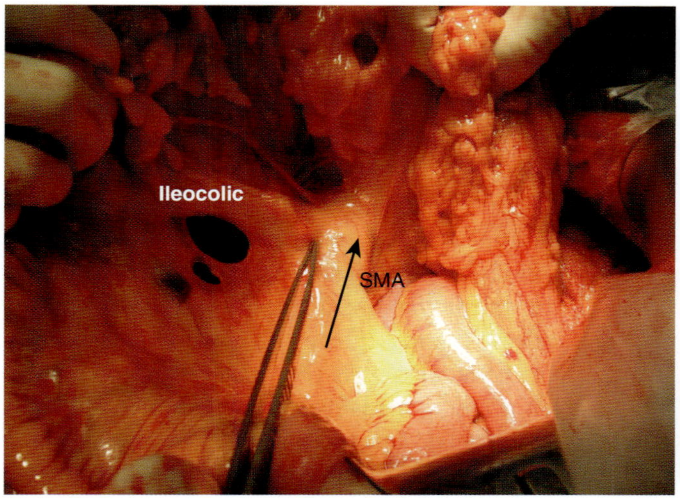

Figure 9-10

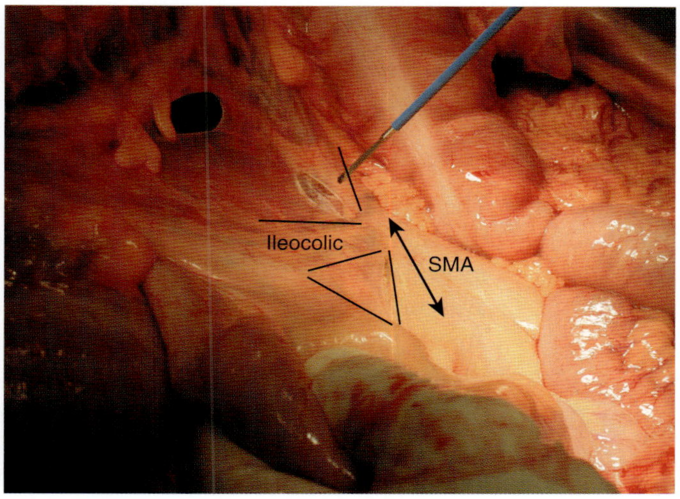

Figure 9-11

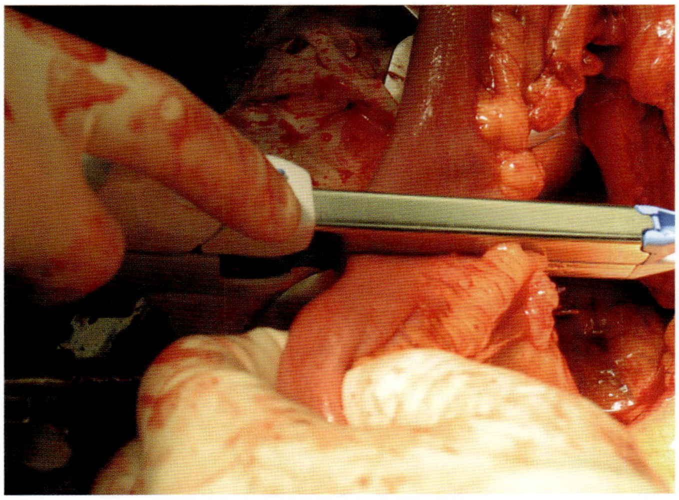
Figure 9-12

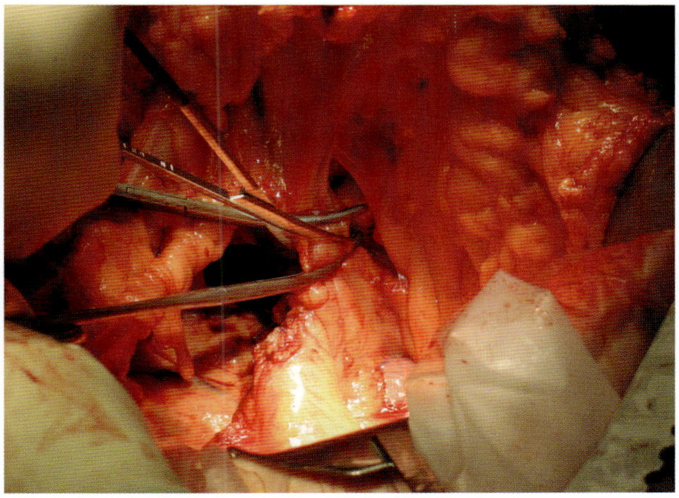
Figure 9-13

- The sigmoid colon and left colon are retracted to the midline to expose the left gutter and the lateral aspect of the left colon (Figure 9-14). The peritoneal surface of the left gutter is incised along the congenital fusion plane at the base of the left colon mesentery to enter an avascular plane from the pelvic brim all the way up to the splenic flexure (Figure 9-15). The areolar tissue plane is developed toward the midline to release the mesentery and colon from the retroperitoneal structures exposing the left ureter and gonadal vessels (Figure 9-16). As the left colon is pushed toward the midline bluntly, the left ureter, gonadal vessels and areolar tissue plane are dropped posteriorly all the way down to the pelvic brim at the sacral promontory and up to the splenic flexure and all the way to the midline at the aorta (Figure 9-17).

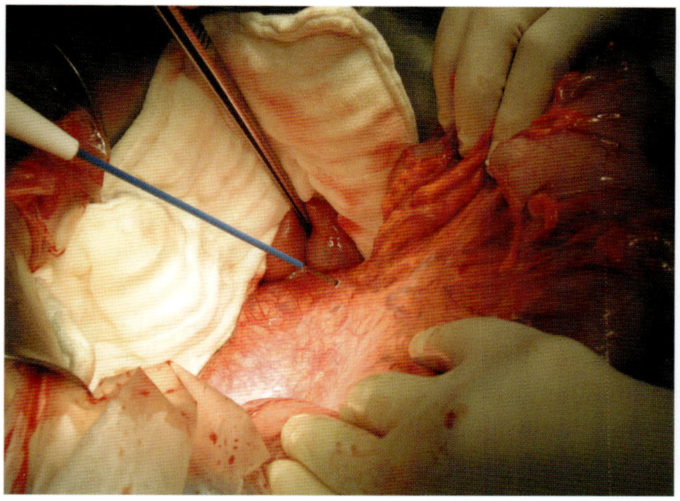
Figure 9-14

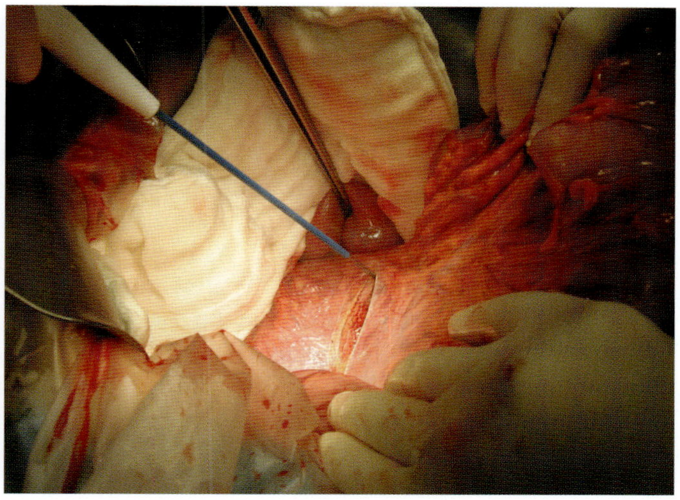
Figure 9-15

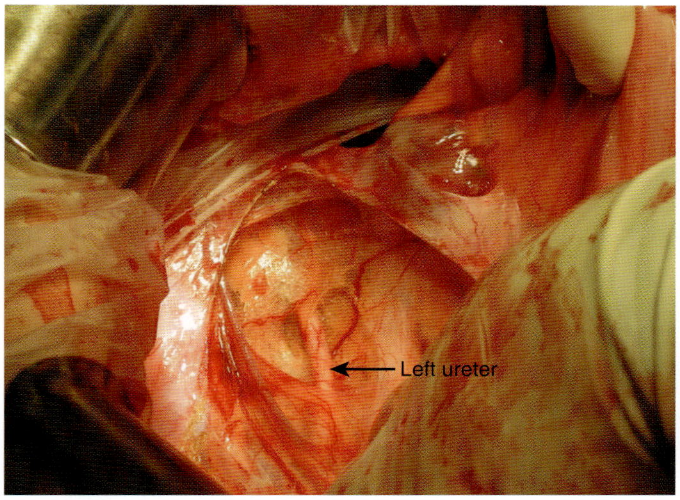

Figure 9-16

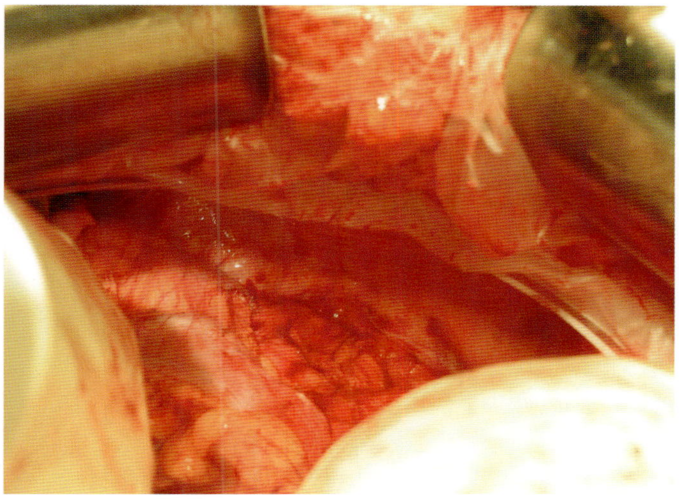
Figure 9-17

- The splenic flexure is released from the left upper quadrant by incising the lateral peritoneal attachments with a finger placed in the avascular tissue plane posteriorly and extended up toward the tip of the spleen. The peritoneum is incised over the finger using the finger as a guide (Figure 9-18). As the splenic flexure is released medially, the dissection turns toward the pancreas, and the attachments of the splenic flexure to the undersurface of the tail of the pancreas are incised with electrocautery over the finger as a guide using electrocautery (Figure 9-19). The splenic flexure attachments, which are occasionally very dense and attached to the spleen, are freed from the tip of the spleen and the vascular pedicle of the spleen to allow the splenic flexure to move toward the midline (Figure 9-20). The omental attachments along the anterior surface of the splenic flexure and transverse colon are incised with electrocautery to preserve the omentum and release the colon from the undersurface of the omentum toward the previously dissected right colon (Figure 9-21).

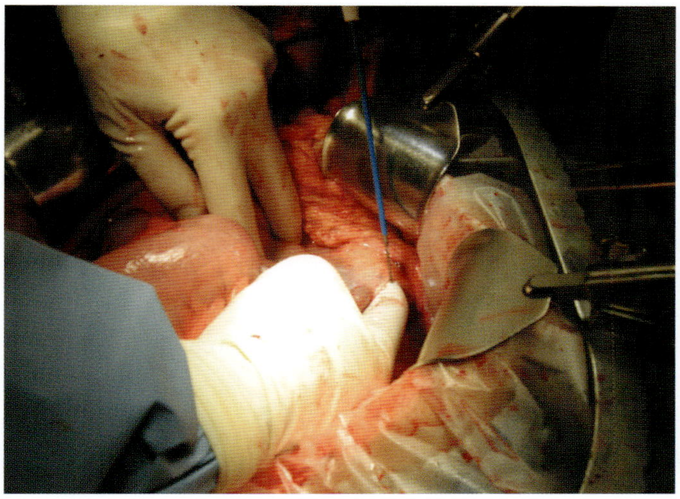
Figure 9-18

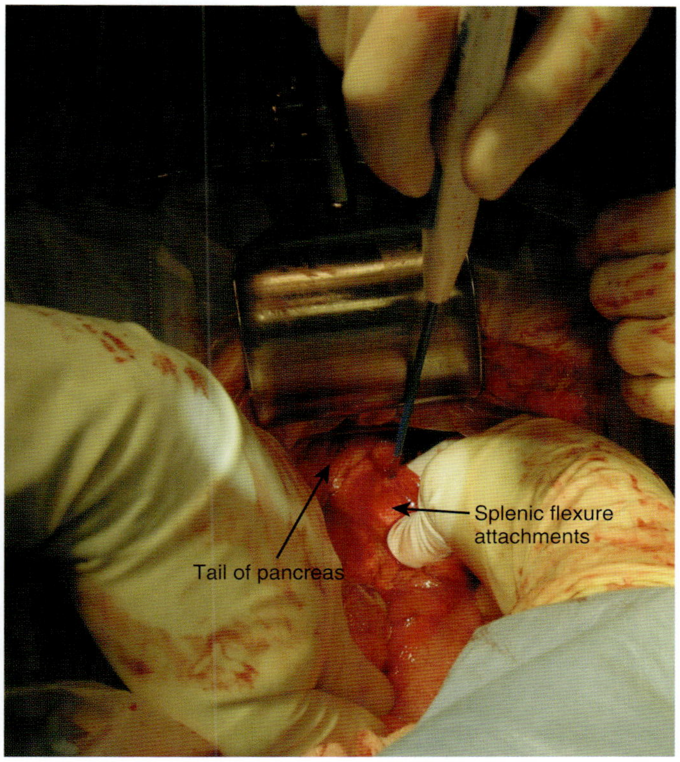

Figure 9-19

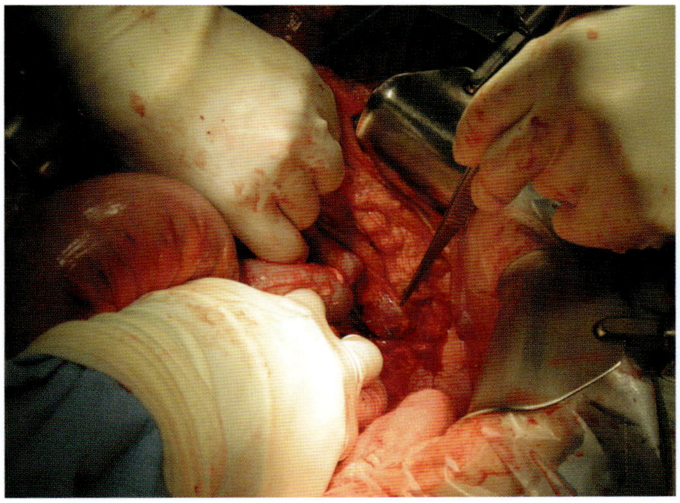
Figure 9-20

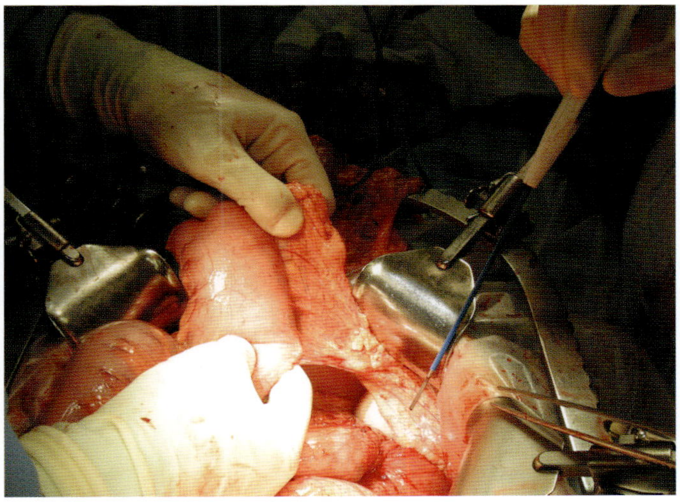
Figure 9-21

- The IMA pedicle or the left colic vessels can be divided at their origin or along the vessel pedicle at a point appropriate for the disease process as the left colon is now mobilized from the retroperitoneal structures (Figure 9-22). The IMV can be ligated at its origin adjacent to the third portion of the duodenum with the left colon retracted anteriorly and the small bowel and right colon retracted to the patient's right (Figure 9-23).
- The small bowel and proximal colon are packed in the upper abdomen, and the pelvic dissection is begun.
- The distal colon is retracted anteriorly, and a pelvic retractor is used to place tension on the mesorectum. The avascular plane of the presacral space is entered with sharp dissection (Figures 9-24 and 9-25). Care is taken to preserve the sympathetic nerves and not violate the mesorectal fascia (Figure 9-26). The posterior dissection is carried from 3 o'clock to

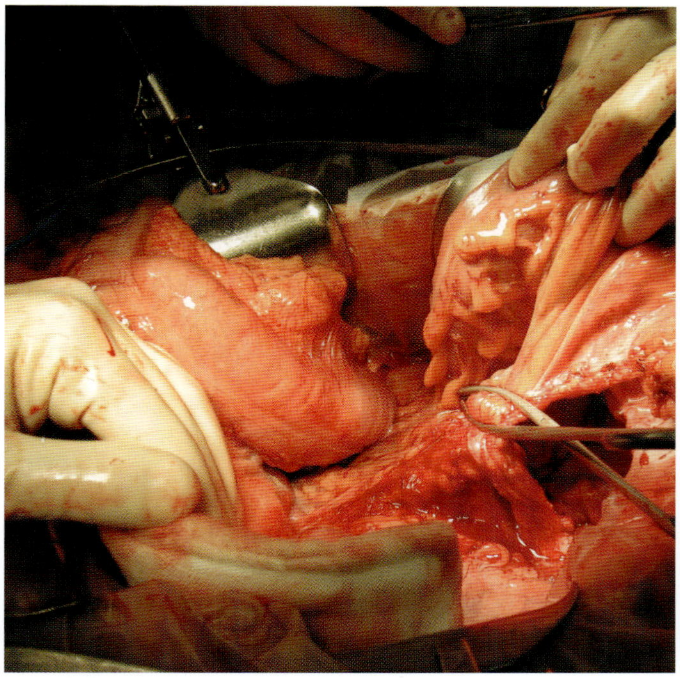

Figure 9-22

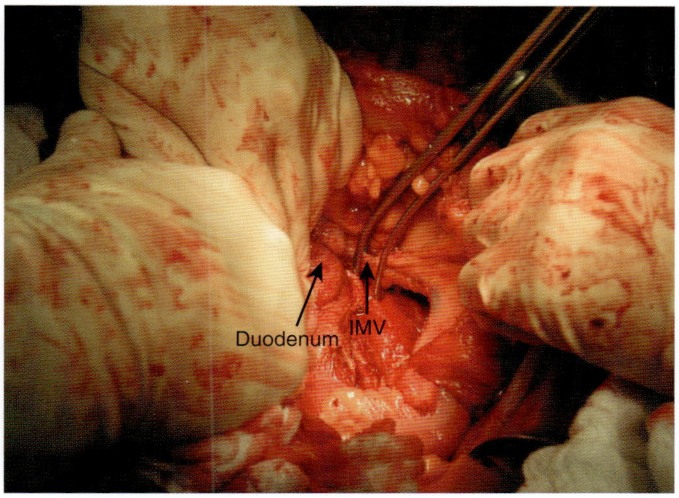

Figure 9-23

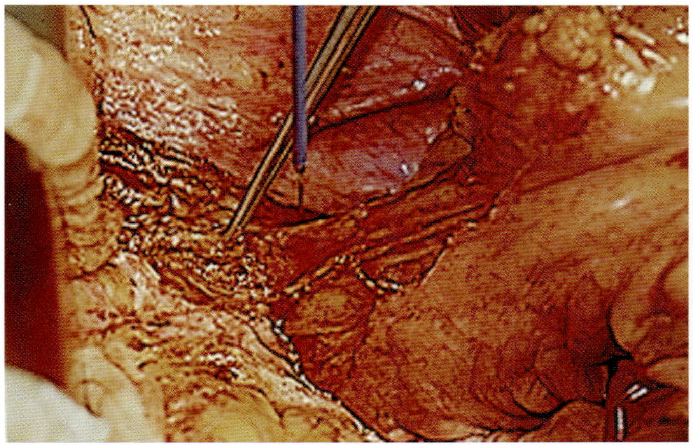

Figure 9-24

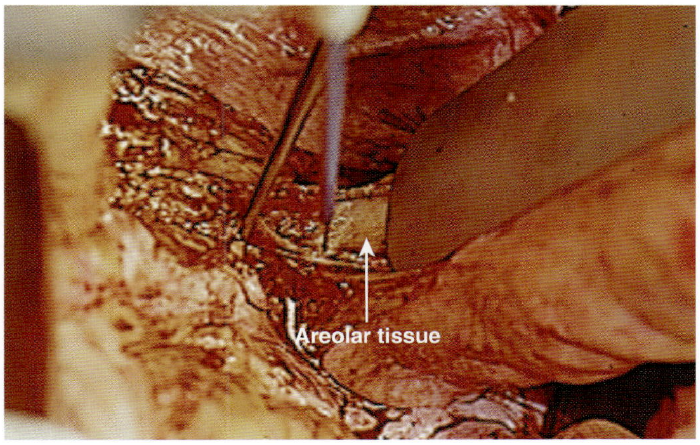

Figure 9-25

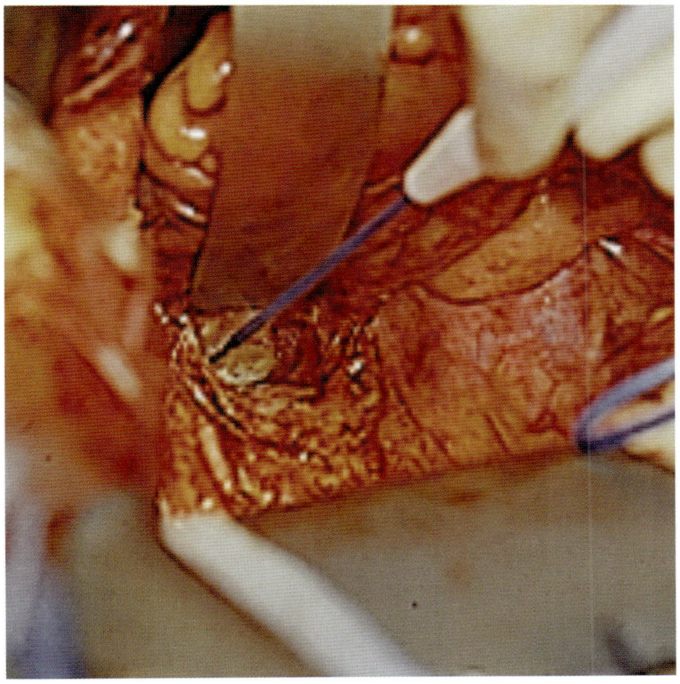

Figure 9-26

9 o'clock all the way down to the pelvic floor (Figures 9-27 and 9-28). A complete and intact mobilization of the mesorectum reveals its bilobed configuration (Figure 9-29).

- The lateral peritoneal attachments are incised down to the anterior peritoneal reflection. The lateral dissection is performed by retracting the rectum medially and sharply dividing the tissue in a posterior-to-anterior fashion (Figure 9-30). When adequate tension is created, the plane of the mesorectal fascia can be seen ensuring that it is completely excised. The

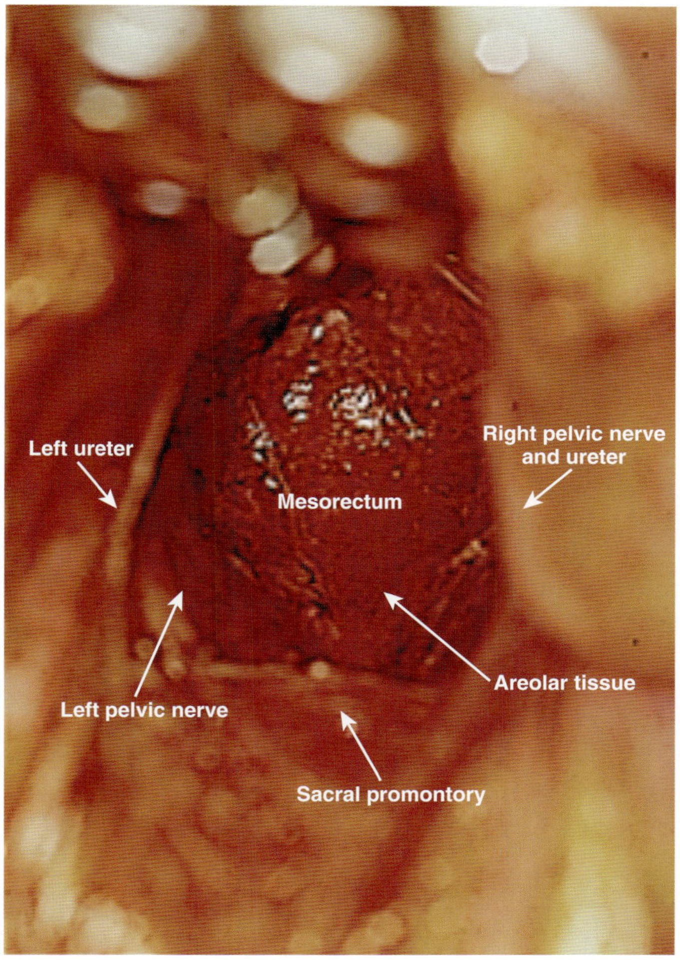

Figure 9-27

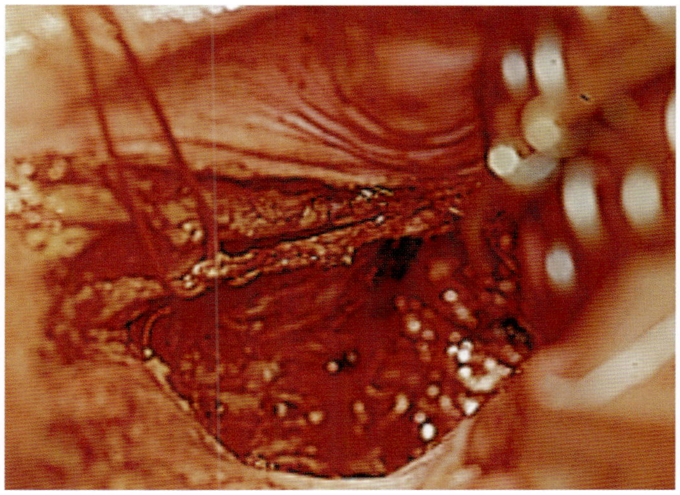

Figure 9-28

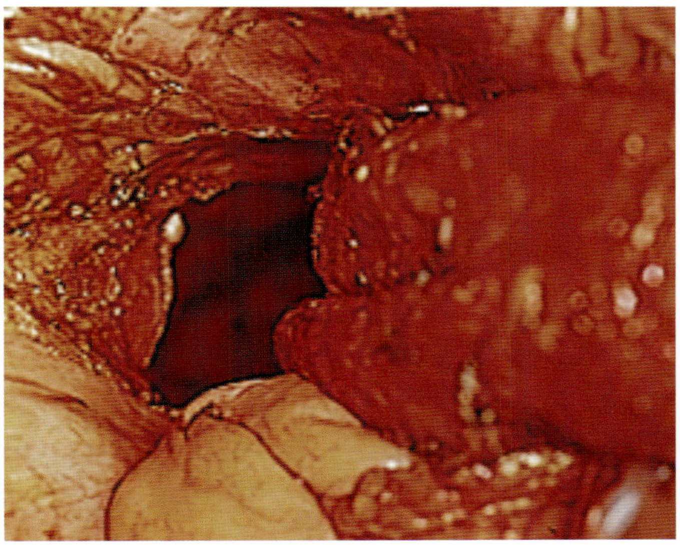

Figure 9-29

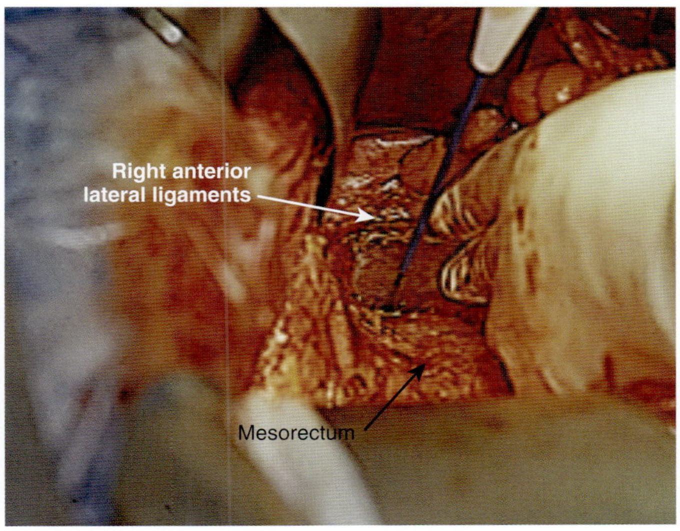

Figure 9-30

anterior peritoneum is incised, the prostate or cervix is retracted anteriorly, and the rectum is retracted posteriorly (Figure 9-31). The anterior dissection is carried down to the pelvic floor, and any remaining lateral attachments are divided.

- The rectum is divided with a linear stapler; the proximal rectum must be occluded to limit spillage as the specimen is removed (Figure 9-32).

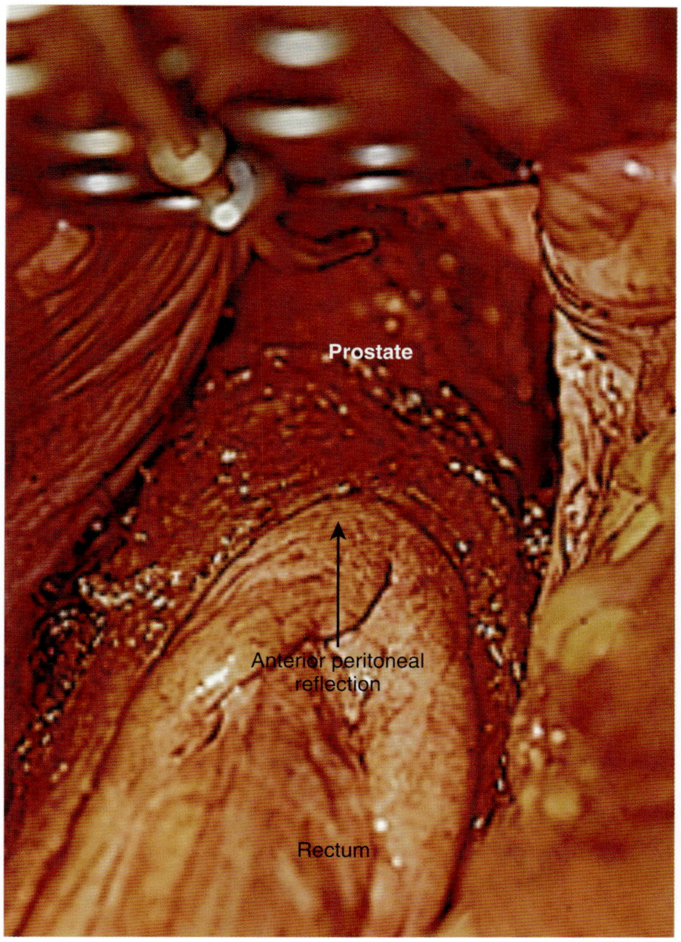

Figure 9-31

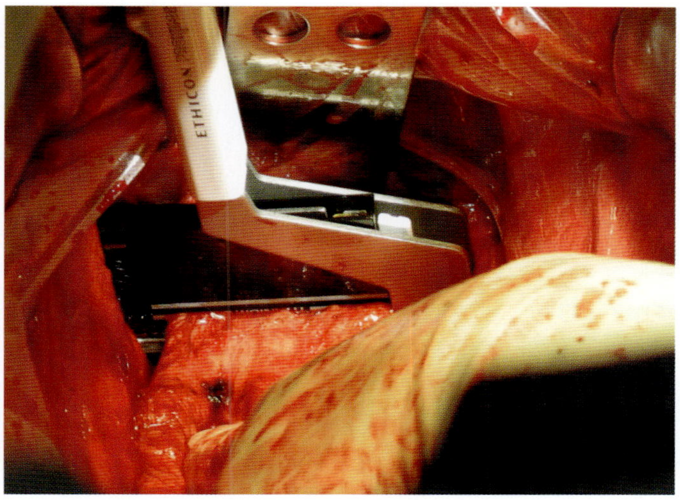

Figure 9-32

J Pouch Construction

- Construction of the 15-cm J pouch is accomplished by folding the terminal 30 cm of the small intestine on itself to create a 15-cm "J" (Figure 9-33*A-C*). The apex of the "J" is opened on the antimesenteric surface for a distance of 1.5 cm, and a 0 polypropylene (Prolene) purse-string suture is placed around the opening (Figure 9-34). The 10-cm linear cutter stapler is fired through the apical opening with the jaws down each limb of the "J" (Figure 9-35). Care must be taken to keep the jaws of the stapler as close to the antimesenteric border as possible to avoid damaging the blood supply to the lateral wall of the pouch. The stapler is fired twice through the apical purse-string to divide the septum completely between the two limbs of the "J" and create a 15-cm-long opening. The transverse staple line of the blind limb of the "J" is secured to the inlet of the pouch using interrupted absorbable suture to invert the transverse staple line and prevent it from twisting (Figure 9-36).

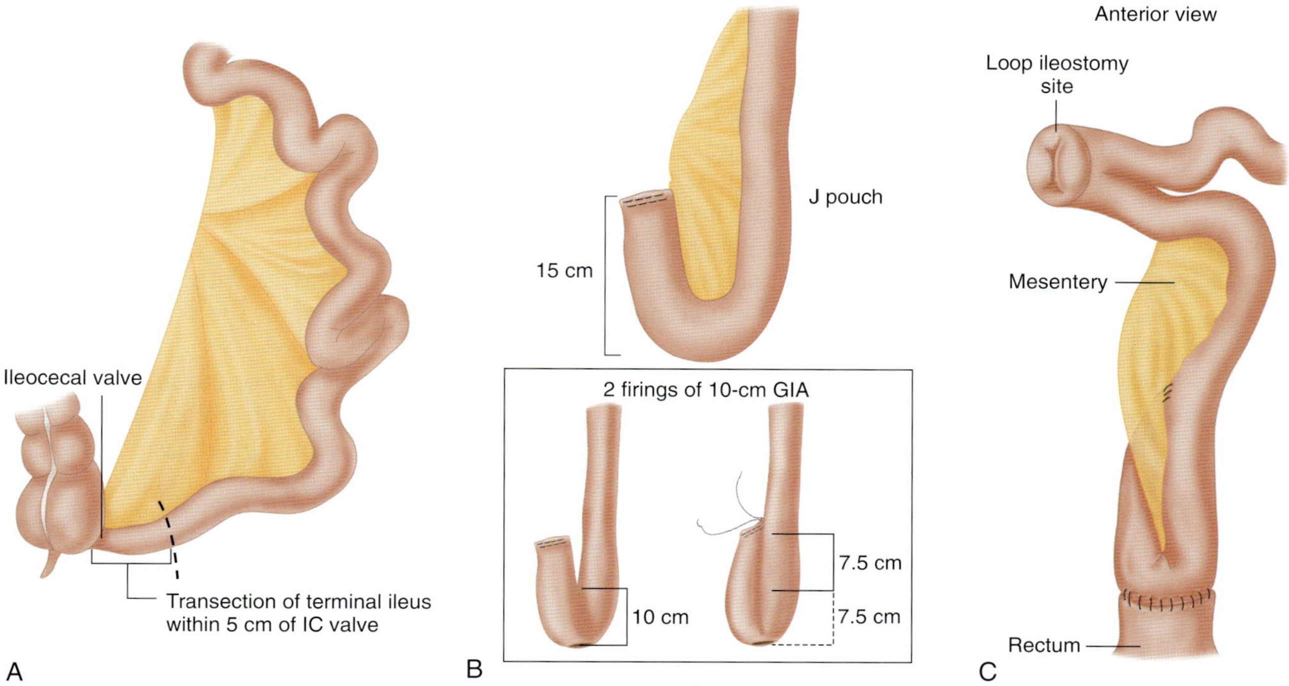

Figure 9-33A-C

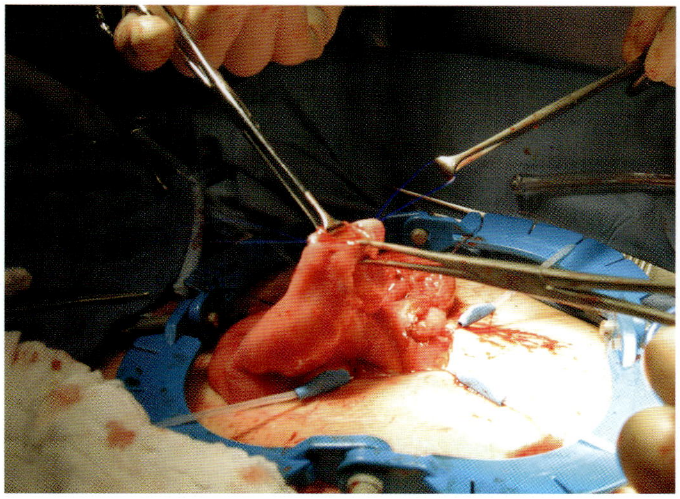

Figure 9-34

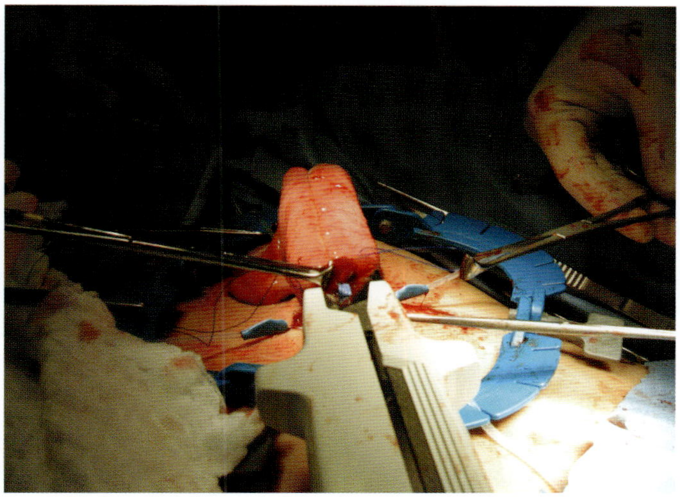

Figure 9-35

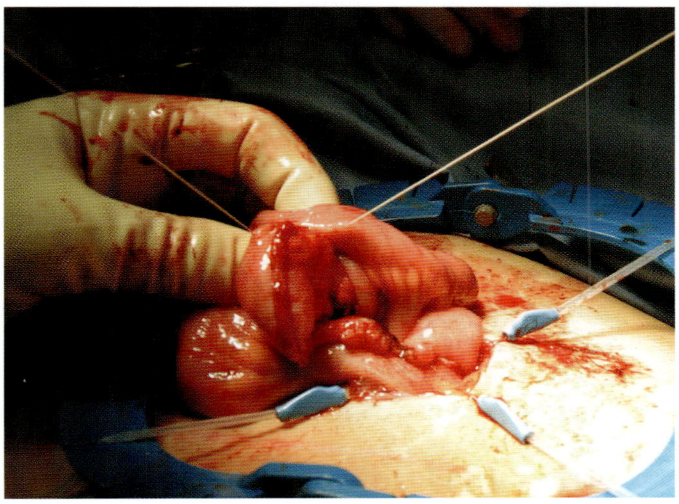

Figure 9-36

- The anvil of the 29-mm circular stapler is secured in the apical purse-string as the last component of constructing the J pouch (Figure 9-37). The J pouch is pulled down into the pelvis with the cut edge of the mesentery to the patient's right, the small bowel falling into the patient's left, the mesentery stretched across the anterior surface of the pelvis, and the posterior wall of the pouch falling into the curve of the sacrum (Figure 9-38). The staple head is reconnected to the post of the stapler, which has been inserted through the anal canal to the level of the transverse staple line. The stapler is closed and fired to create a circular end-to-end, double-stapled, ileal pouch–anal anastomosis.
- The cut edge of the mesentery is secured along the retroperitoneal surface with a running absorbable suture to close the potential internal hernia, prevent twisting of the pouch, and to fix the pouch in the pelvis so that it cannot retract (Figure 9-39).
- A large Blake drain is placed in the pelvis and brought out through a stab wound in the left lower quadrant, secured to the skin with 3-0 nylon, and hooked to suction bulb drainage. The drain is placed behind the pouch all the way down to the level of the anal anastomosis and left in place until drainage has decreased to less than 15 mL per shift. The right lower quadrant ileostomy site is constructed by excising a 3-cm disk of skin and subcutaneous fat in the right lower quadrant on the infraumbilical fat fold in a site previously marked by the enterostomal therapist. The loop ileostomy is brought through the anterior abdominal wall at a site 20 cm proximal to the inlet of the pouch. An adhesion barrier is placed throughout the abdominal cavity and over the loop of small bowel brought out at the ileostomy to prevent adhesion formation. The ileostomy is matured by incising 80% around the circumference of the small bowel at the level of the skin on the distal limb, which is usually inferiorly placed and maturing the mucocutaneous junction at the level of the skin (Figure 9-40). The proximal limb is everted to create a 2.5-cm spigot using three-point sutures of absorbable suture around the circumference of the bowel. A suspensory rod can be used if there is tension on the small bowel or the abdominal wall is thick owing to obesity.
- An ostomy appliance is applied. Care is taken to avoid contamination of the skin sites. The abdomen is closed with a running No. 1 absorbable suture; the subcutaneous tissue is irrigated with antibiotic solution and closed with skin staples; and dressing is applied.

Step 4: Postoperative Care

Patients undergoing open total proctocolectomy, ileal pouch–anal anastomosis, and diverting loop ileostomy require patient-controlled analgesia and deep vein thrombosis chemical and mechanical prophylaxis because of the high risk secondary to inflammatory bowel disease or neoplasia. The patient should be ambulated frequently and given incentive spirometry, and a bladder catheter should be left in place until the patient is fully ambulatory and it is deemed probable that pelvic edema and nerve dysfunction have resolved. A large Blake drain is usually present in the pelvis, and this should remain in place while the output is greater than 15 mL in a shift. The loop ileostomy must be managed with routine emptying at least four times a day. The faceplate adhesive surface must be changed every 4 days. Patient education and management of the ostomy is facilitated by input from an enterostomal therapy nurse.

As mentioned before, avoidance of dehydration and control of ostomy output are essential. Enteral feedings may start as soon as ostomy output is verified. A low-residue postileostomy diet is helpful to avoid a food bolus obstruction proximal to the ostomy. Most patients receive preoperative antibiotics at the time of operation, and the antibiotics are routinely continued for 24 hours postoperatively. The risk of *Clostridium difficile* is low, but this infection is devastating if present. The midline wound is at high risk for infection if there is spillage from the ostomy appliance or leakage beneath the ostomy faceplate onto the midline wound. Caution is important during ostomy changes to prevent contamination and exposure. The patient should be told that after surgery it is common to pass mucus and blood per anum, especially when the patient attempts to empty the bladder on a regular basis.

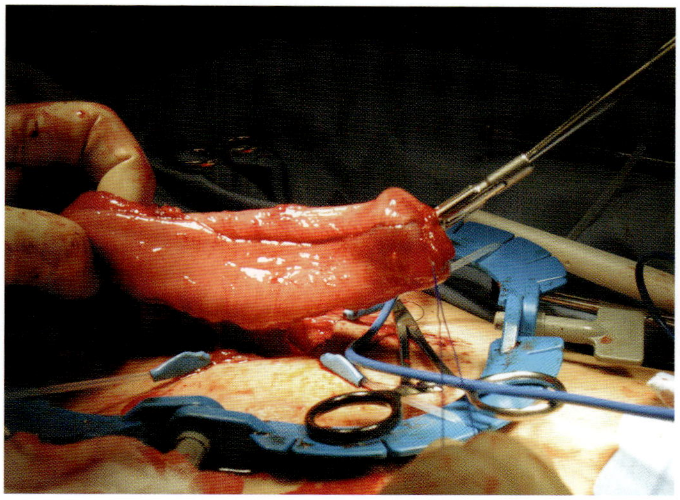

Figure 9-37

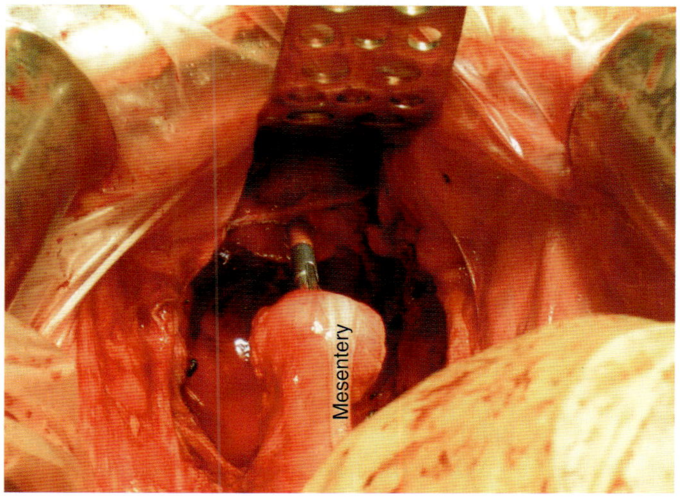

Figure 9-38

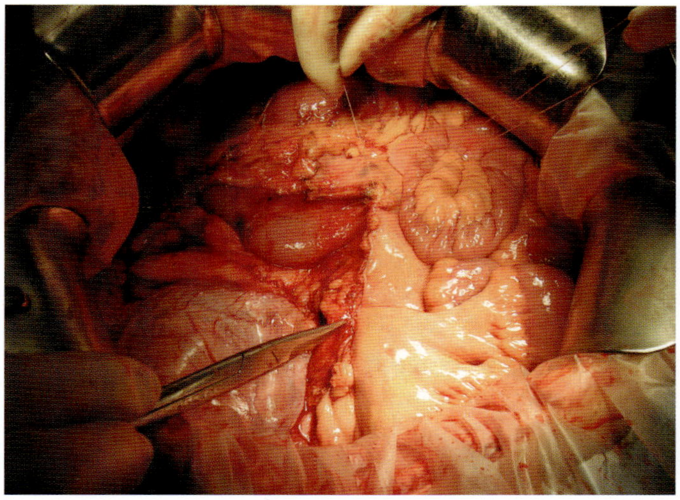

Figure 9-39

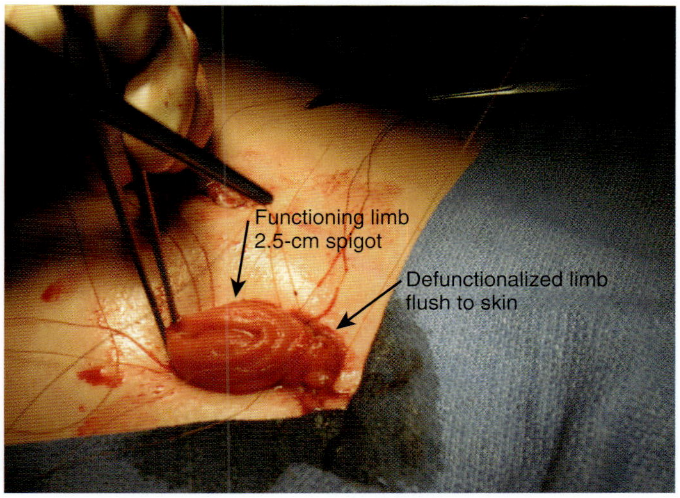

Figure 9-40

Step 5: Pearls and Pitfalls

The incidence of nerve damage and sexual dysfunction can be reduced by following the same areolar tissue planes that are used for accomplishing total mesorectal excision for cancer. However, in a patient with ulcerative colitis and extreme inflammation, this plane may be obliterated and may not be followed easily. In these cases, it may be important to dissect within the mesorectal envelope in the fat, dividing vessels sequentially and leaving a rim of fat in the pelvis that protects the nerves. The anterior lateral ligaments should be divided medially rather than against the lateral side wall of the pelvis to avoid injuring the nerves.

When the pelvis is inspected as the pouch is pulled into the pelvis, the small bowel should be placed to the patient's left, and the cut edge of the mesentery should be placed to the right. Construction of the pouch so that it lays in the curve of the sacrum and the mesentery suspended across the axis of the pelvis anteriorly may provide a better chance of the pouch reaching the pelvic floor without tension. Construction of the J pouch should be designed to allow the pouch always to fall into the pelvis and be suspended by the mesentery anteriorly. This design ultimately causes the inlet of the pouch to be to the patient's left and exit the left side of the pelvis and the blind limb of the "J" to be to the right of the mesentery in the right side of the pelvis.

When the pouch does not reach easily, several measures are possible to lengthen the mesentery. Cross-hatching or transverse incision along the SMA cutting the peritoneum over the fat and preserving the artery gives 1 to 2 cm in length. Care must be taken to free the SMA pedicle from the anterior surface of the duodenum. The ileocolic pedicle sometimes tethers the SMA. Dividing the ileocolic vessel closer to the SMA may provide 1 to 2 cm of length. The window of peritoneum in the terminal ileum mesentery along the terminal branch of the SMA can be opened to allow the distal ileum to reach further. This maneuver relieves some tethering from the apex of the J pouch.

The retention of the ileocolic vascular pedicle has been proposed to allow collateral blood supply to the pouch. A 5-cm horizontal incision crossing several middle-level arcade blood vessels, in the area of the 30 cm of terminal ileum that is used to construct the pouch, allows the mesentery of the terminal ileum to open as the apex of the J pouch advances 5 to 6 cm toward the anal canal. The decision to preserve the ileocolic vessel must be made early in the procedure. It is not routine for our practice to preserve the ileocolic vessel because it causes retraction on the pouch.

On rare occasions, there is a patient in whom the pouch does not reach the pelvis under any circumstance. The pouch can be suspended from the diverting ileostomy in the pelvis with the apex opening closed with either staples or a purse-string. Over time, the mesentery and the bowel may stretch to reach all the way to the pelvic floor; this has occurred only rarely in our 25-year practice.

The cut edge of the mesentery of the small bowel lies along the anterior surface of the aorta after stretching the pouch to the pelvis. It is simple to suture the cut edge of the mesentery to the retroperitoneum to close the peritoneal defect behind the small bowel mesentery to avoid herniation and torsion.

The blind limb of the pouch has been known to expand, twist, and perforate. It is helpful to secure the blind limb of the pouch at the level of the transverse staple line to the lateral side of the inlet of the pouch using a row of interrupted Lembert sutures. This action protects the staple line and protects the pouch from excessive motility at the level of the blind limb and can avoid a late problem.

The loop ileostomy is usually best placed 20 cm proximal to the inlet of the pouch so that there is enough slack on the distal limb of the loop ileostomy to give some freedom for dissection during the procedure to close the ileostomy. The loop ileostomy may require a rod to support the loop ileostomy at the level of the skin when the abdominal wall is thick. Occasionally, the loop ileostomy does not reach the anterior abdominal wall skin because of thickness of the wall. In this circumstance, it is possible to make a divided loop end ileostomy so that the distal limb can be left just inside the abdominal cavity stapled closed, and the proximal end reaches the anterior abdominal wall suspended over a rod and folds back to create the adequate spigot.

It is common for the ileoanal anastomosis to develop a weblike stricture at the anastomosis. At the time of planned ileostomy closure, it is important to perform a digital rectal examination to assess the anastomosis. If the anastomosis cannot be stretched adequately to perform a pouchoscopy with a rigid proctoscope, the patient should undergo examination under anesthesia and dilation of the anal canal. This procedure should be performed carefully with a soft catheter or large proctoscopy swab to dilate the anal canal to open the anastomosis fully. It is important to perform a pouch injection through the distal limb of the ileostomy to fill the pouch and observe evacuation of the contents to rule out staple line or anastomotic leak.

Selected Readings

Fazio VW, Ziv Y, Church JM, et al. Ileal pouch-anal anastomoses complications and function in 1005 patients. Ann Surg 1995;222:120–7.

Fleming FJ, Francone TD, Kim MJ, et al. A laparoscopic approach does reduce short-term complications in patients undergoing ileal pouch-anal anastomosis. Dis Colon Rectum 2011;54:176–82.

Heikens JT, de Vries J, van Laarhoven CJ. Quality of life, health related quality of life and health status in patients having restorative proctocolectomy with ileal pouch-anal anastomosis for ulcerative colitis: a systematic review. Colorectal Dis 2010 Dec 22. doi: 10.1111/j.1463-318.2010.02538.x.

CHAPTER 10

Open Low Anterior Resection of Rectum

Anne Y. Lin

Step 1: Clinical Anatomy

The left colon lies along the left side of the abdomen suspended from the splenic flexure to the pelvic brim by lateral peritoneal attachments. The mesentery of the left colon arises from the midline of the abdomen along the aorta. The sigmoid colon has no lateral peritoneal attachments other than some congenital adhesions that fix the apex of the sigmoid colon to the pelvic brim and the iliac fossa. Otherwise, the sigmoid colon is attached to the retroperitoneum through a midline mesentery arising from the inferior mesenteric artery (IMA) and extending down into the pelvis to the mesorectum. The splenic flexure is attached to the undersurface of the tip of the spleen, the lower edge of the tail of the pancreas, and the anterior surface of the left kidney by various levels of suspensory ligaments and peritoneal extensions. The blood supply to the left colon is based on the IMA, which arises from the anterior surface of the aorta just above the bifurcation of the common iliac arteries. The IMA extends anteriorly and bifurcates to produce the superior rectal artery feeding the sigmoid colon and the rectum. The left colic artery extends cephalad to provide the left colon and distal splenic flexure with blood supply through the arcade at the mesenteric edge known as the marginal artery of Drummond. The retroperitoneum behind the left colon contains the left ureter and the gonadal vessels lying over the psoas muscle. The ureter crosses the iliac vessels at the bifurcation of the iliac vessels into the external and internal iliac branches (Figure 10-1).

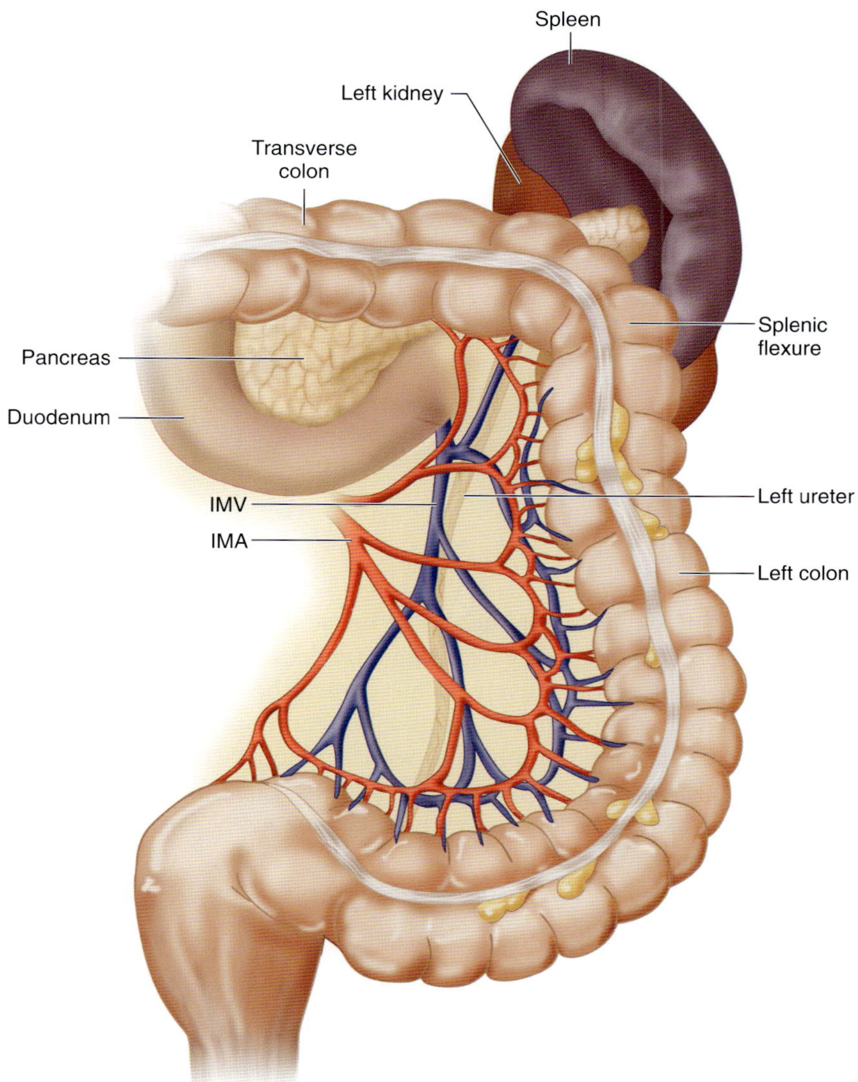
Spleen
Left kidney
Transverse colon
Pancreas
Duodenum
Splenic flexure
IMV
IMA
Left ureter
Left colon

Figure 10-1

The rectum and mesorectum fit within the pelvis as a cylinder within a cylinder (Figure 10-2*A*). They are contained within a fascial envelope that is separated from the surrounding pelvic structures by areolar tissue. Posteriorly, the sympathetic nerves branch just above the sacral promontory and travel laterally. The internal iliac vessels follow the course of the hypogastric nerves but are deep to them as they travel into the pelvis. The ureters enter the pelvis laterally and enter the bladder anterior to the rectum. In males, the seminal vesicles and prostate gland lie below the anterior peritoneal reflection. Denonvilliers' fascia separates the prostate from the anterior surface of the rectum. In females, the cervix and rectovaginal septum lie below the anterior peritoneal reflection. The parasympathetic nerves arise from S2-4 and travel anteriorly to enter the urogenital structures at roughly 2 o'clock and 10 o'clock. The lateral stalks or vasculature to the rectum can be found laterally deep in the pelvis. The mesorectum tapers out as the rectum reaches the levator muscles at the pelvic floor just below the tip of the coccyx (Figure 10-2*B*).

Step 2: Preoperative Considerations

Depending on the level of the tumor, the use of neoadjuvant chemoradiation, or the level of the colorectal anastomosis, a temporary diverting loop ileostomy should be considered, and the patient should be marked preoperatively. A mechanical bowel preparation is recommended because it eliminates formed stool in the distal colon and improves handling and anastomosis formation. Preoperative antibiotic prophylaxis with antibiotics continued for 24 hours postoperatively is preferred. Deep vein thrombosis prophylaxis with sequential compression devices is required and should be supplemented with subcutaneous heparin in patients with cancer. Preoperative tattooing of a neoplastic lesion is very helpful to identify a small lesion intraoperatively.

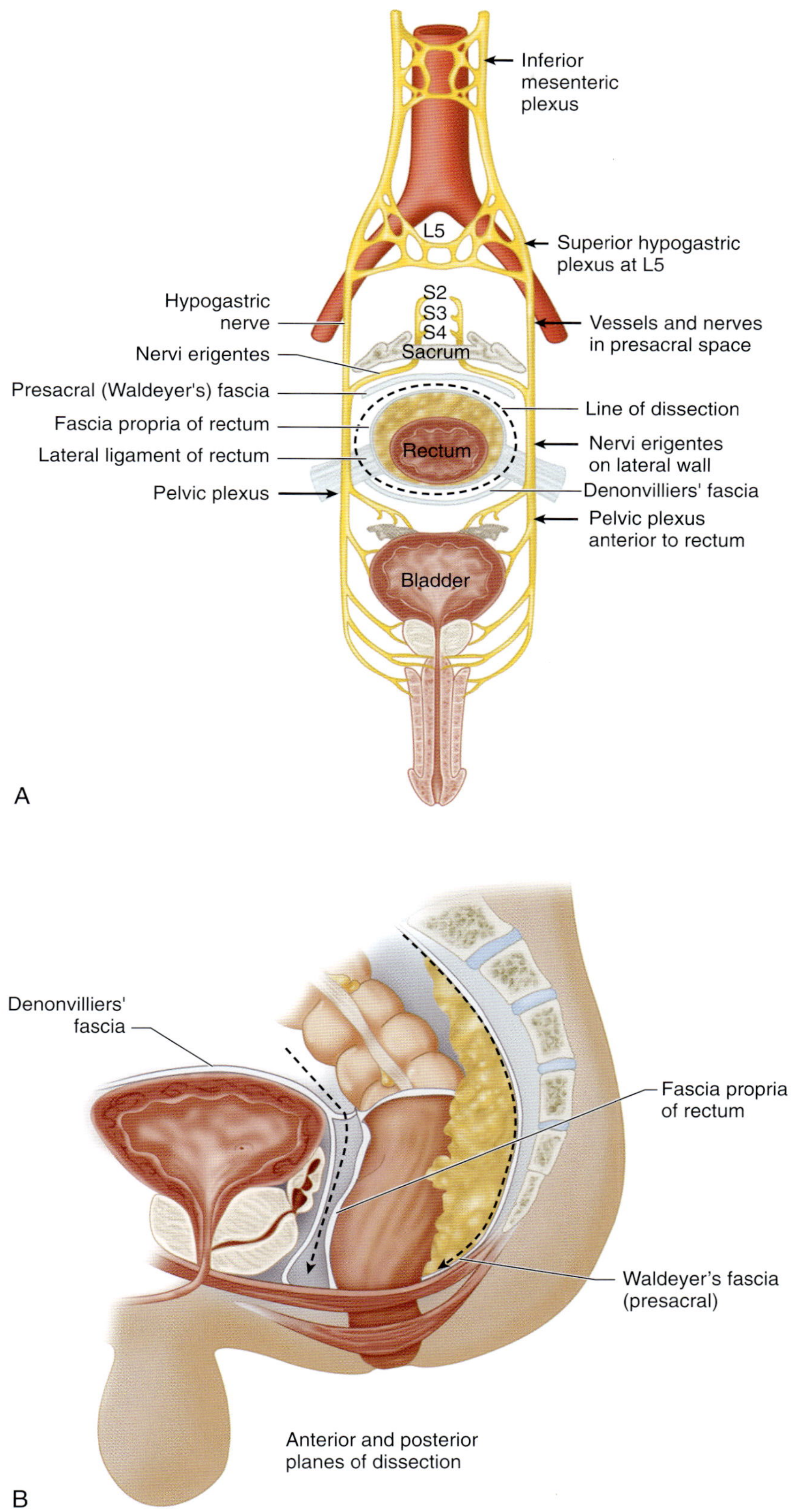

Figure 10-2A-B

Step 3: Operative Steps

- The patient is placed in lithotomy position using Allen's stirrups with sequential compression devices and a bladder catheter in place. The rectum is irrigated with povidone-iodine (Betadine) to clear the rectum of any solid stool and dislodge any free cancer cells. The arms are placed with the left arm extended and the right arm tucked to allow an overhead Mayo stand placed for draping. The abdomen is entered through a vertical midline incision from xiphoid to pubis, and a Bookwalter retractor is placed for exposure and opened widely. The small bowel is retracted to the right upper quadrant and upper midline.
- An incision is made at the base of the lateral aspect of the left colon mesentery along the white line of Toldt with the left colon retracted medially and anteriorly (Figure 10-3). The incision is extended from the pelvis to the left upper quadrant. The exposed areolar tissue plane allows dissection anterior to the retroperitoneum (Figure 10-4). Blunt dissection frees the left colon from the retroperitoneum and exposes the ureter and gonadal vessels within the retroperitoneum (Figure 10-5). The blunt dissection is carried medially to the base of the aorta and cephalad to the splenic flexure level, freeing the left colon from the anterior surface of the kidney (Figure 10-6).

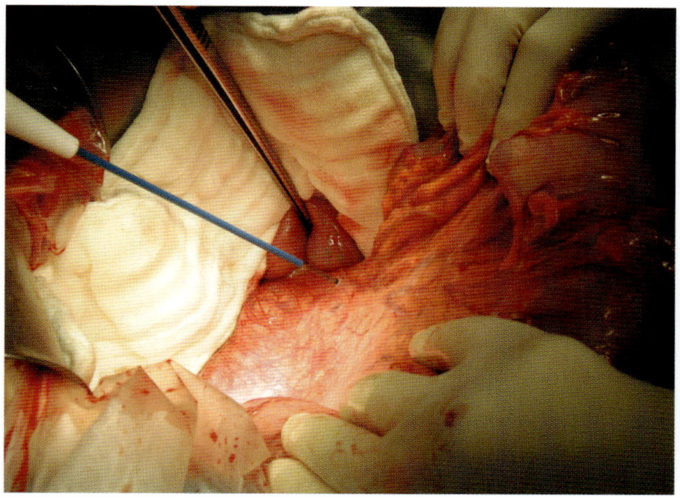

Figure 10-3

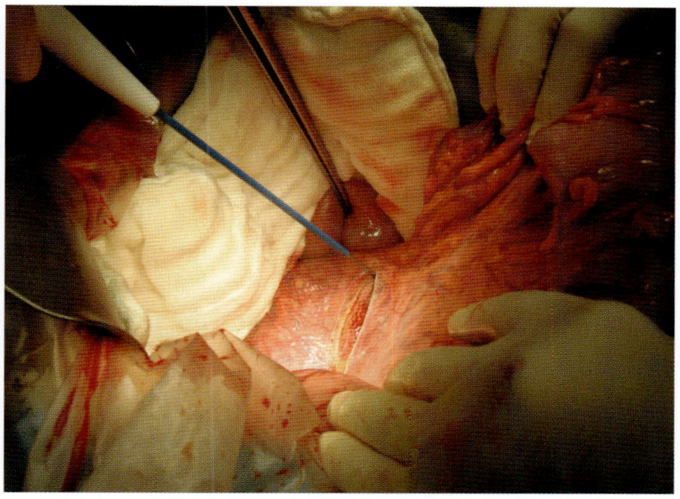

Figure 10-4

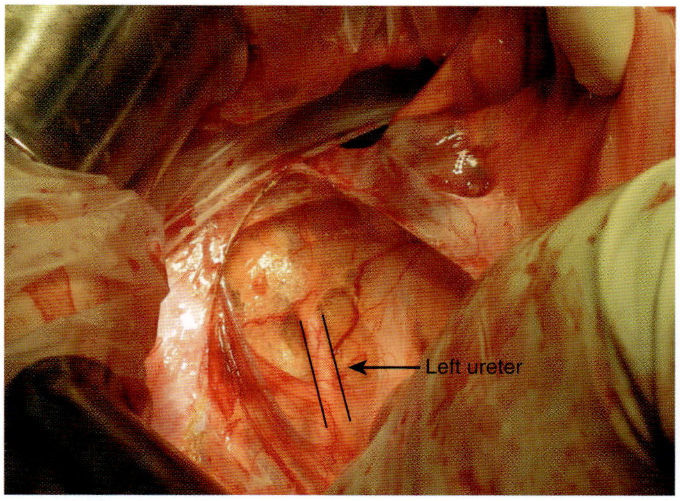

Figure 10-5

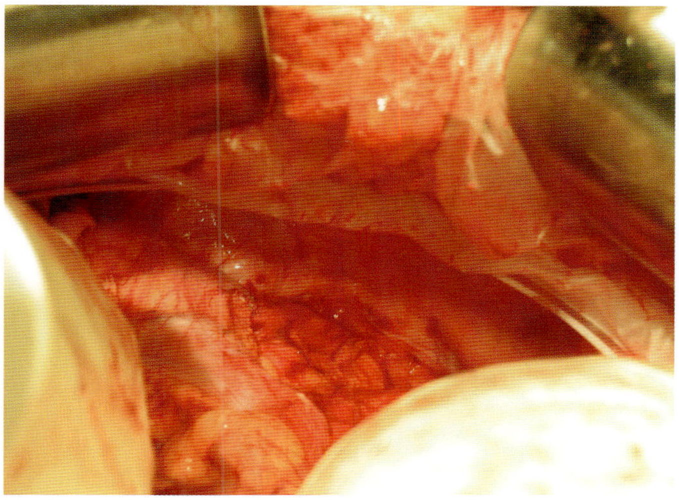

Figure 10-6

- An incision is made on the peritoneal attachments of the splenic flexure using the finger as a guide, incising lateral to medial to release the splenic flexure from the undersurface of the tip of the spleen, the lateral aspect of the abdominal cavity, and the anterior surface of the kidney (Figure 10-7). The tip of the spleen is freed from the splenic flexure, releasing the multiple congenital adhesions and incising the omental attachment to release the splenic flexure toward the midline (Figure 10-8). The attachments of the splenic flexure to the undersurface of the tail of the pancreas and the retroperitoneum are incised all the way to the midline toward the duodenum at the ligament of Treitz (Figures 10-9 and 10-10*A* and *B*).

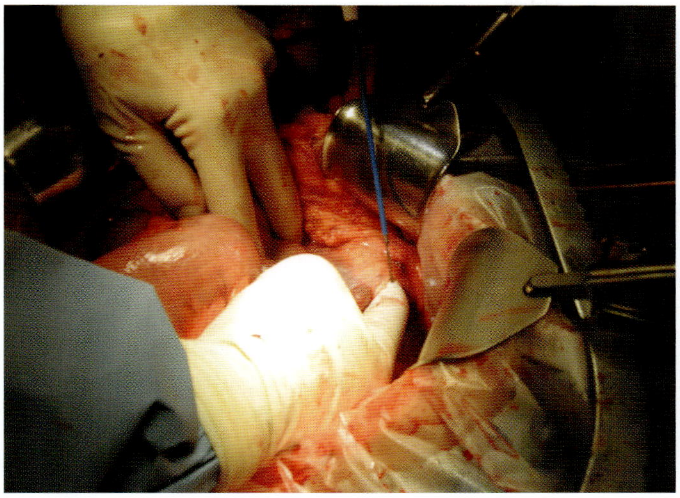

Figure 10-7

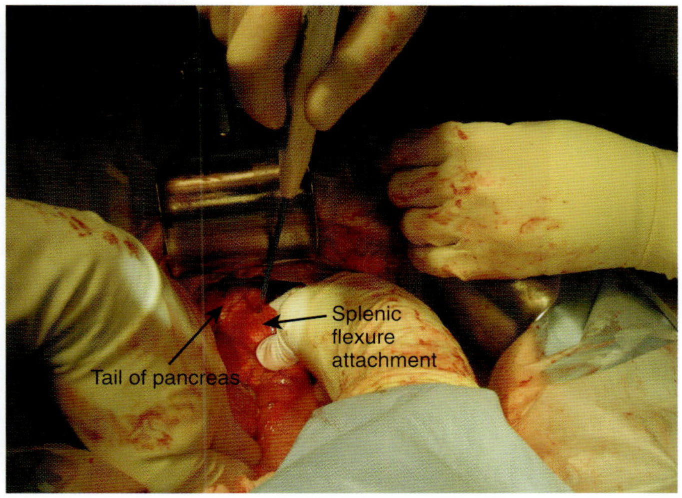

Figure 10-8

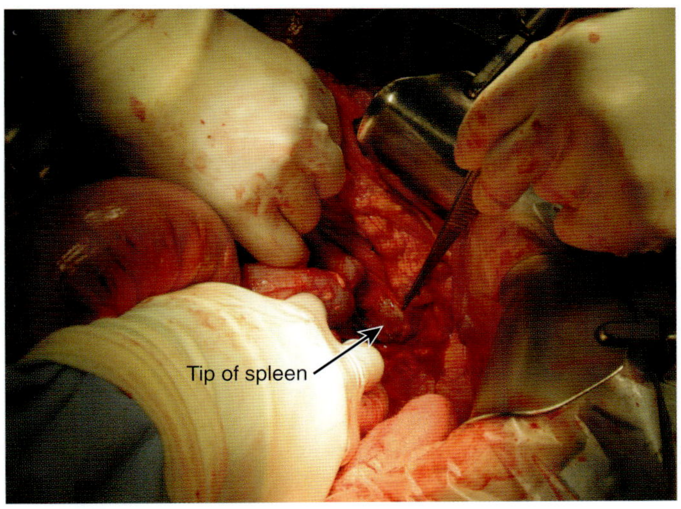

Figure 10-9

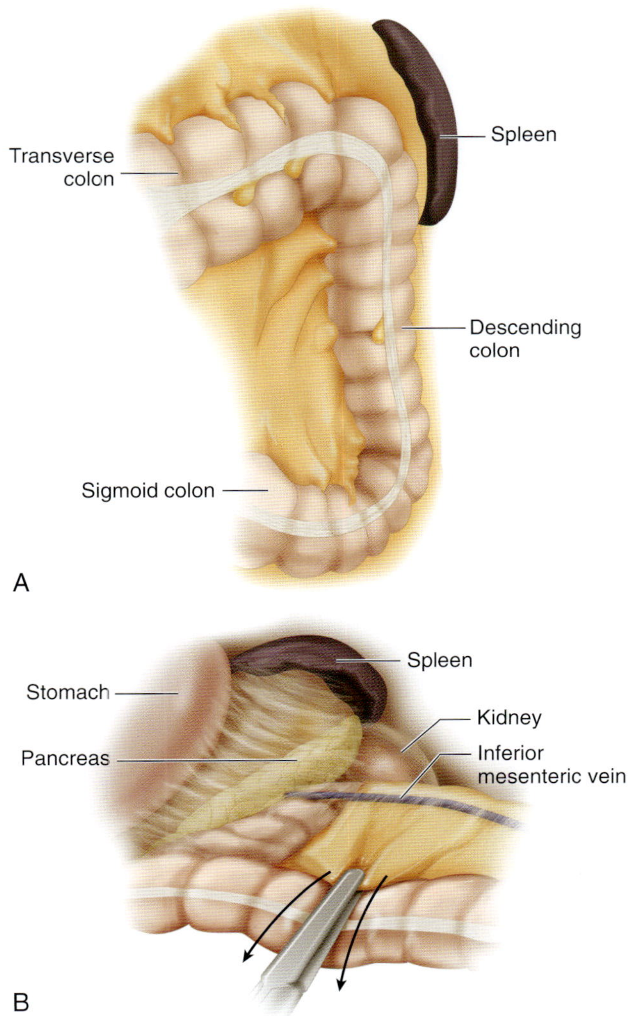

Figure 10-10A-B

- The omental attachments to the anterior surface of the transverse colon are incised releasing the splenic flexure from the left upper quadrant. The omental attachments to the transverse colon are incised all the way to the middle of the transverse colon or to the right colon itself (Figure 10-11).
- The left colon is lifted from the abdomen and is pulled to the patient's left, exposing the medial aspect of the left colon mesentery over the aorta. The IMA is encountered at the level of the aorta just above the bifurcation of the common iliacs. The inferior mesenteric vein (IMV) is identified at the level of the ligament of Treitz at the base of the mesentery of the left colon above a window of clear peritoneum along the anterior surface of the aorta (Figures 10-12 and 10-13). The IMA and vein are isolated at their origins and divided between ties (Figure 10-14).

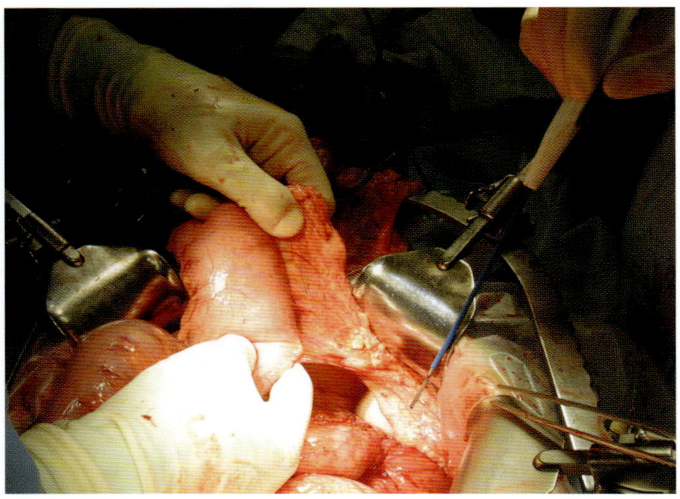

Figure 10-11

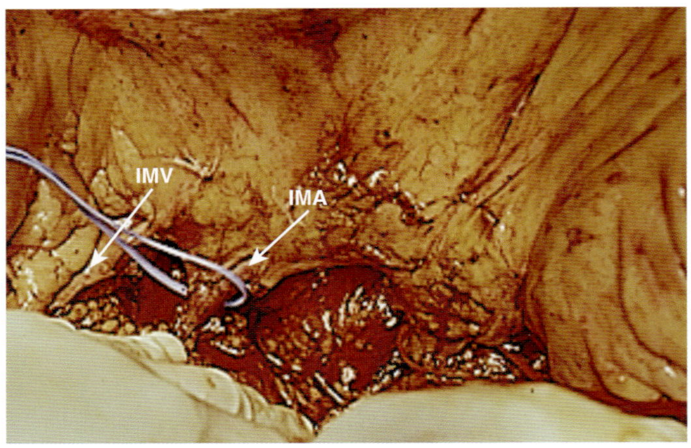

Figure 10-12

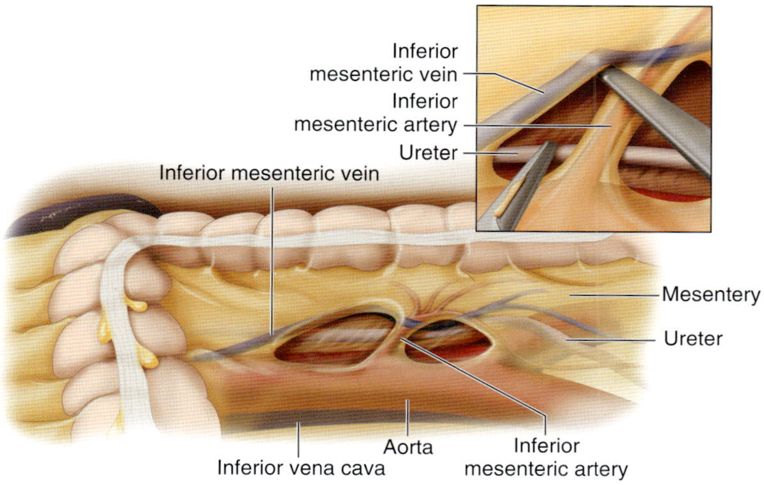

Figure 10-13

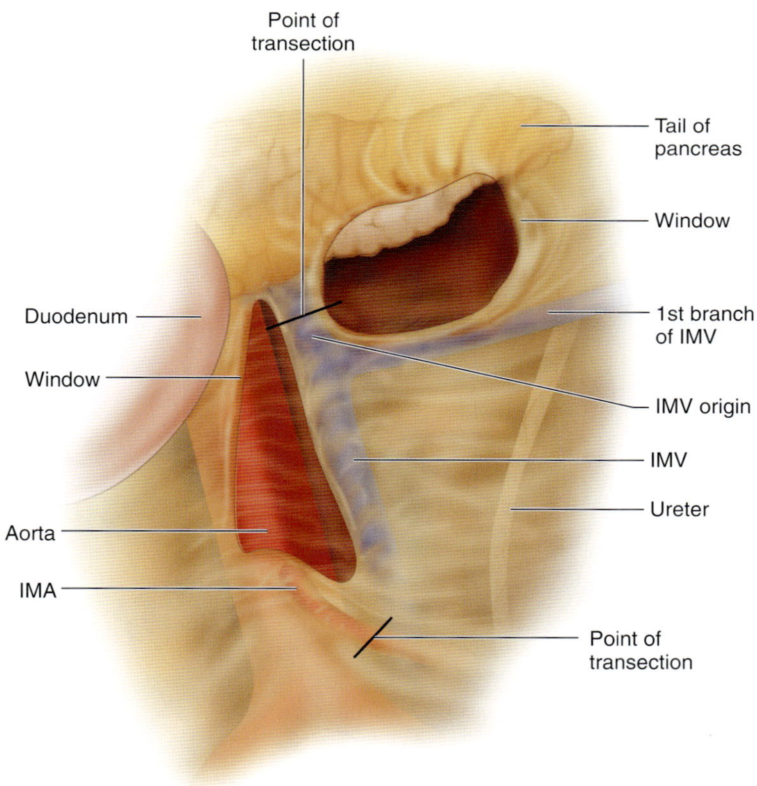

Figure 10-14

- The left colon is stretched all the way to the pelvis bringing the splenic flexure to near the pelvic brim. This maneuver allows the left colon to be evaluated for point of transection to ensure adequate reach into the pelvis for the colorectal anastomosis (Figure 10-15).
- The left colon mesentery is divided so that the IMA pedicle goes with the specimen. A purse-string instrument is used to place a purse-string, or a hand-sewn purse-string is placed at the site of transection after dividing the mesenteric vessels. The purse-string is placed so that adequate blood supply is available and there is no tension or twist (Figure 10-16). The anvil for the stapler is placed into the colotomy, and the purse-string is cinched ensuring that all edges of the colotomy are everted (Figure 10-17).
- The small bowel and proximal colon are packed in the upper abdomen, and the pelvic dissection is begun.

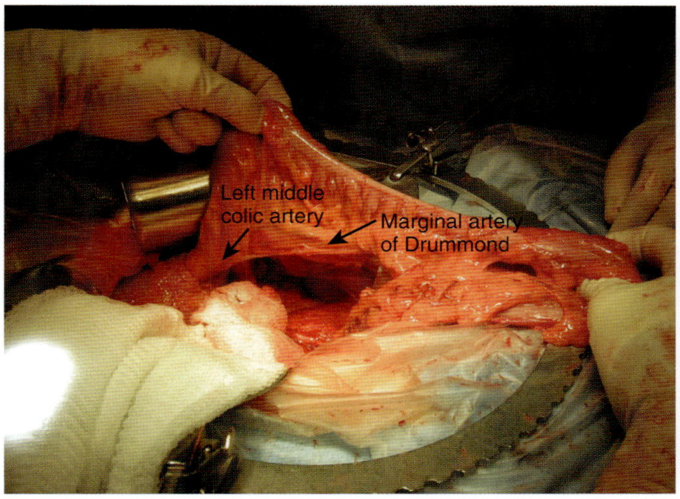

Figure 10-15

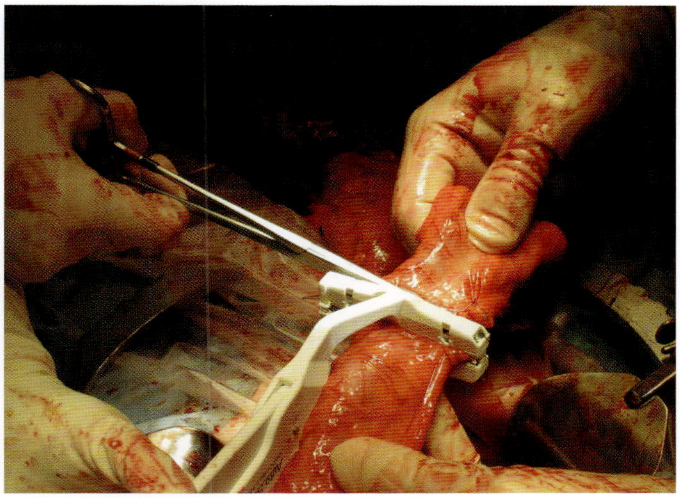

Figure 10-16

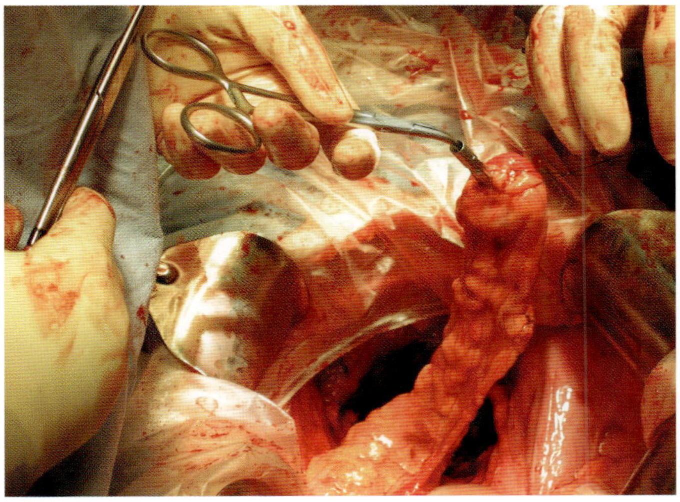

Figure 10-17

- The distal colon is retracted anteriorly, and a pelvic retractor is used to place tension on the mesorectum. The avascular plane of the presacral space is entered with sharp dissection (Figures 10-18 and 10-19). Care is taken to preserve the sympathetic nerves and not violate the mesorectal fascia (Figure 10-20). The posterior dissection is carried from 3 o'clock to

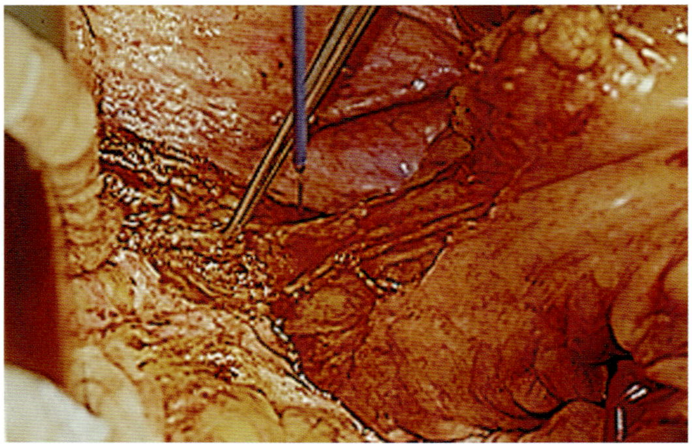

Figure 10-18

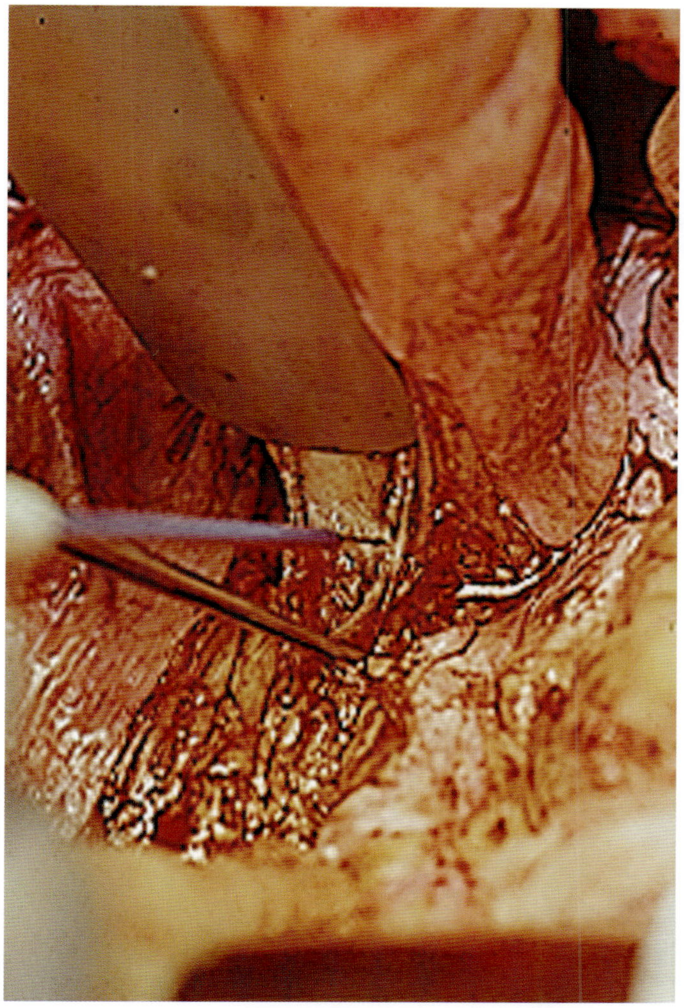

Figure 10-19

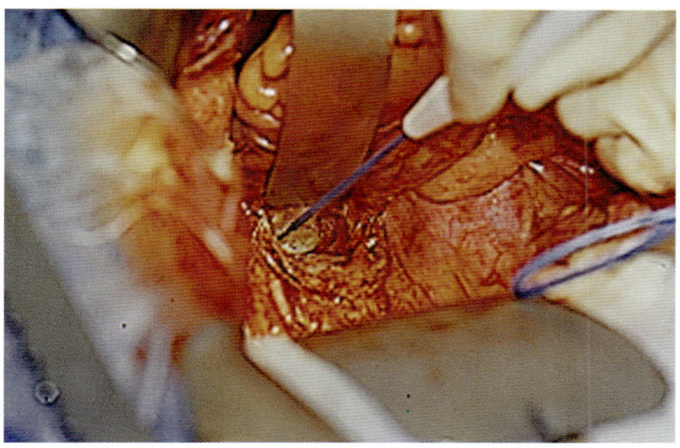

Figure 10-20

9 o'clock all the way down to the pelvic floor or low enough to perform a tumor-specific mesorectal excision (Figures 10-21 and 10-22). A complete and intact mobilization of the mesorectum reveals its bilobed configuration (Figure 10-23).

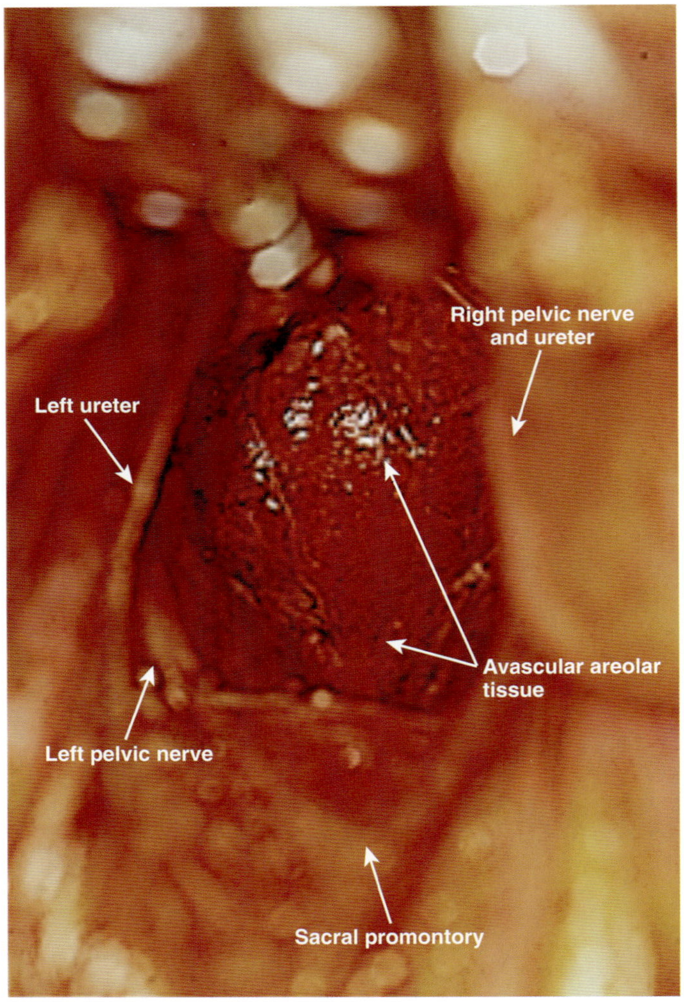

Figure 10-21

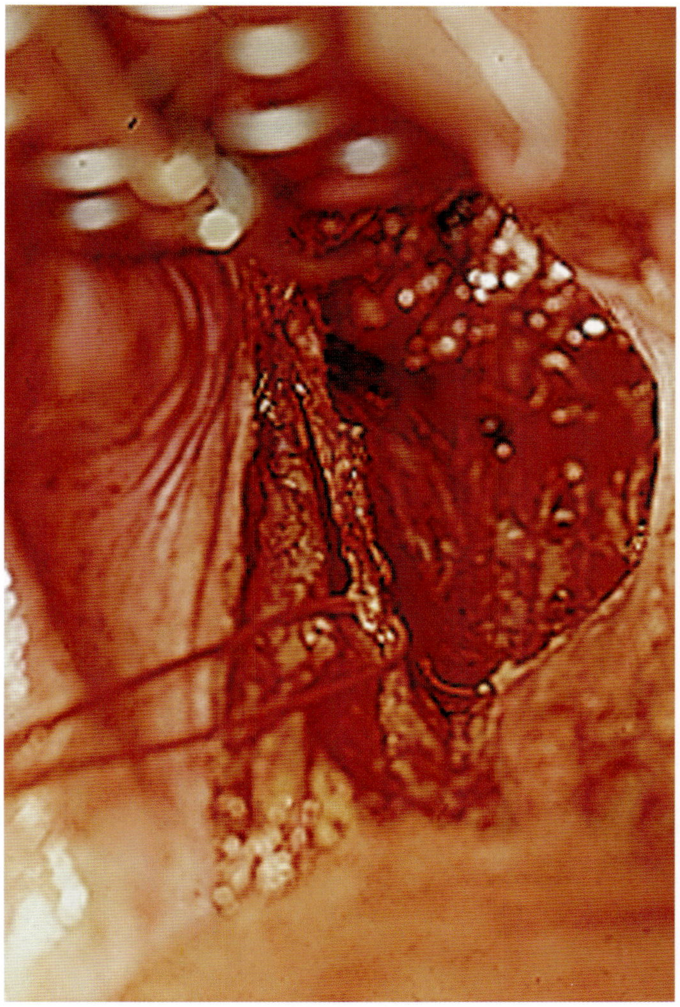

Figure 10-22

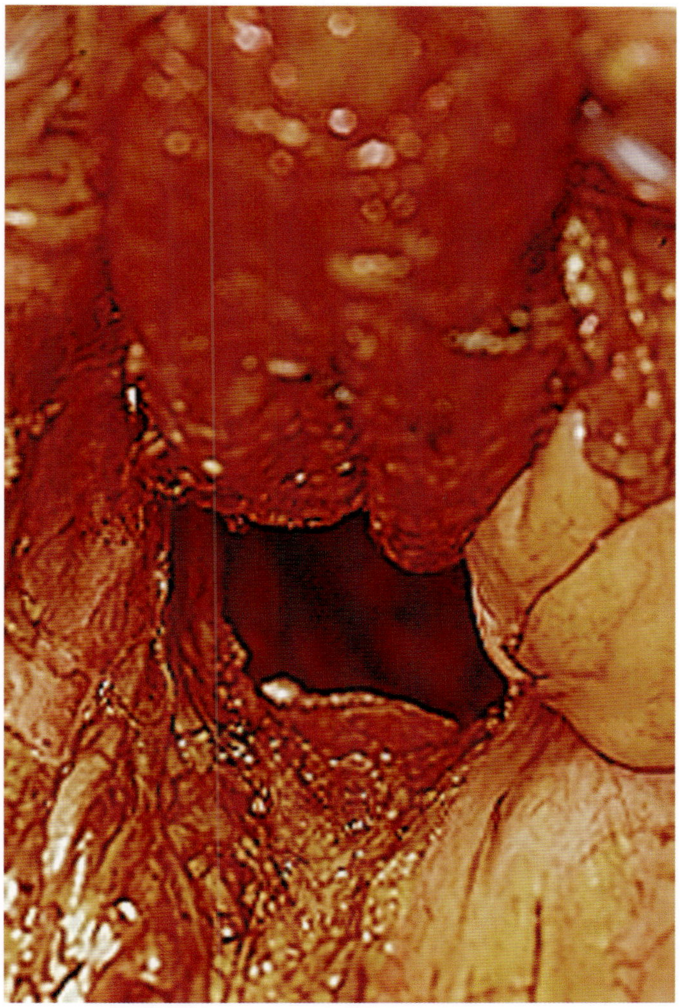

Figure 10-23

- The lateral peritoneal attachments are incised down to the anterior peritoneal reflection. The lateral dissection is performed by retracting the rectum medially and sharply dividing the tissue in a posterior-to-anterior fashion (Figure 10-24). When adequate tension is created, the plane of the mesorectal fascia can be seen ensuring that it is completely excised. The anterior peritoneum is incised, the prostate or cervix is retracted anteriorly, and the rectum is retracted posteriorly (Figure 10-25). The anterior dissection is carried down to the pelvic floor, and any remaining lateral attachments are divided.
- The rectum is divided with a linear cutter stapler; the proximal rectum must be occluded so that tumor cells are not spilled as the specimen is removed (Figure 10-26). If a mesorectal-specific resection is performed, the site of distal resection is identified, and the mesorectum is divided at a right angle, and then the rectum is divided (Figure 10-27).

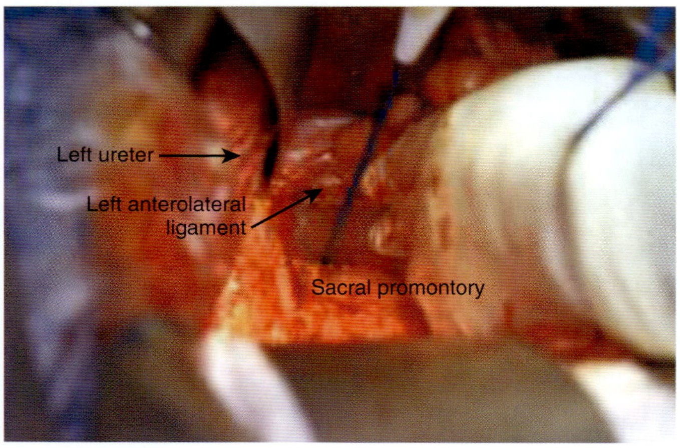

Figure 10-24

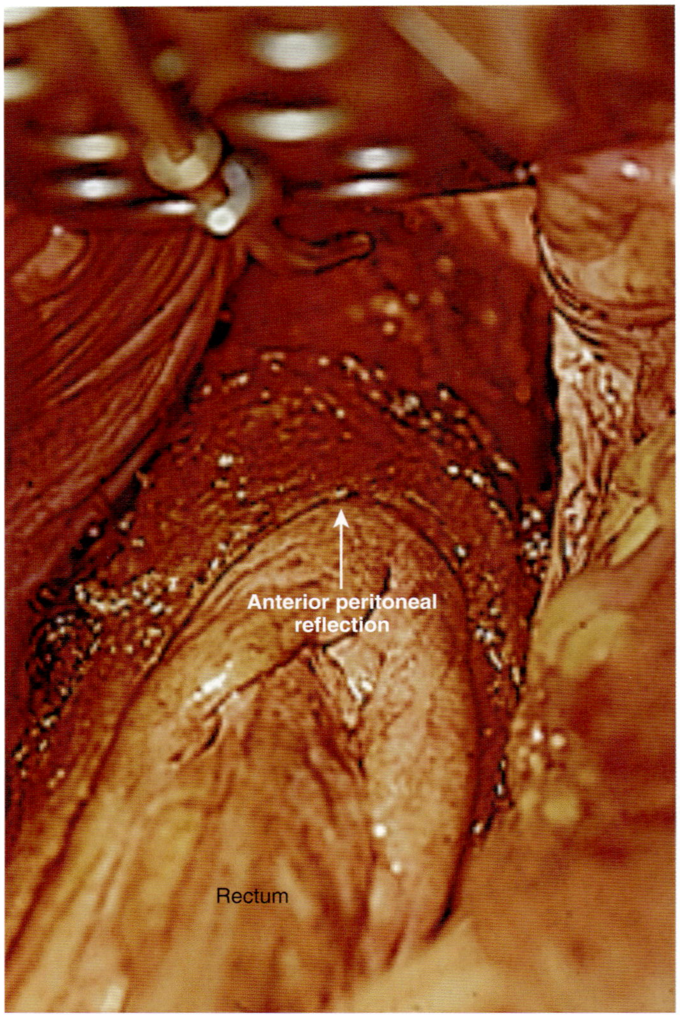

Figure 10-25

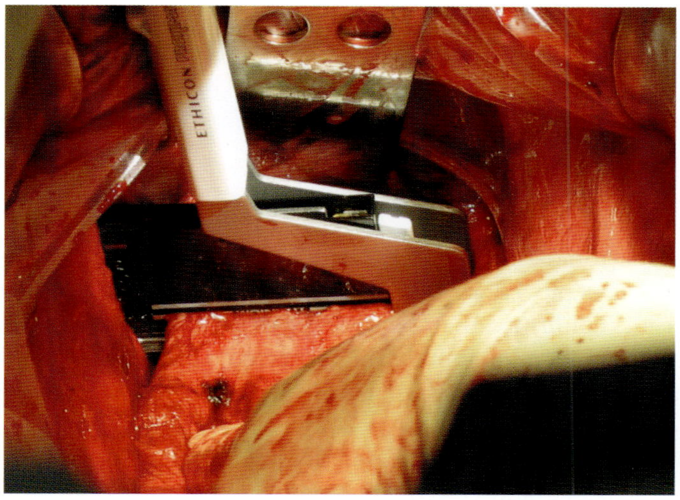

Figure 10-26

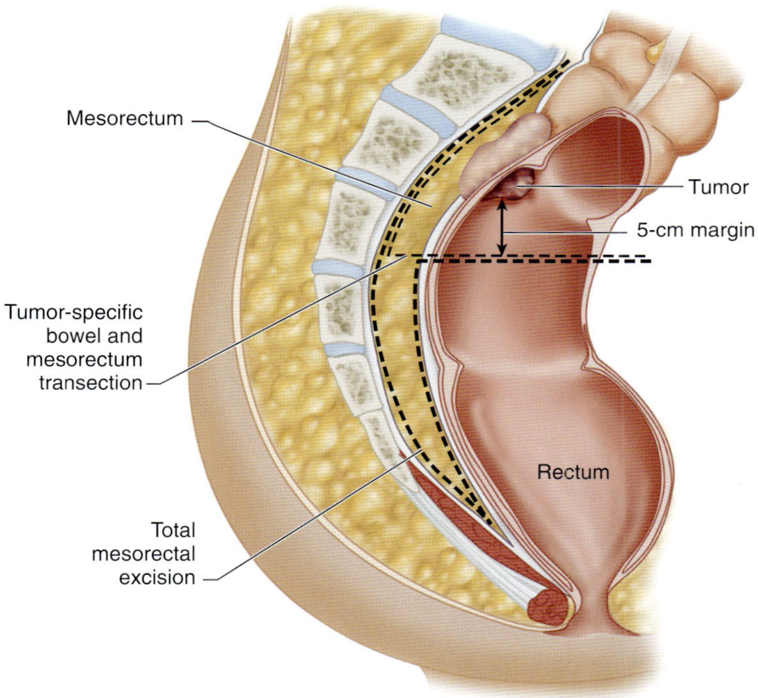

Figure 10-27

- To perform the anastomosis, the stapler head is passed transanally up to the top of the rectal stump. The spike is deployed posterior to the transverse staple line. The anvil is attached to the stapler after it is confirmed that the cut edge of the left colon mesentery is straight (Figure 10-28). The anastomotic doughnuts are inspected, and an air test is performed (Figure 10-29). Typically, a closed suction drain is placed deep in the pelvis for 4 days postoperatively to drain any fluid and blood that may accumulate.
- A diverting loop ileostomy can be created at the discretion of the surgeon (Figure 10-30). The abdomen is irrigated and closed.

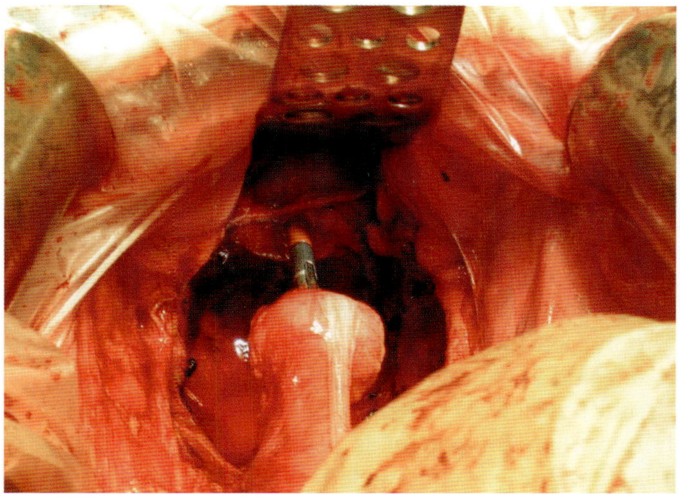

Figure 10-28

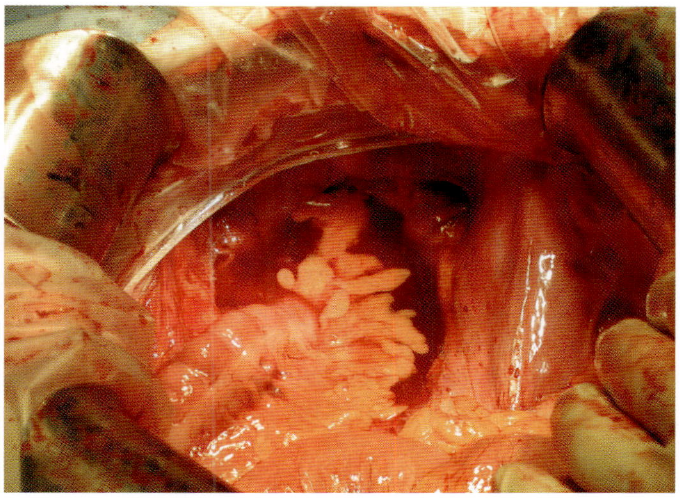

Figure 10-29

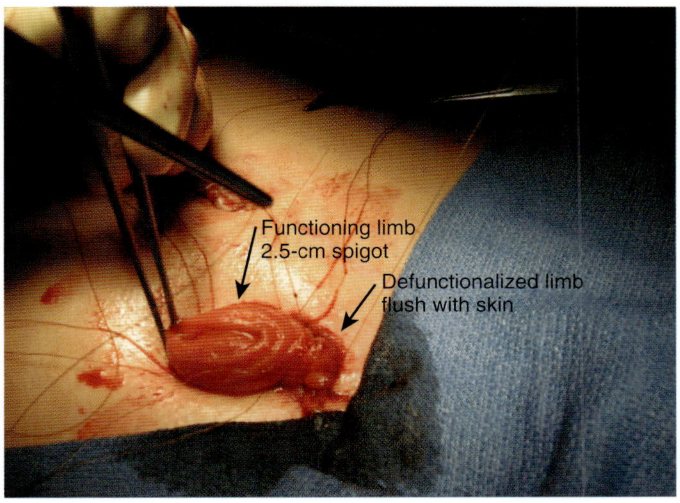

Figure 10-30

Step 4: Postoperative Care

Patients are ambulated early. Intravenous fluid replacement is given to maintain a urine output of greater than 30 mL/hr. Nasogastric decompression is not required unless the patient becomes nauseated. Most patients tolerate clear liquids within 24 to 48 hours, and the diet can be advanced as tolerated. Patients should be given prophylactic antibiotics for 24 hours, incentive spirometry, and deep venous thrombosis prophylaxis and encouraged to ambulate as much as possible during the early postoperative period. Usual hospital stay after an open low anterior resection is 4 to 5 days; the hospital stay is shorter when the patient is placed on an early recovery after surgery (ERAS) program. If a diverting ileostomy is constructed, the patient must receive adequate stoma education. Postoperative pain is usually managed with patient-controlled analgesia narcotics supplemented with intravenous anti-inflammatory agents followed by a switch to oral analgesics.

Step 5: Pearls and Pitfalls

The most critical aspect of a low anterior resection is ensuring an airtight anastomosis with no tension with good blood supply and no twist. Adequate length is ensured by ligation of the IMV at the inferior border of the pancreas and complete mobilization of the splenic flexure by dividing the mesocolic attachments to the inferior border of the pancreas all the way to the midline. The patient may be best served by placement of a pelvic drain if the dissection is carried into the pelvis and there is enough oozing from the surface to justify continued drainage. A pelvic drain does not eliminate the possibility of a leak, but it may be an early indicator of breach of anastomotic integrity. The patient can be fed on an ERAS program.

A complete mesorectal package (complete total mesorectal excision or tumor-specific total mesorectal excision) is the goal of the pelvic dissection. In their *Rectal Cancer Staging Recommendations,* 7th edition, the American Joint Committee on Cancer requires grading of the total mesorectal excision specimen as part of the prognostic summary. The peritoneal surface over all the fat of the mesentery must be intact, or the risk of local recurrence is increased.

Selected Readings

Heald RJ, Moran BJ, Ryall RD, et al. Rectal cancer: the Basingstoke experience of total mesorectal excision, 1978-1997. Arch Surg 1998;133:894–9.

Law WL, Chu KW. Anterior resection for rectal cancer with mesorectal excision: a prospective evaluation of 622 patients. Ann Surg 2004;240:260–8.

CHAPTER 11

Laparoscopic Low Anterior Resection

James W. Fleshman, Jr.

Step 1: Clinical Anatomy

The left colon lies along the left side of the abdomen suspended from the splenic flexure to the pelvic brim by lateral peritoneal attachments (Figure 11-1). The mesentery of the left colon arises from the midline of the abdomen along the aorta. The sigmoid colon has no lateral peritoneal attachments other than some congenital adhesions, which fix the apex of the sigmoid colon to the pelvic brim and the iliac fossa. Otherwise, the sigmoid colon is attached to the retroperitoneum through a midline mesentery arising from the inferior mesenteric artery (IMA) and extending down into the pelvis to the mesorectum. The splenic flexure is attached to the undersurface of the tip of the spleen, the lower edge of the tail of the pancreas, and the anterior surface of the left kidney by various levels of suspensory ligaments and peritoneal extensions. The blood supply to the left colon is based on the IMA, which arises from the anterior surface of the aorta just above the bifurcation of the common iliac arteries. The IMA extends anteriorly and bifurcates to produce the superior rectal artery feeding the sigmoid colon and the rectum. The left colic artery extends cephalad to provide the left colon and distal splenic flexure with blood supply through the arcade at the mesenteric edge known as the marginal artery of Drummond. The retroperitoneum behind the left colon contains the left ureter and the gonadal vessels lying over the psoas muscle. The ureter crosses the iliac vessels at the bifurcation of the iliac vessels into the external and internal iliac branches.

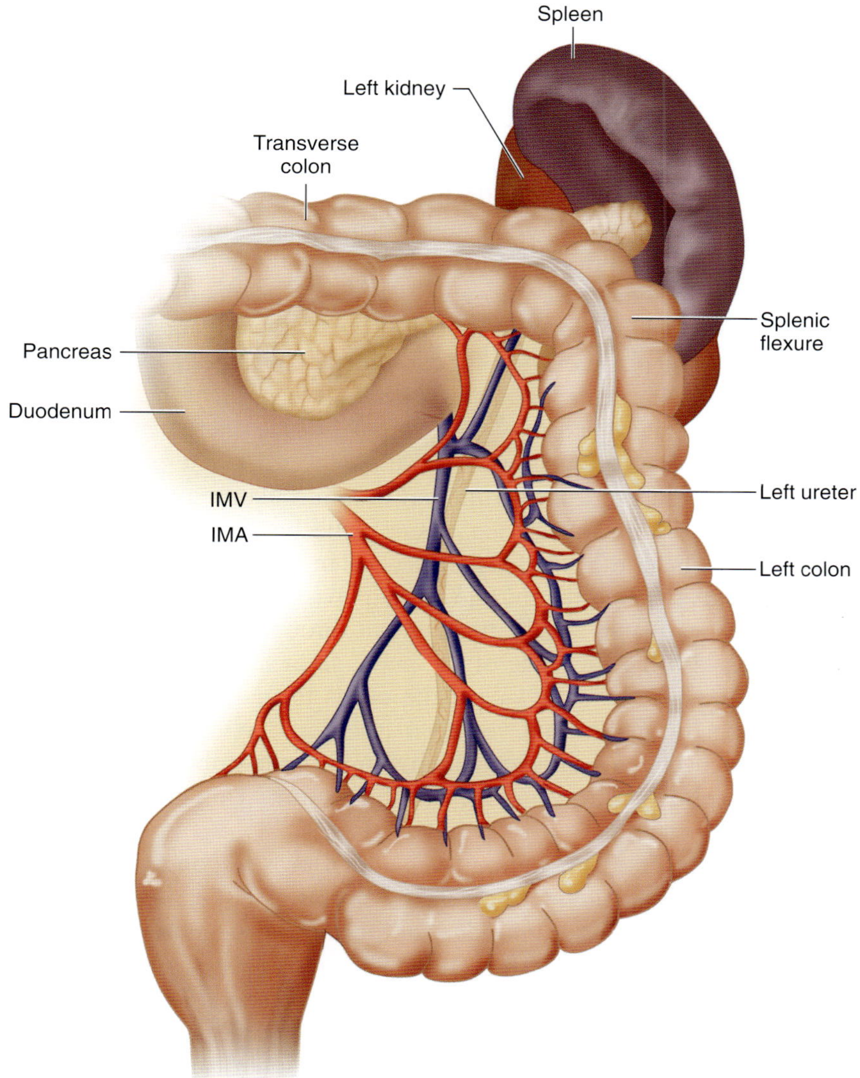

Spleen
Left kidney
Transverse colon
Pancreas
Duodenum
Splenic flexure
IMV
IMA
Left ureter
Left colon

Figure 11-1

Pelvic Anatomy

The pelvic anatomy is complex with interrelationships between the rectum, vagina, uterus, ovaries, bladder, and prostate (Figure 11-2*A*). The anatomy is important for pelvic dissection because of the various structures that are at risk, such as the splanchnic nerves innervating the bladder, the ureters, and the major organs themselves. The anatomy begins at the pelvic brim right at the sacral promontory. The common iliac artery and vein on each side course along the posterior aspect of the pelvic brim. The hypogastric plexus of parasympathetic and sympathetic nerves is found between the bifurcation of the aorta and common iliacs. This plexus coalesces to the right and left as the splanchnic pelvic nerves, which run along the inner aspect of the pelvic side wall to the level of the obturator fossa and the anterolateral ligaments carrying the middle hemorrhoidal vessels. Nerve fibers course from the splanchnic nerve to the rectum through the anterolateral ligaments along the middle hemorrhoidal vessels. Extension of these nerves continues to either the vagina or the prostate as the nervi erigentes. A clear understanding of this nerve anatomy is crucial because it is easily damaged during dissection resulting in sexual dysfunction and urinary bladder dysfunction.

At the level of the sacral promontory, an areolar tissue plane begins behind the superior hemorrhoidal artery. The superior hemorrhoidal artery descends from the bifurcation of the IMA and splits at approximately S1-2 to give two major trunks down the posterior aspect of the rectum. The mesorectal envelope encases the fat, lymphatic, and vascular structures to the rectum. The areolar tissue plane outside the mesorectal envelope is known as the "holy plane" and guides the dissection in the pelvis. A cross-sectional diagram of the pelvis shows the visceral peritoneum encasing the mesorectum with the areolar tissue plane between the visceral peritoneum and the parietal peritoneum posteriorly (Figure 11-2*B*). The parietal peritoneum covers a nerve and venous plexus over the sacrum and the musculature of the side wall of the pelvis. Maintaining dissection within the areolar tissue plane between the parietal and the visceral peritoneal layers protects all of the crucial structures in the pelvis.

The rectum descends through the middle of the pelvis following the curve of the sacrum and at the level of the coccyx makes a right angle to exit through the pelvic floor via the anal canal. The levator ani muscles on either side of the pelvic floor form the support diaphragm of the pelvis and extend up onto the side wall of the pelvis to insert in the ischiospinous ligament attachments covering the nerves and vessels of the deep pelvic floor. The tip of the coccyx attaches to the pubococcygeal ligament, which supports the puborectalis muscle as a semicircular sling from the pubis around the back of the rectum. This muscle closes the top of the anal canal anterior to posterior.

The anterior pelvic structures including the bladder, prostate, and vagina are separated from the rectum by the rectoprostatic or rectovaginal septum. A visceral peritoneal layer known as Denonvilliers' fascia is the posterior boundary of the anterior structures. This fascia protects the seminal vesicles and prostate during dissection. The areolar tissue plane continues around the entire rectum to the anterior surface of the rectum. The plane is found behind or posterior to Denonvilliers' fascia. The anterolateral ligaments carry the middle hemorrhoidal vessels into the mesorectal envelope through the visceral fascia from an anterolateral direction. Dissection and transection of these middle hemorrhoidal vessels reveals the anterior areolar tissue plane behind Denonvilliers' fascia, which can be followed all the way down to the anal canal.

The ureters, which have been described as running into the pelvic area over the pelvic brim crossing the common iliac artery and vein on either side of the pelvis, continue into the pelvis along the side wall of the pelvis toward the posterior aspect of the bladder. In the nonoperated, pristine pelvis, the ureters are higher up along the side wall of the pelvis aiming toward the posterior aspect of the trigone of the bladder. In females, the ureters run between the arterial blood supply of the uterus along the anterior lateral side wall of the pelvis. In males, ureters are not exposed during the distal pelvic dissection. The ureters may be drawn posteriorly after a previous operation but are normally fairly well protected anteriorly and laterally. In a previously operated pelvis, it is always wise to place ureteral stents at the beginning of the procedure to aid in identification of the aberrantly placed ureters.

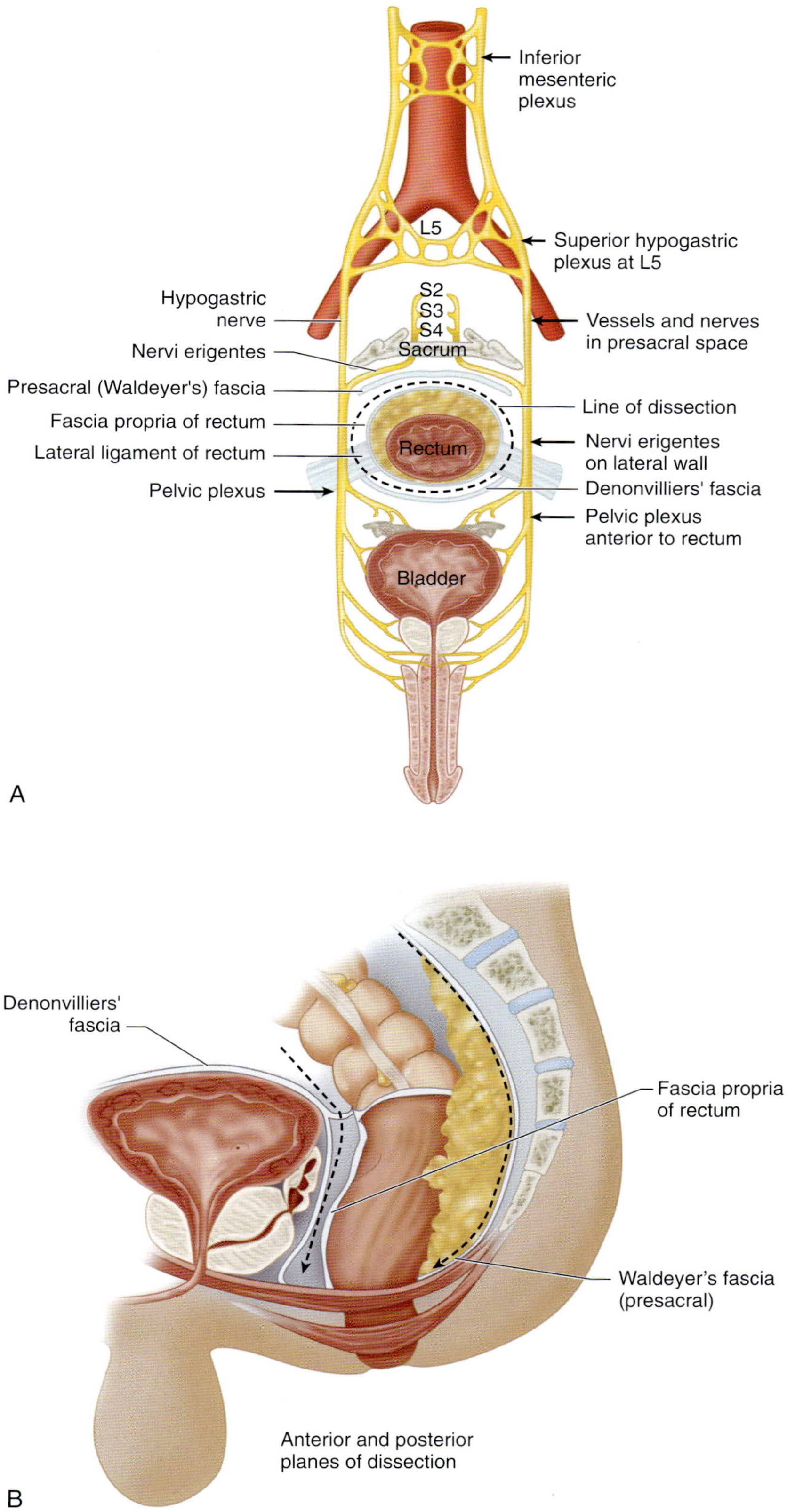

Figure 11-2A-B

The upper anal canal begins at the puborectalis ring or the anorectal ring, which sits at the level of the pelvic floor and can be palpated through the anal canal as a bulge posteriorly. The longitudinal muscles of the rectum continue into the anus as the intersphincteric plane demarcating the line between autonomic internal sphincter and somatic external sphincter fibers all the way down to the level of the anal canal skin where the intersphincteric groove is palpable.

The rectovaginal and rectoprostatic septum descends all the way to the level of the perineum anteriorly. The internal sphincter is the hypertrophied circular muscle of the wall of the rectum. The lowest portion of the internal sphincter can be palpated as a groove where the longitudinal fibers insert on the skin.

Within the anal canal, the dentate line is the junction between the cuboidal epithelium of the anal transition zone, which is the terminal mucosal layer of the rectum, and the squamous epidermal cells of the anal canal skin. Gland openings (or crypts) are found in the dentate line at the base of the columns of Morgagni, which are interdigitating lines of squamous epithelium into the cuboidal and columnar epithelium of the distal rectum. The anal transition zone is the most highly innervated section of the rectum and anal canal containing nerve fibers sensing temperature, vibration, electrical stimulation, pressure, liquid, solid, and gas. The dentate line lies approximately halfway along the surgical anal canal, which extends from the palpable anal verge all the way up to the anorectal ring palpated at the puborectalis sling posteriorly. The anoderm within the anal canal, cephalad to the anal verge, has no hair follicles.

Step 2: Preoperative Considerations

Low anterior resection of the rectum and sigmoid is most commonly performed for rectal cancer. The removal of the entire mesorectum to the level of the pelvic floor is required for all tumors below 7 cm. Upper rectal lesions require a tumor-specific mesorectal excision, which should include 5 cm of length of bowel and mesorectum below the level of the tumor as the transection of the rectum is accomplished. The patient requires a complete bowel preparation and should be marked for a possible loop ileostomy for diversion if the patient has undergone chemoradiation. The patient requires preoperative prophylactic antibiotics and deep vein thrombosis prophylaxis. The level of the tumor should be determined preoperatively with rigid proctoscopy to assist in planning the reconstructive portion of the procedure. A distal margin that is clear of tumor (usually 2 to 5 cm) is necessary before considering reconstruction. If the patient requires a colonic J pouch for reconstruction, this would need to be determined before the operation to plan the extent of resection. A left colon-to-dentate line anastomosis is (practically speaking) the lowest coloanal anastomosis possible.

Step 3: Operative Steps

- The patient is placed in the lithotomy position using Allen's stirrups with the legs flexed 90 degrees at the knees and flexed no more than 10 degrees at the hips (Figure 11-3). The legs point toward the floor to prevent obstruction of the operative field by the knees when the patient is placed in Trendelenburg position. A beanbag is attached to the table with Velcro to fix it in place. The patient is positioned in the beanbag with the arms tucked at the side and incorporated in the beanbag. Tape is placed across the chest to fix the sides of the beanbag and hold the patient as an extra measure of security (Figure 11-4).

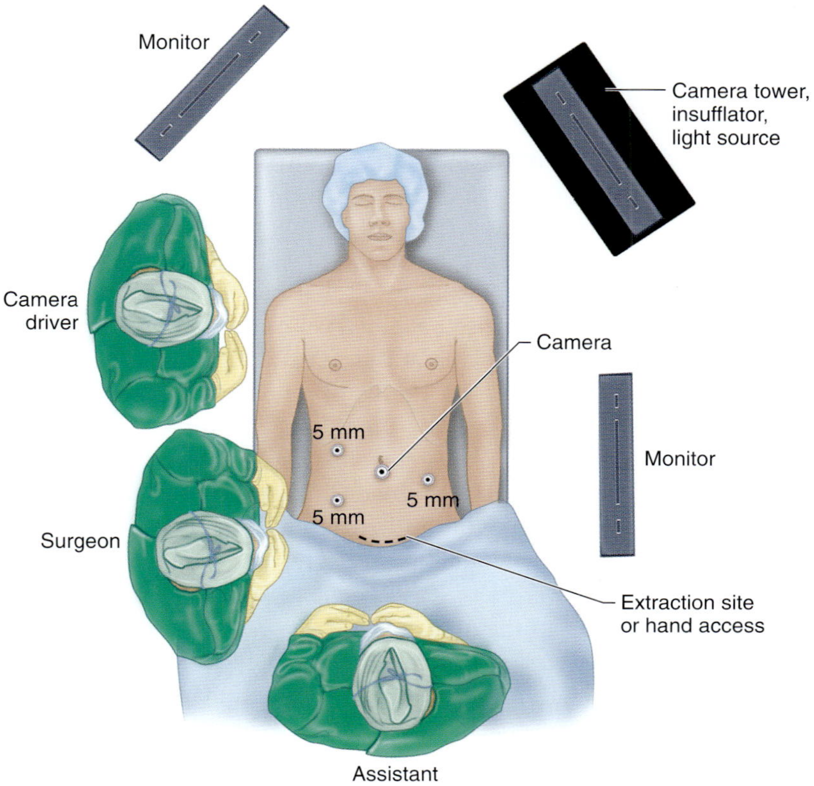

Figure 11-3

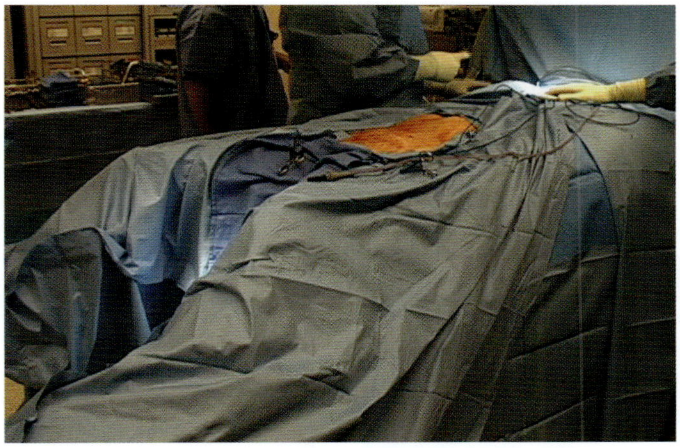

Figure 11-4

- The abdomen is prepared and draped in sterile fashion, and the abdomen is inflated through either an open insertion of a trocar at the umbilicus or a Veress needle at the umbilicus. The trocar is placed above the umbilicus in the vertical midline. The flexible laparoscope is introduced through the trocar at the umbilicus by the camera operator standing at the right shoulder, and the abdomen is explored for metastases or other intra-abdominal disease. The laparoscopic low anterior resection requires a trocar in the right upper and lower quadrants in the anterior axillary line; trocars are placed two fingerbreadths below the costal margin and above the anterior superior iliac spine. A left flank trocar is placed in the anterior axillary line at the level of the umbilicus. A 10-mm trocar is placed in the suprapubic vertical midline, or a hand access port can be placed at this level (Figure 11-5).
- The patient is placed in steep Trendelenburg and airplaned to the right. The sigmoid colon is lifted anteriorly with an endoscopic Babcock clamp through the 10-mm suprapubic port or, alternatively, with the hand of the assistant through the suprapubic hand access (Figure 11-6). The assistant stands between the patient's legs. The operating surgeon stands to the patient's right and grasps a 5-mm grasper in the left hand and an energy source in the right hand. The sigmoid mesentery is incised at the level of the pelvic brim anterior to the sacral promontory to enter the avascular plane at that level. Retraction anteriorly opens this plane and exposes the undersurface of the IMA at its origin (Figure 11-7).
- The left ureter is the first structure to be identified and dissected free from the posterior aspect of the left colon mesentery. The ureter must be visualized before division of the IMA for safety reasons. The hand-assisted approach makes this dissection quite simple. A full laparoscopic approach is more difficult and requires anterior and posterior countertraction and blunt dissection to drop the ureter posteriorly. The surgeon must remember that the dissection plane is angled upward along the pelvic brim as the patient is in right side down and the left leg is actually up in the air.
- The IMA and inferior mesenteric vein (IMV) are isolated at their origins along the anterior surface of the aorta and at the third portion of the duodenum at the ligament of Treitz (Figure 11-8). The medial-to-lateral approach incises the base of the mesentery of the left colon all the way up to the duodenum from the IMA. A window of clear areolar tissue is exposed posterior to the IMV as it runs parallel to the aorta along the base of the left colic mesentery. This window can be developed and the ureter seen in its course toward the hilum of the kidney (Figure 11-9).
- The IMA is divided at its origin using the energy source (Figure 11-10). For cancer, the high ligation of the IMA should be 1 cm above the junction of the aorta. The sympathetic nerves can be dropped posteriorly with blunt dissection to reduce the risk of nerve injury and impotence. The stump of the artery must be visualized carefully after division to ensure there is good hemostasis.

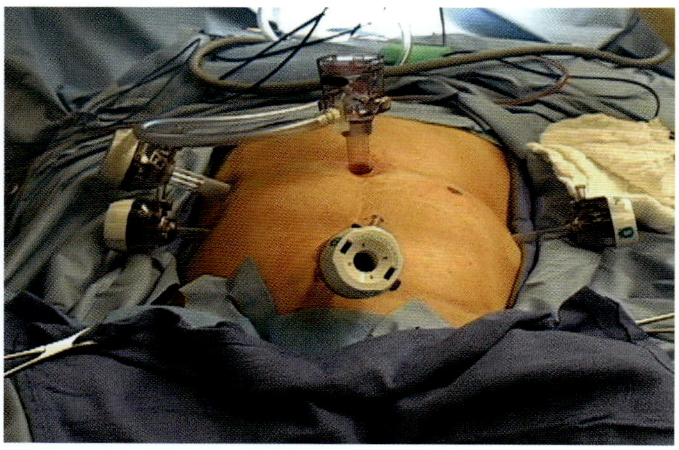

Figure 11-5

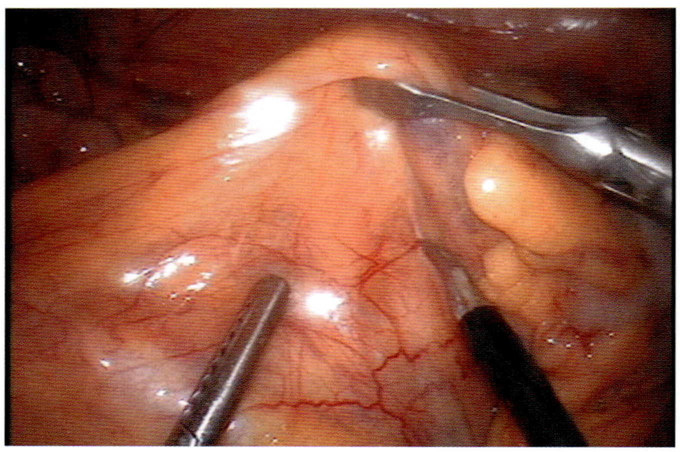

Figure 11-6

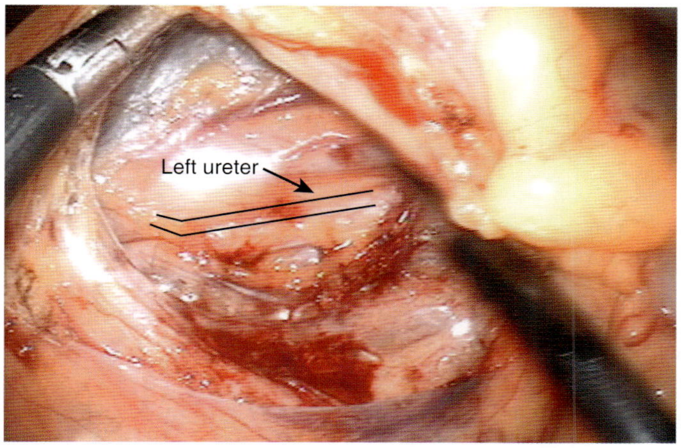

Figure 11-7

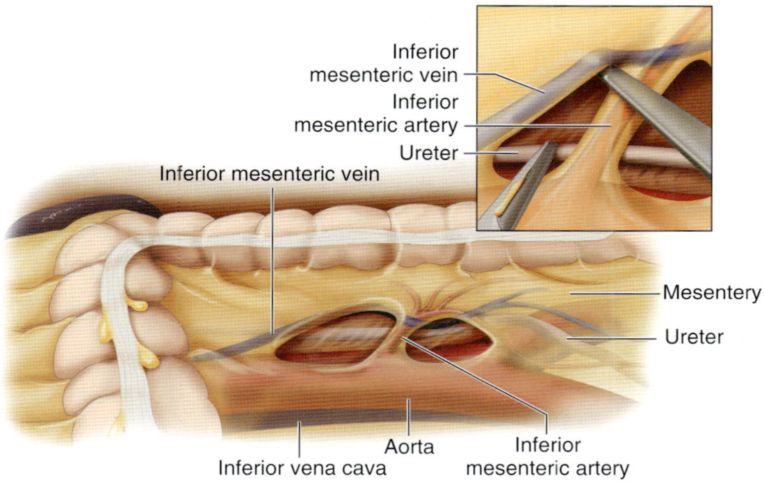

Figure 11-8

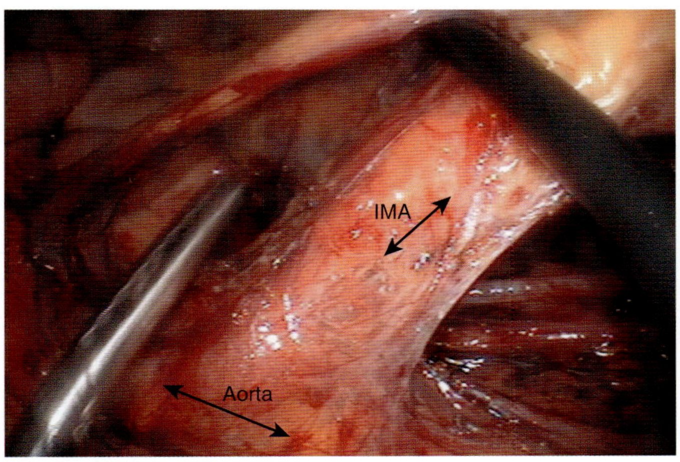

Figure 11-9

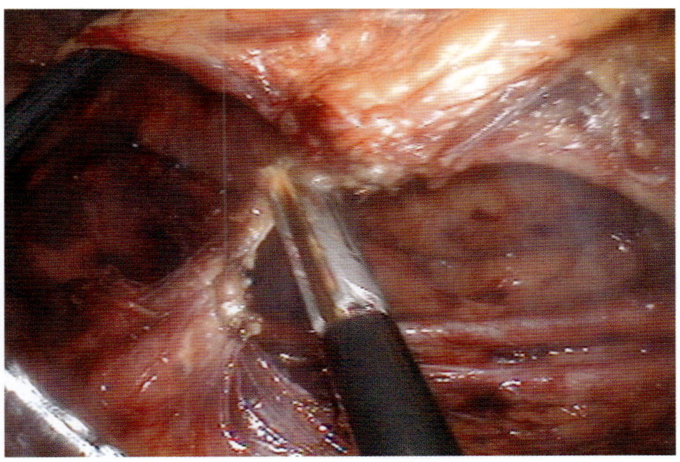

Figure 11-10

- The IMV at the level of the ligament of Treitz has a branch approximately 3 cm caudad to the IMV insertion into the splenic vein. The bifurcation should be included in the specimen by transecting the IMV closer to the ligament of Treitz and the pancreas. The IMV is divided under direct vision after opening the window between the pancreas, the IMV, and the branch (Figure 11-11).
- When the mesenteric vessels have been divided medially, a blunt dissection in the areolar plane can be accomplished all the way out to the lateral aspect of the abdominal wall, dropping the vital structures in the retroperitoneum posteriorly (Figure 11-12). This dissection frees the left colon and its mesentery from the retroperitoneum from the pelvic brim to the splenic flexure. The lateral attachments are incised using the energy source from the pelvic brim up to the splenic flexure (Figure 11-13).

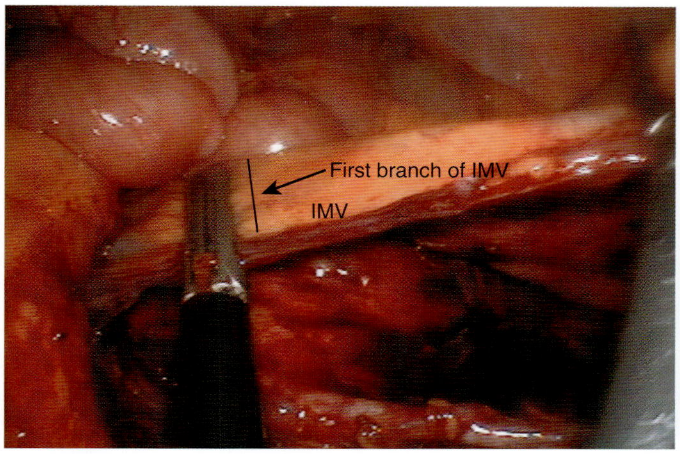

Figure 11-11

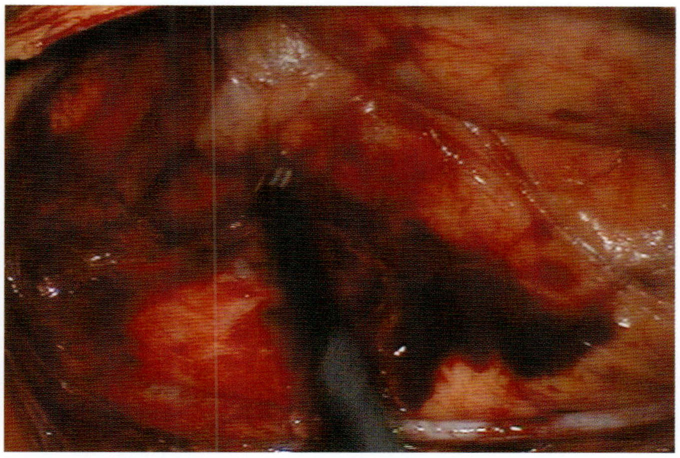
Figure 11-12

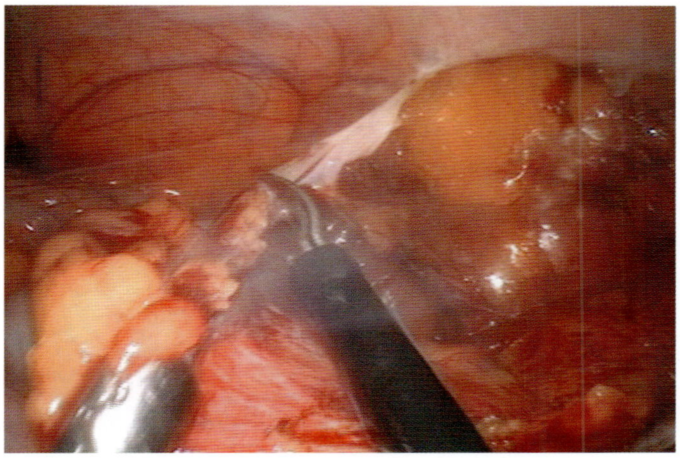
Figure 11-13

- The patient is positioned in steep reverse Trendelenburg and airplaned right. The splenic flexure is released by dividing the lateral attachments of the mesentery of the left colon from the tail of the pancreas, from the lateral side wall, and from the undersurface of the spleen (Figure 11-14*A* and *B*). Electrocautery or other energy source is useful for this maneuver, and combined traction toward the midline and anterior abdominal wall is essential to show the attachments. Simple cross traction would not work (Figure 11-15).
- The division of the suspensory attachments between the pancreas, spleen (Figure 11-16), and omentum along the anterior mesenteric surface of the transverse colon finally releases the left colon from the upper abdomen (Figure 11-17).

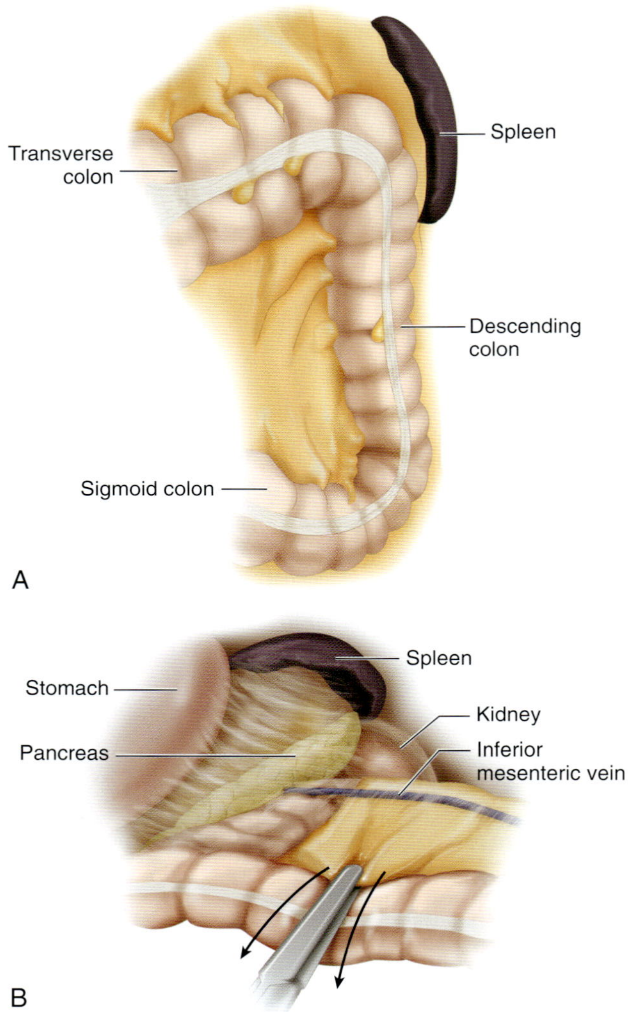

Figure 11-14A-B

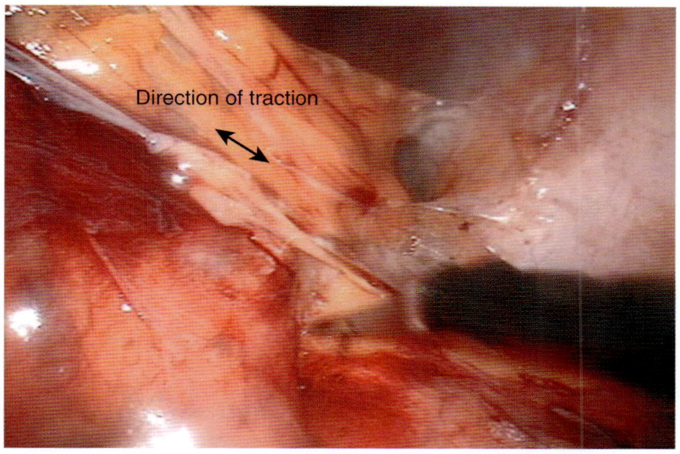

Figure 11-15

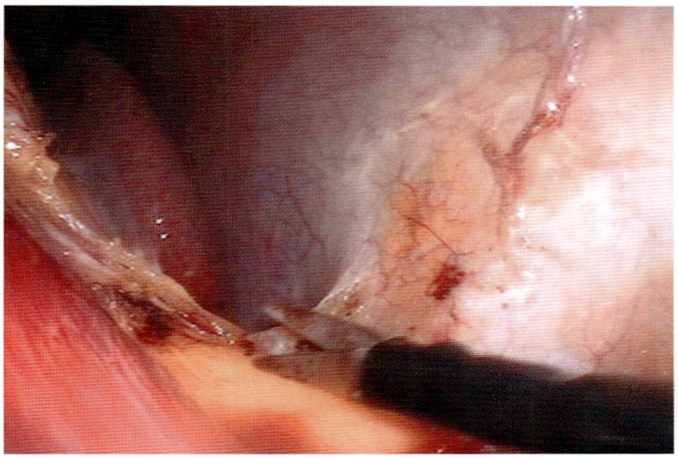
Figure 11-16

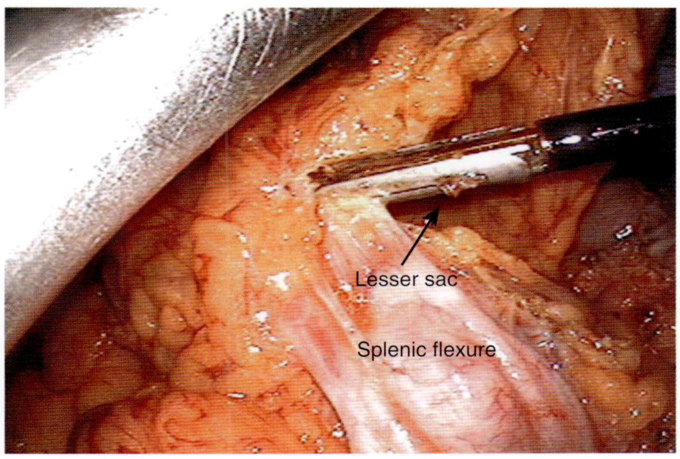

Figure 11-17

- The base of the splenic flexure mesentery is released from the lower edge of the tail of the pancreas, and the lesser sac is opened all the way to the gastroduodenal artery causing the transverse colon to fall toward the pelvis (Figure 11-18). This maneuver reveals the posterior wall of the stomach, the stump of the IMV, and the pancreas after release of the splenic flexure from the left upper quadrant.
- The patient is placed in flat, steep Trendelenburg, and the sigmoid colon is lifted anteriorly by placing a 5-mm grasper beneath the left and sigmoid colon and retracting this toward the anterior abdominal wall. The operating surgeon, still standing on the patient's right, incises the areolar tissue plane posterior to the rectal mesentery and outside the mesenteric envelope (Figure 11-19). The left pelvic side wall is easily seen at the level of the sacral promontory, and the splanchnic pelvic nerve can be protected. Sharp dissection with electrocautery and energy source is important at this level to keep the field clear of blood (Figure 11-20). The right pelvic peritoneal surface is incised to the cul-de-sac to allow the rectum to be retracted to the left.

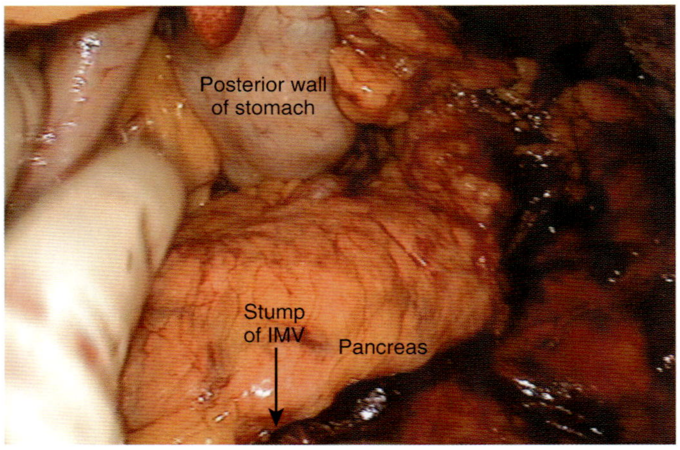

Figure 11-18

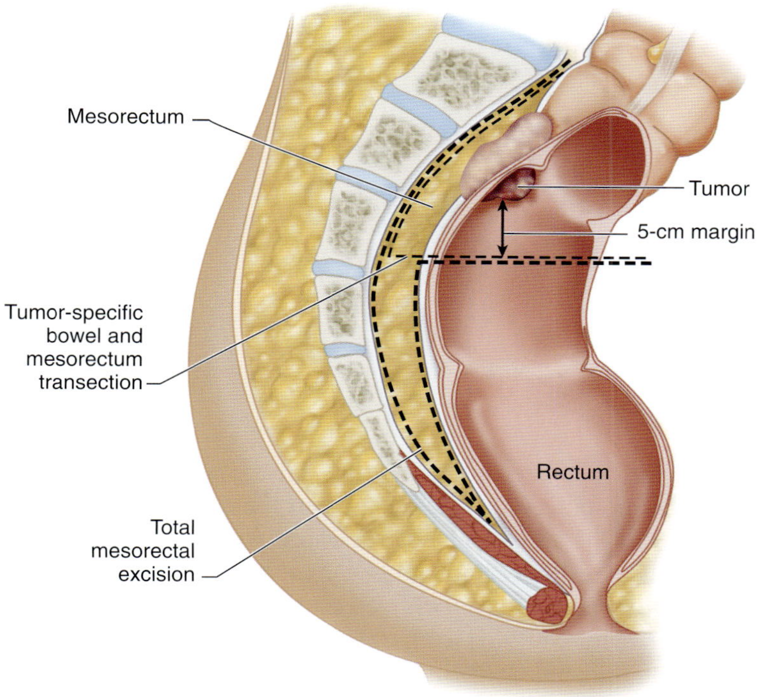

Figure 11-19

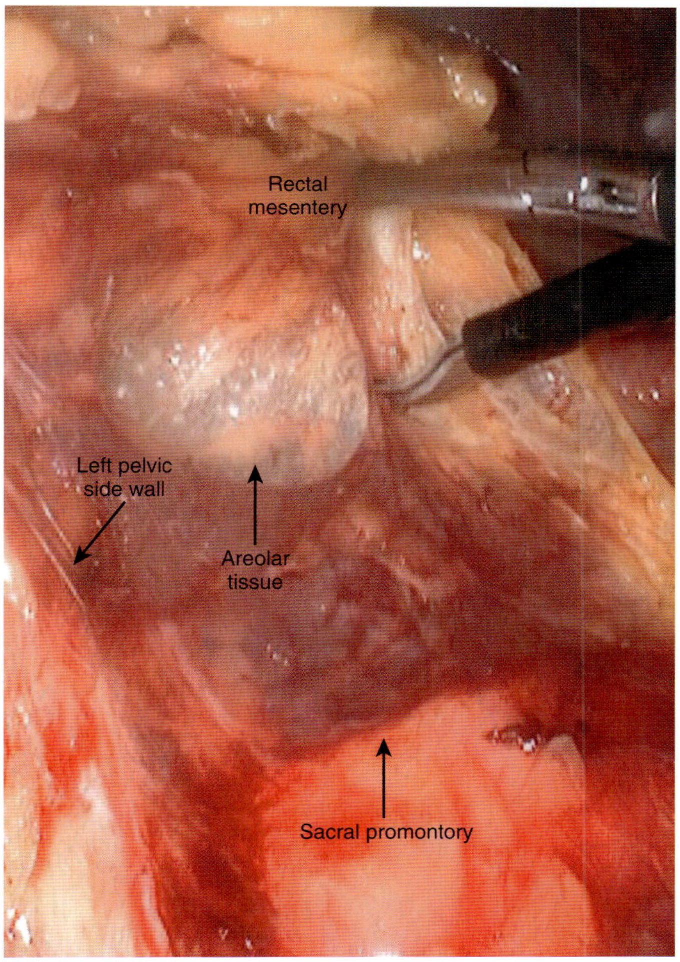

Figure 11-20

- The dissection is carried further into the pelvis, all the way down to the pelvic floor posteriorly to release the mesentery up and away from the sacral curve. The pelvic side wall on the left is cleared, and the attachments are released with sharp and blunt dissection (Figure 11-21). The left pelvic peritoneal surface is incised all the way to the cul-de-sac.
- The left and posterior dissection is completed, and the rectum is retracted to the patient's right. An incision is made anterior to the rectum in the peritoneal surface at the cul-de-sac to expose the left anterolateral ligaments and the rectovaginal or rectoprostatic septum (Figure 11-22). The anterolateral ligaments are divided with the electrocautery hook at the side wall of the pelvis (Figure 11-23).
- The right side of the cul-de-sac incision is accomplished by changing the rectal retraction toward the left side wall. The right anterolateral ligaments are easily stretched across the pelvis (Figure 11-24) and divided from a posterior-to-anterior approach (Figure 11-25).

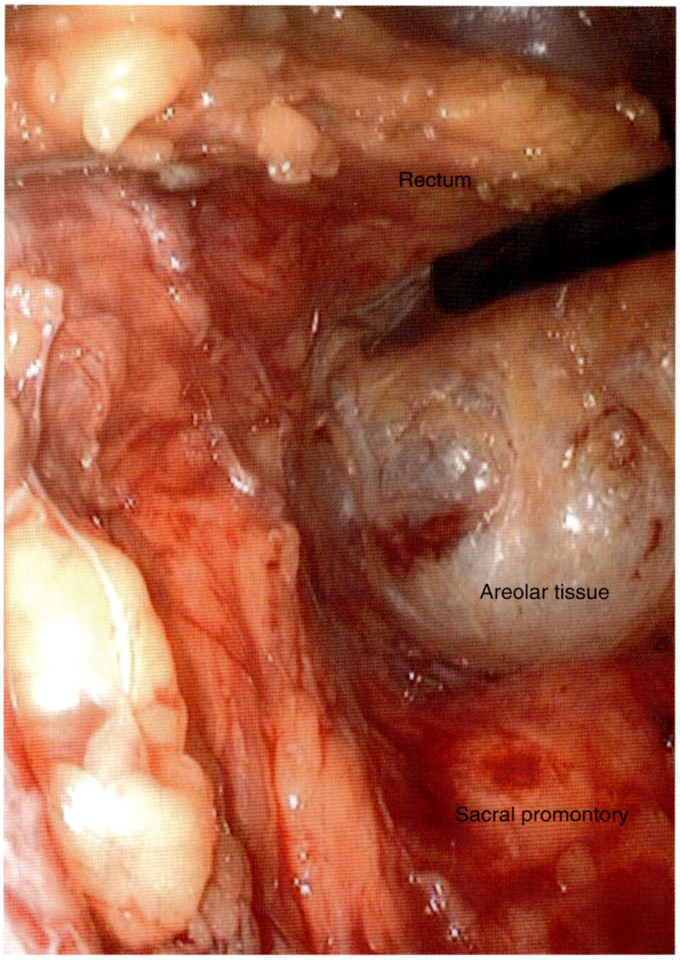

Figure 11-21

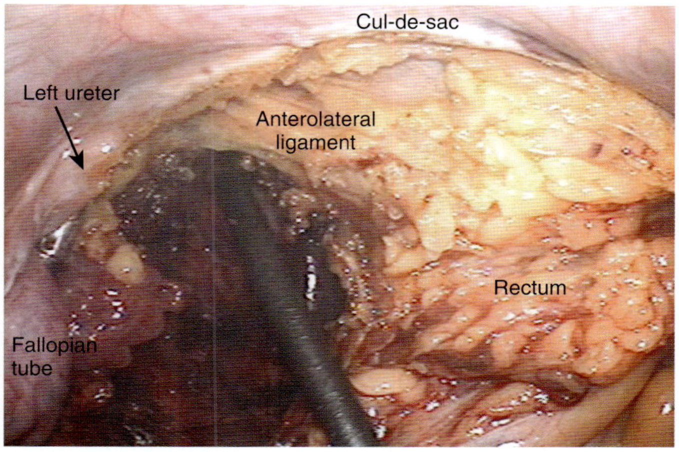

Figure 11-23

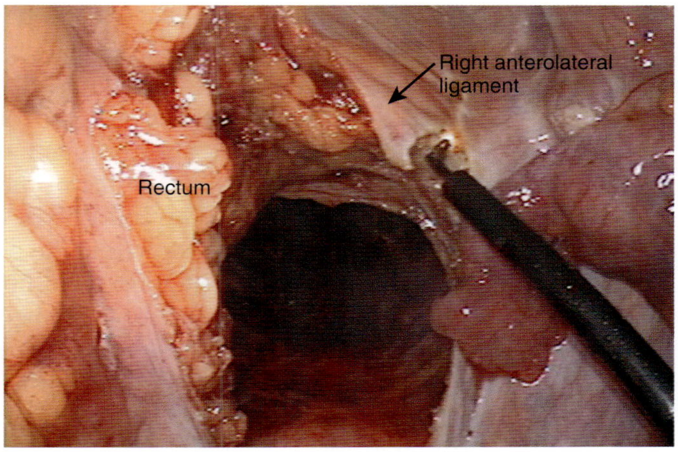

Figure 11-24

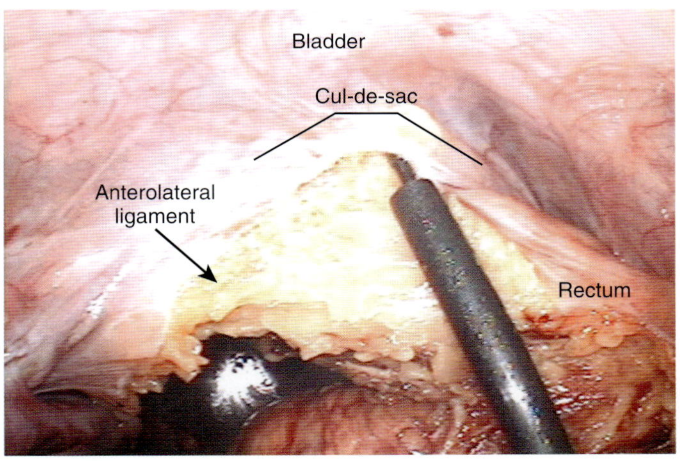

Figure 11-22

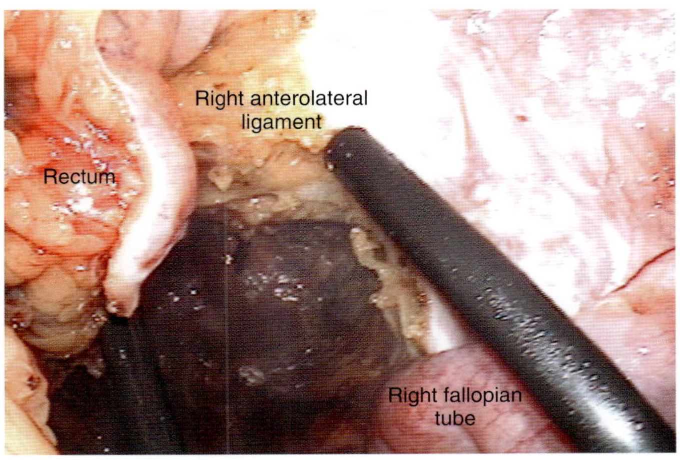

Figure 11-25

- The dissection in the rectovaginal or rectoprostatic septum is accomplished by retracting the posterior aspect of the bladder anteriorly using the left port 5-mm grasper (Figure 11-26). The rectum is pulled posteriorly and cephalad, and the cautery is used to extend the dissection in the areolar tissue plane behind the vagina or prostate all the way down to the level of the anal canal (Figure 11-27). Care must be taken not to enter the vagina. The areolar tissue plane should be easily followed with the flexible scope brought low into the pelvis. The rectum can be transected with laparoscopic staplers or using regular transverse staplers placed through an extraction incision or the hand access port above the pubis. We prefer to use open stapling instruments. The rectum and sigmoid are pulled through the incision. The transverse stapler is placed across the rectum at the level of distal dissection well below the tumor to provide at least a 2-cm margin or as appropriate (Figure 11-28).
- A colonic J pouch is constructed for improved fecal control if indicated. The distal left colon is transected proximal to the sigmoid colon. The colon is folded up on itself, and a 7.5-cm linear cutter stapler is passed through a purse-string placed at the apex of the "J" (Figure 11-29). The transverse staple line of the distal colon is approximated to the inlet of the J pouch with interrupted 3-0 polyglactin 910 (Vicryl) sutures. The anvil of a 29-mm circular stapler anvil and shaft is secured in the purse-string (Figure 11-30). All of this can be accomplished through the suprapubic hand port or extraction site.
- The double-stapled anastomosis can be accomplished between the distal rectal stump and the J pouch and guided through the extraction site or hand site (Figure 11-31). The anastomosis is checked by insufflating air through a rigid proctoscope with the proximal bowel occluded with the pelvis filled with saline. Any leaks of air in the staple line can be repaired with interrupted sutures.

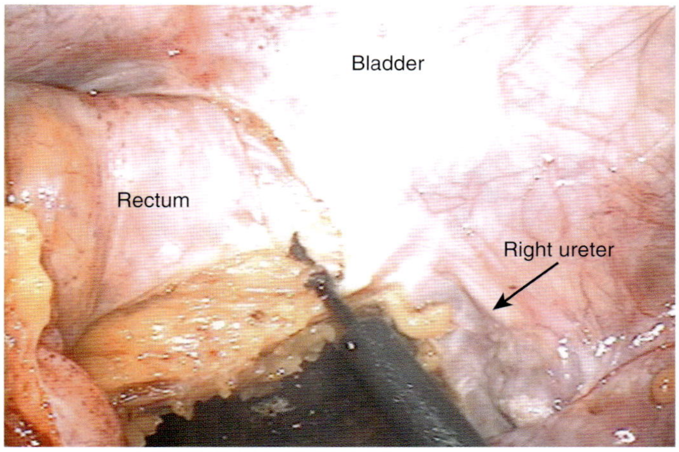

Figure 11-26

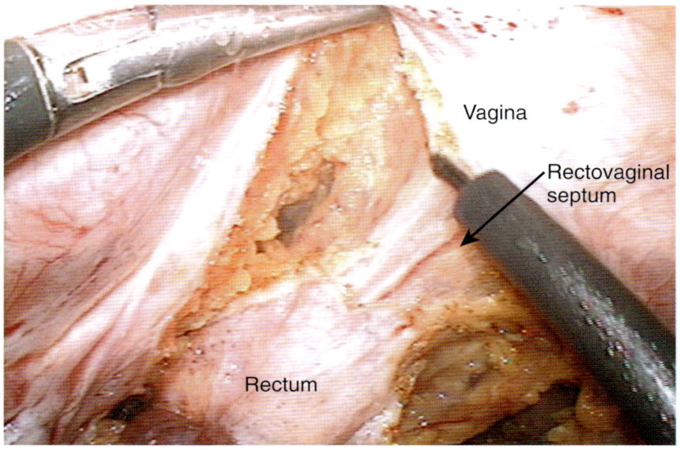

Figure 11-27

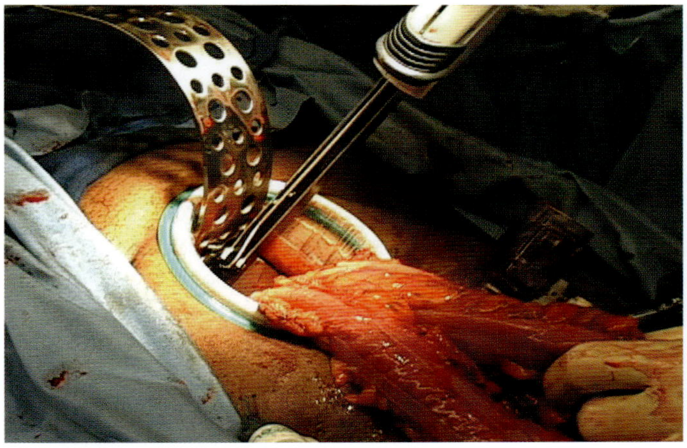
Figure 11-28

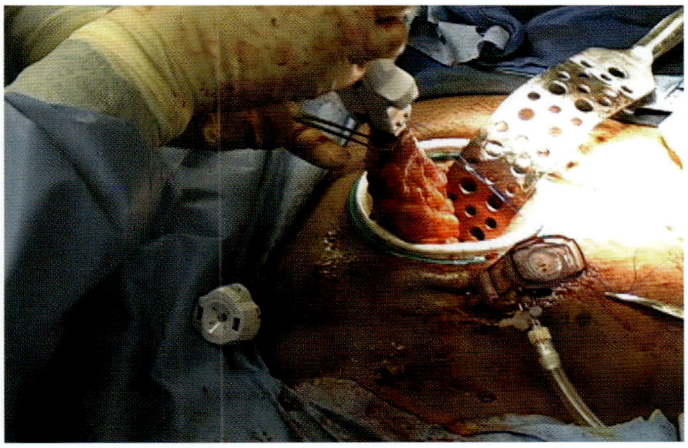
Figure 11-29

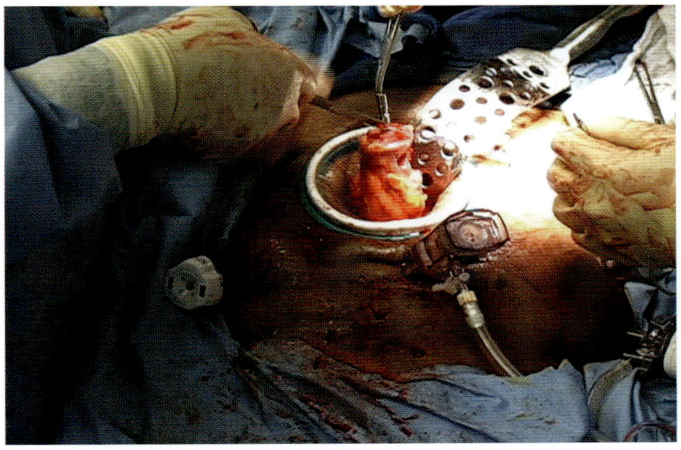
Figure 11-30

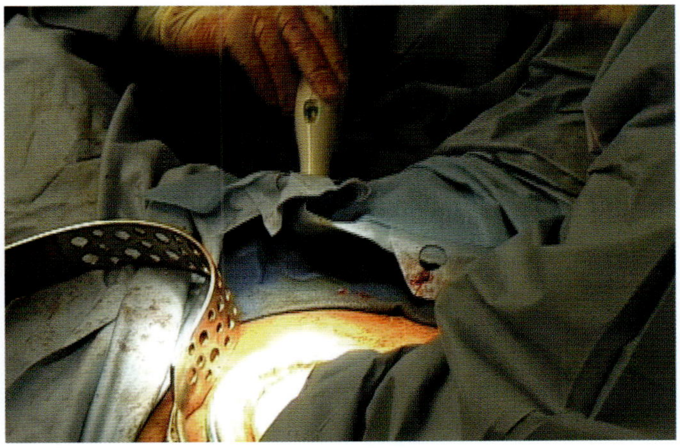
Figure 11-31

- A loop ileostomy is constructed if the patient has received neoadjuvant chemoradiation or if there is any question regarding the integrity of the anastomosis (Figure 11-32).

Step 4: Postoperative Care

The Pfannenstiel incision is closed with running No. 1 absorbable suture in the fascia. The patient recovers on the ward. An enterostomal therapy nurse is involved in the postoperative care and education of the patient. Early ambulation and early feeding are the practice for these patients. Patients require incentive spirometry, patient-controlled analgesia supplemented by nonsteroidal anti-inflammatory drugs, and deep vein thrombosis prophylaxis with sequential compression devices and subcutaneous anticoagulant. A drain can be placed in the pelvis through one of the trocar sites, to be removed when the drainage has decreased to less than 15 mL/hr in a 24-hour period.

Step 5: Pearls and Pitfalls

The most important and most feared complication after a low anterior resection with colorectal reconstruction is anastomotic leak, which occurs in approximately 10% of low rectal anastomosis procedures. If the loop ileostomy is in place, management of the anastomotic leak is simple with either interventional radiology drainage of an abscess or antibiotic treatment and maintenance of the Blake drain to provide management of the output. The loop ileostomy should be left in place until radiologic confirmation is obtained that the leak has healed. Transanal repair of the leak is sometimes possible, or simple observation is sufficient to allow the leak to heal.

Ileostomy difficulties may arise after creation of a loop ileostomy in an obese patient. Difficulty with maintaining an appliance can be overcome with the help of an enterostomal therapy nurse using a belt with concavity insertion and with local revision of the stoma as needed. Ileostomy closure should be considered after 6 to 8 weeks of recovery if no postoperative chemotherapy is required. Otherwise, the patient is most appropriately treated with continued diversion during chemotherapy because of the risk of severe diarrhea during the chemotherapy phase.

The patient should be warned that postoperative bowel function is not going to approach preoperative function because the rectal reservoir and the sigmoid have been removed. The patient normally has four to five small, rapidly occurring bowel movements on a daily basis as the colonic J pouch or the straight colorectal anastomosis matures. However, this rate of bowel movements may slow to a more reasonable rate, and the patient may gain control and the ability to defer bowel movement with time.

Selected Reading

Jayne DG, Thorpe HC, Copeland J, et al. Five-year follow-up of the Medical Research Council CLASICC trial of laparoscopically assisted versus open surgery for colorectal cancer. Br J Surg 2010;97:1638–45.

Kang SB, Park JW, Jeong SY, et al. Open versus laparoscopic surgery for mid or low rectal cancer after neoadjuvant chemoradiotherapy (COREAN trial): short-term outcomes of an open-label randomised controlled trial. Lancet Oncol 2010;11:637–45.

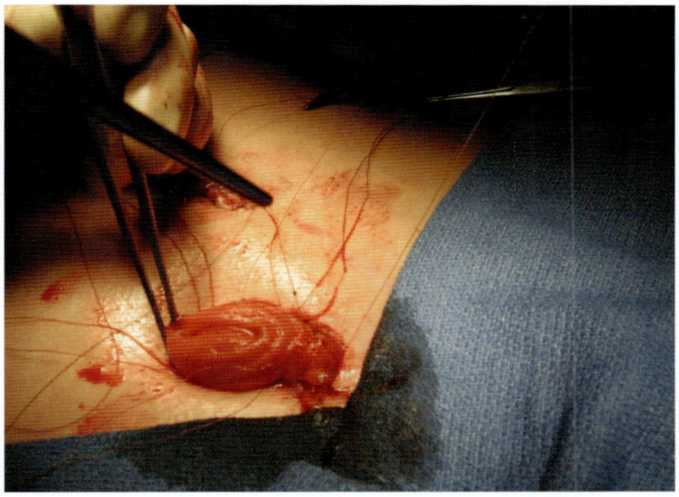

Figure 11-32

CHAPTER 12

Open Abdominal Perineal Resection

James W. Fleshman, Jr.

Step 1: Clinical Anatomy

The left colon lies along the left side of the abdomen suspended from the splenic flexure to the pelvic brim by lateral peritoneal attachments. The mesentery of the left colon arises from the midline of the abdomen along the aorta. The sigmoid colon has no lateral peritoneal attachments other than some congenital adhesions, which fix the apex of the sigmoid to the pelvic brim and the iliac fossa. Otherwise, the sigmoid colon is attached to the retroperitoneum through a midline mesentery arising from the inferior mesenteric artery (IMA) and extending down into the pelvis to the mesorectum. The splenic flexure is attached to the undersurface of the tip of the spleen, the lower edge of the tail of the pancreas, and the anterior surface of the left kidney by various levels of suspensory ligaments and peritoneal extensions. The blood supply to the left colon is based on the IMA, which arises from the anterior surface of the aorta just above the bifurcation of the common iliac arteries. The IMA extends anteriorly and bifurcates to produce the superior rectal artery feeding the sigmoid colon and the rectum. The left colic artery extends cephalad to provide the left colon and distal splenic flexure with blood supply through the arcade at the mesenteric edge known as the marginal artery of Drummond. The retroperitoneum behind the left colon contains the left ureter and the gonadal vessels lying over the psoas muscle. The ureter crosses the iliac vessels at the bifurcation of the iliac vessels into the external and internal iliac branches (Figure 12-1).

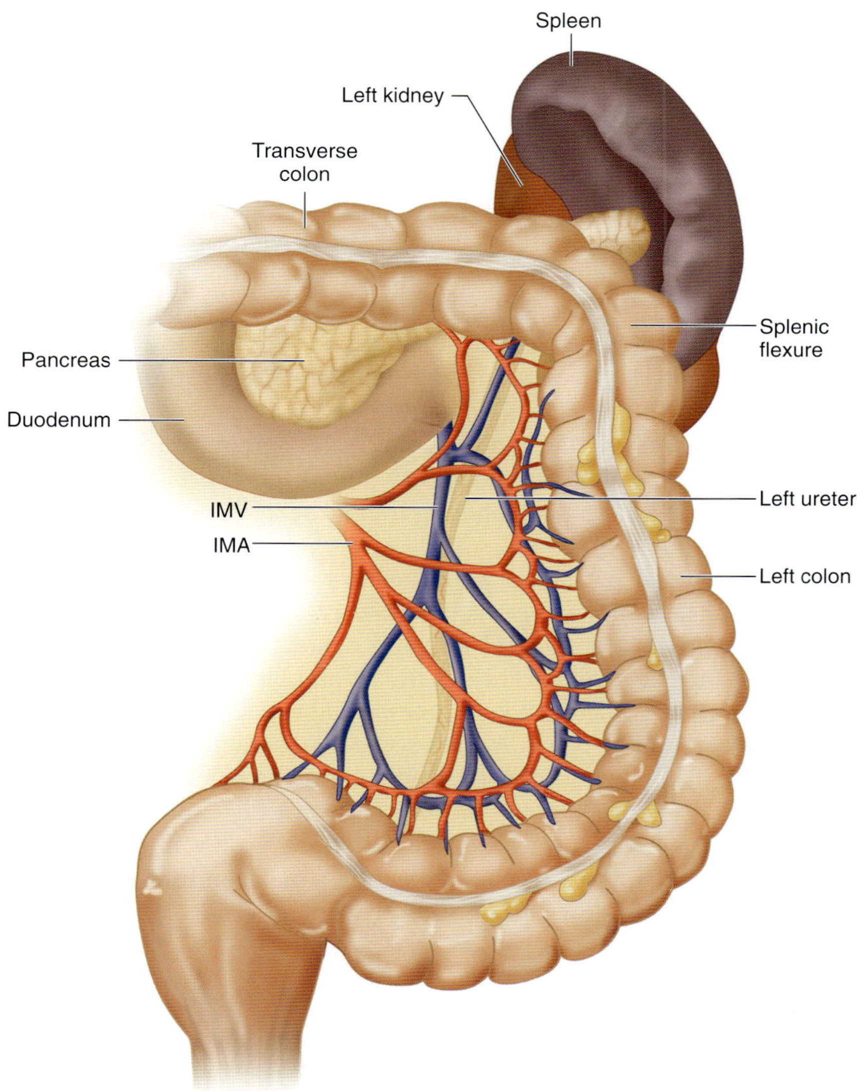
Spleen
Left kidney
Transverse colon
Pancreas
Duodenum
Splenic flexure
Left ureter
IMV
IMA
Left colon

Figure 12-1

Pelvic Anatomy

The pelvic anatomy is complex and has interrelationships between the rectum, vagina, uterus, ovaries, bladder, and prostate. The anatomy is important for pelvic dissection because of the various structures that are at risk, such as the splanchnic nerves, innervating the bladder, the ureters, and the organs themselves. The common iliac artery and vein on each side of the sacral promontory course along the posterior aspect of the pelvic brim. The hypogastric plexus of parasympathetic and sympathetic nerves is found between the bifurcation of the aorta and common iliacs. This plexus coalesces to the right and left to become the splanchnic pelvic nerves, which run along the inner aspect of the pelvic side wall to the level of the obturator fossa, and the anterolateral ligaments carrying the middle hemorrhoidal vessels. Nerve fibers course from the splanchnic nerve to the rectum through the anterolateral ligaments along the middle hemorrhoidal vessels. Extension of these nerves continues to either the vagina or the prostate as the nervi erigentes. A clear understanding of this nerve anatomy is crucial because it is easily damaged during dissection resulting in both sexual dysfunction and urinary bladder dysfunction (Figure 12-2*A*).

At the level of the sacral promontory, an areolar tissue plane begins behind the superior hemorrhoidal artery. The superior hemorrhoidal artery descends from the bifurcation of the IMA and splits at approximately S1-2 to give two major trunks down the posterior aspect of the rectum. The mesorectal envelope encases the fat and lymphatic and vascular supply to the rectum. The areolar tissue plane outside the mesorectal envelope is known as the "holy plane" and guides the dissection in the pelvis. A cross-sectional diagram of the pelvis shows the visceral peritoneum encasing the mesorectum with the areolar tissue plane between the visceral peritoneum and the parietal peritoneum posteriorly. The parietal peritoneum covers a nerve and venous plexus over the sacrum and the musculature of the side wall of the pelvis. Maintaining dissection within the areolar tissue plane between the parietal and the visceral peritoneal layers protects all of the crucial structures in the pelvis (Figure 12-2*B*).

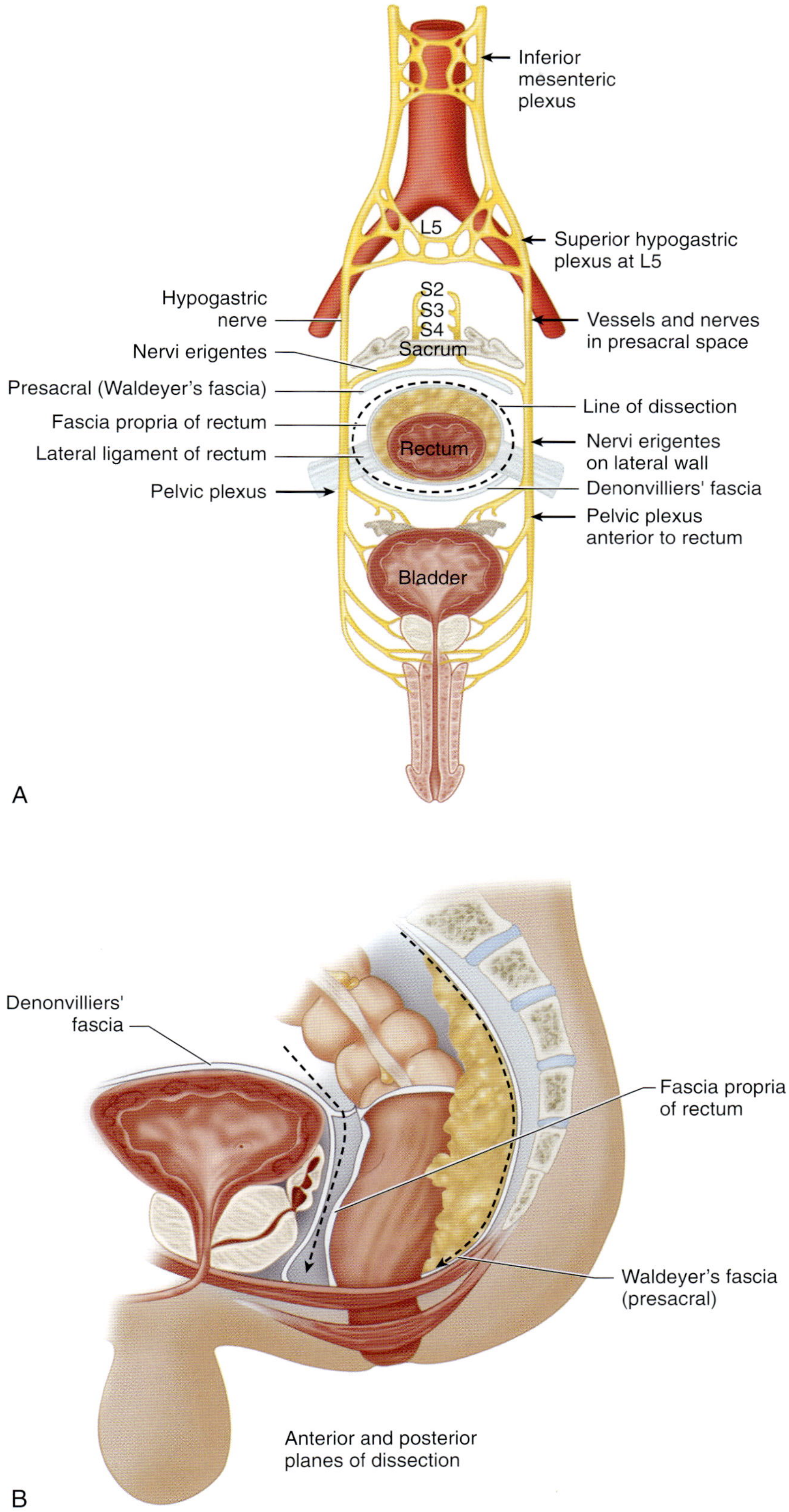

Figure 12-2A-B

The rectum descends through the middle of the pelvis following the curve of the sacrum and at the level of the coccyx makes a right angle to exit through the pelvic floor via the anal canal. The levator ani muscles on either side of the pelvic floor form the support diaphragm of the pelvis and extend up onto the side wall of the pelvis to insert in the ischiospinous ligament attachments covering the nerves and vessels of the deep pelvic floor. The tip of the coccyx attaches to the pubococcygeal ligament, which supports the puborectalis muscle as a semicircular sling from the pubis around the back of the rectum. This muscle closes the top of the anal canal anterior to posterior (Figure 12-3).

The anterior pelvic structures including the bladder, prostate, and vagina are separated from the rectum by the rectoprostatic or rectovaginal septum. A visceral peritoneal layer known as Denonvilliers' fascia is the posterior boundary of the anterior structures. This fascia protects the seminal vesicles and prostate during dissection. The areolar tissue plane surrounding the mesorectum fat continues around the entire rectum to the anterior surface of the rectum below the cul-de-sac of the pelvis. The plane is found behind or posterior to Denonvilliers' fascia. The anterolateral ligaments of the rectum carry the middle hemorrhoidal vessels into the mesorectal envelope through the visceral fascia from an anterolateral direction. Dissection and transection of these middle hemorrhoidal vessels reveals the anterior areolar tissue plane behind Denonvilliers' fascia, which can be followed all the way down to the anal canal.

The ureters, which have been described as running into the pelvic area over the pelvic brim crossing the common iliac artery and vein on either side of the pelvis, continue into the pelvis along the side wall of the pelvis toward the posterior aspect of the bladder. In the nonoperated, pristine pelvis, the ureters are higher up along the side wall of the pelvis aiming toward the posterior aspect of the trigone of the bladder. In females, the ureters run between the arterial blood supply of the uterus along the anterior lateral side wall of the pelvis. In males, ureters are not exposed during the distal pelvic dissection. The ureters may be drawn posteriorly after a previous operation but are normally well protected anteriorly and laterally. In a previously operated pelvis, it is always wise to place ureteral stents at the beginning of the procedure to aid in identification of the aberrantly placed ureters.

Anal Anatomy

The upper anal canal begins at the puborectalis sling or the anorectal ring, which sits at the level of the pelvic floor and can be palpated through the anal canal as a bulge posteriorly (Figure 12-3, *inset*). The longitudinal muscles of the rectum continue into the anus as the intersphincteric plane demarcating the line between autonomic internal sphincter and somatic external sphincter fibers all the way down to the level of the anal canal skin where the intersphincteric groove is palpable. Outside the circular fibers of the external sphincter that encircle the rectum, the ischiorectal fossa fat is found. The pudendal nerve and vessels traverse the ischiorectal fat from each ischial spine through Alcock's canal to the posterolateral aspect of the anal canal. During the perineal portion of a procedure, the pudendal nerves and vessels must be controlled.

The rectovaginal and rectoprostatic septum descends all the way to the level of the perineum anteriorly. The transverse perineal muscle separates the anterior and posterior perineum. The terminal fibers of the longitudinal muscle of the rectum insert into the skin of the anal canal just outside the anal verge as the corrugator cutanei ani and cause the ridges that are noticed around the anal canal. The internal sphincter is the hypertrophied circular muscle of the wall of the rectum. The lowest portion of the internal sphincter can be palpated as a groove where the longitudinal fibers insert on the skin.

Within the anal canal, the dentate line is the junction between the cuboidal epithelium of the anal transition zone, which is the terminal mucosal layer of the rectum, and the squamous epidermal cells of the anal canal skin. Gland openings (or crypts) are found in the dentate line

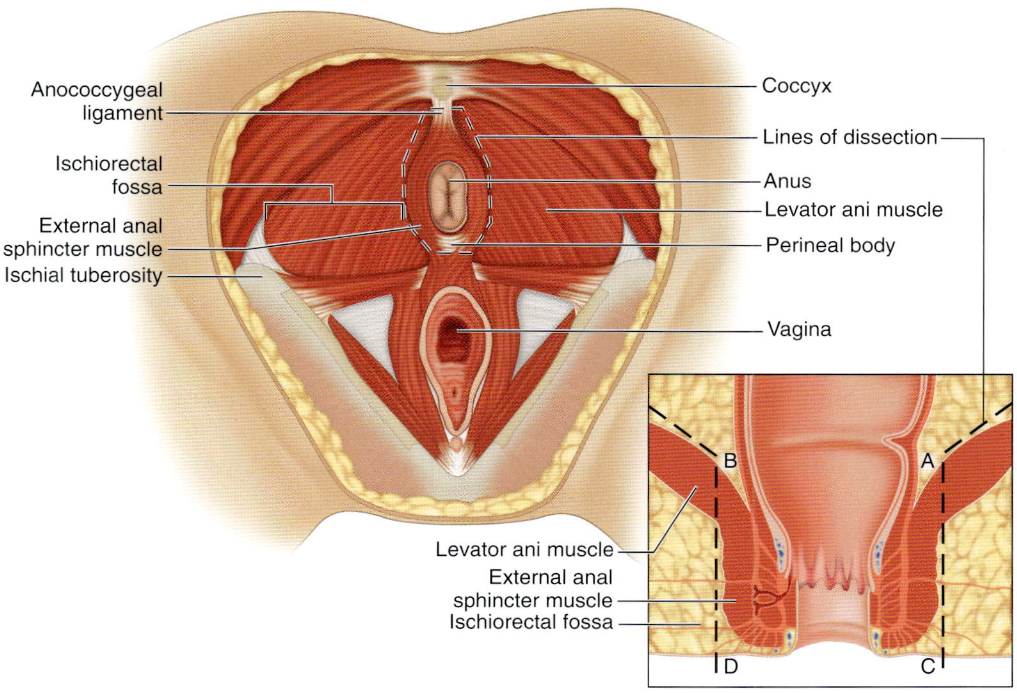
Anococcygeal ligament
Ischiorectal fossa
External anal sphincter muscle
Ischial tuberosity
Coccyx
Lines of dissection
Anus
Levator ani muscle
Perineal body
Vagina
Levator ani muscle
External anal sphincter muscle
Ischiorectal fossa
A
B
C
D

Figure 12-3

at the base of the Morgagni columns, which are interdigitating lines of squamous epithelium into the cuboidal and columnar epithelium of the distal rectum. The anal transition zone is the most highly innervated section of the rectum and anal canal containing nerve fibers sensing temperature, vibration, electrical stimulation, pressure, liquid, solid, and gas. The dentate line lies approximately halfway along the surgical anal canal, which extends from the palpable anal verge all the way up to the anorectal ring palpated at the puborectalis sling posteriorly. The anoderm within the anal canal, cephalad to the anal verge, has no hair follicles.

Step 2: Preoperative Considerations

Open abdominal perineal resection of the rectum is commonly performed for patients with large rectal cancers extending into the external sphincter or locally advanced tumors that prevent a deep pelvic reconstruction because of tumor features. The preparation for an abdominal perineal resection is very simple. Clear liquids for several days beforehand and a single enema the day before surgery is adequate preparation. It is easier to operate on these patients if they do not have a rectum full of solid stool. The patient requires preoperative antibiotics, compression and chemical deep vein thrombosis prophylaxis, and enterostomal therapy consultation for marking of the left lower quadrant colostomy site. Almost all of these patients will have had chemoradiation for either anal cancer or rectal cancer and may require vacuum-assisted closure (VAC) at the end of the procedure for wound management. Patients who have large tumors and require excision of the entire pelvic floor musculature require reconstruction of the pelvic floor with biologic mesh at the time of the perineal portion of the procedure. Ureteral stent placement is necessary only if the tumor is large and the patient has had previous surgery.

Step 3: Operative Steps

- The abdomen is explored through an open abdominal midline incision with the patient in modified lithotomy position using Allen's stirrups. A Bookwalter retractor and ring drape are used for exposure. The sigmoid colon and left colon are retracted toward the midline (Figures 12-4 and 12-5*A*), and the incision is made along the base of the left colon mesentery along the left gutter to enter the avascular plane behind the mesentery of the left colon anterior to the retroperitoneal structures (Figure 12-6). This incision exposes the left ureter in its course along the left gutter (Figure 12-7). The blunt dissection can be used to develop the plane in a medial and a cephalad direction to protect the ureter (Figures 12-5*B* and 12-8).

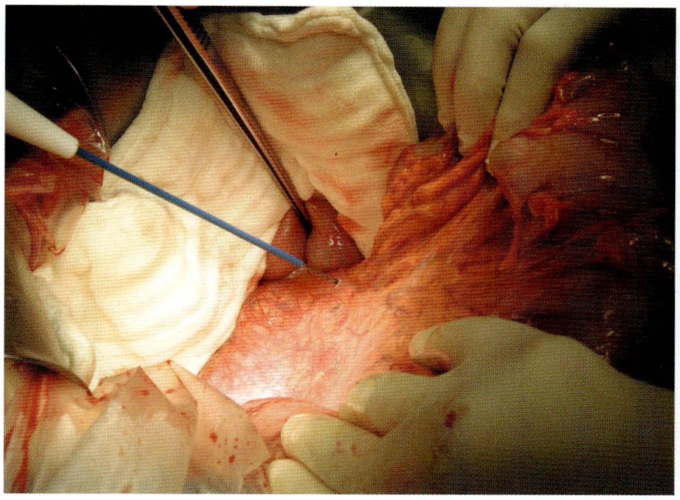
Figure 12-4

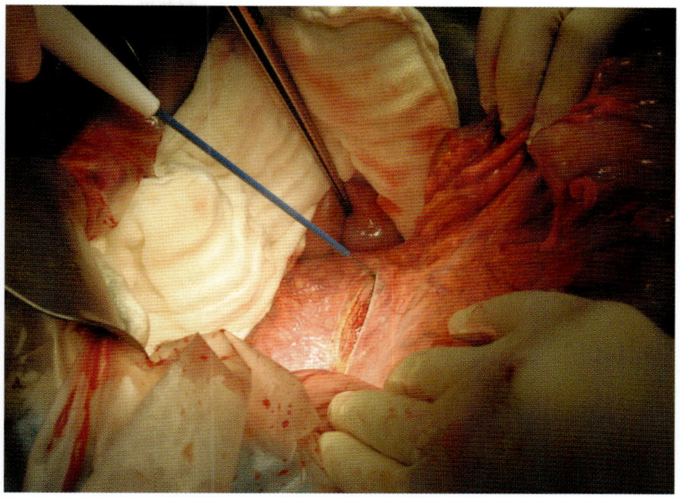
Figure 12-6

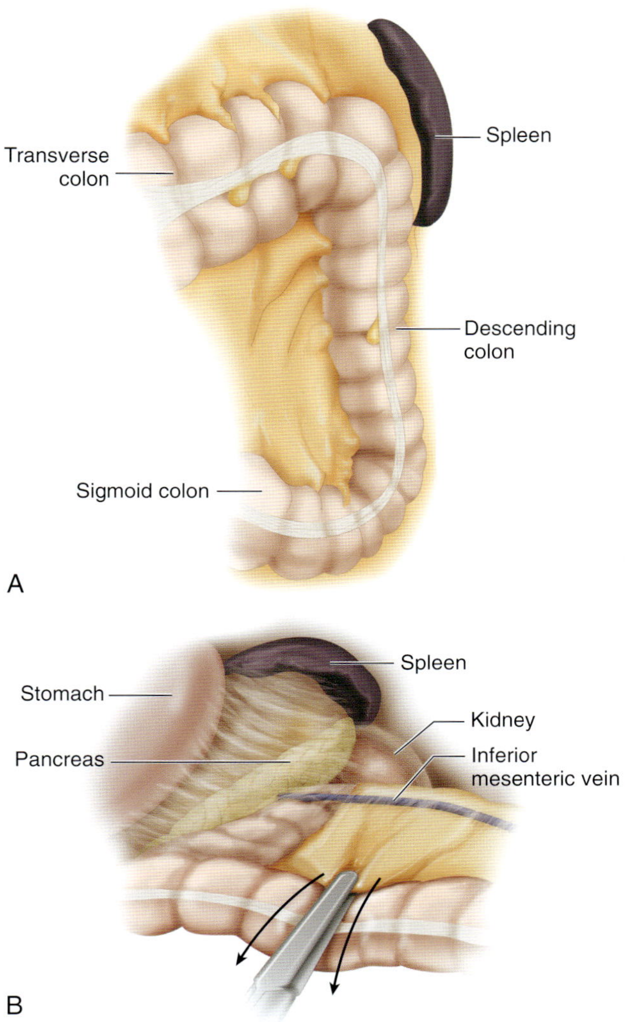

Figure 12-5A-B

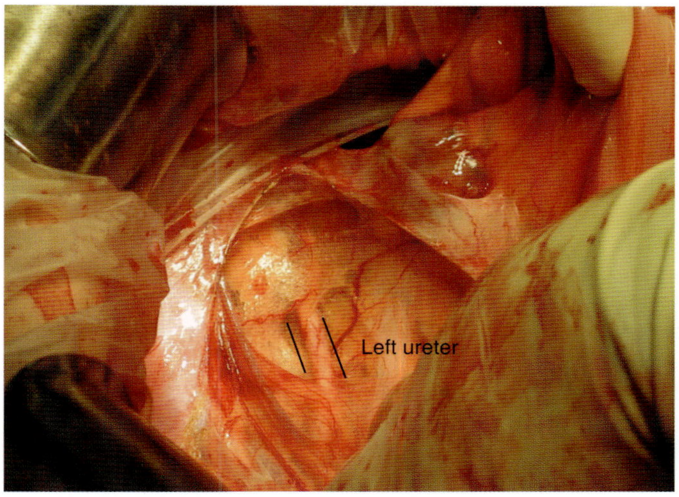

Figure 12-7

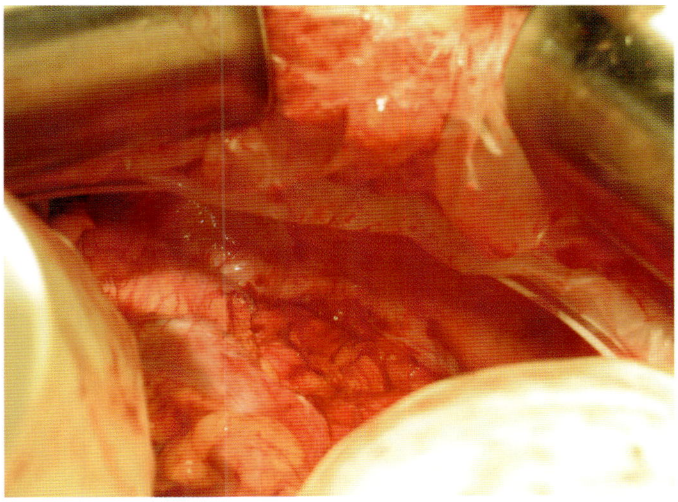
Figure 12-8

- The splenic flexure is mobilized from the anterior surface of the kidney. An incision is made over the dissecting finger to release the lateral attachments (Figure 12-9). The base of the splenic flexure mesentery is released from the tail of the pancreas (Figure 12-10) and the tip of the spleen (Figure 12-11). The transverse colon is released from the overlying omentum by incising the avascular attachments on the antimesenteric surface to release the splenic flexure completely (Figure 12-12).

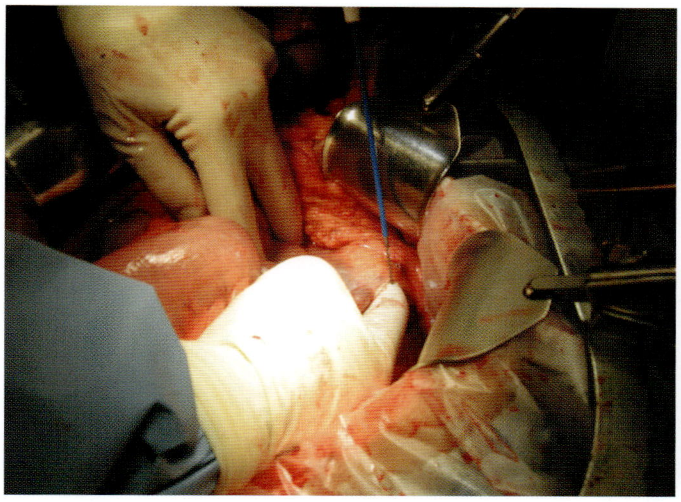

Figure 12-9

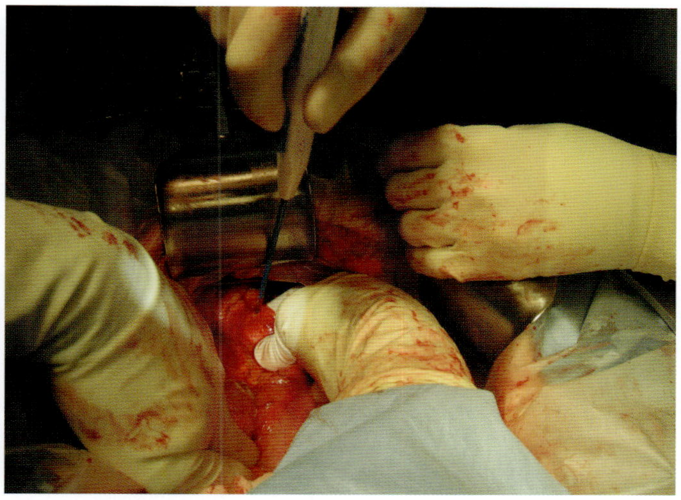

Figure 12-10

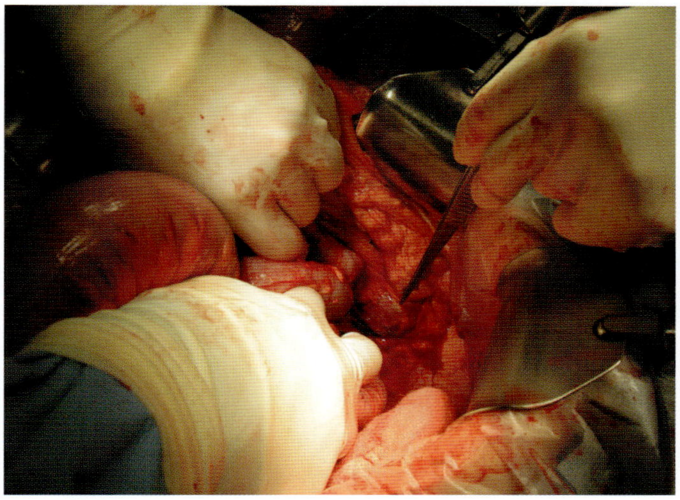

Figure 12-11

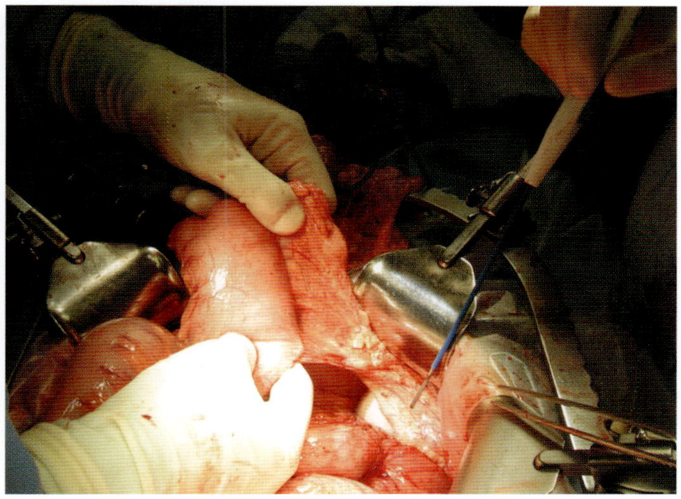

Figure 12-12

- The IMA and inferior mesenteric vein (IMV) are isolated at their origin along the aorta at the base of the left colon mesentery (Figures 12-13 through 12-15). The vessels are identified, ligated, and divided; this results in a complete release of the left colon mesentery to the pelvis and full exposure of the retroperitoneum from the splenic flexure to the pelvic brim (Figure 12-16).

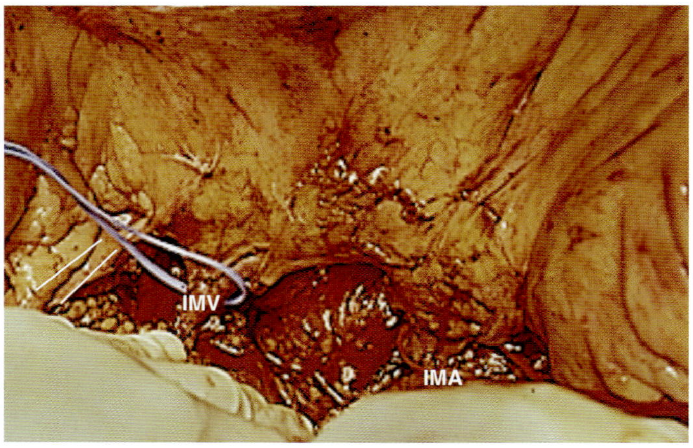

Figure 12-13

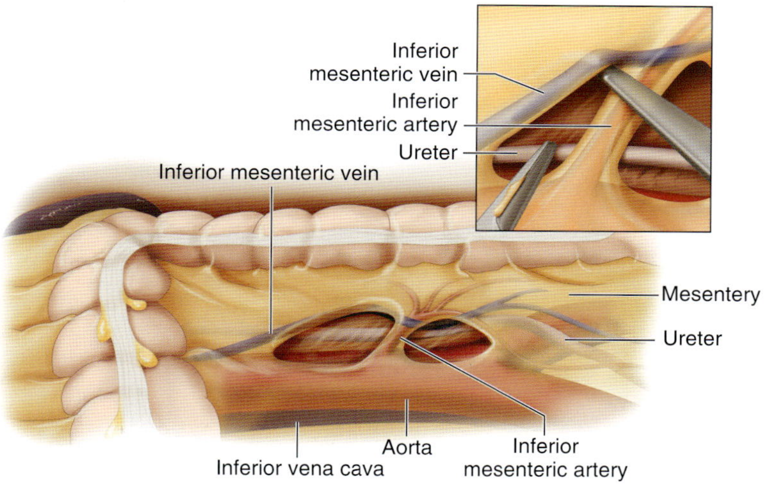

Figure 12-14

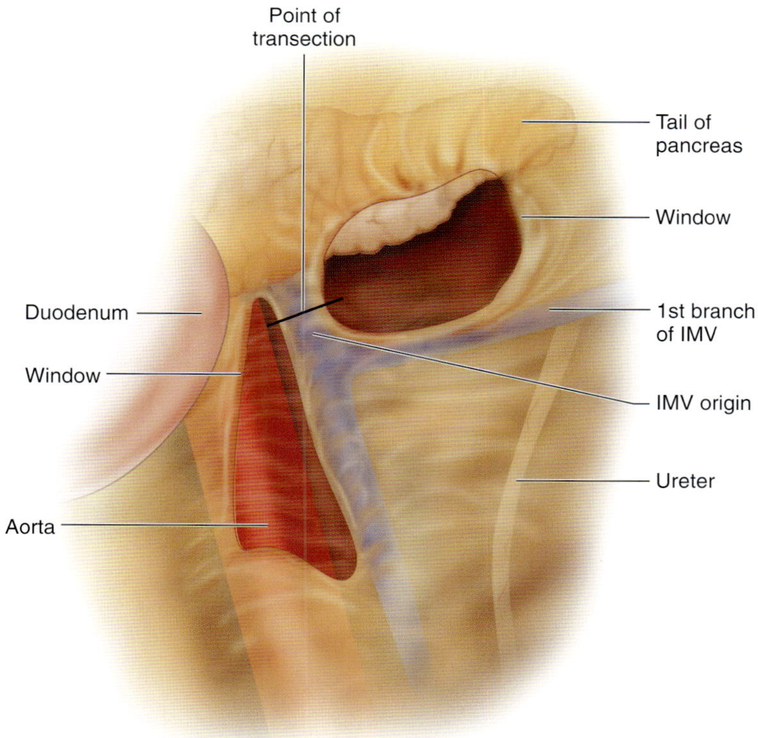

Figure 12-15

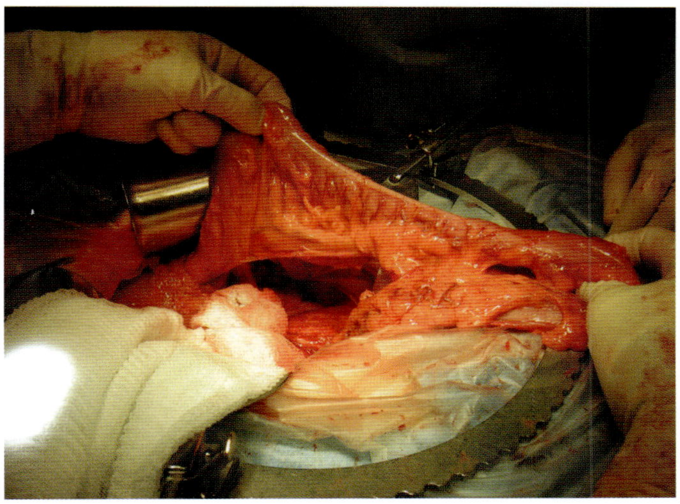

Figure 12-16

- The rectum is retracted anteriorly to expose the avascular areolar tissue plane at the sacral promontory (Figure 12-17). The splanchnic nerves are protected at the pelvic brim (Figure 12-18). The areolar tissue plane is followed all the way to the pelvis protecting the hypogastric nerve plexus (Figure 12-19), the splanchnic nerves, and the ureters on both sides of the pelvis (Figure 12-20).

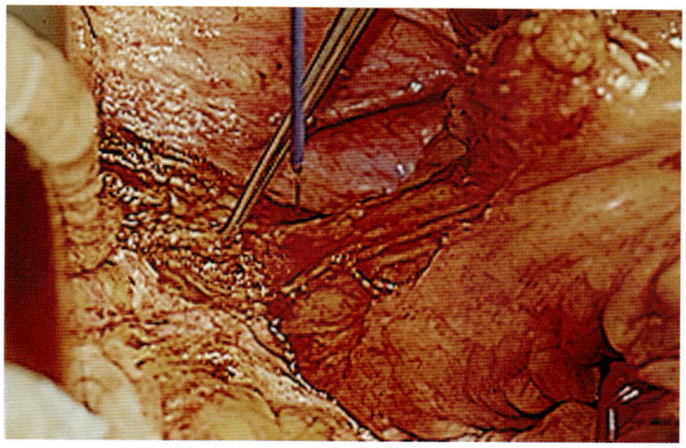

Figure 12-17

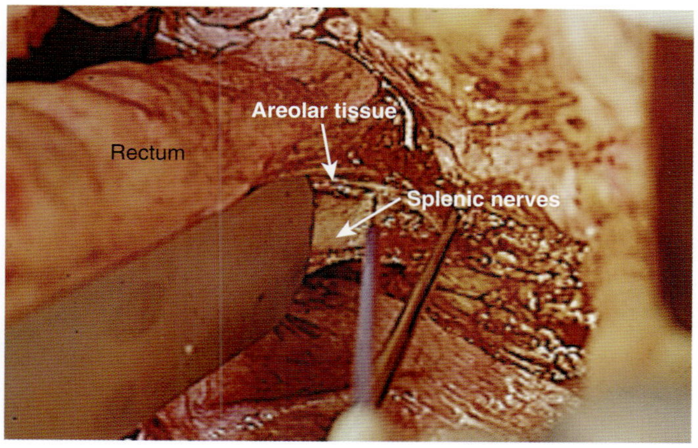

Figure 12-18

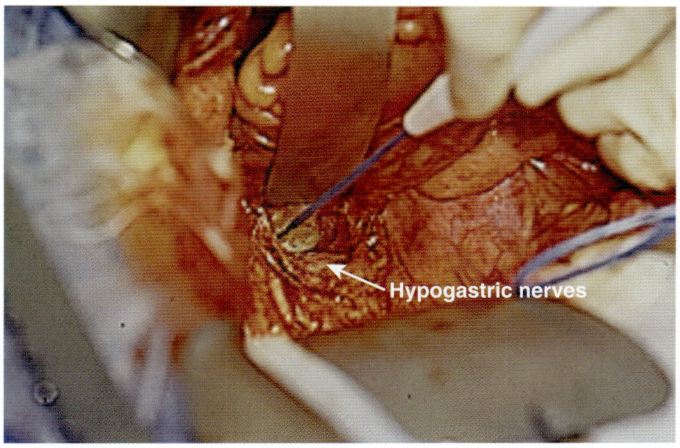

Figure 12-19

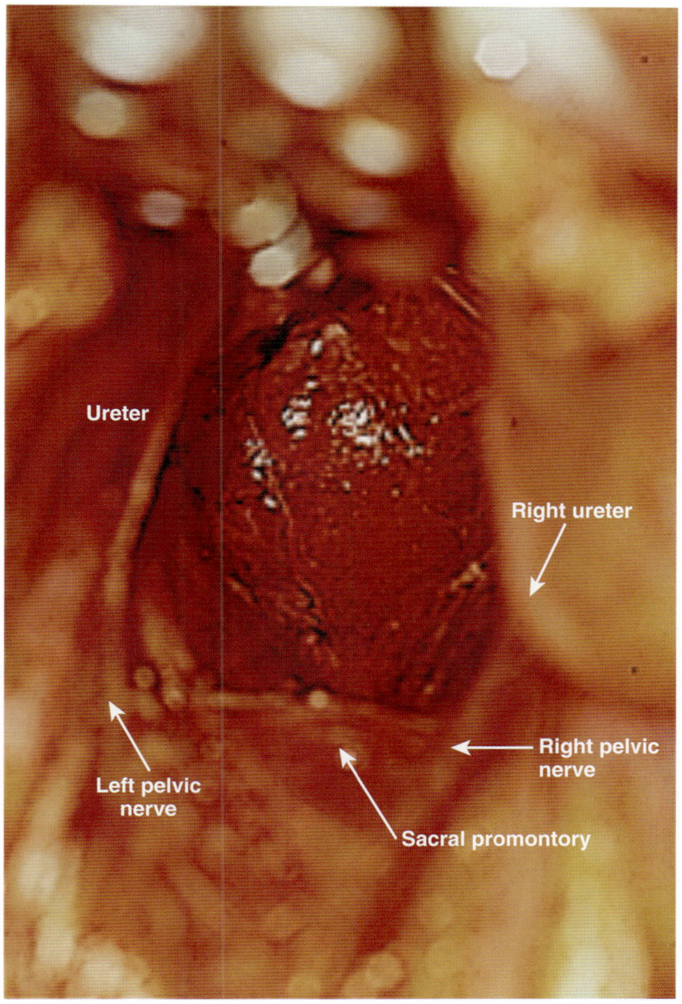

Figure 12-20

- The dissection is carried into the pelvis, releasing the mesorectum in toto from the sacrum, exposing the entire pelvis, and resulting in a double-lobed mesentery of the rectum retracted anteriorly (Figure 12-21). This maneuver allows the lateral pelvic nerves and the ureters to be seen in detail and protected (Figure 12-22).
- The anterior dissection of the rectum is begun at the cul-de-sac. An incision is made behind the bladder, and a Thorlakson retractor can be used to lift the bladder anteriorly to open the rectoprostatic or rectovaginal septum. The areolar tissue plane is followed all the way to the anal canal (Figure 12-23). The anterolateral ligaments on either side of the rectum can be divided with electrocautery to release the rectum from the deep pelvic side walls (Figure 12-24). During this dissection, it is important to know where the left ureter is and to protect any other structures. Medial traction on the rectum exposes the areolar tissue along the left pelvic brim.

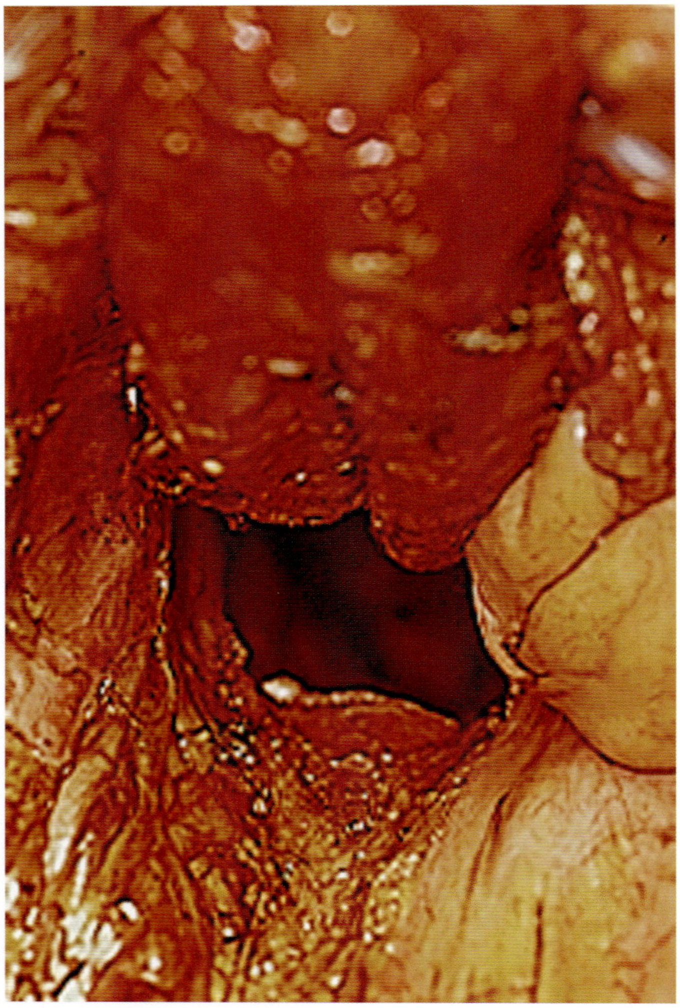

Figure 12-21

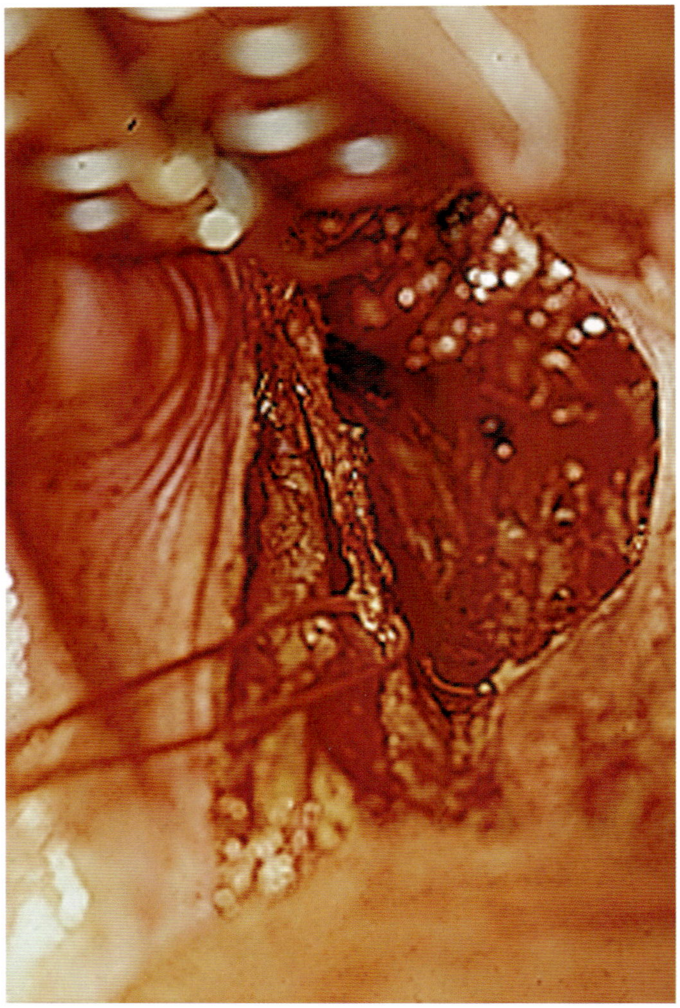

Figure 12-22

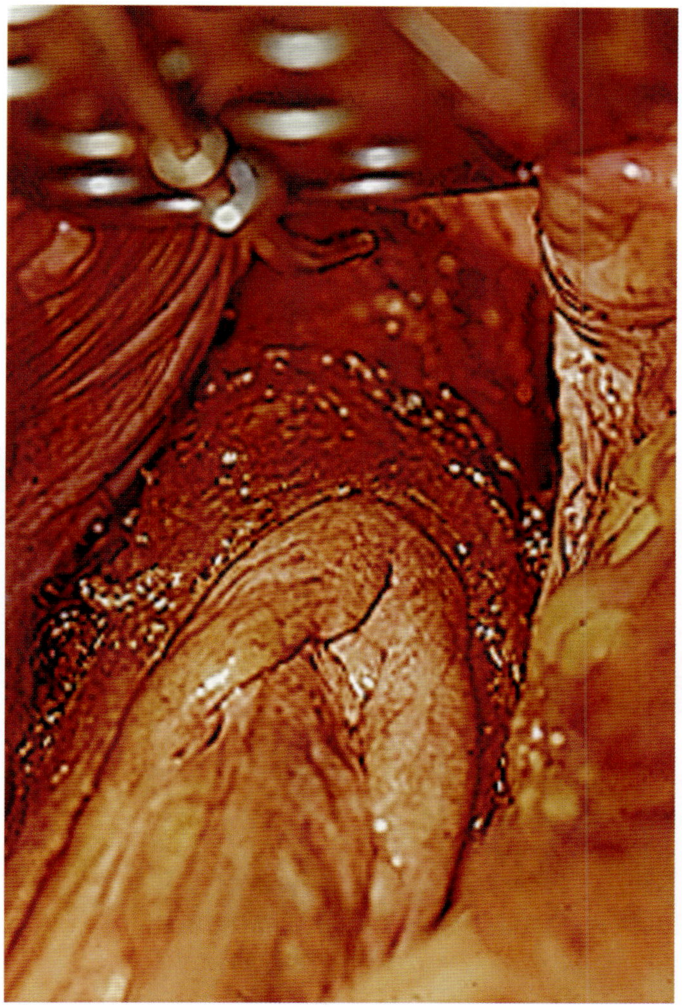

Figure 12-23

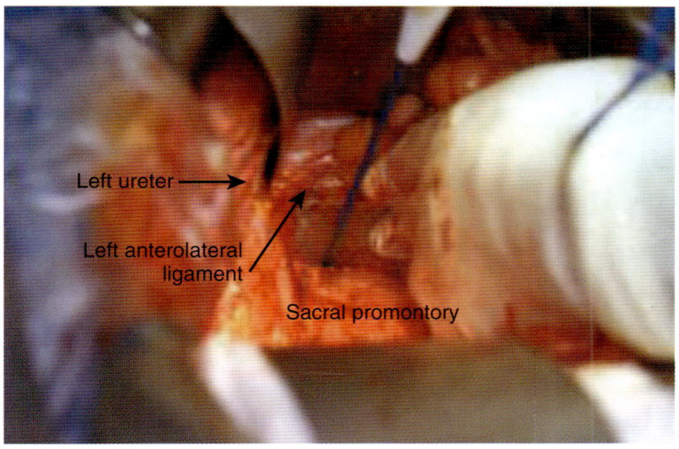

Figure 12-24

- The descending sigmoid colon junction is divided with a 75-mm linear cutter stapler at the site for the planned colostomy (Figure 12-25). The left lower quadrant colostomy site is constructed by excising a 3-cm disk of skin (Figures 12-26 and 12-27*A-C*) and splitting the

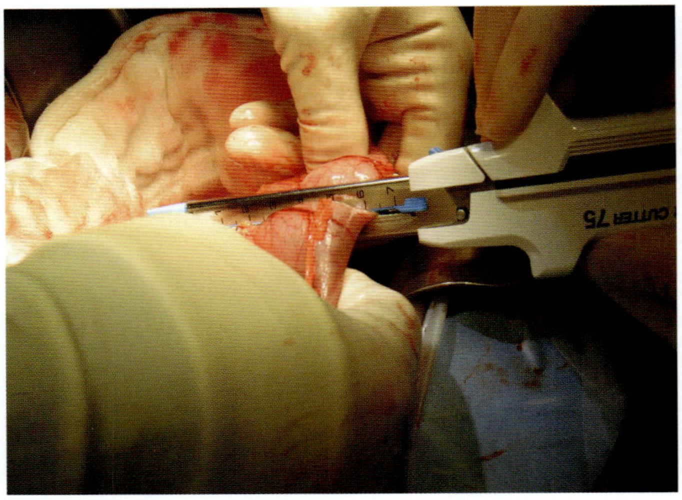

Figure 12-25

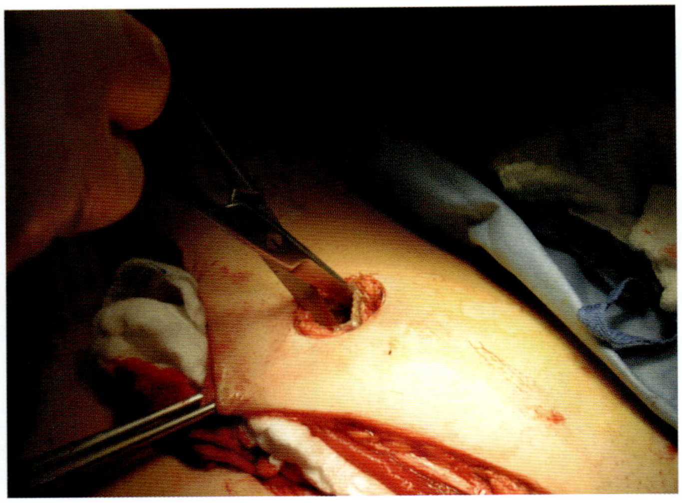

Figure 12-26

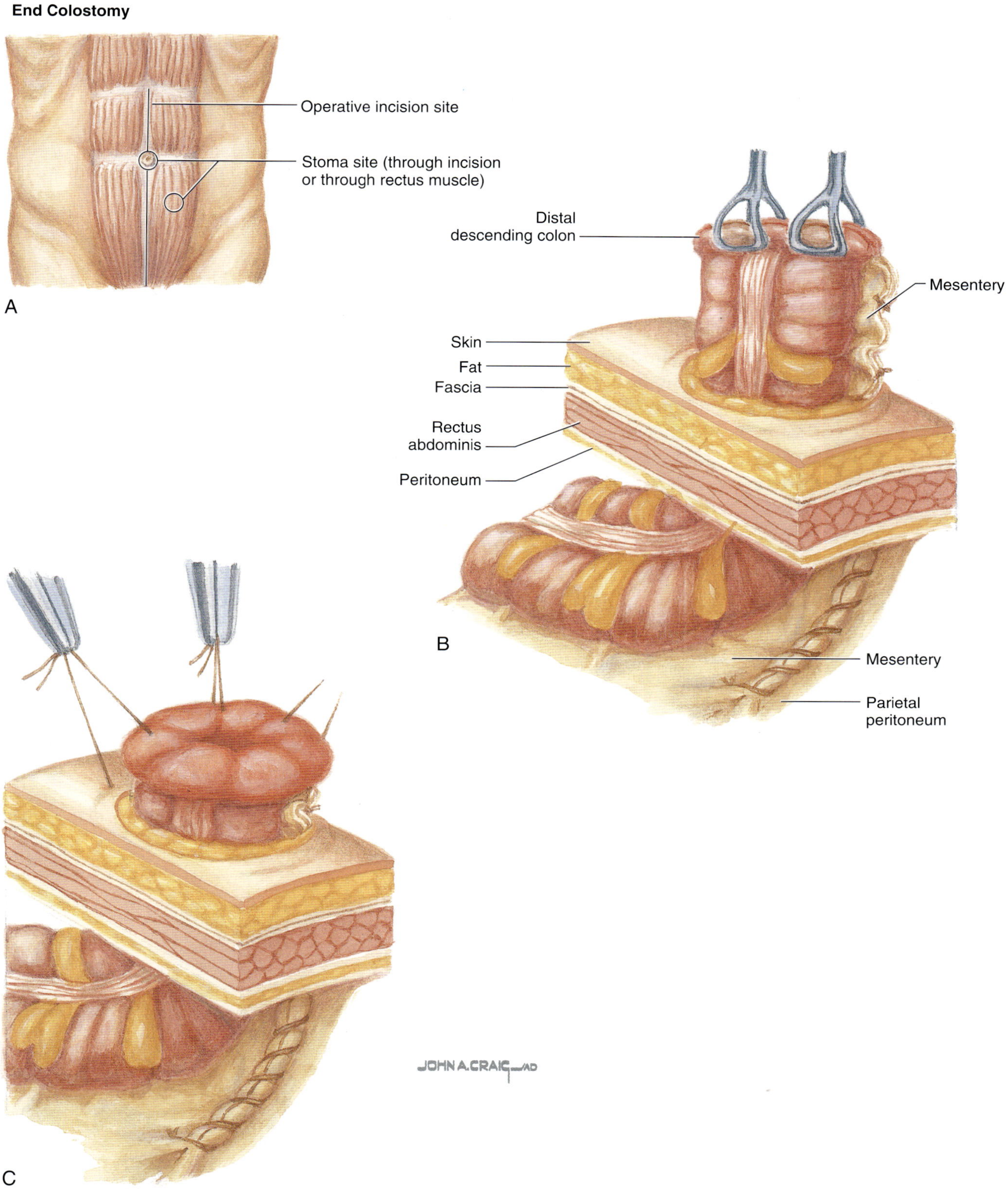

Figure 12-27A-C *Netter illustration from www.netterimages.com.*

rectus muscle in the middle of the bundle to deliver two fingerbreadths (Figure 12-28). The cut end of the bowel is brought out through the anterior abdominal wall and "matured" to the skin with circumferential interrupted 3-0 absorbable suture (Figure 12-29). The large Blake drain is brought out through a stab wound in the lower abdomen, and the abdominal wall is closed with a running absorbable suture. The skin is closed with skin staples, and the ostomy appliance and dressing are applied.

- The patient is moved to a stretcher and rolled back onto the operating table to the prone-jackknife position with a roll under the hips and rolls under the chest, with the buttocks taped apart (Figure 12-30). The perineum is prepared and draped, and the anal canal is closed with a subcutaneous circumanal suture at the anal verge (Figure 12-31).

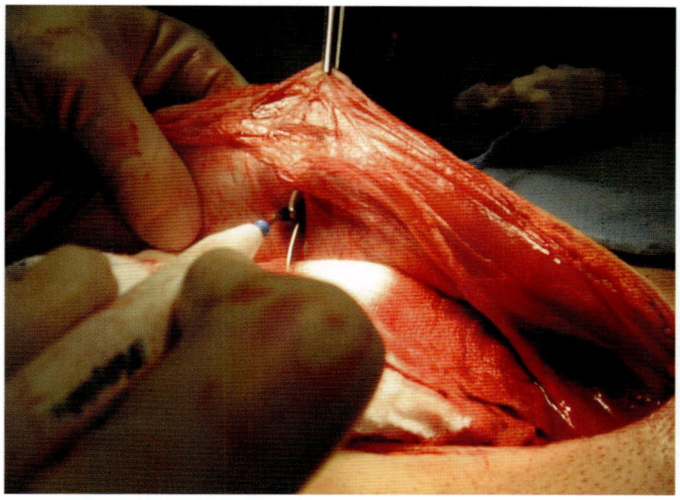

Figure 12-28

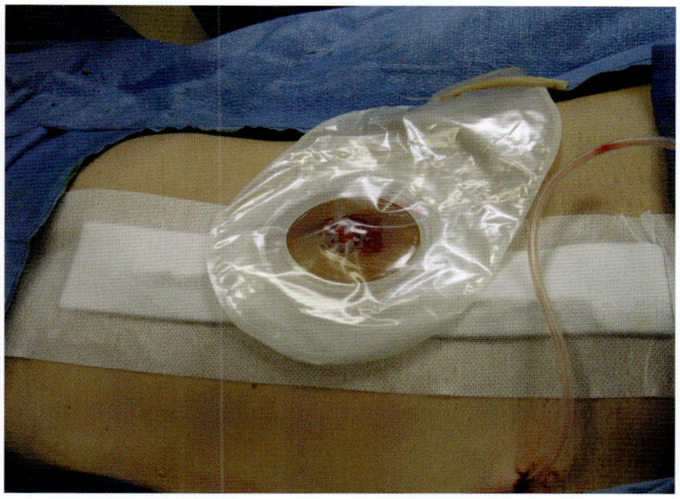

Figure 12-29

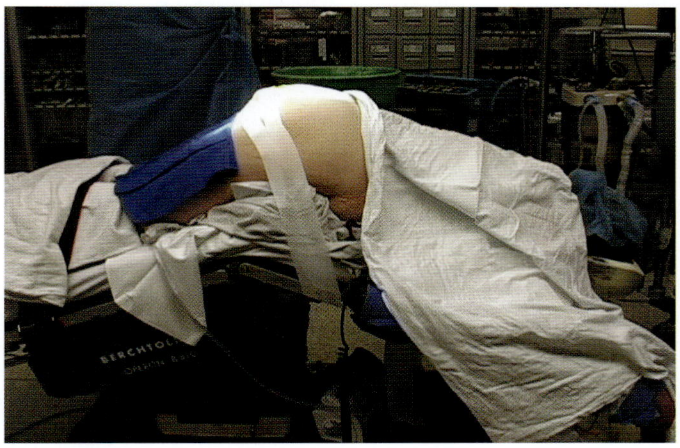

Figure 12-30

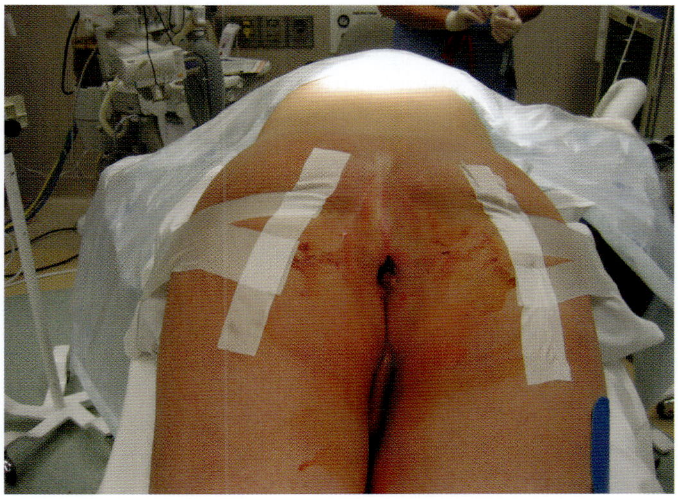

Figure 12-31

- An elliptical incision is made on the perineal skin from the tip of the coccyx to the anterior perineal body outside the external sphincter and carried into the ischial rectal fossa (Figure 12-32). The dissection in the ischial rectal fossa extends up to the undersurface of the levator muscles separating the fat from the outer aspect of the external sphincter. The bear claw St. Mark's retractor is useful to maintain exposure during this portion of the dissection (Figure 12-33). The pudendal nerves and vessels are identified and controlled in the lateral aspects of the ischiorectal fossa space. The tip of the coccyx is either incised and removed or exposed for the transverse incision made in the pelvic floor anterior to the tip of the coccyx (Figure 12-34). The posterior pelvic space is entered, and the previously dissected space is easily exposed (Figure 12-35).
- The muscles of the levator plate are incised along each side of the rectum over a finger placed into the pelvic cavity through the posterior incision (Figures 12-3 and 12-36). Depending on the size of the tumor, a cuff of muscle can be left, or the entire muscle can be removed. As the dissection moves anteriorly, the posterior aspect of the vagina or prostate is eventually encountered. The vagina, or a portion thereof, can be excised to provide anterior clear margins (Figure 12-37). The dissection must be maintained in the vagina posterior to the lateral aspect of the vagina where the nerves and vessels are found. A portion of the coccyx can be removed during this dissection to provide clear margins for a posteriorly placed tumor. This removal is easily accomplished with an incision along the edges of the coccyx and transection of the osteocartilaginous junction with rongeurs (bone cutters). This maneuver also facilitates total excision of the pelvic floor.

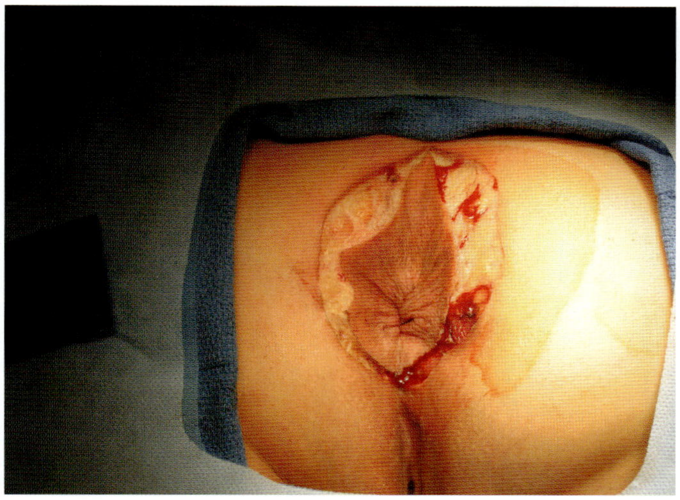
Figure 12-32

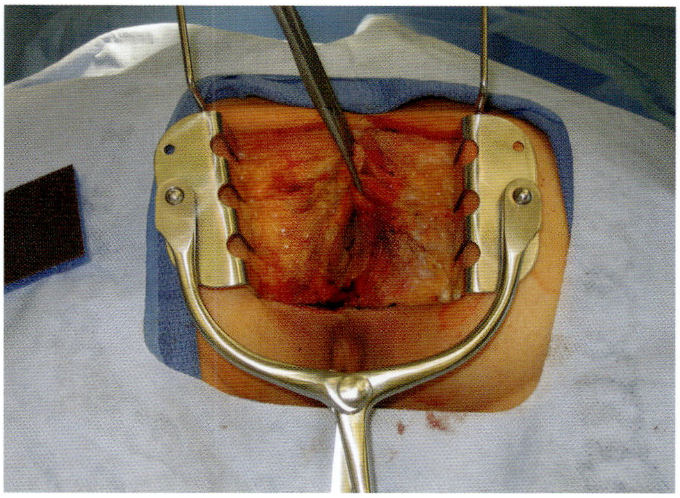
Figure 12-33

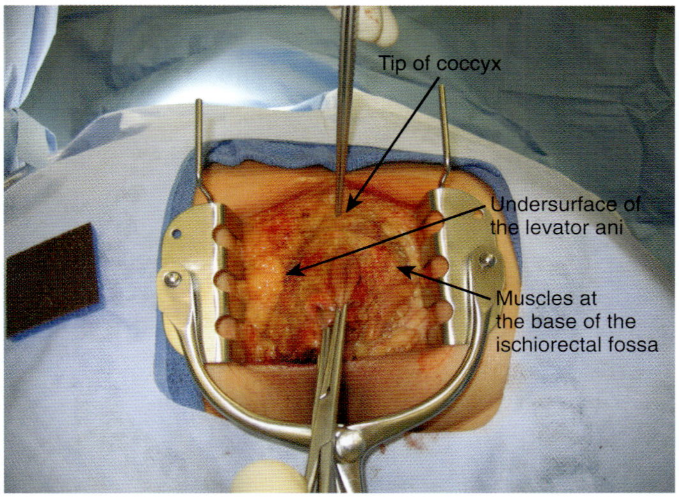

Figure 12-34

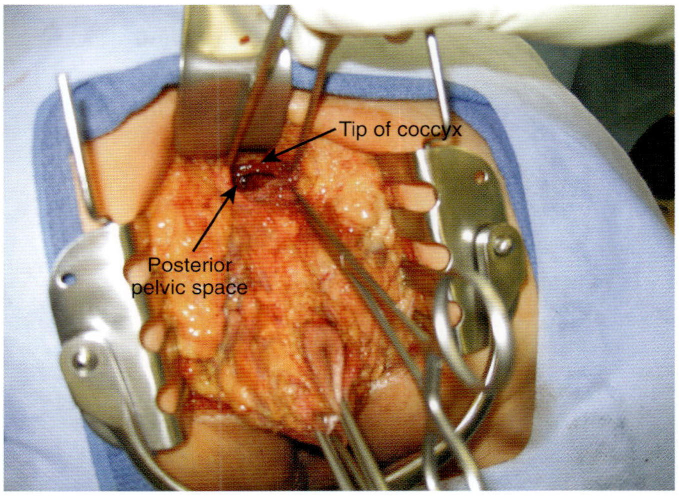

Figure 12-35

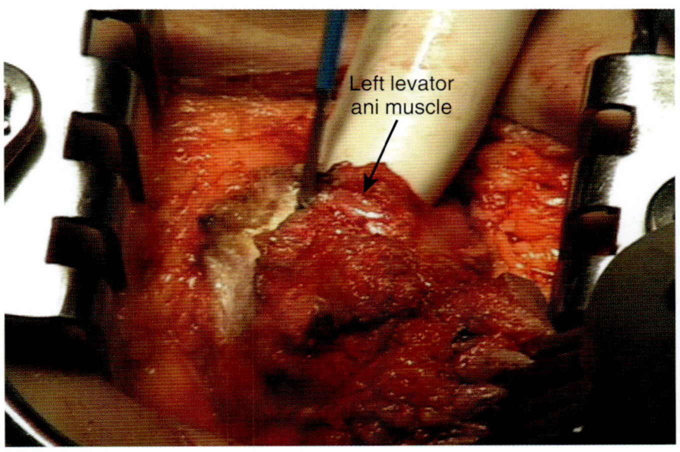

Figure 12-36

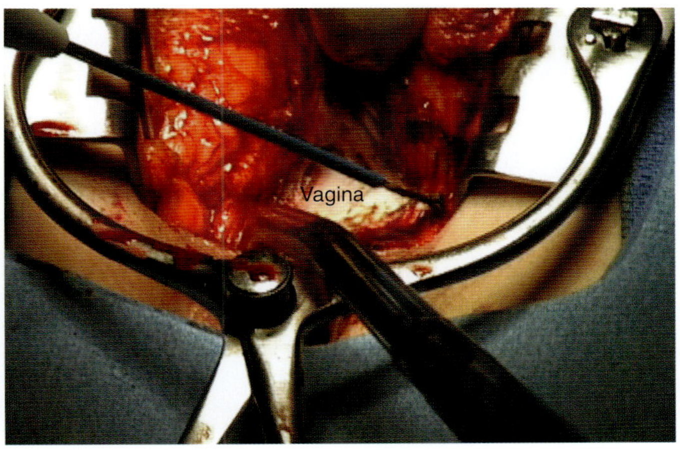

Figure 12-37

- The rectum and sigmoid colon are delivered through the posterior aspect of the pelvic floor opening (Figure 12-38). The posterior aspect of the bladder and the deep pelvis are now exposed (Figure 12-39). The Blake drain from within the abdominal cavity is brought down into the pelvis. The decision is made whether the closure can be accomplished with sutures to approximate the muscle cuff in the midline or whether a biomesh replacement is needed (Figure 12-40).
- The subcutaneous fat of the ischiorectal fossa is reapproximated in the midline with layers of interrupted horizontal mattress sutures of absorbable suture to the level of the subcuticular layer, which is left open. Polysporin ointment and a 4 × 4 gauze are applied (Figure 12-41).

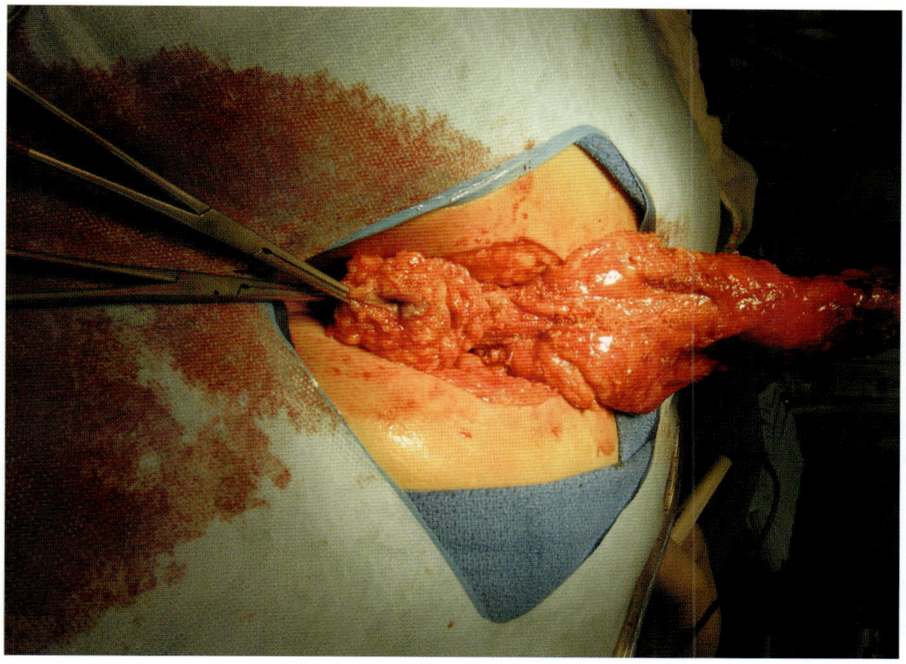
Figure 12-38

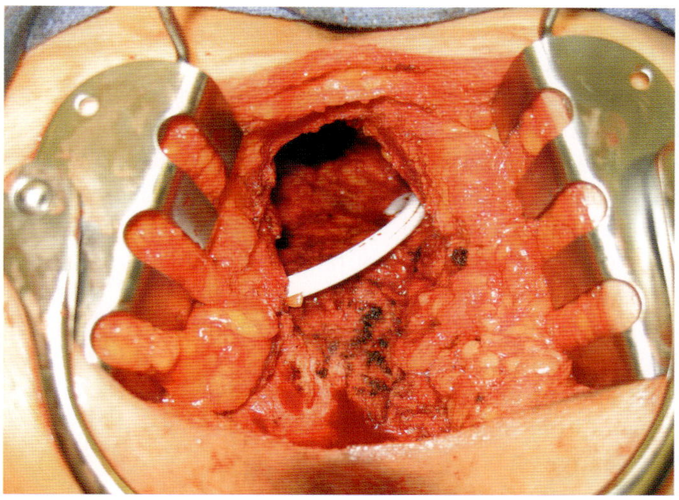
Figure 12-39

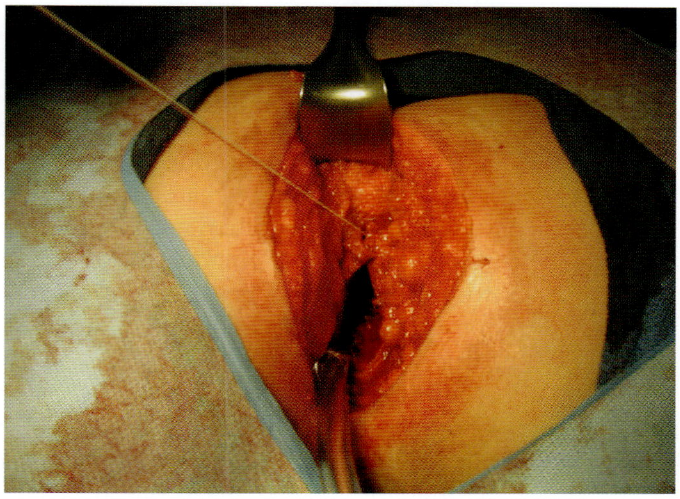
Figure 12-40

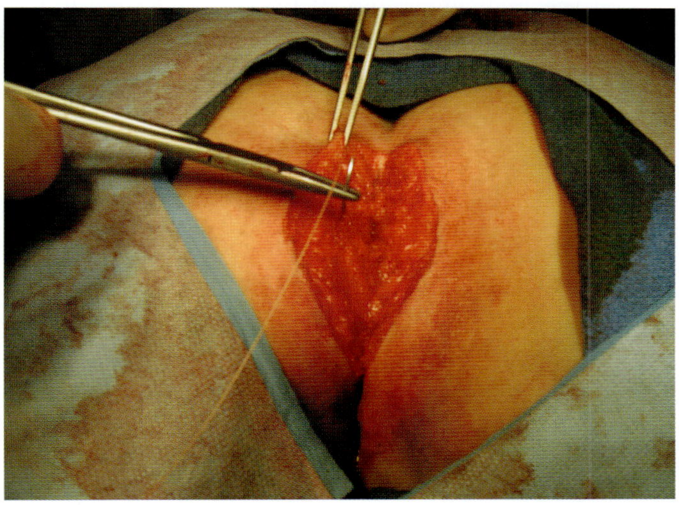
Figure 12-41

- In cases where the coccyx is to be removed, this should be accomplished first (Figure 12-42). The edge of the coccyx is cauterized, and the osteocartilaginous junction is transected to allow the rectum and sigmoid to be pulled through the pelvic floor with the coccyx attached. If a portion of the vagina is to be excised, the rectum is removed from the vagina as the final maneuver (Figure 12-43). The posterior vagina is closed with a running full-thickness absorbable suture from the apex of the cuff out to the introitus (Figure 12-44). Over time, the vagina restretches to accommodate space. The rest of the pelvic floor closure proceeds as previously described.

Step 4: Postoperative Care

Instruction in enterostomal therapy and appliance change is very helpful for a new ostomate. Patients require significant analgesia with patient-controlled narcotic and nonsteroidal anti-inflammatory drug administration.

The perineum becomes a major concern and focus of the patient after this procedure. The patient should not sit, scoot, or ride in a car sitting for at least 2 weeks. A shower or tub soak is sometimes helpful to relieve some of the pain and to clean the area. There is a significant amount of serous drainage in the first 2 weeks until the wound begins to seal. Patients who have undergone chemoradiation for squamous cell cancer have an extremely high risk of wound breakdown. This condition is easily treated with placement of a wound VAC in the wound after it separates. In many circumstances, if the wound raises any suspicions of potential problems, a wound VAC could be placed primarily at the time of the operation to begin healing and improve tissue oxygenation and contraction. The Blake drain is left in the pelvis until the drainage has decreased to less than 50 mL/day and is clear serous in nature.

The patient can be started on a clear liquid diet and advanced quickly to a regular diet as soon as nausea and bloating are gone. The patient should be able to care for the colostomy and be having semiformed bowel movements before discharge.

Venous thromboembolism prophylaxis and patient-controlled analgesia are required for all of these patients because they are at high risk for coagulopathy with a diagnosis of cancer and pelvic dissection. The bladder catheter is left in the bladder in most male patients for at least 4 to 5 days because of the high likelihood of urinary retention and need for reinsertion if removed earlier. Female patients can have the bladder catheter removed earlier and tend to do well with voiding despite the pelvic dissection.

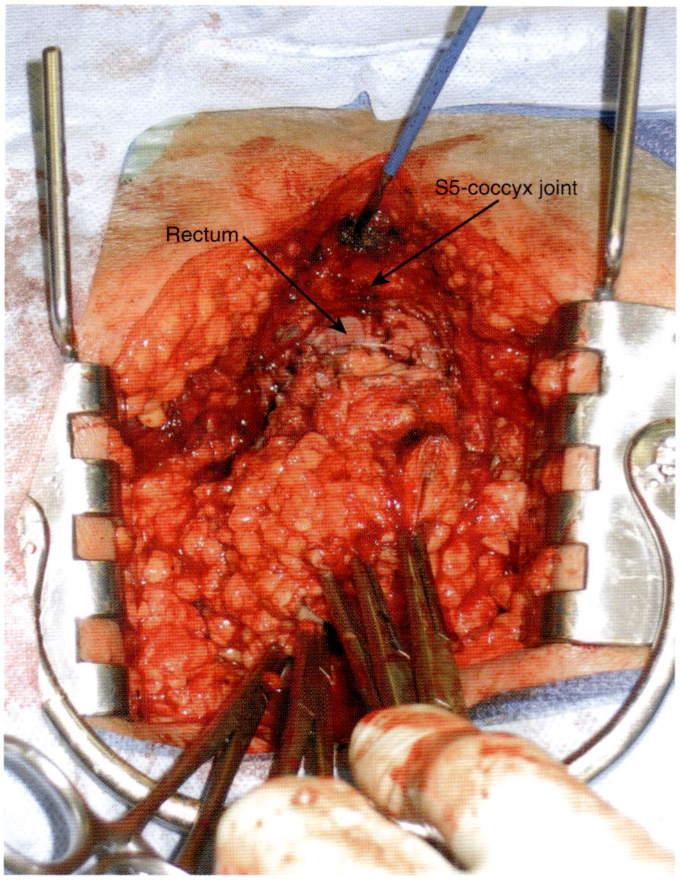

Figure 12-42

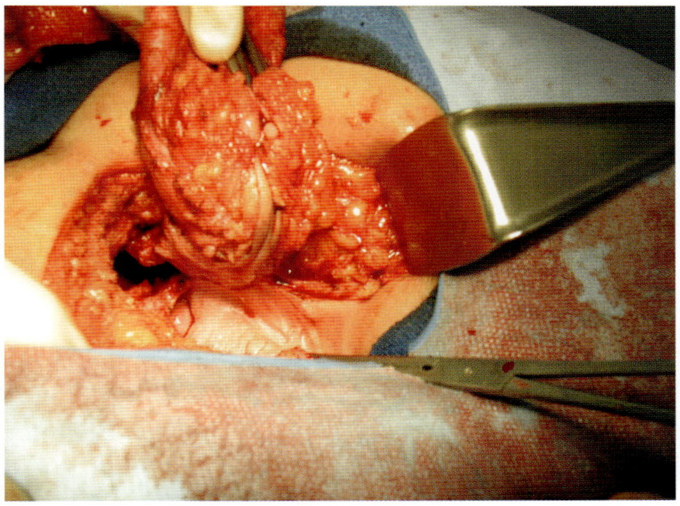

Figure 12-43

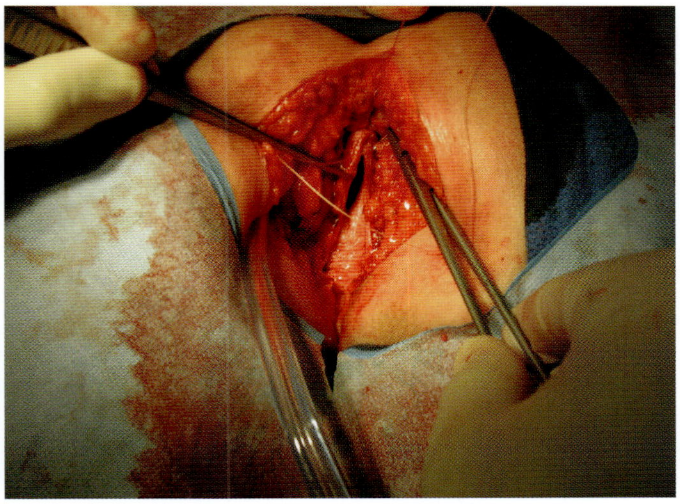

Figure 12-44

Step 5: Pearls and Pitfalls

The colostomy represents a major source of complications because of blood supply, the possibility of retraction, and the difficulty of maintaining an appliance if poorly placed on the abdominal wall. Preoperative marking can avoid most of these problems if the patient is placed in the sitting position, standing position, and lying position and asked to visualize the ostomy site (Figure 12-27). Doing this with the patient dressed in his or her usual clothes may also help identify the path of the belt. Most of the time, it is better to ask the patient to change his or her clothes style rather than move the ostomy to the upper abdomen.

As mentioned earlier, the perineal wound is the most likely site of complication. Close attention to avoiding sitting, scooting, or any lateral traction to the perineal wound can reduce the risk of breakdown of the wound, infection, and future complications of perineal hernia. If an abscess forms in the pelvis, a computed tomography (CT) scan can aid in the diagnosis, and placement of a drain by a vascular interventional radiologist can be performed to eliminate the collection. The pelvic drain placed at the time of operation can be left in place for longer periods if there is an extremely high volume of lymphatic and serous fluid collecting in the now empty pelvis.

The patient should be told that the perineum will be numb and that different sensations will be present. The skin requires at least 2 to 6 weeks to heal completely because of the previous radiation and the ongoing drainage that frequently occurs because of the deep fat plane with poor blood supply.

Selected Readings

Dozois EJ, Privitera A, Holubar SD, et al. High sacrectomy for locally recurrent rectal cancer: can long-term survival be achieved? J Surg Oncol 2011;103:105–9.

D'Souza DN, Pera M, Nelson H, et al. Vaginal reconstruction following resection of primary locally advanced and recurrent colorectal malignancies. Arch Surg 2003;138:1340–3.

Marr R, Birbeck K, Garvican J, et al. The modern abdominoperineal excision: the next challenge after total mesorectal excision. Ann Surg 2005;242:74–82.

CHAPTER 13

Laparoscopic Abdominal Perineal Resection

James W. Fleshman, Jr.

Step 1: Clinical Anatomy

The left colon lies along the left side of the abdomen suspended from the splenic flexure to the pelvic brim by lateral peritoneal attachments. The mesentery of the left colon arises from the midline of the abdomen along the aorta. The sigmoid colon has no lateral peritoneal attachments other than some congenital adhesions, which fix the apex of the sigmoid to the pelvic brim and the iliac fossa. Otherwise, the sigmoid colon is attached to the retroperitoneum through a midline mesentery arising from the inferior mesenteric artery (IMA) and extending down into the pelvis to the mesorectum. The splenic flexure is attached to the undersurface of the tip of the spleen, the lower edge of the tail of the pancreas, and the anterior surface of the left kidney by various levels of suspensory ligaments and peritoneal extensions. The blood supply to the left colon is based on the IMA, which arises from the anterior surface of the aorta just above the bifurcation of the common iliac arteries. The IMA extends anteriorly and bifurcates to produce the superior rectal artery feeding the sigmoid colon and the rectum. The left colic artery extends cephalad to provide the left colon and distal splenic flexure with blood supply through the arcade at the mesenteric edge known as the marginal artery of Drummond. The retroperitoneum behind the left colon contains the left ureter and the gonadal vessels lying over the psoas muscle. The ureter crosses the iliac vessels at the bifurcation of the iliac vessels into the external and internal iliac branches (Figure 13-1).

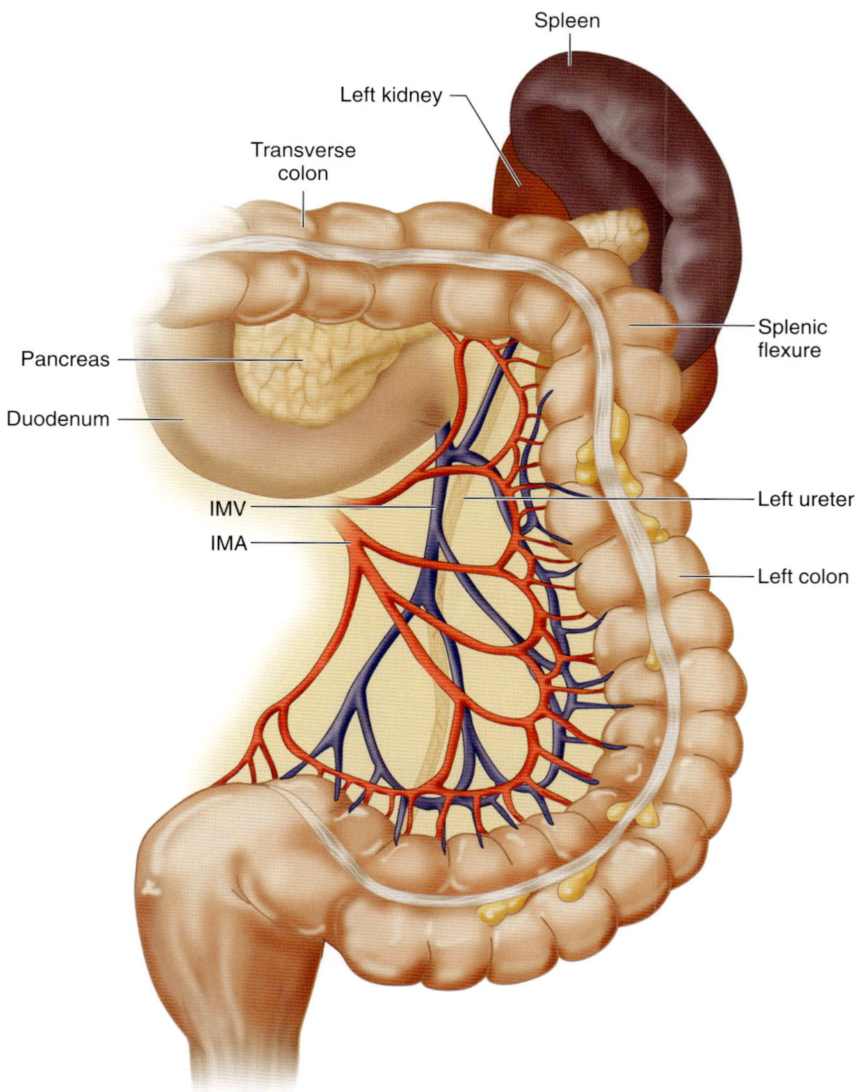
Spleen
Left kidney
Transverse colon
Splenic flexure
Pancreas
Duodenum
Left ureter
IMV
IMA
Left colon

Figure 13-1

Pelvic Anatomy

The pelvic anatomy is complex and has interrelationships between the rectum, vagina, uterus, ovaries, bladder, and prostate. The anatomy is important for pelvic dissection because of the various structures that are at risk, such as the splanchnic nerves, innervating the bladder, the ureters, and the organs themselves. The anatomy begins at the pelvic brim right at the sacral promontory. The common iliac artery and vein on each side course along the posterior aspect of the pelvic brim. The hypogastric plexus of parasympathetic and sympathetic nerves is found between the bifurcation of the aorta and common iliacs. This plexus coalesces to the right and left as the splanchnic pelvic nerves, which run along the inner aspect of the pelvic side wall to the level of the obturator fossa and the anterolateral ligaments carrying the middle hemorrhoidal vessels. Nerve fibers course from the splanchnic nerve to the rectum through the anterolateral ligaments along the middle hemorrhoidal vessels. Extension of these nerves continues to either the vagina or the prostate as the nervi erigentes. A clear understanding of this nerve anatomy is crucial because it is easily damaged during dissection and results in both sexual dysfunction and urinary bladder dysfunction (Figure 13-2*A*).

At the level of the sacral promontory, an areolar tissue plane begins behind the superior hemorrhoidal artery. The superior hemorrhoidal artery descends from the bifurcation of the IMA and splits at approximately S1-2 to give two major trunks down the posterior aspect of the rectum. The mesorectal envelope encases the fat and lymphatic and vascular structures to the rectum. The areolar tissue plane outside the mesorectal envelope is known as the "holy plane" and guides the dissection in the pelvis. A cross-sectional diagram of the pelvis shows the visceral peritoneum encasing the mesorectum with the areolar tissue plane between the visceral peritoneum and the parietal peritoneum posteriorly. The parietal peritoneum covers a nerve and venous plexus over the sacrum and the musculature of the side wall of the pelvis. Maintaining dissection within the areolar tissue plane between the parietal and the visceral peritoneal layers protects all of the crucial structures in the pelvis (Figure 13-2*B*).

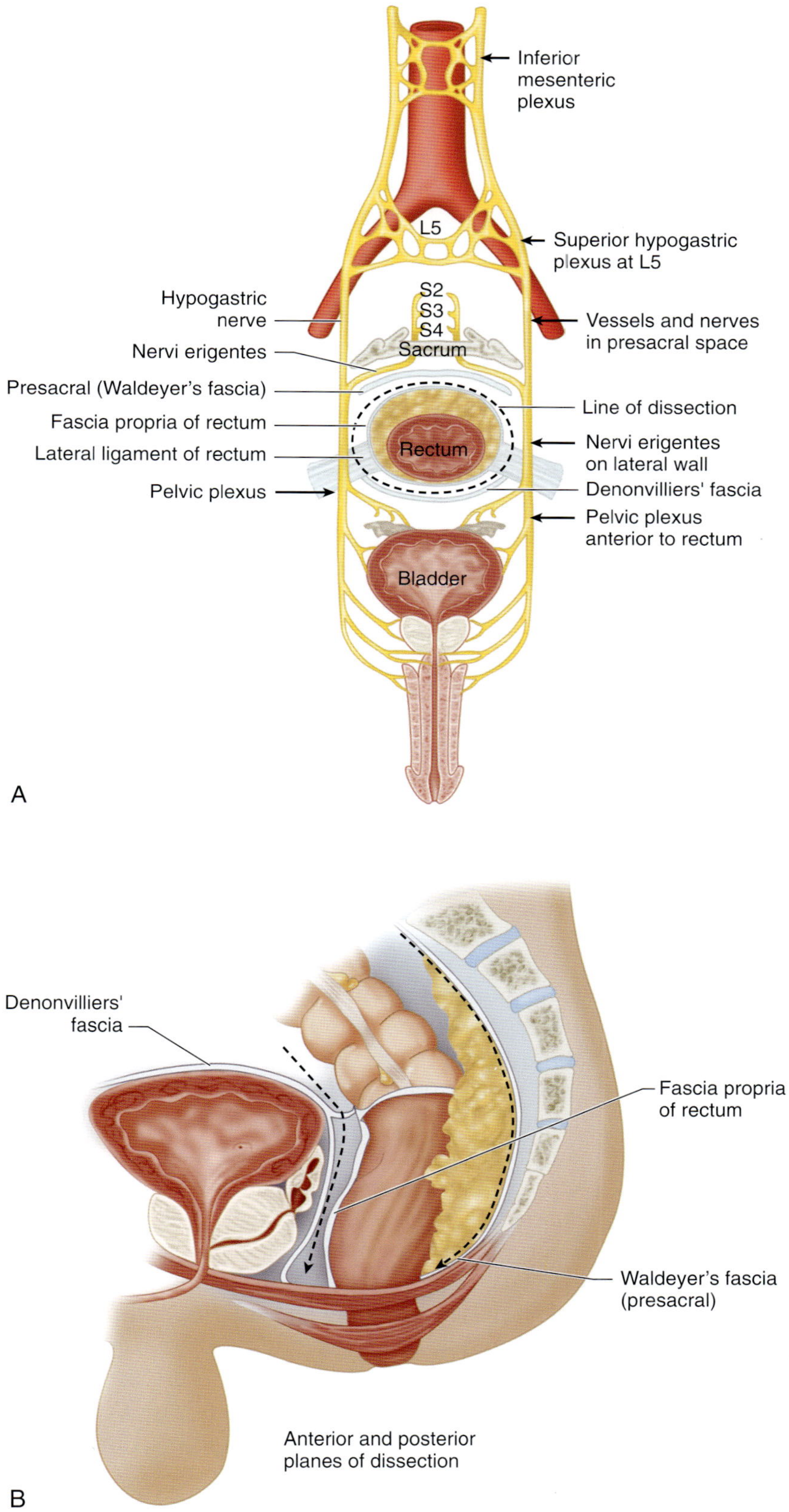

Figure 13-2A-B

The rectum descends through the middle of the pelvis following the curve of the sacrum and at the level of the coccyx makes a right angle to exit through the pelvic floor via the anal canal. The levator ani muscles on either side of the pelvic floor form the support diaphragm of the pelvis and extend up onto the side wall of the pelvis to insert in the ischiospinous ligament attachments covering the nerves and vessels of the deep pelvic floor. The tip of the coccyx attaches to the pubococcygeal ligament, which supports the puborectalis muscle as a semicircular sling from the pubis around the back of the rectum. This muscle closes the top of the anal canal anterior to posterior (Figure 13-3).

The anterior pelvic structures including the bladder, prostate, and vagina are separated from the rectum by the rectoprostatic or rectovaginal septum. A visceral peritoneal layer known as Denonvilliers' fascia is the posterior boundary of the anterior structures. This fascia protects the seminal vesicles and prostate during dissection. The areolar tissue plane continues around the entire rectum to the anterior surface of the rectum. The plane is found behind or posterior to Denonvilliers' fascia. The anterolateral ligaments carry the middle hemorrhoidal vessels into the mesorectal envelope through the visceral fascia from an anterolateral direction. Dissection and transection of these middle hemorrhoidal vessels reveals the anterior areolar tissue plane behind Denonvilliers' fascia, which can be followed all the way down to the anal canal.

The ureters, which have been described as running into the pelvic area over the pelvic brim crossing the common iliac artery and vein on either side of the pelvis, continue into the pelvis along the side wall of the pelvis toward the posterior aspect of the bladder. In the nonoperated, pristine pelvis, the ureters are higher up along the side wall of the pelvis aiming toward the posterior aspect of the trigone of the bladder. In females, the ureters run between the arterial blood supply of the uterus along the anterior lateral side wall of the pelvis. In males, ureters are not exposed during the distal pelvic dissection. The ureters may be drawn posteriorly after a previous operation but are normally well protected anteriorly and laterally. In a previously operated pelvis, it is always wise to place ureteral stents at the beginning of the procedure to aid in identification of the aberrantly placed ureters.

Anal Canal Anatomy

The upper anal canal begins at the puborectalis ring or the anorectal ring, which sits at the level of the pelvic floor and can be palpated through the anal canal as a bulge posteriorly (Figure 13-3, *insert*). The longitudinal muscles of the rectum continue into the anus as the intersphincteric plane demarcating the line between autonomic internal sphincter and somatic external sphincter fibers all the way down to the level of the anal canal skin where the intersphincteric groove is palpable. The ischiorectal fossa fat is found outside the circular fibers of the external sphincter that encircle the rectum. The pudendal nerve and vessels traverse the ischiorectal fat from each ischial spine to the posterolateral aspect of the anal canal. During the perineal portion of a procedure, the pudendal nerves and vessels must be controlled.

The rectovaginal and rectoprostatic septum descends all the way to the level of the perineum anteriorly. The transverse perineal muscle separates the anterior and posterior perineum. The terminal fibers of the longitudinal muscle of the rectum insert into the skin of the anal canal just outside the anal verge as the corrugator cutanei ani and cause the ridges that are noticed around the anal canal. The internal sphincter is the hypertrophied circular muscle of the wall of the rectum. The lowest portion of the internal sphincter can be palpated as a groove where the longitudinal fibers insert on the skin.

Within the anal canal, the dentate line is the junction between cuboidal epithelium of the anal transition zone, which is the terminal mucosal layer of the rectum, and the squamous epidermal cells of the anal canal skin. Gland openings (or crypts) are found in the dentate line at the base of the Morgagni columns, which are interdigitating lines of squamous epithelium into the cuboidal and columnar epithelium of the distal rectum. The anal transition zone is the

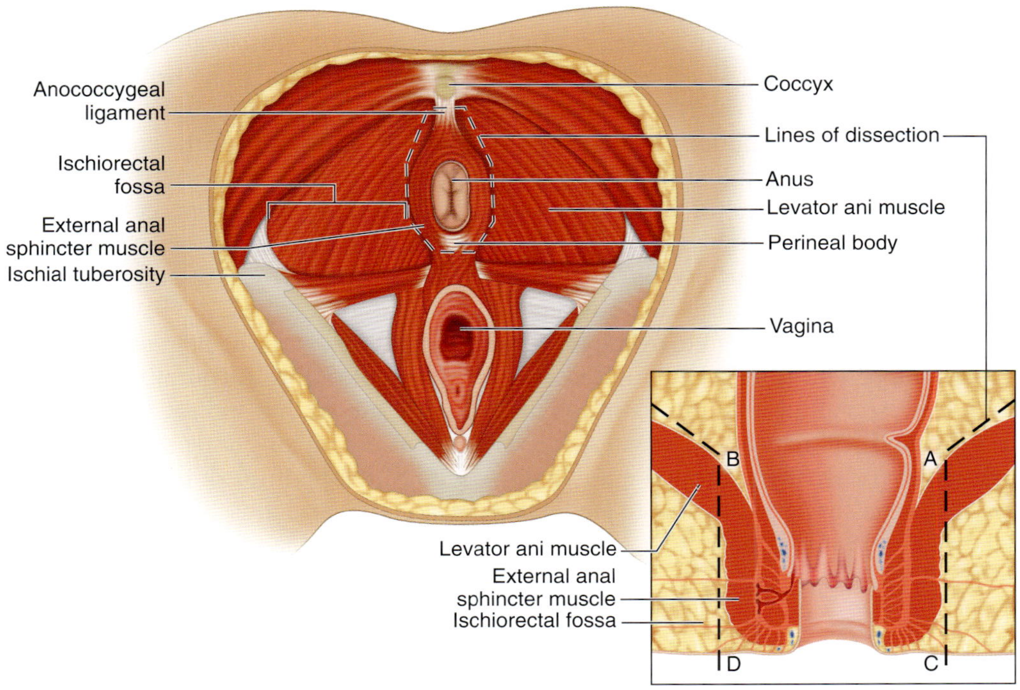

Anococcygeal ligament
Ischiorectal fossa
External anal sphincter muscle
Ischial tuberosity
Coccyx
Lines of dissection
Anus
Levator ani muscle
Perineal body
Vagina
B
A
Levator ani muscle
External anal sphincter muscle
Ischiorectal fossa
D
C

Figure 13-3

most highly innervated section of the rectum and anal canal containing nerve fibers sensing temperature, vibration, electrical stimulation, pressure, liquid, solid, and gas. The dentate line lies approximately halfway along the surgical anal canal, which extends from the palpable anal verge all the way up to the anorectal ring palpated at the puborectalis sling posteriorly. The anoderm within the anal canal, cephalad to the anal verge, has no hair follicles.

Step 2: Preoperative Considerations

Abdominal perineal resection of the rectum is most commonly performed for rectal cancers or anal cancers involving the low rectum or anal canal or both. Removal of the entire anal canal is required when the tumor has invaded the sphincter complex. The tumors require a total mesorectal excision, which should also include a portion of the pelvic floor musculature. More recent data suggest that complete removal of the pelvic floor muscle all the way out to the ischial spines reduces the risk of local recurrence. However, the use of neoadjuvant therapy for these tumors may reduce the need to remove all of the pelvic floor and allow the removal of only a cuff. The tumor should not be exposed during mobilization of the mesorectum if the tumor is posterior and lying at the level of the pelvic floor. In cases where the tumor is large and fills the pelvis, removal of the coccyx with the pelvic floor may be necessary. The laparoscopic approach is appropriate for this portion of the procedure but may become more difficult as the tumor gets larger and invades adjacent structures. The perineal dissection may be used to achieve radial margins up in the low pelvis.

The patient should undergo marking for a permanent stoma with the help of an enterostomal therapist. The patient should be educated on care of the colostomy. A complete bowel preparation is unnecessary, but it is important to empty the rectum so that spillage is minimized. The perineal wound will require closure in some way, and arranging for plastic surgery consultation preoperatively is usually appropriate if a large portion of the perineal skin and muscle is to be removed. Plastic surgeons are able to swing flaps of skin, fat, and muscle to help fill the defect. The use of biomesh for pelvic floor reconstruction is now possible and may eliminate the need for larger flap procedures.

Step 3: Operative Steps

- The patient is placed in the lithotomy position using Allen's stirrups with the legs flexed 90 degrees at the knees and flexed no more than 10 degrees at the hips. The legs point toward the floor to prevent obstruction of the operative field by the knees when the patient is placed in the Trendelenburg position. A beanbag is attached to the table with Velcro to fix it in place. The patient is positioned in the beanbag with the arms tucked at the side and incorporated in the beanbag. As an extra measure of security, tape is placed across the chest to fix the sides of the beanbag and hold the patient (Figure 13-4).

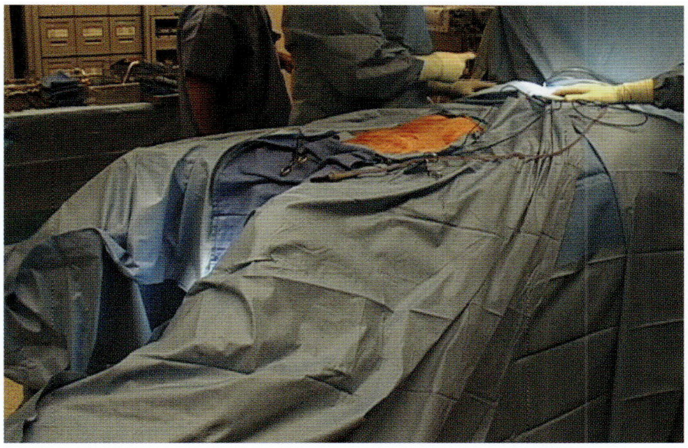

Figure 13-4

- The abdomen is prepared and draped sterilely, and the abdomen is inflated through either an open insertion of a trocar at the umbilicus or a Veress needle at the umbilicus. The trocar is placed above the umbilicus in the vertical midline. The flexible laparoscope is introduced through the trocar at the umbilicus by the camera operator standing at the right shoulder, and the abdomen is explored for metastases or other intra-abdominal disease. Laparoscopic proctectomy requires trocars in the right upper and lower quadrants in the anterior axillary line; the trocars are placed two fingerbreadths below the costal margin and above the anterior superior iliac spine. A left flank trocar is placed in the anterior axillary line at the level of the umbilicus. A 10-mm trocar is placed in the suprapubic vertical midline, or a hand access port can be placed at this level (Figure 13-5). The goal should be to perform a completely laparoscopic procedure with no other incision on the abdomen besides the colostomy.
- The patient is placed in steep Trendelenburg and airplaned to the right. The sigmoid colon is lifted anteriorly with a Babcock clamp through the 10-mm suprapubic port or alternatively with the hand of the assistant through the suprapubic hand access port. The assistant stands between the legs. The operating surgeon stands to the patient's right and holds a 5-mm grasper in the left hand and an energy source in the right. The sigmoid mesentery is incised at the level of the pelvic brim anterior to the sacral promontory to enter the avascular plane at that level (Figure 13-6). Retraction anteriorly opens this plane and exposes the undersurface of the IMA at its origin.
- The left ureter is the first structure to be identified and dissected free from the posterior aspect of the left colon mesentery. The ureter must be visualized before division of the IMA for safety reasons. A full laparoscopic approach is more difficult and requires anterior and posterior countertraction and blunt dissection to drop the ureter posteriorly. The surgeon must remember that the dissection plane is angled upward along the pelvic brim as the patient is in right-side-down position, and the left leg is actually up in the air (Figure 13-7).
- The IMA and inferior mesenteric vein (IMV) are isolated at their origins along the anterior surface of the aorta and at the third portion of the duodenum at the ligament of Treitz (Figure 13-8). The medial to lateral approach incises the base of the mesentery of the left colon all the way up to the duodenum from the IMA. A window of clear areolar tissue is exposed posterior to the IMV as it runs parallel to the aorta along the base of the left colic mesentery. This window can be developed, and the ureter can be seen in its course toward the hilum of the kidney (Figure 13-9).
- The IMA is divided at its origin using the energy source (Figure 13-10). For cancer, high ligation of the IMA should be 1 cm above the junction of the aorta. The sympathetic nerves can be dropped posteriorly with blunt dissection to reduce the risk of nerve injury and impotence. The stump of the artery must be visualized carefully after division to ensure there is good hemostasis.

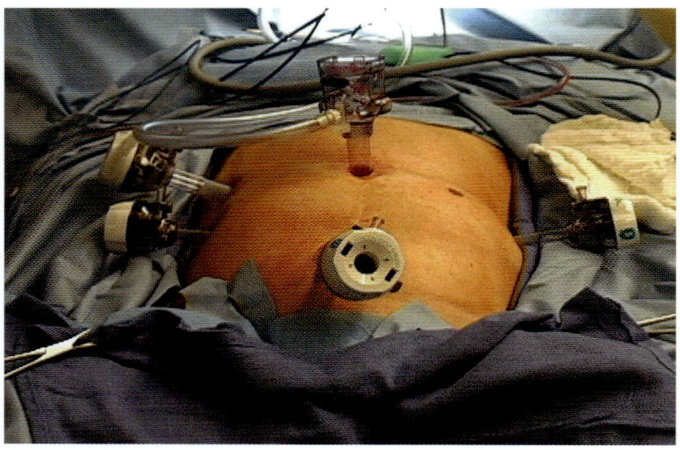

Figure 13-5

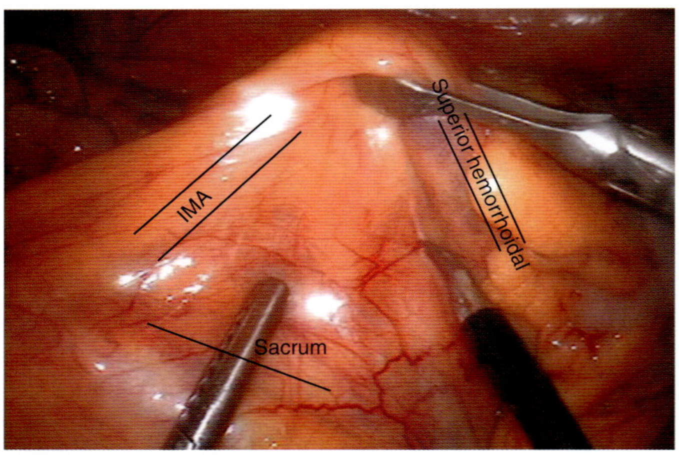

Figure 13-6

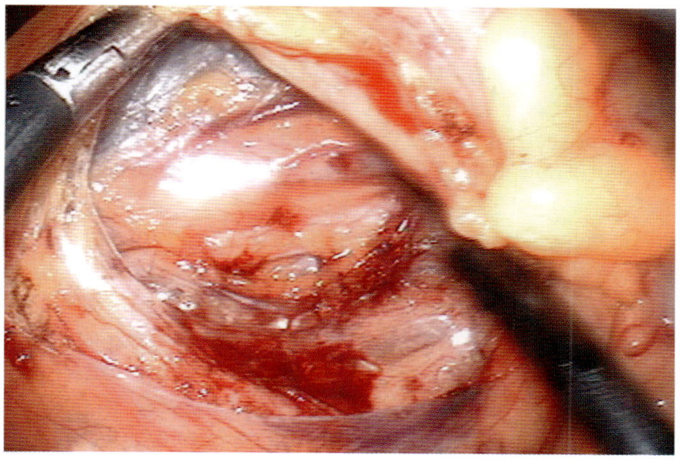

Figure 13-7

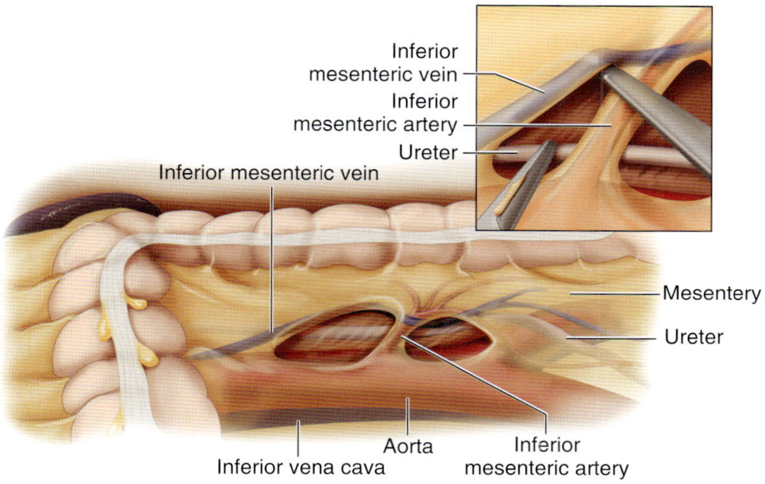

Figure 13-8

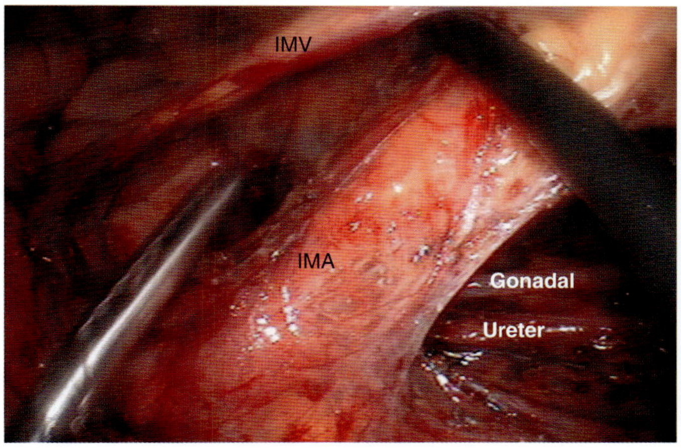

Figure 13-9

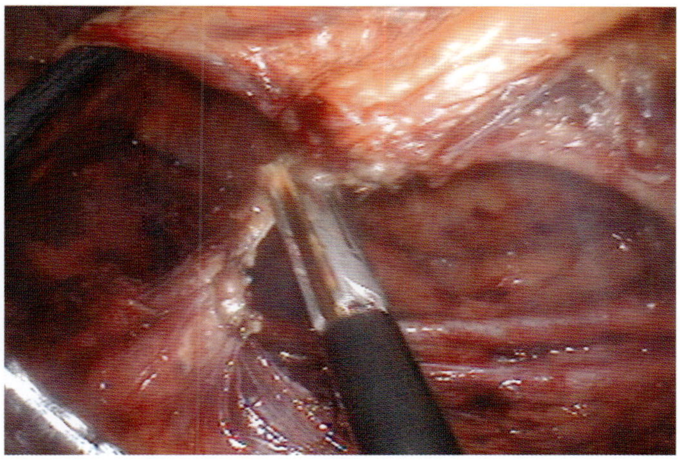

Figure 13-10

- The IMV at the level of the ligament of Treitz has a branch approximately 3 cm caudad to the IMV insertion into the splenic vein (Figure 13-11). The bifurcation should be included in the specimen by transecting the IMV closer to the ligament of Treitz and the pancreas. The IMV is divided under direct vision after opening the window between the pancreas, the IMV, and the branch (Figure 13-12).
- After the mesenteric vessels have been divided medially, a blunt dissection in the areolar plane can be accomplished all the way out to the lateral aspect of the abdominal wall, dropping the vital structures in the retroperitoneum posteriorly (Figure 13-13). This maneuver frees the left colon and its mesentery from the retroperitoneum from the pelvic brim to the splenic flexure. The lateral attachments are incised using the energy source from the pelvic brim up to the splenic flexure (Figure 13-14). If the splenic flexure must be mobilized, the lateral attachments and suspensory ligaments from the pancreas and spleen are divided (Figures 13-15 and 13-16) This maneuver is facilitated by placing the patient in reverse Trendelenburg and airplaned to the right.

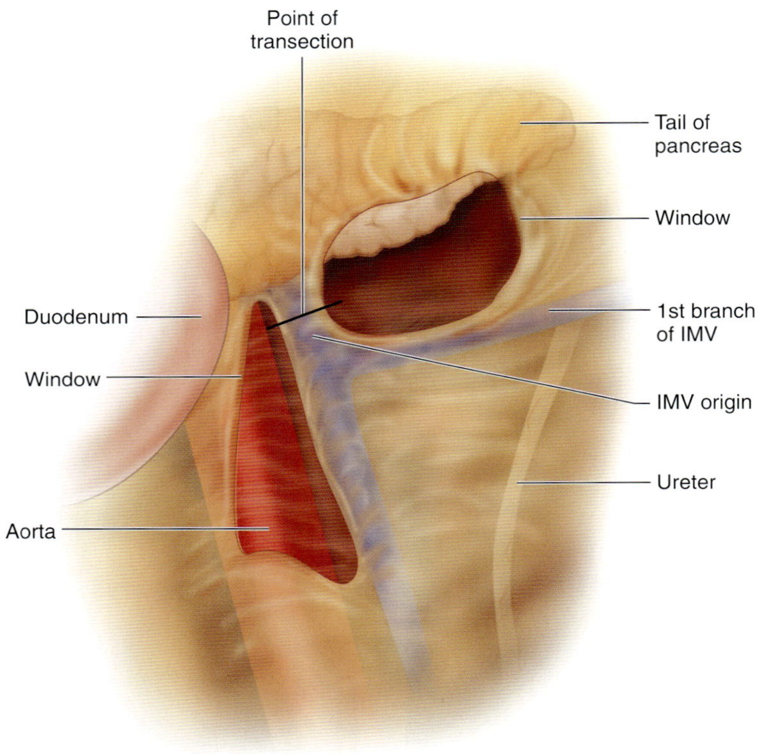

Figure 13-11

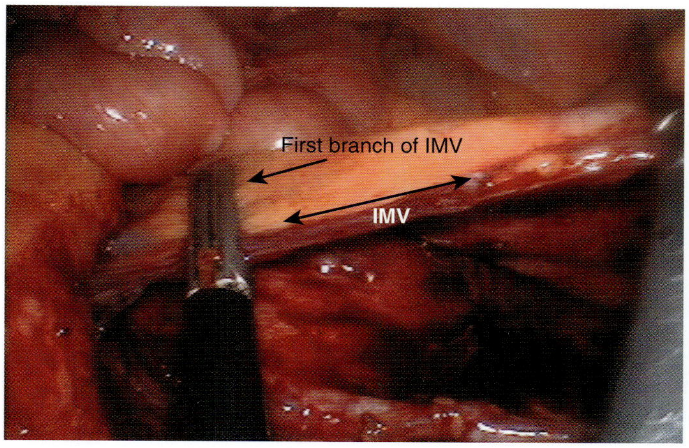

Figure 13-12

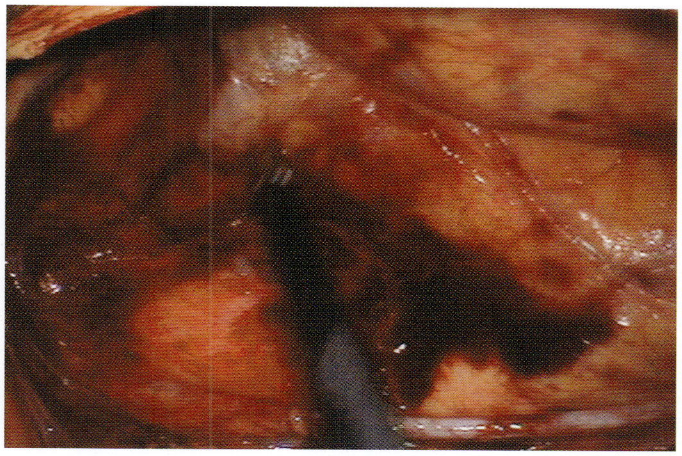

Figure 13-13

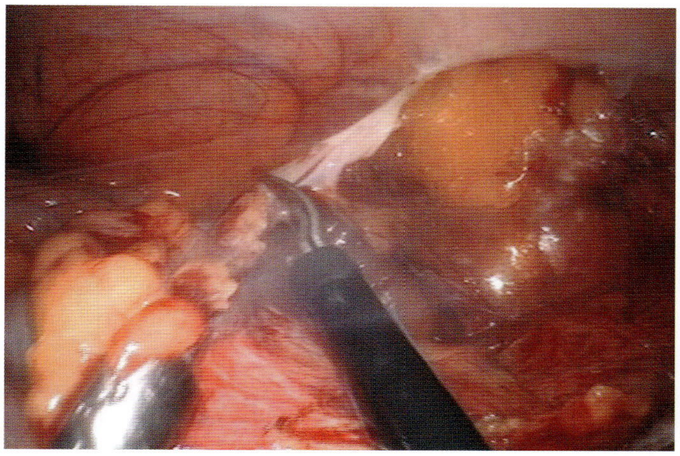

Figure 13-14

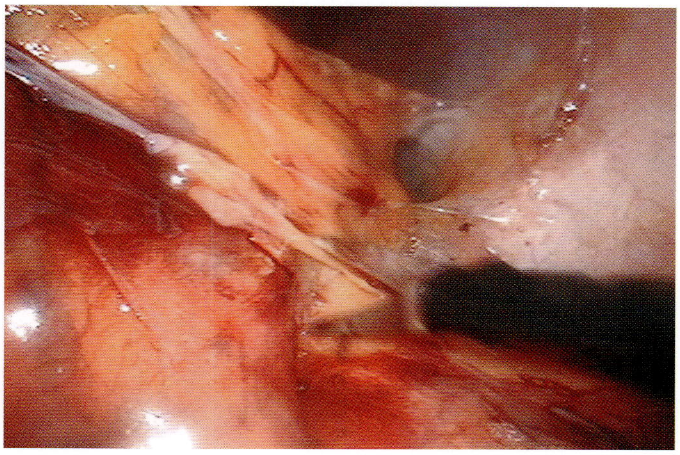

Figure 13-15

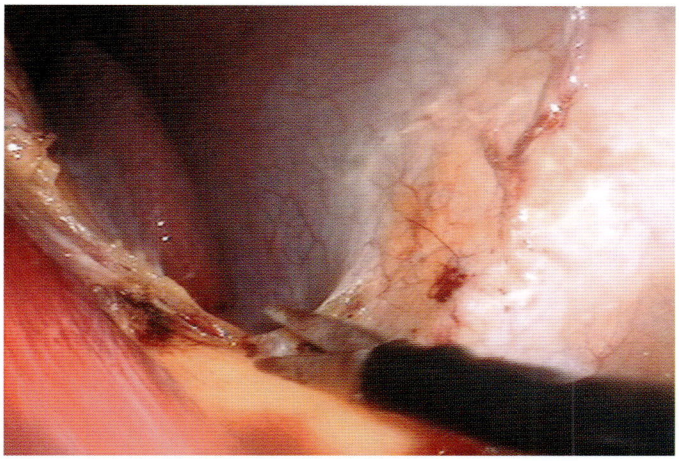

Figure 13-16

- The patient is placed in flat, steep Trendelenburg, and the sigmoid colon is lifted anteriorly by placing a 5-mm grasper beneath the left and sigmoid colon and retracting this toward the anterior abdominal wall (Figure 13-17). The operating surgeon still standing on the patient's right incises the areolar tissue plane posterior to the rectal mesentery and outside the mesenteric envelope (Figure 13-18). The left pelvic side wall is easily seen at the level of the sacral promontory, and the splanchnic nerve can be protected. Sharp dissection with electrocautery and an energy source is important at this level to keep the field clear of blood. The right pelvic peritoneal surface is incised to the cul-de-sac to allow the rectum to be retracted to the left (Figure 13-19), and the anterolateral ligaments are divided (Figure 13-20).

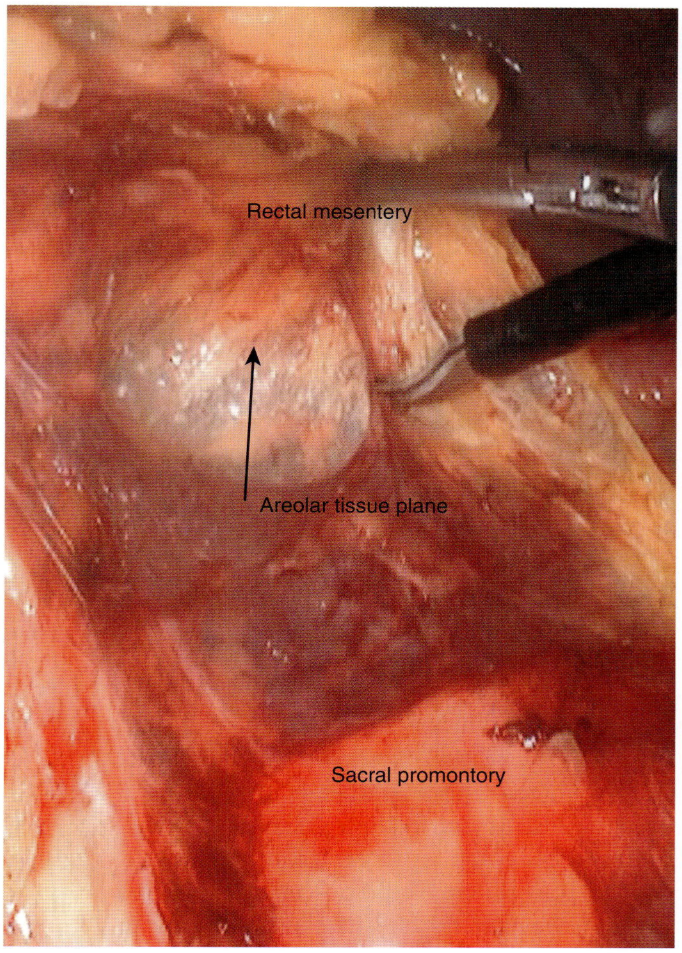

Figure 13-17

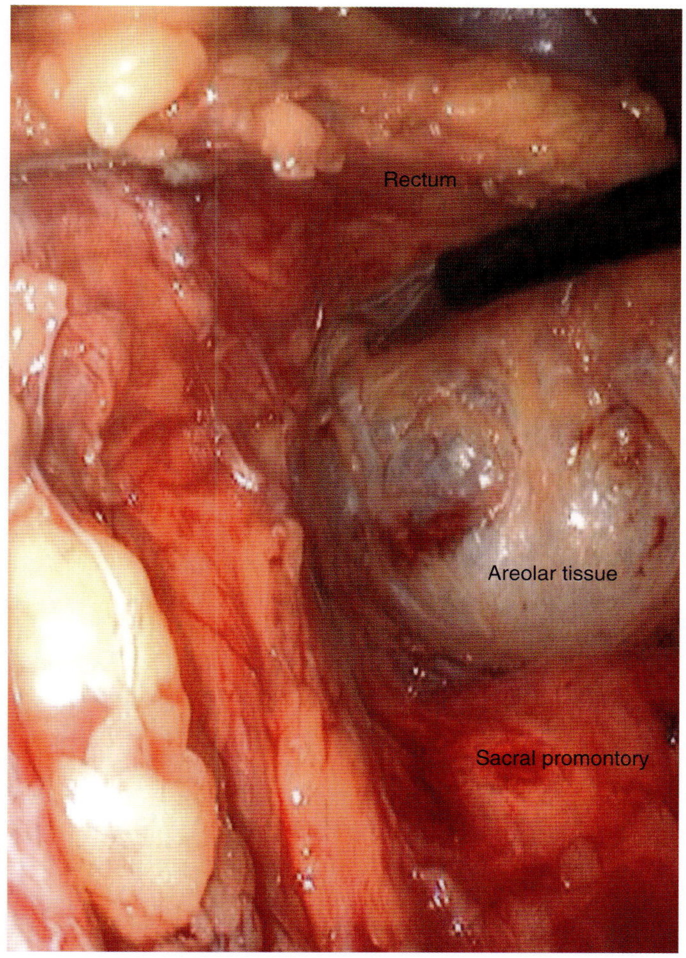

Figure 13-18

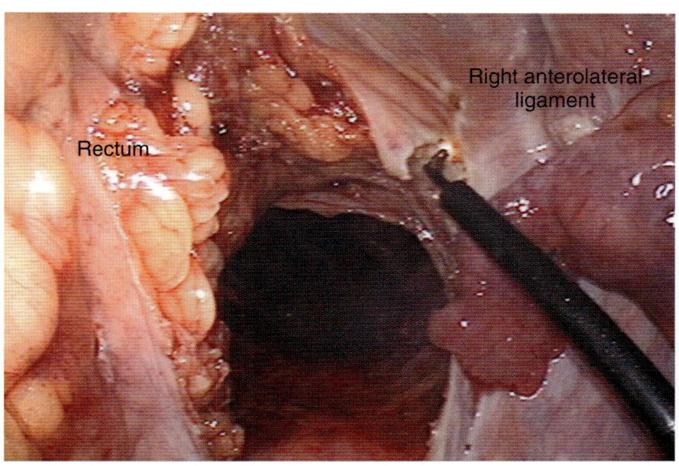

Figure 13-19

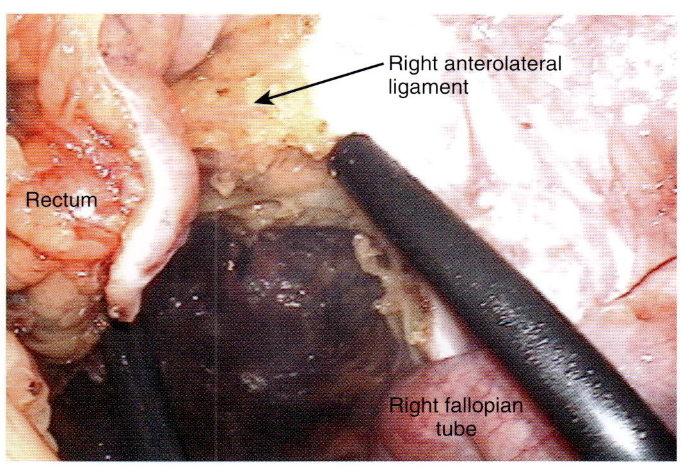

Figure 13-20

- The dissection is carried further into the pelvis, all the way down to the pelvic floor posteriorly to release the mesentery up and away from the sacral curve. The pelvic side wall on the left is cleared, and the attachments are released with sharp and blunt dissection (Figure 13-21).
- The left pelvic peritoneal surface is incised all the way to the cul-de-sac. The left and posterior dissection is completed, and the rectum is retracted to the patient's right. An incision is made anterior to the rectum in the peritoneal surface at the cul-de-sac to expose the left anterolateral ligaments and the rectovaginal or rectoprostatic septum. The anterolateral ligaments are divided with the electrocautery hook at the side wall of the pelvis (Figure 13-22).
- The right side of the cul-de-sac incision is accomplished by changing the rectal retraction toward the left side wall (Figure 13-23).
- The dissection in the rectovaginal or rectoprostatic septum is accomplished by retracting the posterior aspect of the bladder anteriorly using the left port 5-mm grasper (Figure 13-24). The rectum is pulled posteriorly and cephalad, and the cautery is used to extend the dissection in the areolar tissue plane behind the vagina or prostate all the way down to the level of the anal canal. Care must be taken not to enter the vagina or tumor. The areolar tissue plane should be easily followed with the flexible scope brought low into the pelvis.
- With the pelvic rectum mobilized to the pelvic floor, the rectum is now left in place. The descending sigmoid colon junction is identified. With the 5-mm grasper in the left hand through the right upper quadrant trocar and sealing instrument in the right hand through the right lower quadrant trocar, the mesentery of the left colon is transected from the level of the IMV all the way up to the point of planned transection of the descending sigmoid colon junction (Figure 13-25). The assistant stands on the patient's left with the 5-mm grasper or between the legs through the 10-mm trocar to lift the colon toward the anterior abdominal wall. The mesentery can be divided in a straight line from the cut end of the IMV up to the level of the colon at the descending sigmoid colon junction.

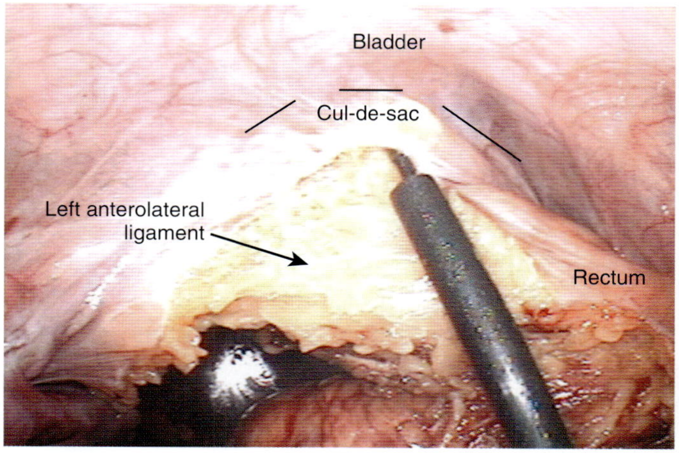

Figure 13-21

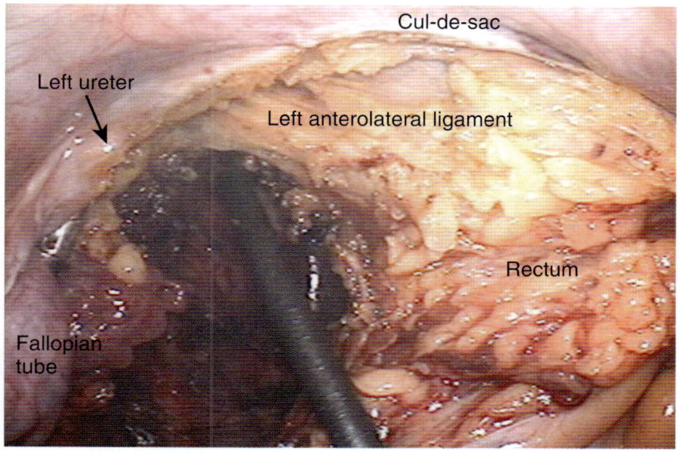

Figure 13-22

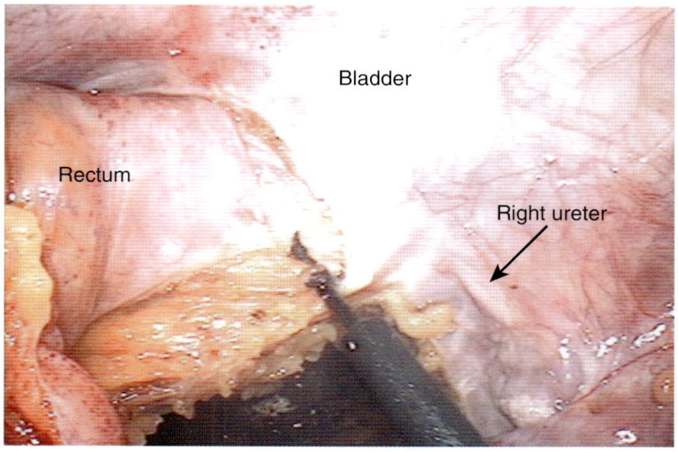

Figure 13-23

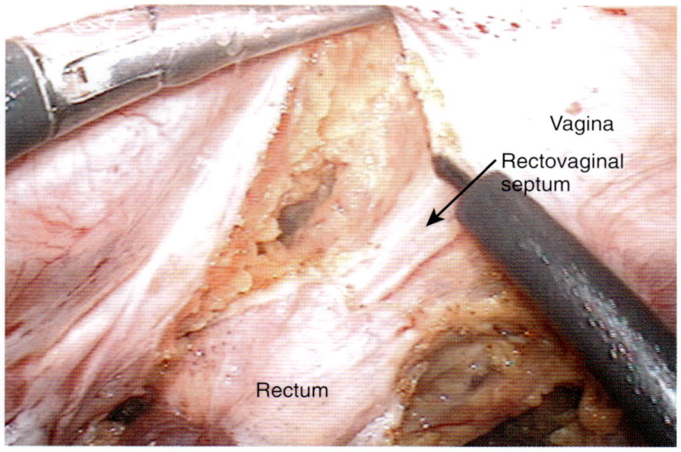

Figure 13-24

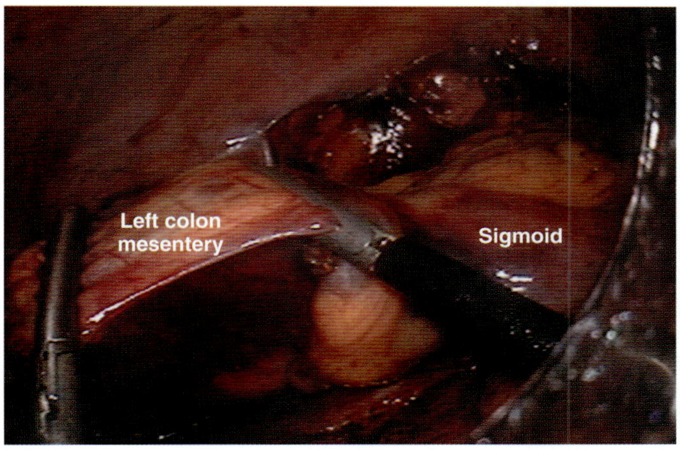

Figure 13-25

- A 3-cm-diameter disk of skin and subcutaneous fat is removed from the previously marked site of the left lower quadrant. A 3-cm vertical incision is made in the base of the colostomy site in the anterior fascia, and the rectus muscle is split with a large clamp to expose the posterior fascia and peritoneum. The internal fascia is incised externally through the ostomy site to deliver two fingerbreadths through the anterior abdominal wall. A Babcock clamp is placed through the opening in the anterior abdominal wall. The proximal end of the descending sigmoid colon junction is grasped, and this is pulled through the anterior abdominal wall. A 75-mm linear cutter stapler is used to transect the colon in an antimesenteric to mesenteric direction (Figures 13-26 and 13-27).

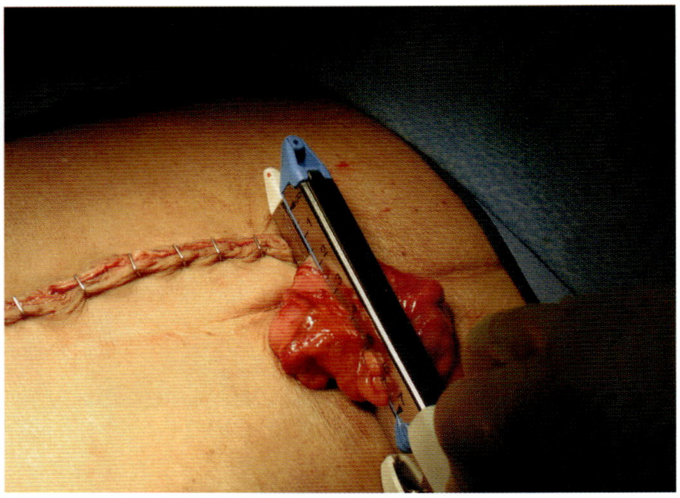

Figure 13-26

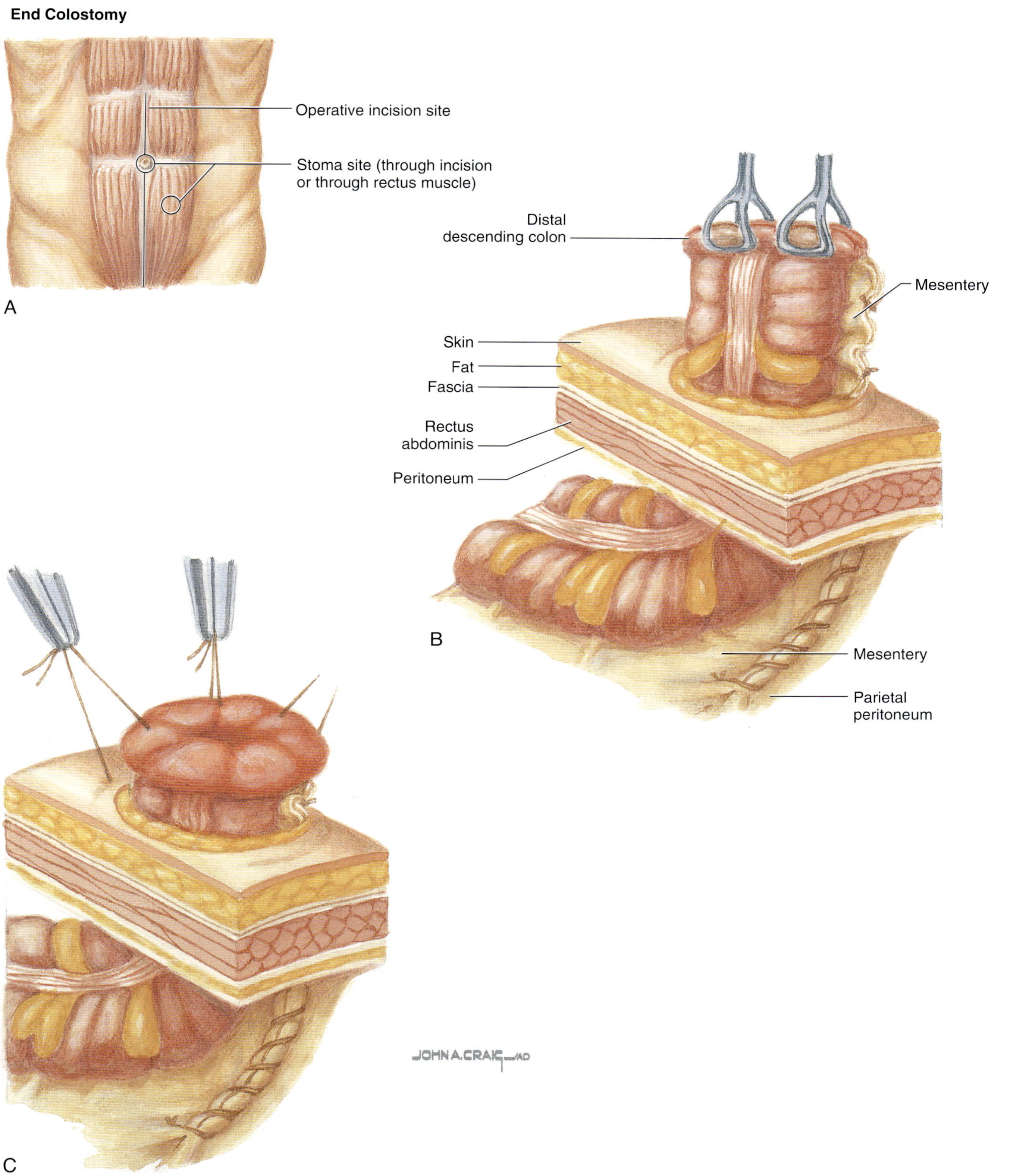

Figure 13-27A-C *Netter illustration from* www.netterimages.com. *©* *Elsevier Inc. All rights reserved.*

- If the abdominal wall is too thick for this maneuver to occur easily through the colostomy site, the colon can be transected internally by using an Endo GIA stapler (Covidien, Mansfield, Mass.) placed through a 10-mm trocar at the suprapubic site (Figure 13-28). The stapled end of the bowel is brought out through the anterior abdominal wall. The opening is enlarged to accommodate the size of the mesentery in an obese patient. The transverse staple line is excised, and the ostomy is matured at the level of the skin to create a flush stoma by placing interrupted 3-0 absorbable sutures interspersed around the circumference of the colon (Figure 13-29). The colon should be oriented to maintain the anatomic position of the mesentery and the antimesenteric border.
- The sigmoid colon and rectum with the mesentery are allowed to fall into the pelvis. The abdomen is deflated of carbon dioxide after placing a Blake drain through the suprapubic port and out through the right lower quadrant port (Figure 13-30). Occasionally, the ports have to be removed to get the drain in, and the drain is then placed down into the pelvis alongside the rectum and sigmoid. The drain is secured to the skin with 3-0 nylon and hooked to a suction bulb drainage. The umbilical incision is closed with a figure-eight suture on the fascia, subcutaneous tissue is irrigated with an antibiotic saline solution at all sites, and the skin is closed with skin staples or subcuticular sutures and covered with plastic bandages. An ostomy appliance is applied.
- The patient is rolled to the prone-jackknife position on the operating table with a roll under the hips and under the chest. The airway is secured during the move and while the patient is in the prone-jackknife position (Figure 13-31).
- The buttocks are taped apart, and the perineum is prepared and draped sterilely with antisepsis solution (Figure 13-32). The anal canal is closed with a No. 1 suture placed to encircle the anal verge in the intersphincteric groove and tied securely. The incision is planned by placing marks at the tip of the coccyx and the anterior portion of the perineal body at the back of the vagina or at the base of the scrotum. The lateral marks are placed on the inner aspect of the buttock outside the external sphincter muscle. The incision is made to connect the dots as an ellipse incising the skin and exposing the ischial rectal fat (Figure 13-33). The dissection is carried down outside the external sphincter to the level of the levator muscles in the upper regions of the ischiorectal fossa. Hemostasis should be complete. A bear claw St. Mark's self-retaining retractor can be used for exposure. The anal skin and anal canal are grasped with Kocher clamps as a device for holding and moving the distal rectum and anal canal (Figures 13-34 and 13-35).

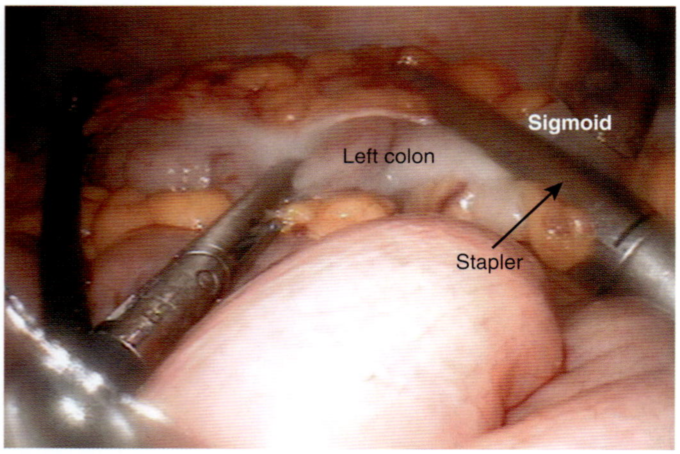

Figure 13-28

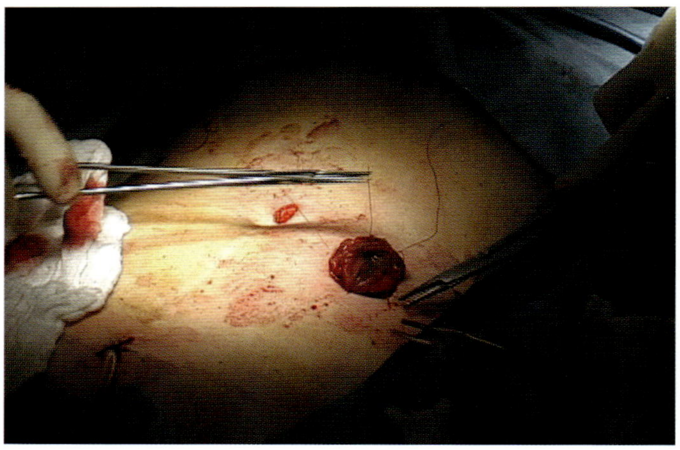
Figure 13-29

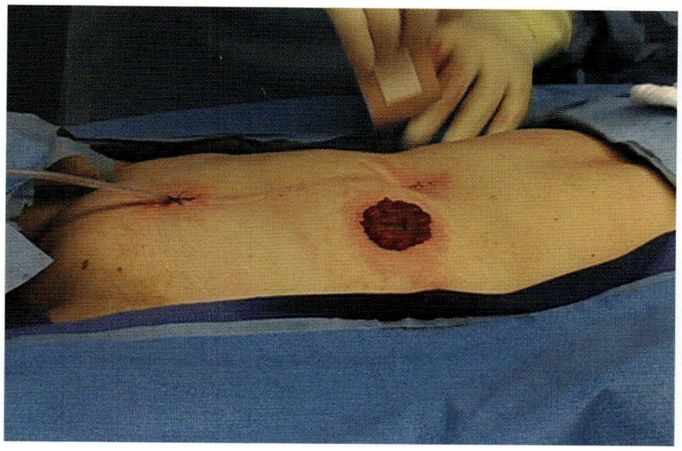

Figure 13-30

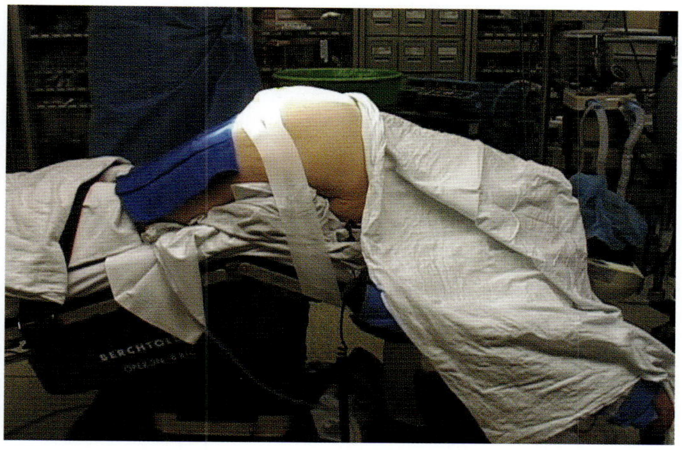

Figure 13-31

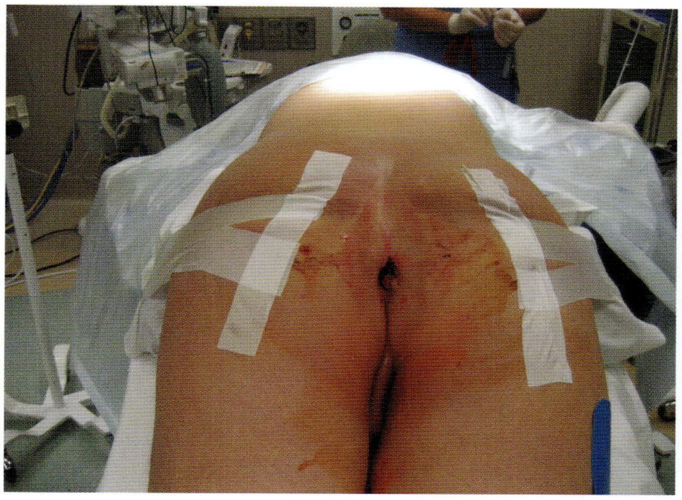

Figure 13-32

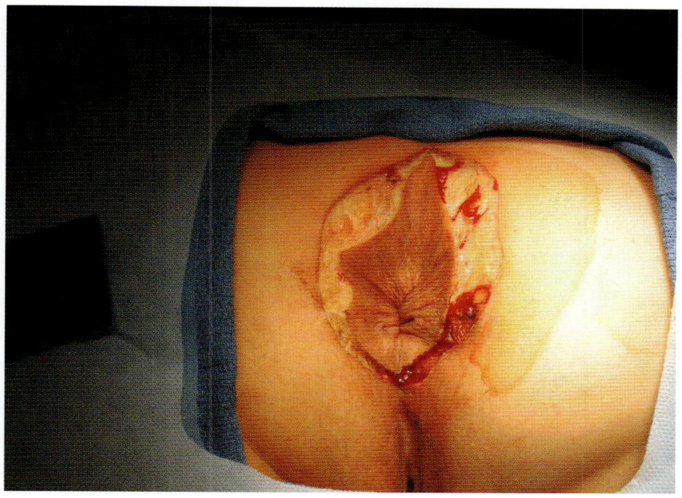

Figure 13-33

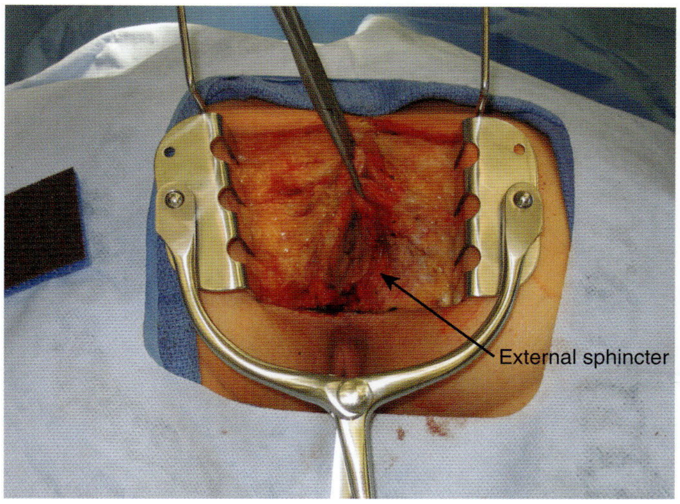

Figure 13-34

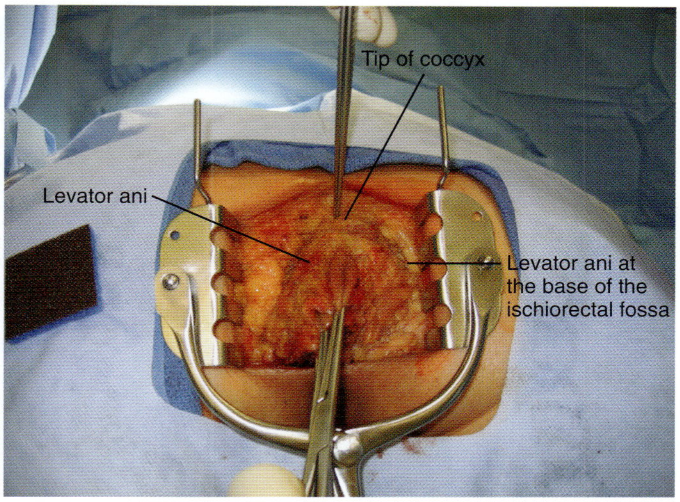

Figure 13-35

- An incision is made anterior to the tip of the coccyx full-thickness through the pelvic floor muscle to enter the previously dissected pelvis posteriorly (Figure 13-36). A finger is inserted into the pelvic space and curled over the levator ani plate on each side of the anal canal. The tumor or tumor mass can be palpated, and then an incision should be made far enough outside the mass to leave a cuff of the pelvic floor attached to the tumor to prevent exposure of the tumor during the incision. The incision is carried from the posterior aspect to the pelvic floor all the way up to the anterior aspect on both sides of the anal canal (Figure 13-37). The rectum and sigmoid colon are delivered through the pelvic floor opening, which is usually quite generous at this point (Figure 13-38).
- The dissection of the rectum from the posterior aspects of the vagina or the prostate and seminal vesicles is sometimes quite difficult, especially in the case of an anteriorly placed tumor growing through the rectal wall and sphincter mechanism into the rectovaginal or rectoprostatic septum (Figure 13-39). In this case, a wide enough margin removing a portion of the adjacent tissue is necessary to achieve clear circumferential radial margins. The issue of hemostasis is very relevant at this point because the prostate and the vagina are extremely well vascularized. Occasionally, suture ligation is required to preclude the venous lakes found in this area.
- The final attachments of the anterior rectum from the perineal body are incised and the entire specimen can be delivered. The pelvis is inspected and irrigated, and hemostasis is completed (Figure 13-40). The Blake drain is pulled down into the pelvis. At this point, a decision needs to be made whether the muscle in the pelvic floor can reach across to the midline and provide adequate tissue for primary closure of the pelvic floor or whether a biomesh is needed to fill the gap. Pelvic floor reconstruction with primary sutures is almost always possible using this technique (Figure 13-41). Application of figure-eight sutures of No. 1 Vicryl to approximate the cut edges of the muscle in the midline beginning at the coccyx and moving forward to the back of the anterior structures gives a good, strong closure. The ischiorectal fossa fat is irrigated copiously, and layers of horizontal mattress sutures of 0 absorbable suture are used to approximate the fat across the midline and obliterate the dead space in the ischiorectal fossa (Figure 13-42). As the layers get closer to the skin, the buttocks begin moving toward the midline. The final layer for closure is the most superficial subcutaneous fat, leaving the skin open along the entire length of the wound to heal by secondary intention. A gauze pad and mesh underwear are used as the preferred dressing for the perineal wound closure.

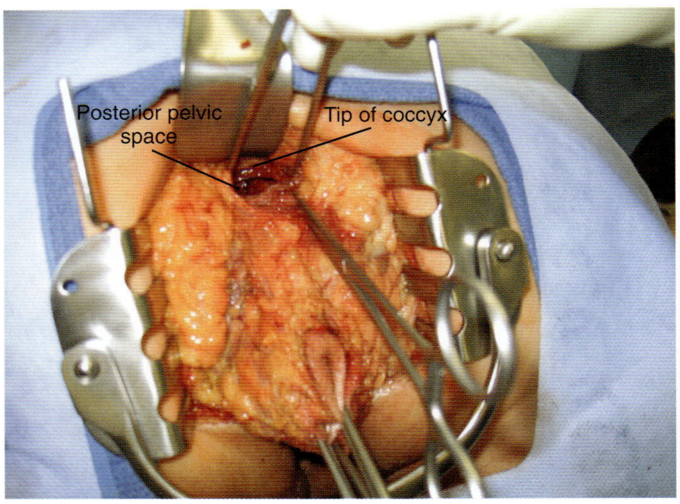

Figure 13-36

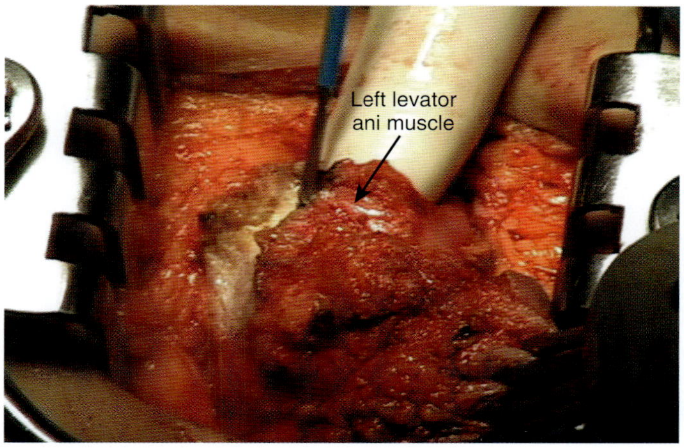

Figure 13-37

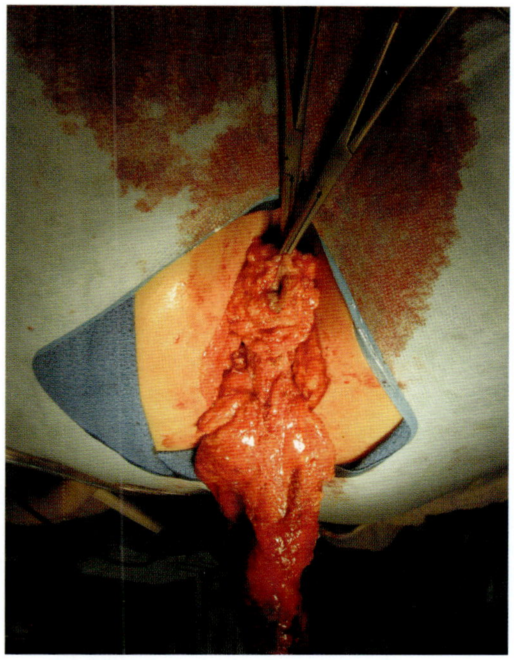
Figure 13-38

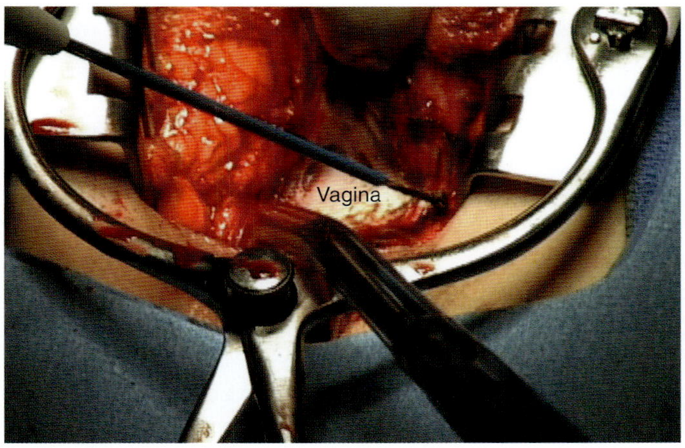

Figure 13-39

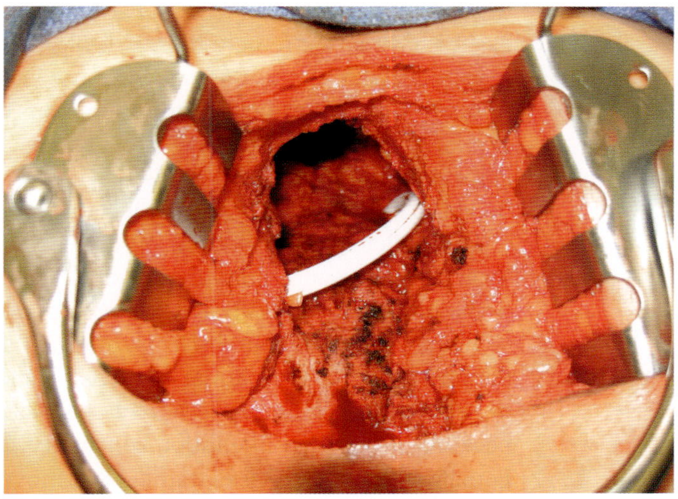
Figure 13-40

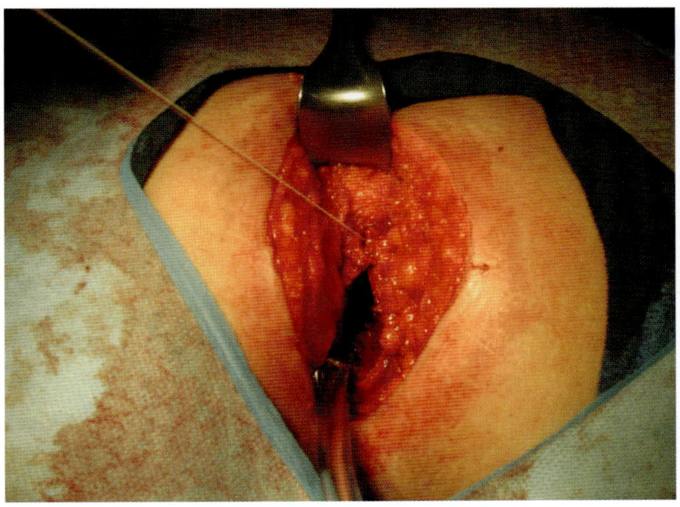
Figure 13-41

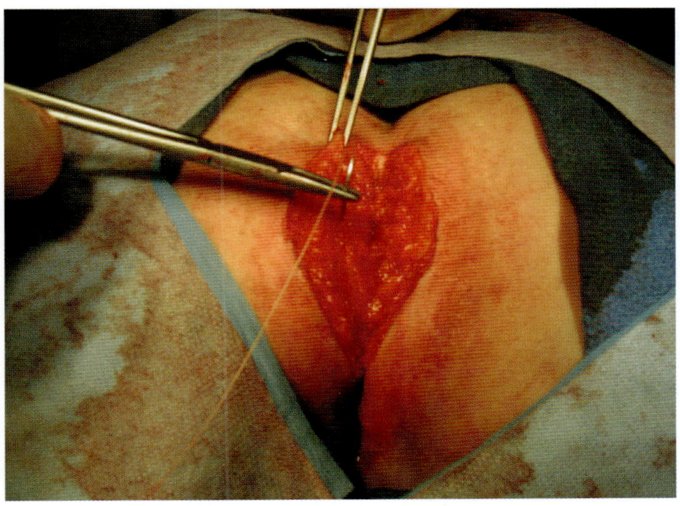
Figure 13-42

Step 4: Postoperative Care

Complications of the perineal wound are the most common complications of laparoscopic abdominal perineal resections. Because the abdominal portion is performed completely laparoscopically and the only incision is the colostomy and the trocar sites, very few wound complications are noted, and the abdominal portion of the care in the postoperative setting is minor. Instruction in enterostomal therapy and appliance change is very helpful for the new ostomate.

The perineum becomes the major concern and focus of the patient because it generates most of the pain encountered after this procedure. The patient should not sit, scoot, or ride in a car sitting for at least 2 weeks. A shower or tub soak is sometimes helpful to relieve some of the pain and to clean the area. There is a significant amount of serous drainage in the first 2 weeks until the wound begins to seal. Patients who have undergone chemoradiation for squamous cell cancer have an extremely high risk of wound breakdown. This condition is easily treated with placement of a vacuum-assisted closure (VAC) in the wound after it separates. In many circumstances, if the wound raises any suspicions of potential problems, a wound VAC could be placed primarily at the time of the operation to begin healing and improve tissue oxygenation and contraction. The Blake drain is left in the pelvis until the drainage has decreased to less than 50 mL/day and is clear serous in nature.

The patient can be started on a clear liquid diet and advanced quickly to a regular diet as soon as nausea and bloating are gone. The patient should be able to care for the colostomy and be having semiformed bowel movements before discharge.

Venous thromboembolism prophylaxis and patient-controlled analgesia are required for all patients because they are at high risk for coagulopathy with a diagnosis of cancer and pelvic dissection. The catheter is left in the bladder in most male patients for at least 4 to 5 days because of the high likelihood of urinary retention and need for reinsertion if removed earlier. Female patients can have catheters removed earlier and tend to do well with voiding despite the pelvic dissection.

Step 5: Pearls and Pitfalls

The colostomy represents a major source of complications because of blood supply, the possibility of retraction, and the difficulty of maintaining an appliance if poorly placed on the abdominal wall. Preoperative marking can avoid most of these problems if the patient is placed in the sitting position, standing position, and lying position and asked to visualize the ostomy site. Doing this with the patient dressed in his or her usual clothes may also help identify the path of the belt. Most of the time, it is better to ask the patient to change his or her clothes style rather than move the ostomy to the upper abdomen.

As mentioned earlier, the perineal wound is the most likely site of complication. Close attention to avoiding sitting, scooting, or any lateral traction to the perineal wound can reduce the risk of breakdown of the wound, infection, and future complications of perineal hernia. If an abscess forms in the pelvis, a computed tomography (CT) scan can aid in the diagnosis, and placement of a drain by a vascular interventional radiologist can be performed to eliminate the collection. The pelvic drain placed at the time of operation can be left in place for longer periods if there is an extremely high volume of lymphatic and serous fluid collecting in the now empty pelvis.

The patient should be told that the perineum will be numb and that different sensations will be present. The skin requires at least 2 to 6 weeks to heal completely because of the previous radiation and the ongoing drainage that frequently occurs because of the deep fat plane with poor blood supply.

Selected Readings

Fleshman JW, Wexner SD, Anvari M, et al. Laparoscopic vs. open abdominoperineal resection for cancer. Dis Colon Rectum 1999;42:930–9.

Ng SS, Leung KL, Lee JF, et al. Laparoscopic-assisted versus open abdominoperineal resection for low rectal cancer: a prospective randomized trial. Ann Surg Oncol 2008;15:2418–25.

CHAPTER 14

Perineal Proctectomy for Prolapse (Altmeier/Prassad Technique)

Anne Y. Lin

Step 1: Clinical Anatomy

The left colon lies along the left side of the abdomen suspended from the splenic flexure to the pelvic brim by lateral peritoneal attachments. The mesentery of the left colon arises from the midline of the abdomen along the aorta. The sigmoid colon has no lateral peritoneal attachments other than some congenital adhesions, which fix the apex of the sigmoid to the pelvic brim and the iliac fossa. Otherwise, the sigmoid colon is attached to the retroperitoneum through a midline mesentery arising from the inferior mesenteric artery (IMA) and extending down into the pelvis to the mesorectum. The splenic flexure is attached to the undersurface of the tip of the spleen, the lower edge of the tail of the pancreas, and the anterior surface of the left kidney by various levels of suspensory ligaments and peritoneal extensions. The blood supply to the left colon is based on the IMA, which arises from the anterior surface of the aorta just above the bifurcation of the common iliac arteries. The IMA extends anteriorly and bifurcates to produce the superior rectal artery feeding the sigmoid colon and the rectum. The left colic artery extends cephalad to provide the left colon and distal splenic flexure with blood supply through the arcade at the mesenteric edge known as the marginal artery of Drummond. The retroperitoneum behind the left colon contains the left ureter and the gonadal vessels lying over the psoas muscle. The ureter crosses the iliac vessels at the bifurcation of the iliac vessels into the external and internal iliac branches (Figure 14-1).

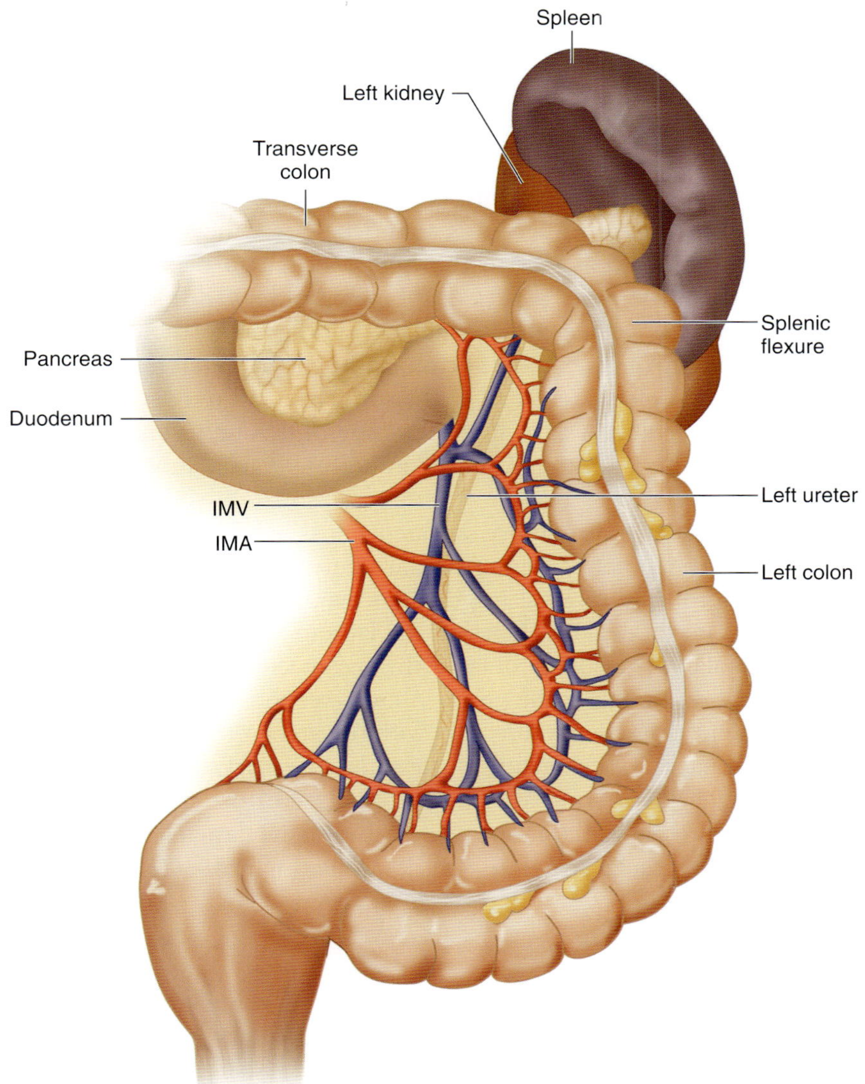
Spleen
Left kidney
Transverse colon
Splenic flexure
Pancreas
Duodenum
IMV
IMA
Left ureter
Left colon

Figure 14-1

Pelvic Anatomy

The pelvic anatomy is complex and has interrelationships between the rectum, vagina, uterus, ovaries, bladder, and prostate. The anatomy is important for pelvic dissection because of the various structures that are at risk, such as the splanchnic nerves, innervating the bladder, the ureters, and the organs themselves. The common iliac artery and vein on each side of the sacral promontory course along the posterior aspect of the pelvic brim. The hypogastric plexus of parasympathetic and sympathetic nerves is found between the bifurcation of the aorta and common iliacs. This plexus coalesces to the right and left to become the splanchnic pelvic nerves, which run along the inner aspect of the pelvic side wall to the level of the obturator fossa and the anterolateral ligaments carrying the middle hemorrhoidal vessels. Nerve fibers course from the splanchnic nerve to the rectum through the anterolateral ligaments along the middle hemorrhoidal vessels. Extensions of these nerves continue to either the vagina or the prostate as the nervi erigentes. A clear understanding of this nerve anatomy is crucial because it is easily damaged during dissection resulting in both sexual dysfunction and urinary bladder dysfunction (Figure 14-2*A*).

At the level of the sacral promontory, an areolar tissue plane begins behind the superior hemorrhoidal artery. The superior hemorrhoidal artery descends from the bifurcation of the IMA and splits at approximately S1-2 to give two major trunks down the posterior aspect of the rectum. The mesorectal envelope encases the fat and lymphatic and vascular structures of the rectum. The areolar tissue plane outside the mesorectal envelope is known as the "holy plane" and guides the dissection in the pelvis. A cross-sectional diagram of the pelvis shows the visceral peritoneum encasing the mesorectum with the areolar tissue plane between the visceral peritoneum and the parietal peritoneum posteriorly. The parietal peritoneum covers a nerve and venous plexus over the sacrum and the musculature of the side wall of the pelvis. Maintaining dissection within the areolar tissue plane between the parietal and the visceral peritoneal layers protects all of the crucial structures in the pelvis (Figure 14-2*B*).

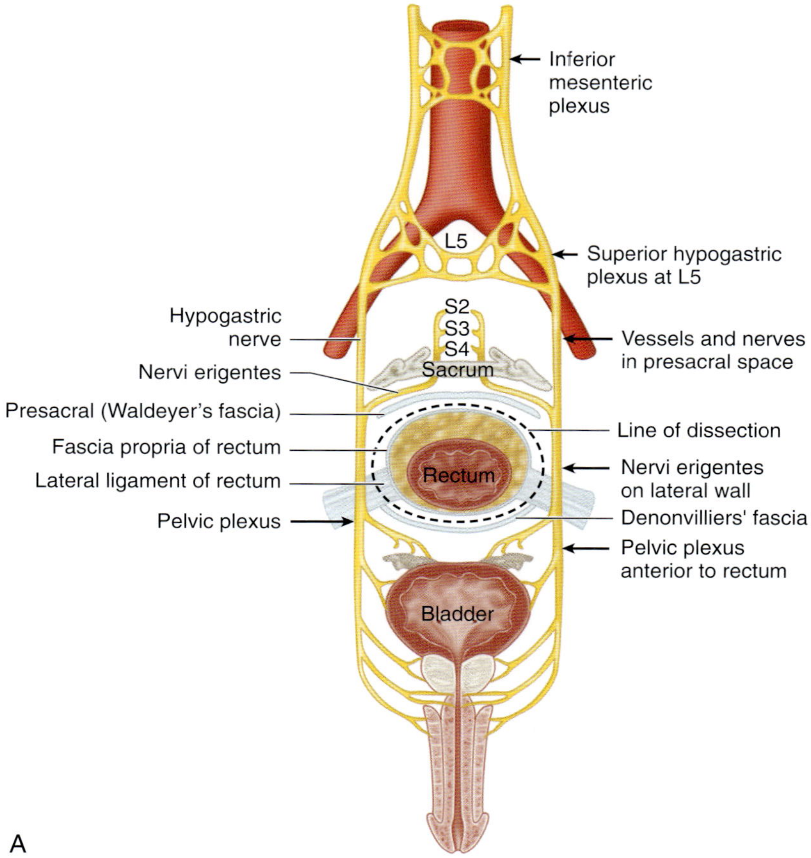

A

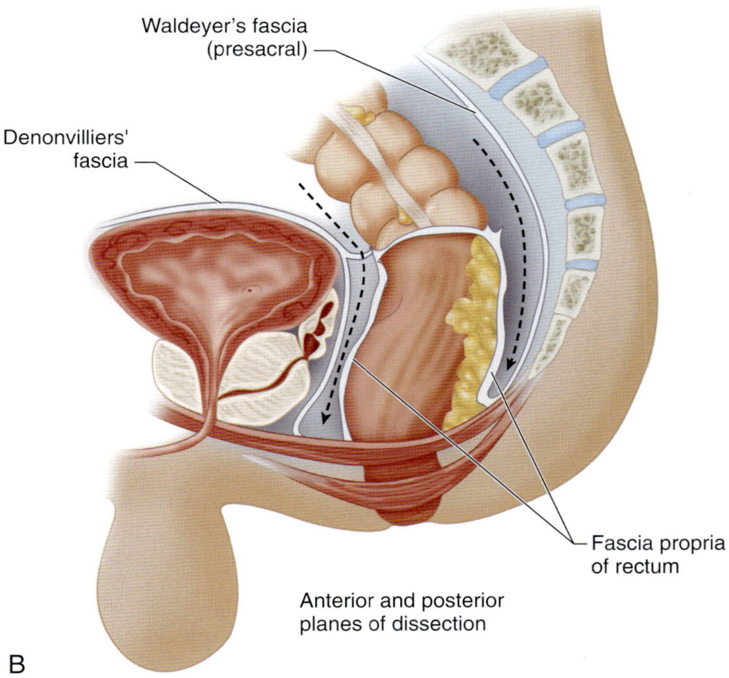

B

Figure 14-2A-B

The rectum descends through the middle of the pelvis following the curve of the sacrum and at the level of the coccyx makes a right angle to exit through the pelvic floor via the anal canal. The levator ani muscles on either side of the pelvic floor form the support diaphragm of the pelvis and extend up onto the side wall of the pelvis to insert in the ischiospinous ligament attachments covering the nerves and vessels of the deep pelvic floor. The tip of the coccyx attaches to the pubococcygeal ligament, which supports the puborectalis muscle as a semicircular sling from the pubis around the back of the rectum. This muscle closes the top of the anal canal anterior to posterior (Figure 14-3).

The anterior pelvic structures including the bladder, prostate, and vagina are separated from the rectum by the rectoprostatic or rectovaginal septum. A visceral peritoneal layer known as Denonvilliers' fascia is the posterior boundary of the anterior structures. This fascia protects the seminal vesicles and prostate during dissection. The areolar tissue plane surrounding the fat of the mesorectum continues around the entire rectum to the anterior surface of the rectum below the cul-de-sac of the pelvis. The plane is found behind or posterior to Denonvilliers' fascia. The anterolateral ligaments of the rectum carry the middle hemorrhoidal vessels into the mesorectal envelope through the visceral fascia from an anterolateral direction. Dissection and transection of these middle hemorrhoidal vessels reveals the anterior areolar tissue plane behind Denonvilliers' fascia, which can be followed all the way down to the anal canal.

The ureters, which have been described as running into the pelvic area over the pelvic brim crossing the common iliac artery and vein on either side of the pelvis, continue into the pelvis along the side wall of the pelvis toward the posterior aspect of the bladder. In the nonoperated, pristine pelvis, the ureters are higher up along the side wall of the pelvis aiming toward the posterior aspect of the trigone of the bladder. In females, the ureters run between the arterial blood supply of the uterus along the anterolateral side wall of the pelvis. In males, ureters are not exposed during the distal pelvic dissection. The ureters may be drawn posteriorly after a previous operation but are normally well protected anteriorly and laterally. In a previously operated pelvis, it is always wise to place ureteral stents at the beginning of the procedure to aid in identification of the aberrantly placed ureters.

Anal Anatomy

The upper anal canal begins at the puborectalis sling or the anorectal ring, which sits at the level of the pelvic floor and can be palpated through the anal canal as a bulge posteriorly (Figures 14-2*A* and *B* and 14-3) The longitudinal muscles of the rectum continue into the anus as the intersphincteric plane demarcating the line between autonomic internal sphincter and somatic external sphincter fibers all the way down to the level of the anal canal skin where the intersphincteric groove is palpable. The ischiorectal fossa fat is found outside the circular fibers of the external sphincter that encircle the rectum. The pudendal nerve and vessels traverse the ischiorectal fat from each ischial spine through Alcock's canal to the posterolateral aspect of the anal canal. During the perineal portion of a procedure, the pudendal nerves and vessels must be controlled.

The rectovaginal and rectoprostatic septum descends all the way to the level of the perineum anteriorly. The transverse perineal muscle separates the anterior and posterior perineum. The terminal fibers of the longitudinal muscle of the rectum insert into the skin of the anal canal just outside the anal verge as the corrugator cutanei ani and cause the ridges that are noticed around the anal canal. The internal sphincter is the hypertrophied circular muscle of the wall of the rectum. The lowest portion of the internal sphincter can be palpated as a groove where the longitudinal fibers insert on the skin.

Within the anal canal, the dentate line is the junction between cuboidal epithelium of the anal transition zone, which is the terminal mucosal layer of the rectum, and the squamous epidermal cells of the anal canal skin. Gland openings (or crypts) are found in the dentate line

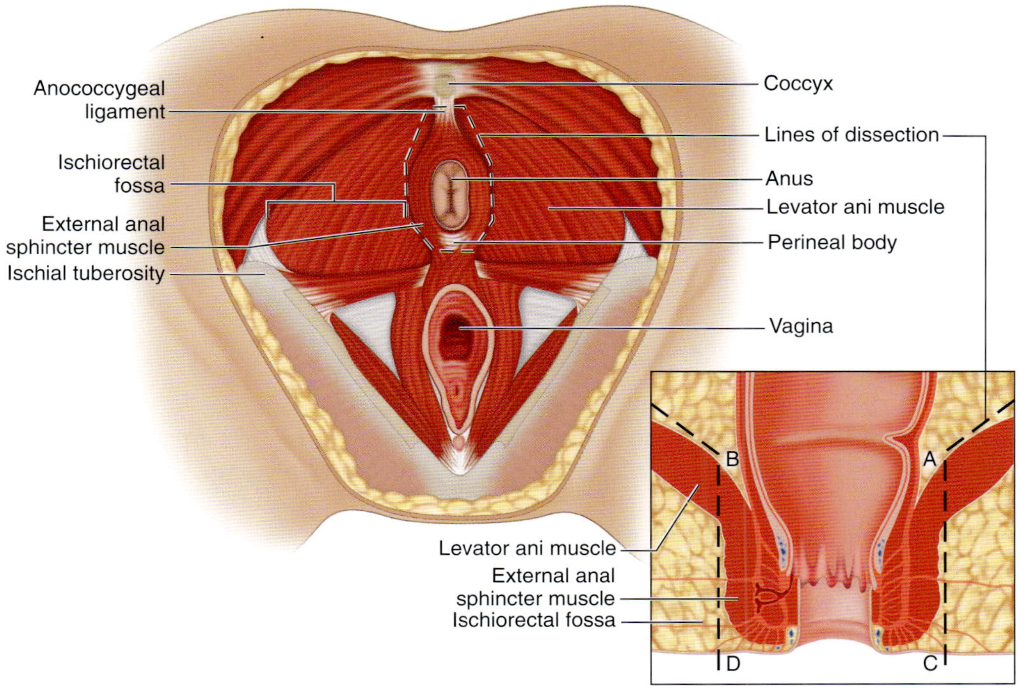
Anococcygeal ligament
Ischiorectal fossa
External anal sphincter muscle
Ischial tuberosity
Coccyx
Lines of dissection
Anus
Levator ani muscle
Perineal body
Vagina
Levator ani muscle
External anal sphincter muscle
Ischiorectal fossa
A
B
C
D

Figure 14-3

at the base of the Morgagni columns, which are interdigitating lines of squamous epithelium into the cuboidal and columnar epithelium of the distal rectum. The anal transition zone is the most highly innervated section of the rectum and anal canal containing nerve fibers sensing temperature, vibration, electrical stimulation, pressure, liquid, solid, and gas. The dentate line lies approximately halfway along the surgical anal canal, which extends from the palpable anal verge all the way up to the anorectal ring palpated at the puborectalis sling posteriorly. The anoderm within the anal canal, cephalad to the anal verge, has no hair follicles.

Step 2: Preoperative Considerations

Colonoscopy should be performed before the operation. Testing to determine sphincter function and anatomy can also be performed to evaluate potential for sphincter function recovery after the operation. All patients should undergo a full mechanical bowel preparation. Patients should receive preoperative antibiotics and deep vein thrombosis chemical prophylaxis and sequential compression devices. A bladder catheter should be placed.

Step 3: Operative Steps

- The patient is placed in the prone-flexed position (Figure 14-4). The perineum is prepared and draped in the standard sterile fashion. A self-retaining retractor is used for retraction (Figure 14-5).
- The redundant distal rectum is prolapsed through the anal canal (Figure 14-6). The rectal wall is circumferentially infiltrated with local anesthetic containing epinephrine approximately 1 cm proximal to the dentate line (Figure 14-6).
- A full-thickness circumferential incision is made in the rectum until the perirectal fat is reached. It is helpful to score the mucosa initially before the full-thickness incision to maintain a consistent rectal cuff distance. Four quadrant stay sutures are placed in the anal cuff (Figure 14-7).
- Rectal dissection is performed in the areolar tissue plane proximally until the bowel cannot be easily prolapsed further. The anterior peritoneum at the cul-de-sac is encountered at this time. The apex of the peritoneum anteriorly is tagged with sutures to facilitate closure of the peritoneum later in the procedure (Figure 14-8).

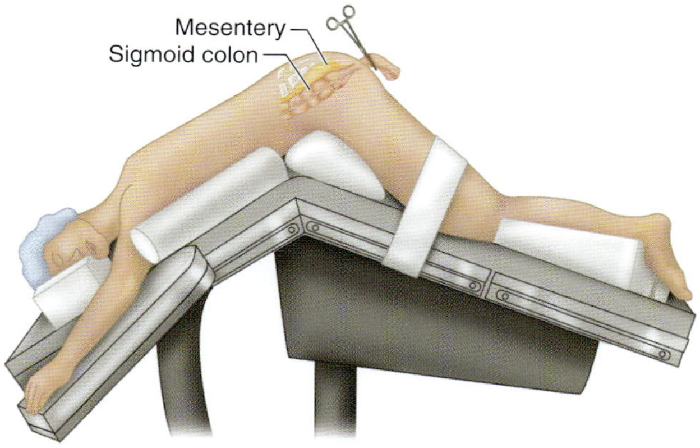

Figure 14-4

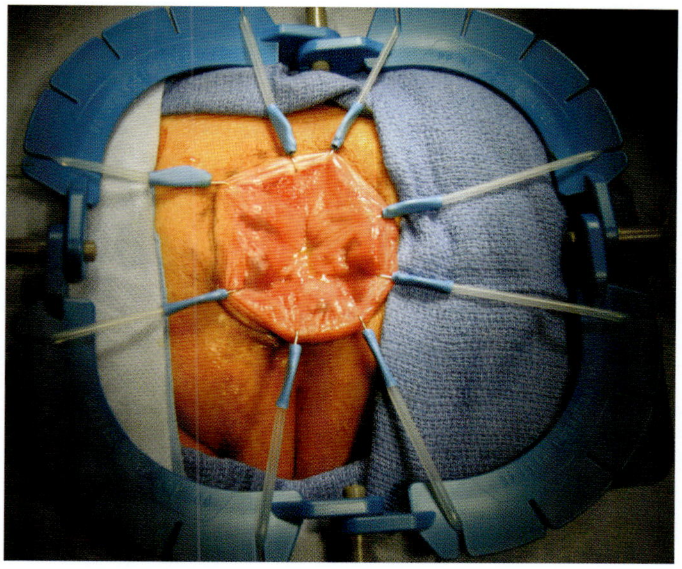

Figure 14-5

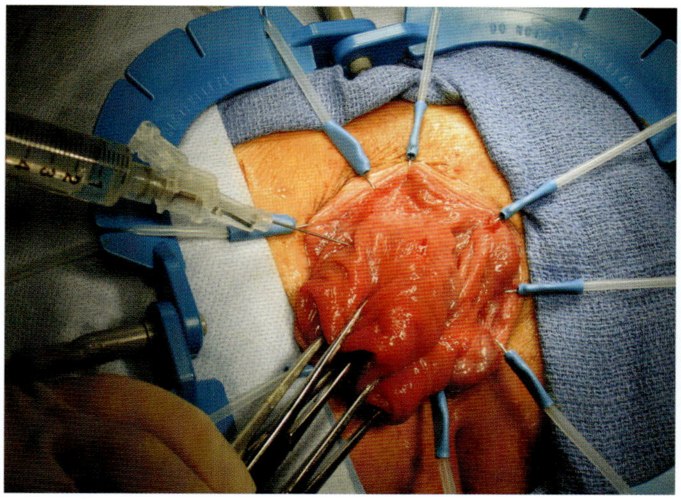

Figure 14-6A

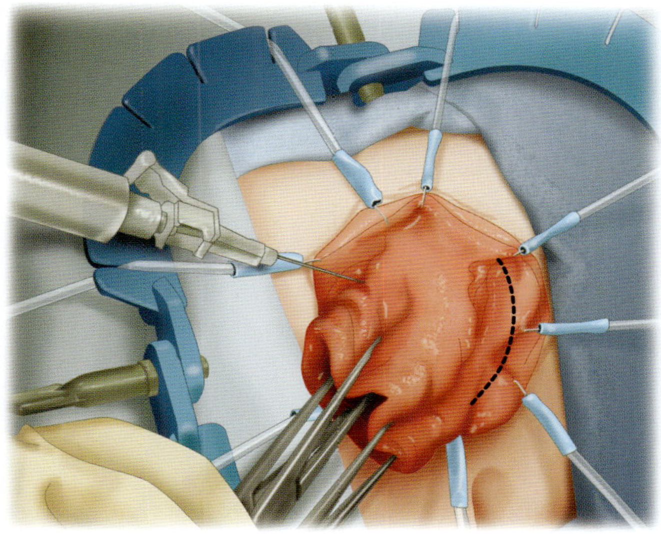

Figure 14-6B

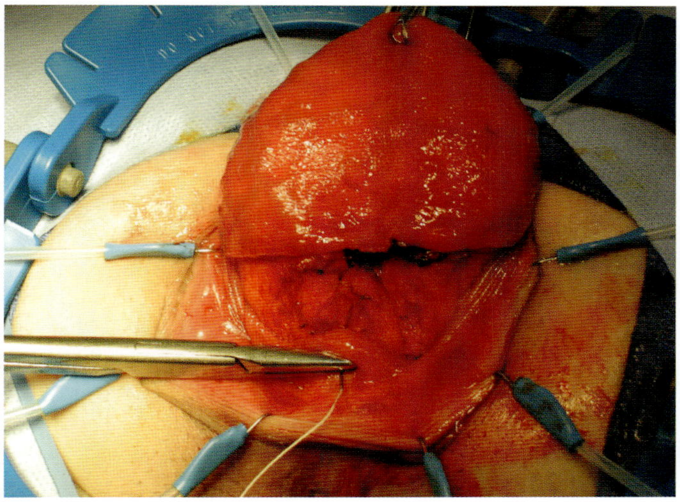

Figure 14-7

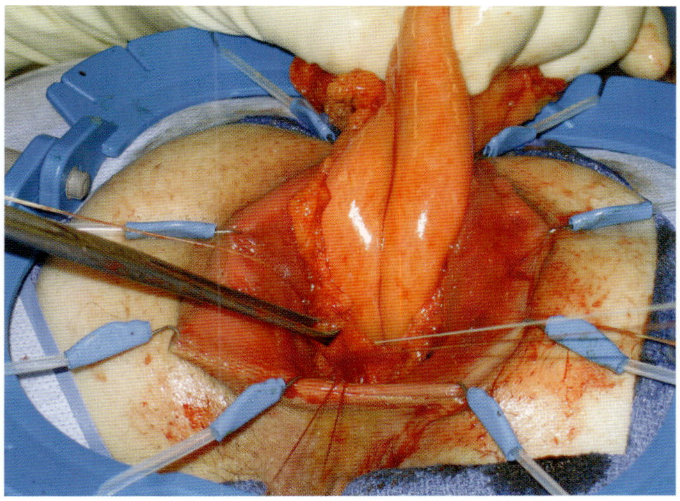

Figure 14-8

- Attention is given to careful ligation of the posterior mesorectal and sigmoid vessels all the way up to the sacral promontory (Figure 14-9).
- The point of proximal colon transection is usually at the left colon–sigmoid junction (Figure 14-10). The resection is performed at the limit of adequate blood supply and at the extent of mobilization of the proximal segment, which allows a left colon-to-anal canal anastomosis under slight tension. The anastomosis should spontaneously return to the pelvis at the level of the puborectalis muscle (Figure 14-11).
- Reefing of the levator muscles may be performed anterior or posterior to the rectum to make the anorectal angle more acute and to reduce the opening of the pelvic floor outlet. It should be just loose enough to allow admittance of a finger (Figures 14-12 and 14-13).

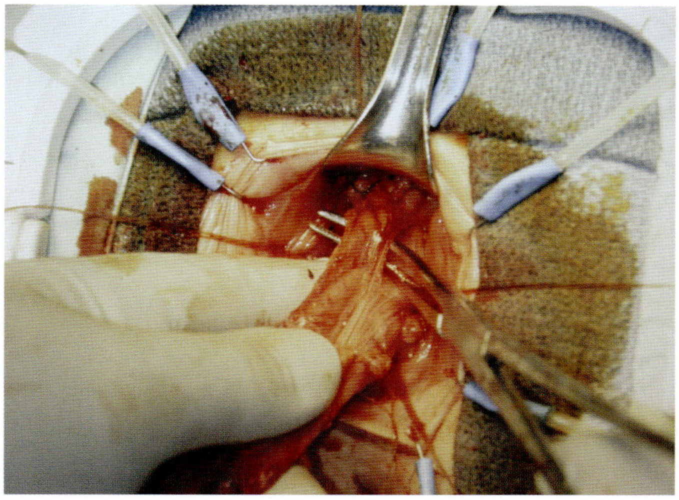

Figure 14-9

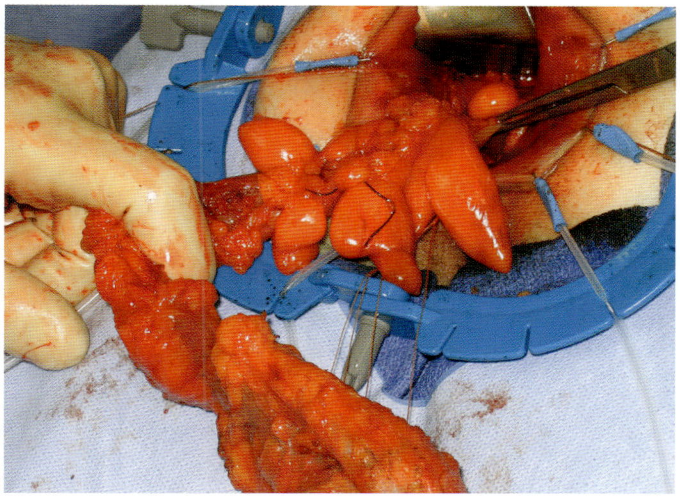

Figure 14-10

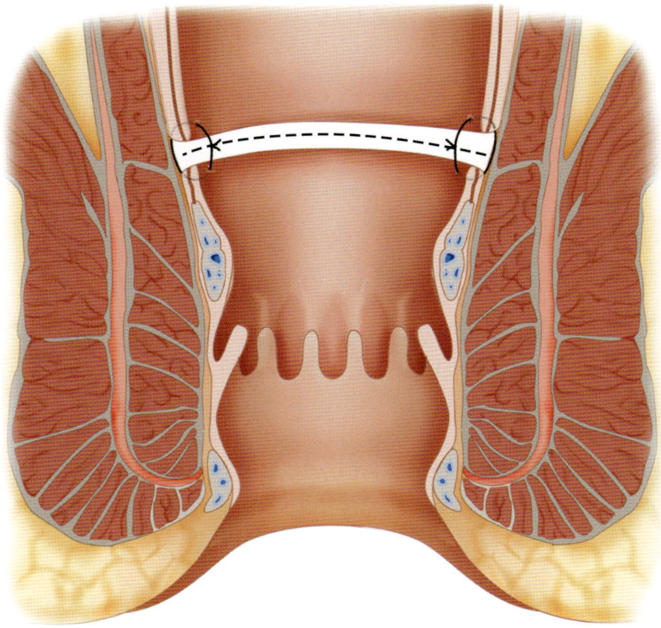

Figure 14-11

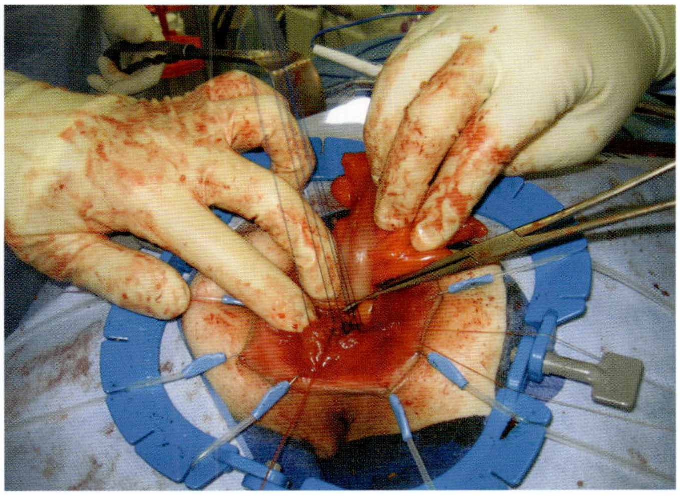

Figure 14-12

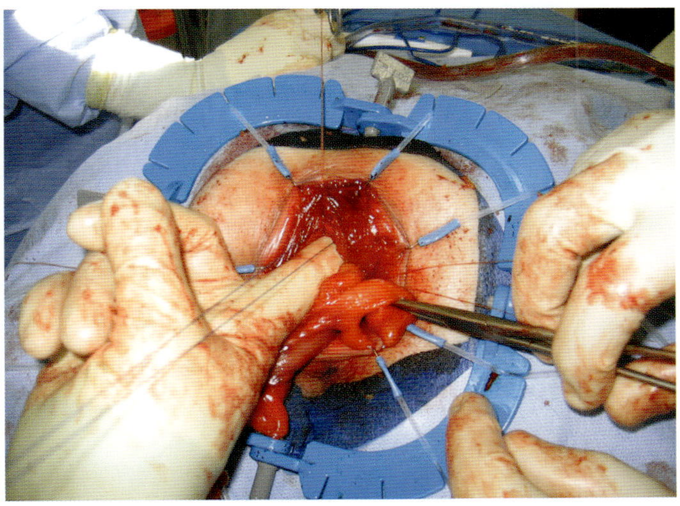

Figure 14-13

- The left colon is sequentially resected at the level of the anal canal as sutures are placed full-thickness through the bowel using the four previously placed anal cuff quadrant sutures (Figures 14-14 and 14-15). The intervening spaces are filled with full-thickness sutures until a complete coloanal anastomosis is obtained (Figure 14-16).

Step 4: Postoperative Care

Pain is usually minimal. Diet may be resumed after 2 days of bowel rest. The patient may be discharged after return of bowel function.

Step 5: Pearls and Pitfalls

Careful attention must be given to ligation or energy sealing of the posterior mesorectal and sigmoid vessels because these may retract into the pelvis before establishing hemostasis. Also, care must be taken to avoid too-proximal ligation of the mesentery, which causes a shortened length of proximal bowel and tension at the anastomosis. Resection of the proximal bowel and suture placement should be performed in segments to prevent retraction of the proximal bowel into the pelvis.

Selected Readings

Glasgow SC, Birnbaum EH, Kodner IJ, et al. Recurrence and quality of life following perineal proctectomy for rectal prolapse. J Gastrointest Surg 2008;12:1446–51.

Riansuwan W, Hull TL, Bast J, et al. Comparison of perineal operations with abdominal operations for full-thickness rectal prolapse. World J Surg 2010;34:1116–22.

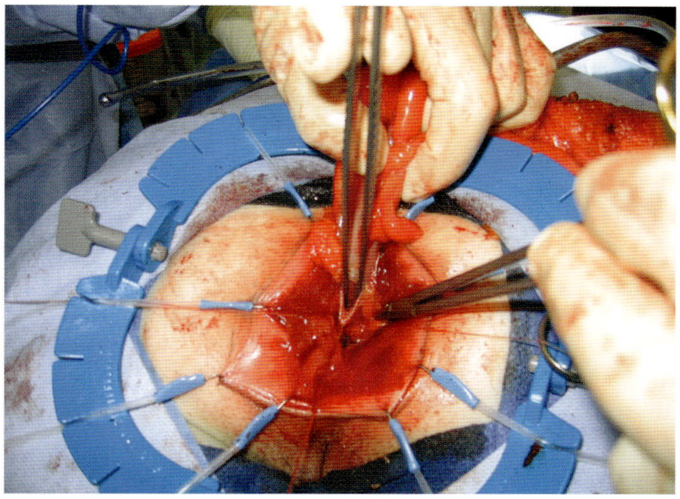
Figure 14-14

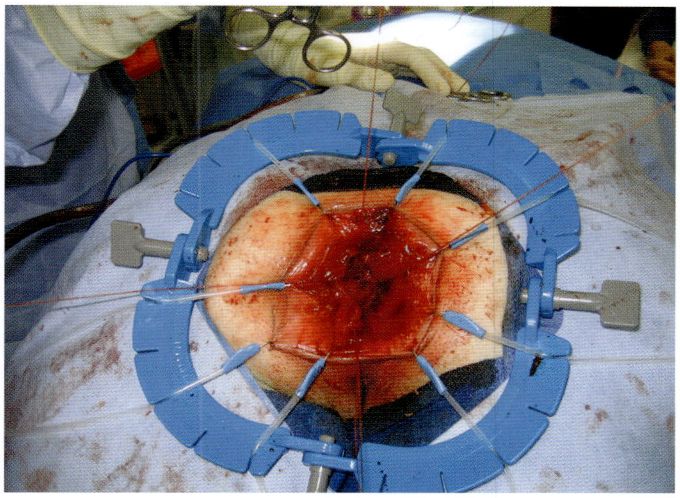
Figure 14-15

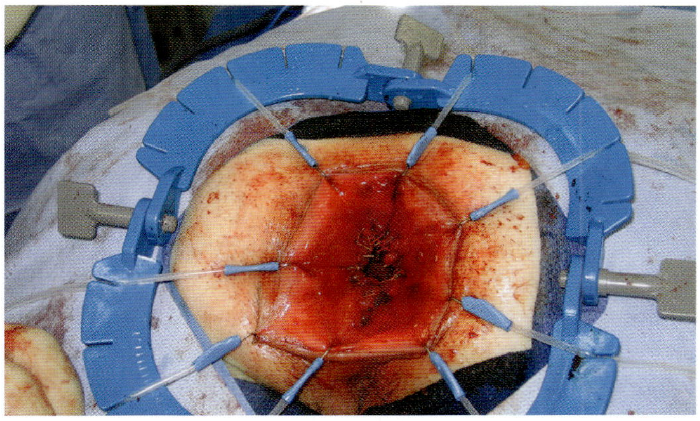
Figure 14-16

CHAPTER 15

Open Resection Rectopexy for Rectal Prolapse

Elisa H. Birnbaum

Step 1: Clinical Anatomy

The left colon is adherent to the retroperitoneum along the left gutter via an avascular filmy tissue plane. The left colon and its mesentery attach to the posterior retroperitoneum where the ureter and gonadal vessels are found. There is also an avascular peritoneal surface attaching the left colon to the left and posterior abdominal wall from the splenic flexure to the sigmoid colon. The peritoneal attachments along the left gutter suspend the left colon from the left side of the abdomen from the pelvic rim all the way up to the splenic flexure. At the pelvic rim, the colon becomes free from pelvic side wall attachments and assumes a sigmoid shape and at this point is known as the sigmoid colon. The sigmoid colon lies free within the abdominal cavity and pelvis attached posteriorly to its vascular pedicle arising from the aorta. It is common to see a redundant sigmoid colon with a narrow vascular pedicle. The sigmoid colon continues distally into the pelvis where at the level of the sacral promontory the three taenia coalesce and become the top of the rectum. The upper portion of the rectum is intraperitoneal. The exact limits of the rectum are controversial. The rectosigmoid junction is considered to be at the level of S3 by anatomists, but most surgeons regard the sacral promontory as the landmark for the upper rectum (Figure 15-1). The rectum is approximately 12 to 15 cm long. There is an absence of taenia at the epiploic appendices and diverticulum. The mesentery can be ill-defined, and the posterior aspect of the rectum is extraperitoneal and closely adherent to the sacral hollow. This peritonealized mesorectum becomes elongated in patients with prolapse. This posterior tissue is perirectal areolar tissue containing the terminal branches of the inferior mesenteric artery (IMA). The upper third of the rectum is intraperitoneal, exposed to the peritoneum anteriorly and laterally. The middle third of the rectum is exposed to the peritoneum in its anterior aspect only, and the lower one third of the rectum is entirely extraperitoneal. The anterior peritoneal reflection can be variable but generally occurs at 7 to 9 cm from the anal verge in men and 5 to 7.5 cm from the anal verge in women.

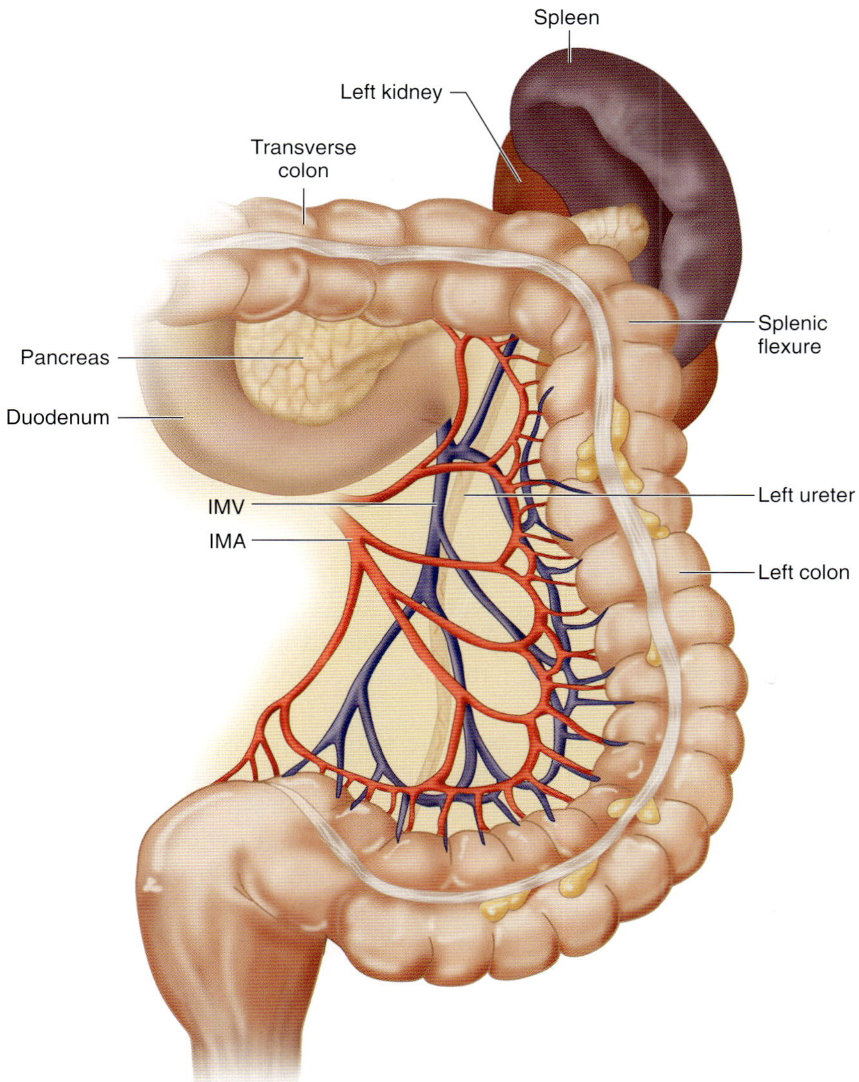
Spleen
Left kidney
Transverse colon
Splenic flexure
Pancreas
Duodenum
Left ureter
IMV
IMA
Left colon

Figure 15-1

Step 2: Preoperative Considerations

Resection rectopexy is indicated for young patients with full rectal prolapse and occasionally patients with significant internal intussusception. A mechanical bowel preparation is typically performed, and prophylactic antibiotics appropriate for colectomy are given within 1 hour of the incision to reduce the risk of wound infection. Patients require routine deep vein thrombosis prophylaxis. Preoperative counseling should include the risk of rectal prolapse recurrence and the possibility of persistent fecal incontinence. Patients with normal sphincter tone are better candidates for abdominal rectopexy because perineal proctectomy requires the anal sphincter to be lax and completely everted during prolapse.

Step 3: Operative Steps

- General endotracheal anesthesia is required. An oral gastric tube helps decompress the stomach during the procedure. The patient is placed in the lithotomy position. Sequential compression devices and deep vein thrombosis chemical prophylaxis are applied, and a bladder catheter is placed.
- A Pfannenstiel incision is used for exposure into the pelvis. Alternatively, a lower midline incision can be made from the umbilicus to the pubis. A body wall retractor is placed for abdominal wall retraction.
- The patient is placed in the Trendelenburg position, and the small bowel is packed out of the pelvis allowing access to the redundant rectosigmoid junction (Figure 15-2).
- A peritoneal incision is made from the lateral ligaments to the sacral promontory along the left peritoneal reflection, and a similar incision is made along the right peritoneal reflection (Figure 15-3).

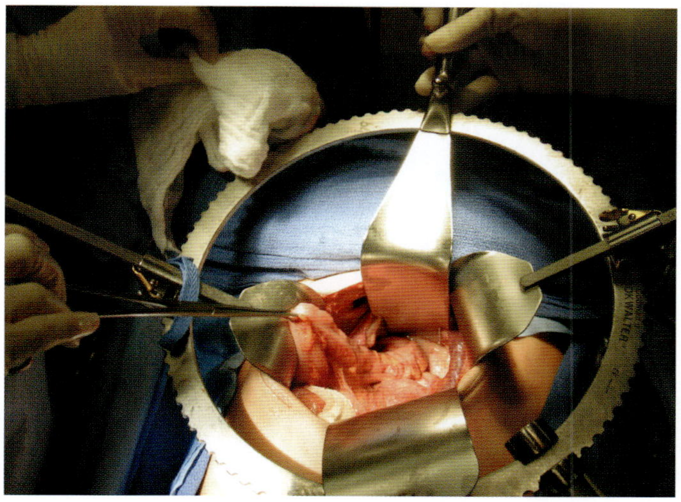

Figure 15-2

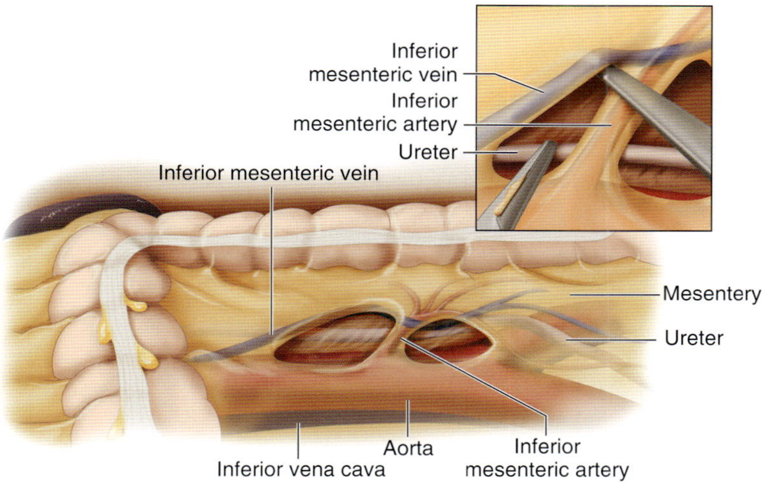

Figure 15-3

- The presacral space is entered at the sacral promontory, and the areolar tissue is divided down to the pelvic floor along the mesorectum (Figure 15-4). Dissection in this areolar tissue plane (Figure 15-5) allows release of the mesorectum in its envelope around the circumference of the pelvis (Figure 15-6). A Thorlakson retractor is useful for maintaining traction of the redundant mesorectum (Figures 15-7 and 15-8).

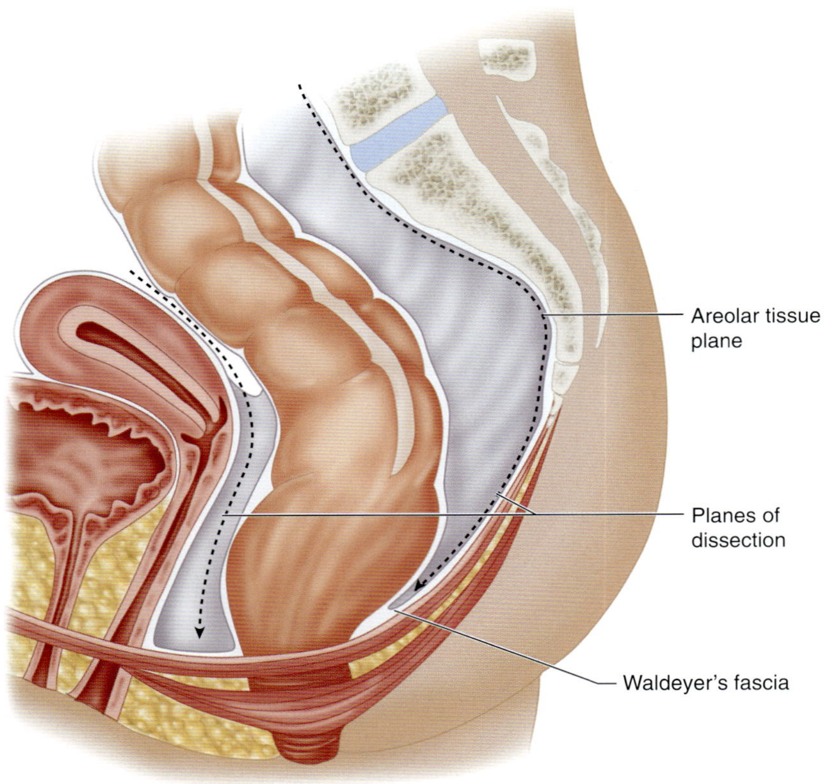

Figure 15-4

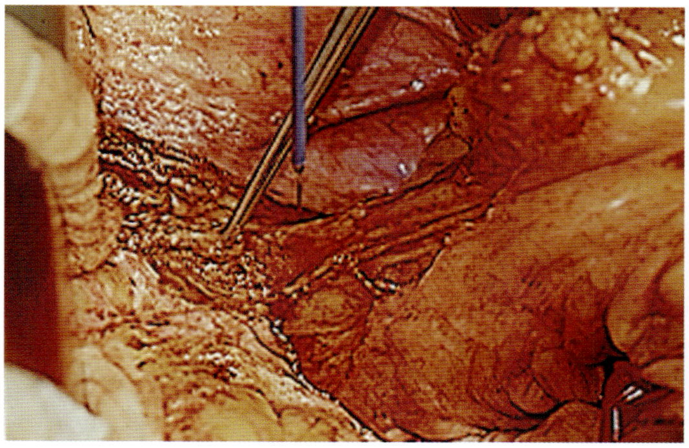
Figure 15-5

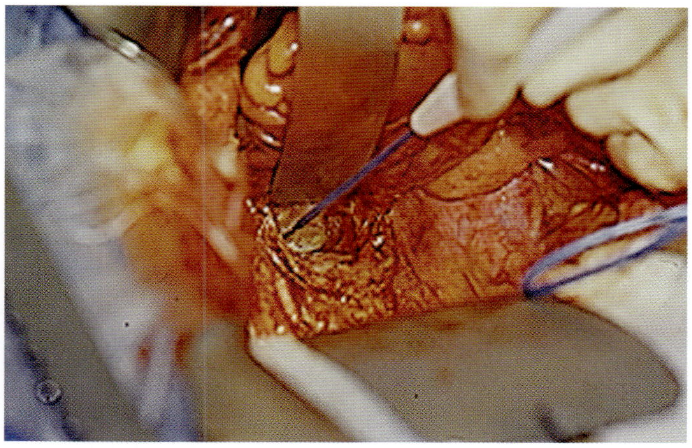
Figure 15-7

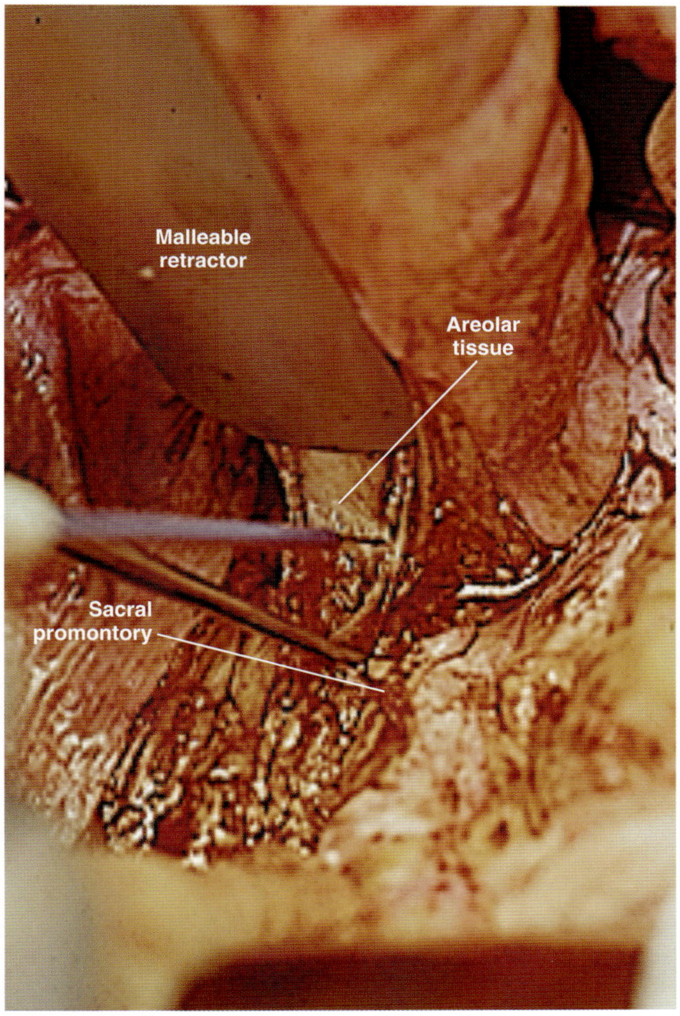

Figure 15-6

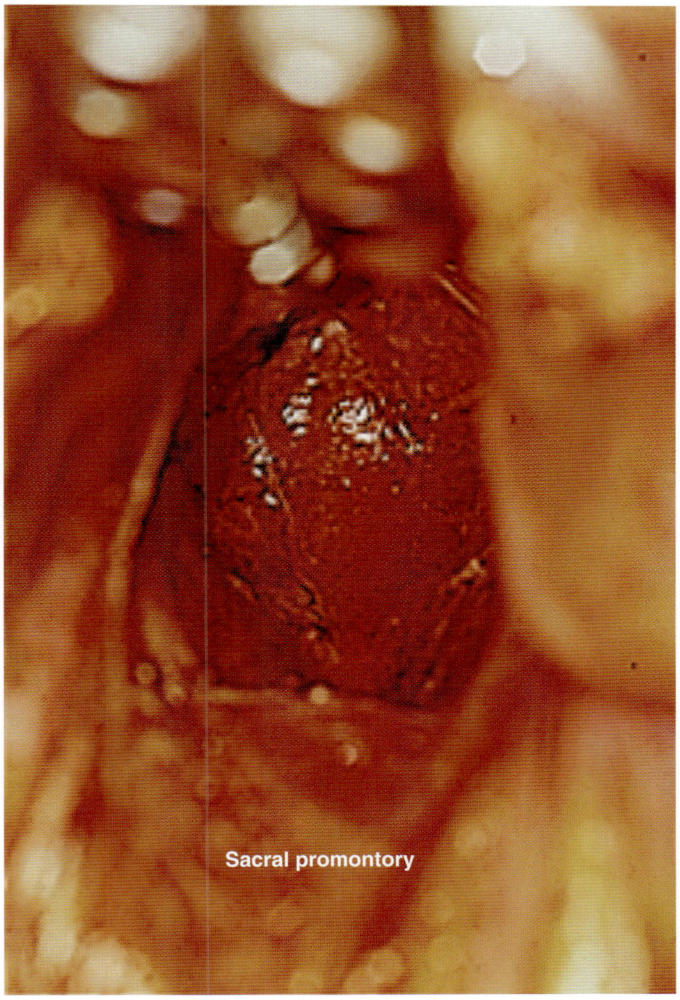

Figure 15-8

- The anterior rectovaginal septum is identified. It is frequently thickened owing to chronic prolapse. An incision is made along the anterior surface of the rectum through the rectovaginal peritoneal reflection, and dissection is done in this areolar plane (Figure 15-9) down to the level of the pelvic floor. The anterolateral ligaments entering from the pelvic side walls are preserved to protect the splanchnic nerves and middle rectal vessels within the fatty structure.
- The distance of dissection in the anterior and posterior plane is checked by placing a gloved finger within the anal canal to assess mobilization to the pelvic floor.
- The redundant rectosigmoid is resected. Because the descending colon is typically not redundant and is a retroperitoneal organ, the proximal resection margin is chosen just distal to this point. The mesentery of the distal descending colon is mobilized along the left gutter (Figure 15-10). The left colon mesentery is ligated and divided up to the edge of the colon. A proximal purse-string suture is placed at the distal descending colon junction, a Kocher clamp is placed distally, and the bowel is divided (Figure 15-11).
- A 29-mm circular stapler head is placed within the purse-string suture, and the purse-string is tied.
- The redundant rectum is retracted toward the sacral promontory, and the distal resection margin is chosen at a point where the anastomosis can be done without redundancy but also without tension. This point is typically in the upper rectum.
- The mesentery is divided and ligated to this point, and the rectal wall is isolated and divided with a linear cutter stapler (Figure 15-12).
- The circular stapler is passed through the rectal stump, and the point is brought out just anterior to the staple line. The instrument is coupled, engaged, and then fired.
- After removal of the circular stapler, the pelvis is filled with fluid, and air is insufflated through the rectum via a proctoscope. The anastomosis is checked for air leakage and repaired with 3-0 polyglactin Lembert sutures as needed.

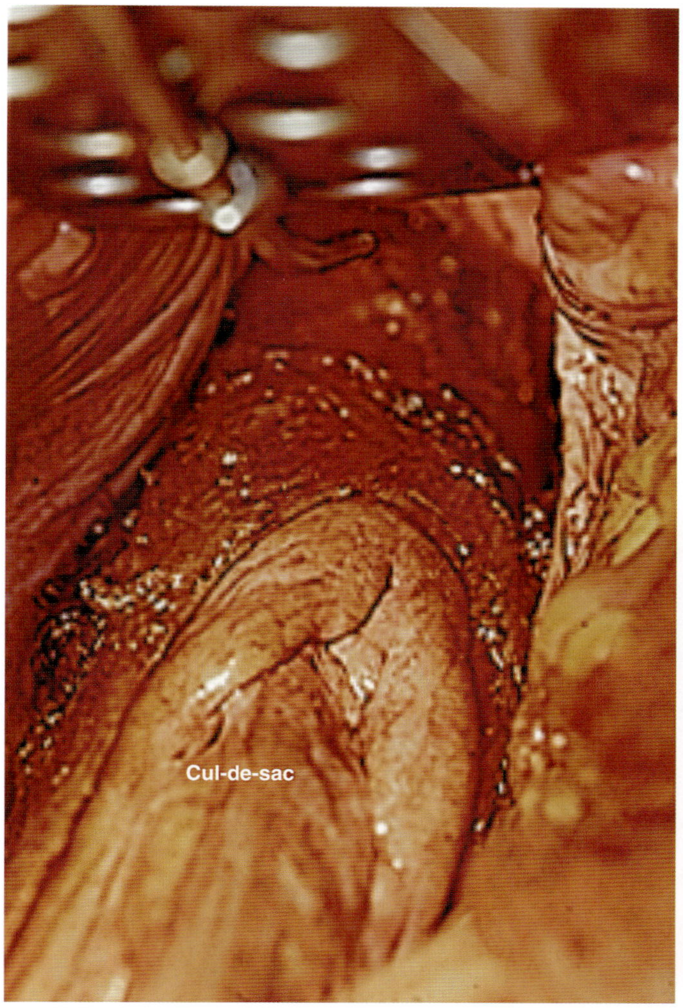

Figure 15-9

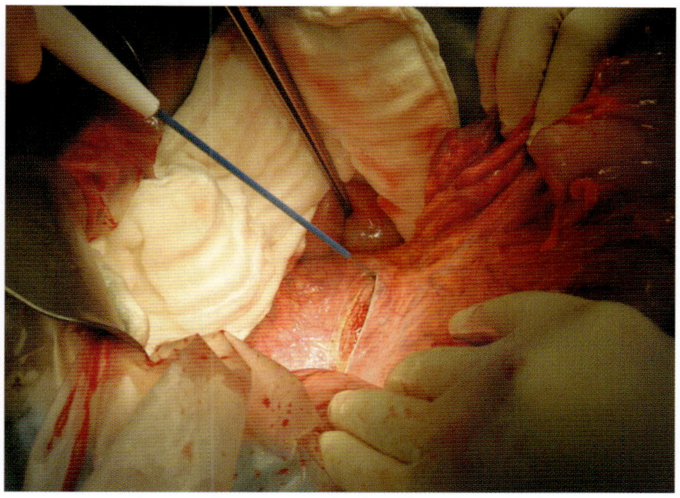
Figure 15-10

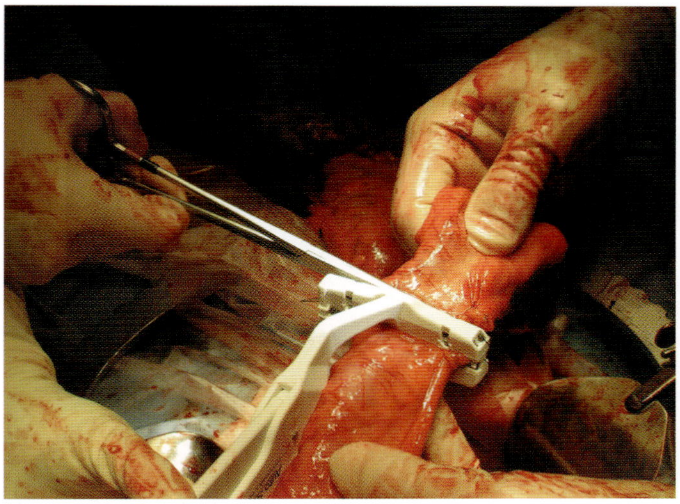
Figure 15-11

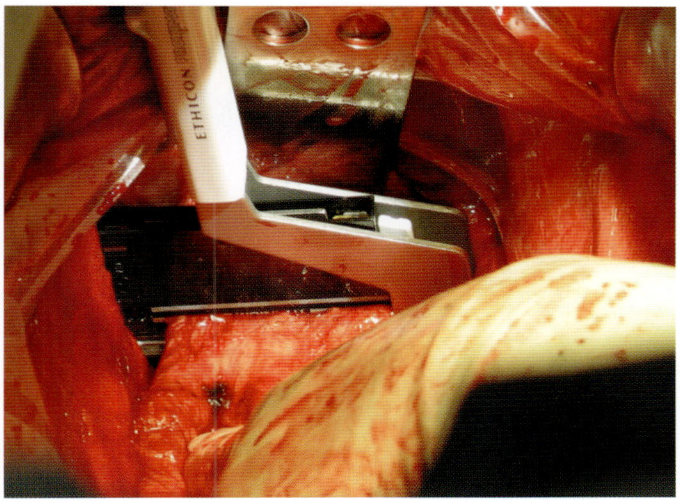

Figure 15-12

- A sutured rectopexy is performed at the sacral promontory with No. 1 polypropylene suture (Figure 15-13). The suture is placed through the left lateral ligament (Figure 15-14) and then through the periosteum at the level of the sacral promontory (Figure 15-15). Care must be taken to avoid the left internal iliac vein. The suture is passed back through the left lateral ligament. The right lateral ligament is affixed in a similar fashion (Figure 15-16). The sutures are tied snuggly, and the pelvis is irrigated with saline (Figure 15-17). A drain is typically not used. The abdominal fascia is closed with No. 1 absorbable suture.

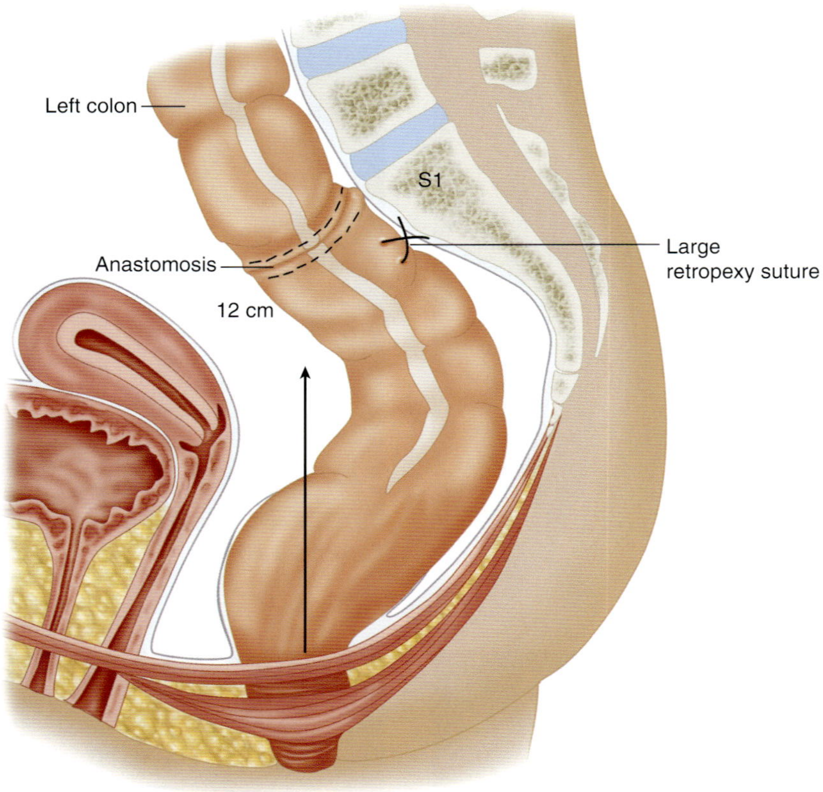

Figure 15-13

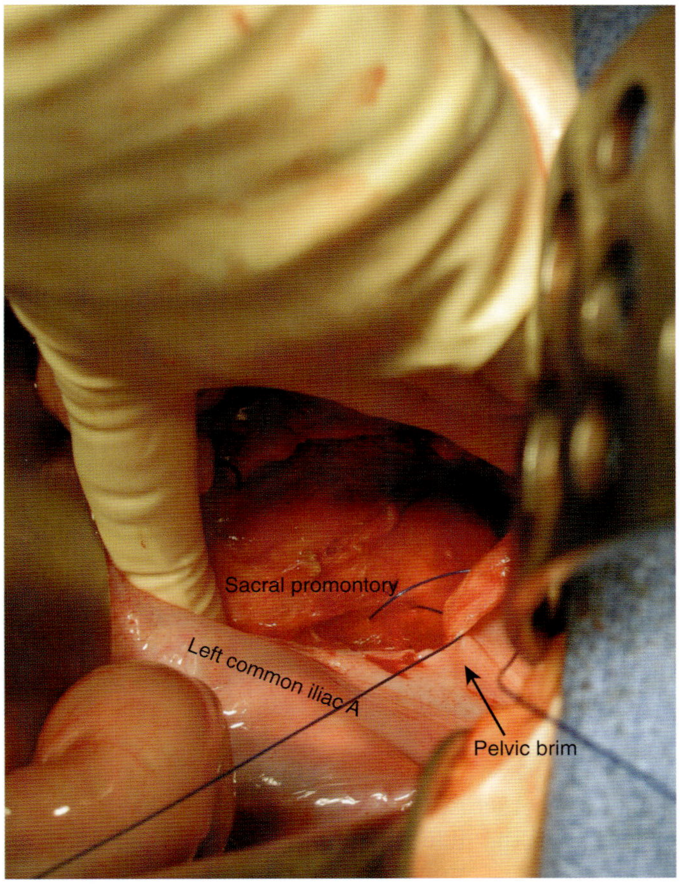

Figure 15-14

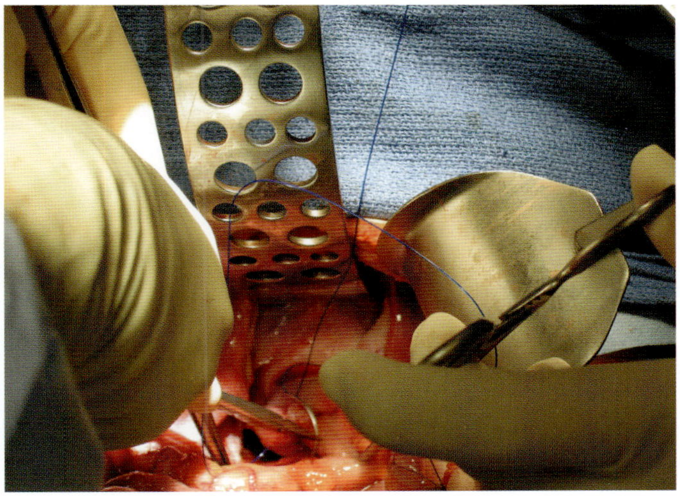

Figure 15-15

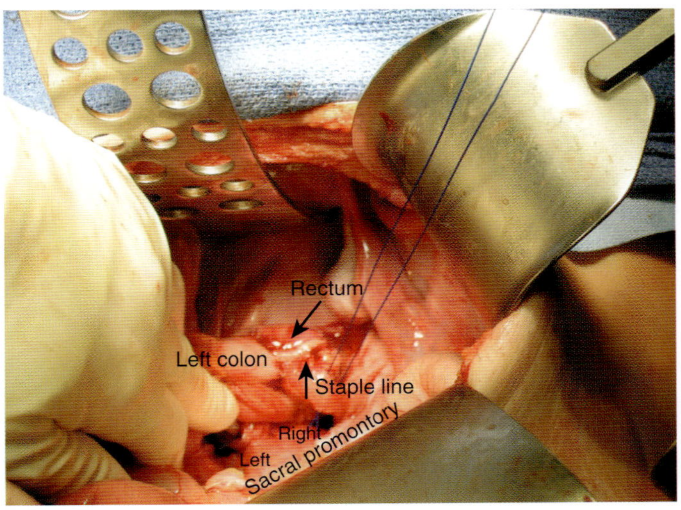

Figure 15-16

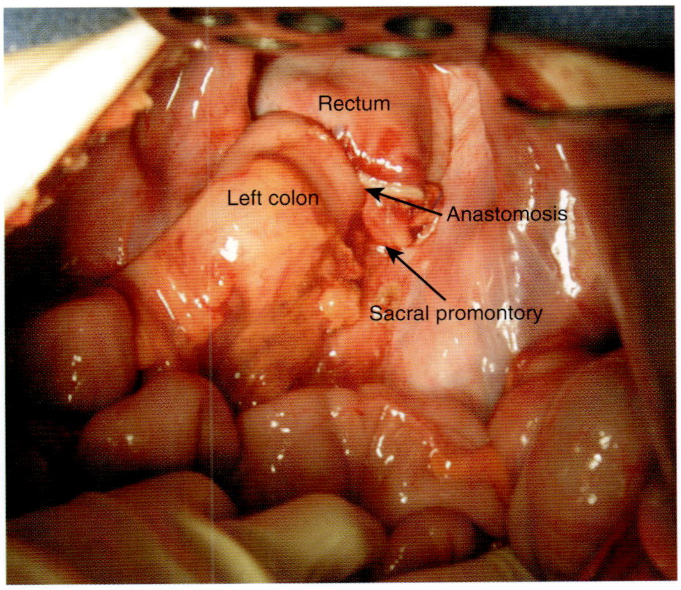

Figure 15-17

Step 4: Postoperative Care

Intravenous fluid replacement is given to maintain a urine output of approximately 30 mL/hr. Nasogastric decompression is not required unless the patient becomes nauseated. Patients are ambulated early, and deep vein thrombosis prophylaxis should be given. Antibiotics are given for the first 24 hours, and patients are encouraged to use incentive spirometry. Postoperative analgesia is usually maintained with patient-controlled analgesia followed by oral analgesics. Patients are initially given a liquid diet and advanced as tolerated. The usual hospital stay is approximately 4 to 5 days.

Step 5: Pearls and Pitfalls

The risk of anastomotic leak can be minimized by ensuring the use of well-vascularized tissue in the descending colon and rectum. Although resection of the redundant colon is one of the goals of this procedure, the anastomosis should be done under minimal tension. Checking for an air leak may not eliminate the risk of anastomotic leakage but helps to identify trouble spots that can be repaired at the time of operation.

Placing the rectopexy suture is best accomplished with a single pass through the periosteum of the central sacral promontory. If bleeding is encountered, it often stops when the suture is tied. Lateral placement of the suture risks injury to the internal iliac vessels. Sharp or cautery dissection of the rectal mesentery in the areolar tissue plane under direct vision helps to minimize the tearing of presacral veins that can occur with blunt dissection.

Most patients have frequent, loose bowel movements when their bowel function returns. Reduced rectal vault capacity and absence of the sigmoid "brake" results in urgency. Stretch injury to the anal sphincter from chronic prolapse may prevent complete return of fecal continence.

Selected Readings

Karas JR, Uranues S, Altomare DF, et al. No rectopexy versus rectopexy following rectal mobilization for full-thickness rectal prolapse: a randomized controlled trial. Dis Colon Rectum 2011;54:29–34.

Riansuwan W, Hull TL, Bast J, et al. Comparison of perineal operations with abdominal operations for full-thickness rectal prolapse. World J Surg 2010;34:1116–22.

CHAPTER 16

Laparoscopic Rectopexy

Matthew G. Mutch

Step 1: Clinical Anatomy

The left colon lies along the left side of the abdomen suspended from the splenic flexure to the pelvic brim by lateral peritoneal attachments. The mesentery of the left colon arises from the midline of the abdomen along the aorta. The sigmoid colon has no lateral peritoneal attachments other than some congenital adhesions, which fix the apex of the sigmoid to the pelvic brim and the iliac fossa. Otherwise, the sigmoid colon is attached to the retroperitoneum through a midline mesentery arising from the inferior mesenteric artery (IMA) and extending down into the pelvis to the mesorectum. The splenic flexure is attached to the undersurface of the tip of the spleen, the lower edge of the tail of the pancreas, and the anterior surface of the left kidney by various levels of suspensory ligaments and peritoneal extensions. The blood supply to the left colon is based on the IMA, which arises from the anterior surface of the aorta just above the bifurcation of the common iliac arteries (see Figure 16-3). The IMA extends anteriorly and bifurcates to produce the superior rectal artery feeding the sigmoid colon and the rectum. The left colic artery extends cephalad to provide the left colon and distal splenic flexure with blood supply through the arcade at the mesenteric edge known as the marginal artery of Drummond. The retroperitoneum behind the left colon contains the left ureter and the gonadal vessels lying over the psoas muscle. The ureter crosses the iliac vessels at the bifurcation of the iliac vessels into the external and internal iliac branches (Figure 16-1).

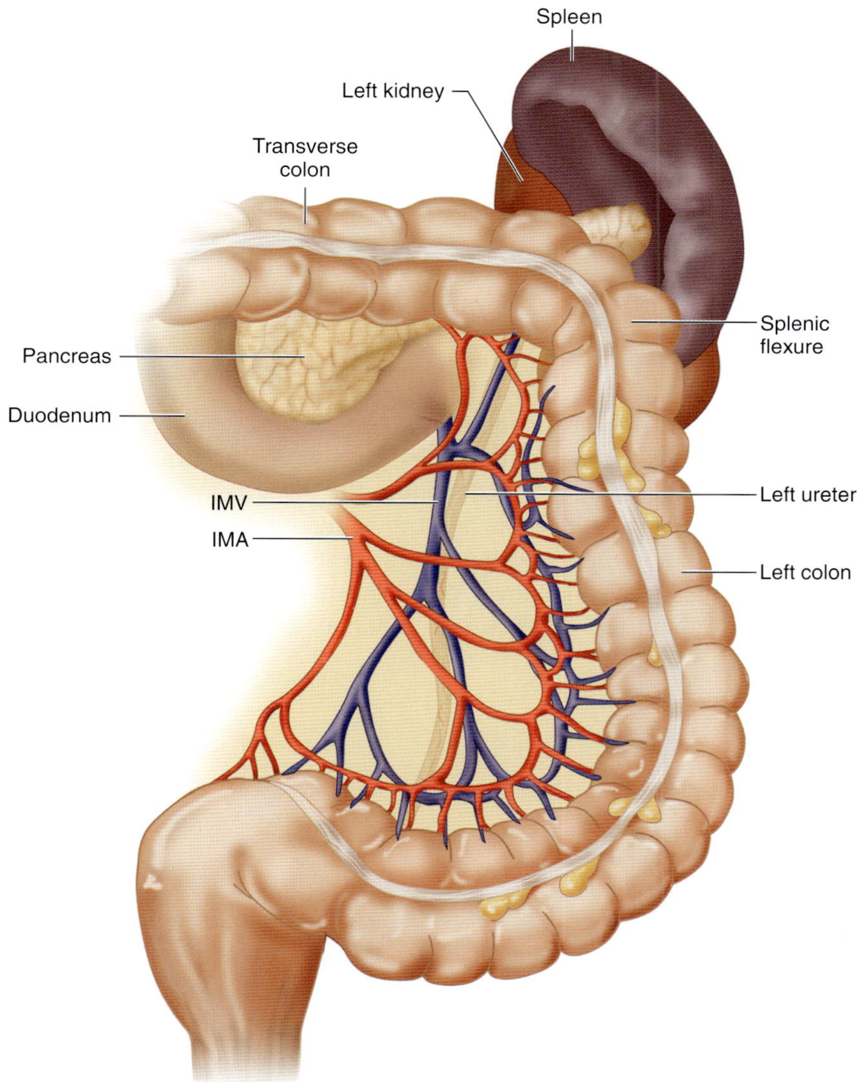
Spleen
Left kidney
Transverse colon
Splenic flexure
Pancreas
Duodenum
Left ureter
IMV
IMA
Left colon

Figure 16-1

Pelvic Anatomy

The rectum and mesorectum fit within the pelvis as a cylinder within a cylinder. They are contained within a fascial envelope that is separated from the surrounding pelvic structures by areolar tissue. Posteriorly, the sympathetic nerves branch just above the sacral promontory and travel laterally. The internal iliac vessels follow the course of the hypogastric nerves but are deep to them as they travel into the pelvis. The ureters enter the pelvis laterally and enter the bladder anterior to the rectum. In males, the seminal vesicles and prostate gland lay below the anterior peritoneal reflection. Denonvilliers' fascia separates the prostate from the anterior surface of the rectum. In females, the cervix and rectovaginal septum lay below the anterior peritoneal reflection. The parasympathetic nerves arise from S2-4, traveling anteriorly to enter the urogenital structures at roughly 2 o'clock and 10 o'clock. The lateral stalks or vasculature to the rectum can be found laterally deep in the pelvis. The mesorectum tapers out as the rectum reaches the levator muscles at the pelvic floor just below the tip of the coccyx.

Step 2: Preoperative Considerations

Patients must have a total colon examination. Attention to the presence of constipation as part of the patient's symptoms is necessary to ensure success. A mechanical bowel preparation may be beneficial because it eliminates formed stool in the distal colon and improves handling and anastomosis formation. It may be more important in this setting to minimize postoperative constipation and pressure on the rectopexy sutures. Antibiotic prophylaxis begun preoperatively that continues for 24 hours postoperatively is preferred. Deep vein thrombosis prophylaxis with sequential compression devices is required and may be supplemented with subcutaneous heparin.

Step 3: Operative Steps

- For laparoscopic colorectal surgery, a mechanical bed should always be used to allow for extremes of patient position, which facilitates the use of gravity as a retractor to help keep the small bowel out of the way. The patient is placed on a beanbag and in the lithotomy position. Both of the patient's arms are tucked to the side with thumbs up and palms facing the patient's hips. The beanbag is used to cocoon the patient to minimize movement when the patient is placed in steep positions. Some surgeons advocate padding the shoulders. The most important point about patient positioning is the angle of flexion of the hips. The angle of flexion should be less than 10 degrees and with minimal abduction. When operating in the left upper quadrant, the surgeon's hand and instrument will hit the thigh; this is minimized by keeping the flexion and abduction as limited as possible.
- The camera port is placed below the umbilicus. Two working ports are placed on the right side of the abdomen, lateral to the rectus muscle. The two ports are centered around the umbilical port and are spaced a hand's width apart. A second working port is placed in the left lower quadrant as low as possible and lateral to the rectus muscle.
- The pelvis is exposed to assess the pelvic structures and how deep the cul-de-sac is positioned (Figure 16-2).

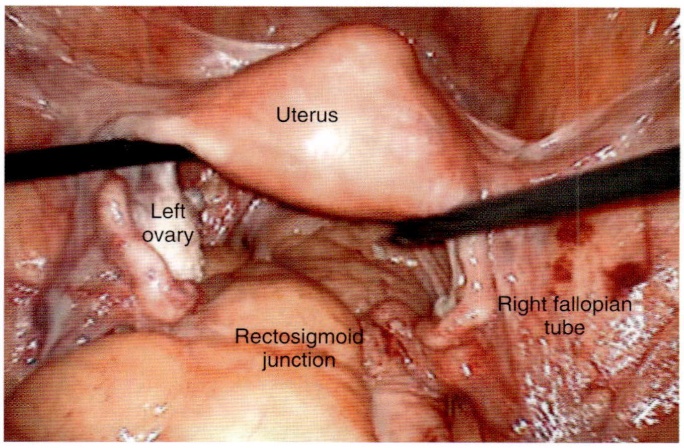
Uterus
Left ovary
Rectosigmoid junction
Right fallopian tube

Figure 16-2

- The retroperitoneum and presacral space are entered by retracting the superior rectal artery at the level of the sacral promontory (Figure 16-3). The peritoneum is scored from deep down into the pelvis up to the origin of the IMA (Figure 16-4). When the retroperitoneum is entered, the left ureter is identified and swept into the retroperitoneum. The dissection is carried out laterally beyond the sigmoid colon.
- The rectum can be retracted anteriorly so that it can be mobilized posteriorly down to the pelvic floor. The avascular plane of the presacral space is entered (Figure 16-5). This dissection is carried all the way to the pelvic floor (Figures 16-6 and 16-7).
- The lateral peritoneal attachments are divided to the level of the anterior peritoneal reflection (Figure 16-8).

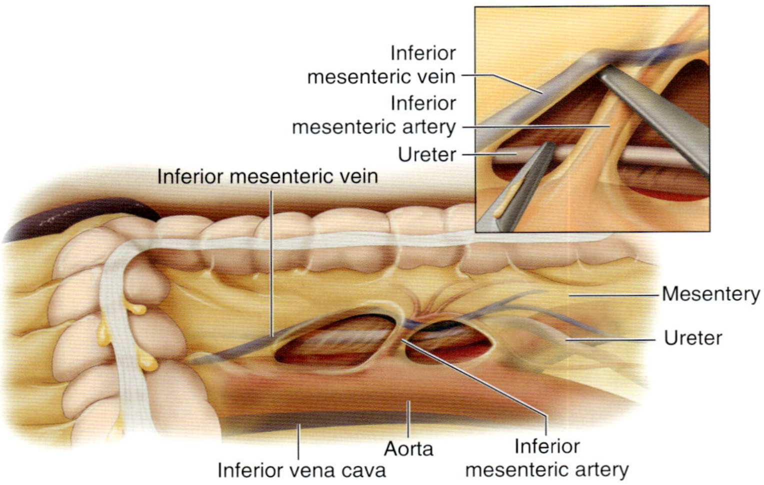

Figure 16-3

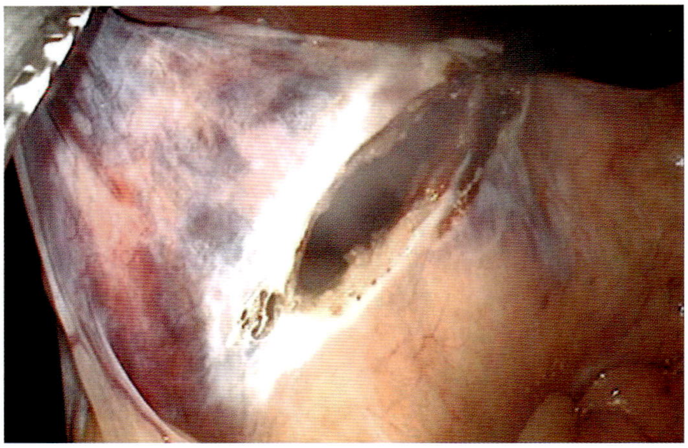

Figure 16-4

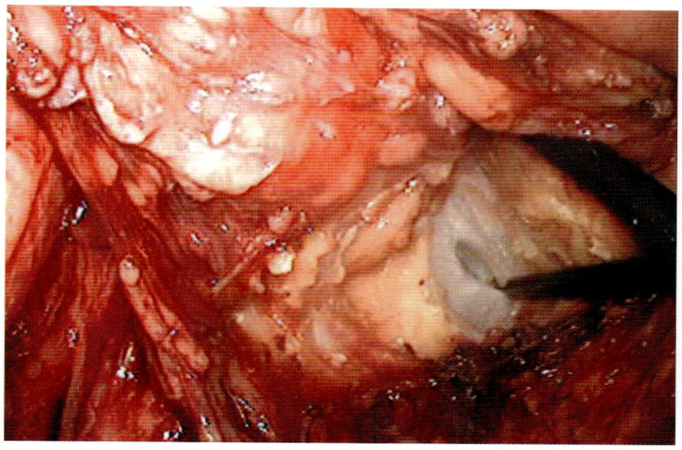

Figure 16-5

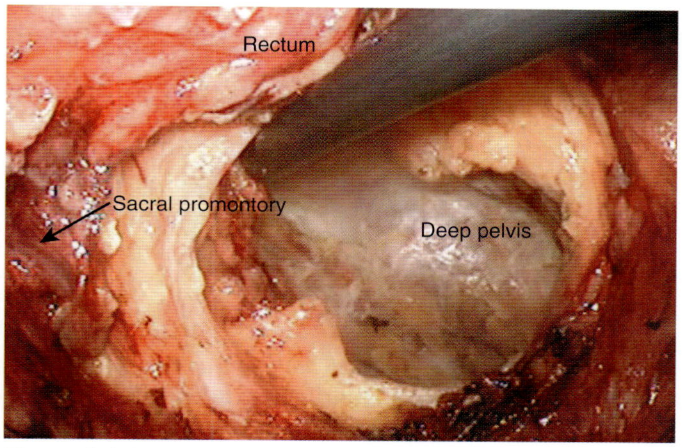

Figure 16-6

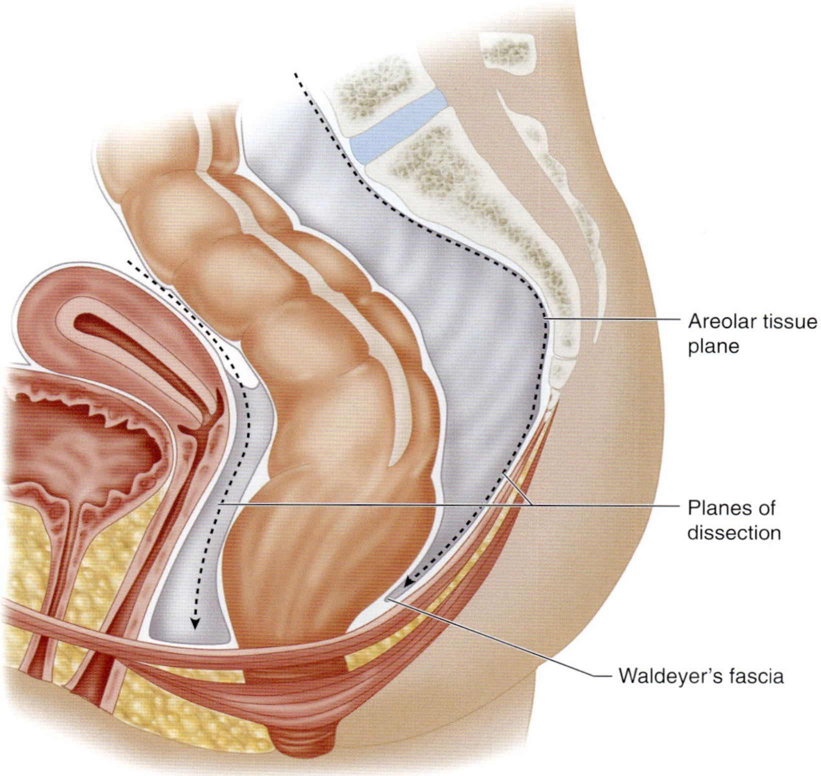

Figure 16-7

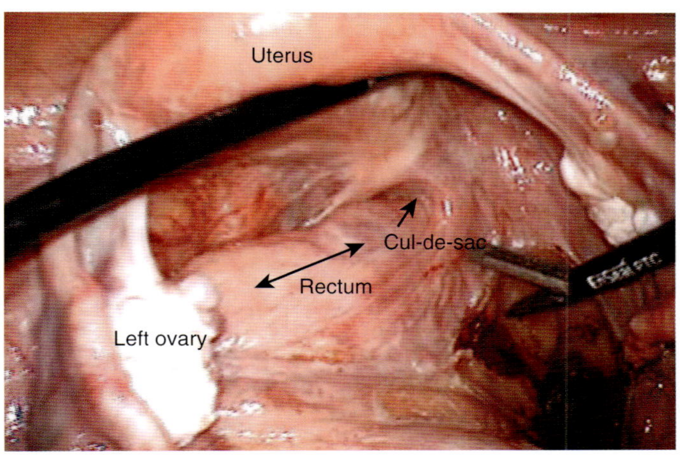

Figure 16-8

- By incising the anterior peritoneum, the anterior rectum can be mobilized down to the pelvic floor (Figures 16-9 and 16-10). The rectovaginal septum is developed by blunt and cautery dissection and carried down to the level of the pelvic floor (Figure 16-11). The lateral stalks typically are not divided to preserve the vascular supply of the distal rectum.
- With the rectum completely mobilized, it can be sutured to the sacral promontory (Figure 16-12). Using a 2-0 permanent, monofilament suture, two stitches are placed through the lateral peritoneal wings of the rectum into the periosteum of the sacral promontory (Figures 16-13 and 16-14). When the needle is passed into the periosteum, it should not be removed because of the risk of significant bleeding from sacral veins. The point of peritoneal attachment to the sacral promontory should stretch the rectum over the curve of the sacrum.

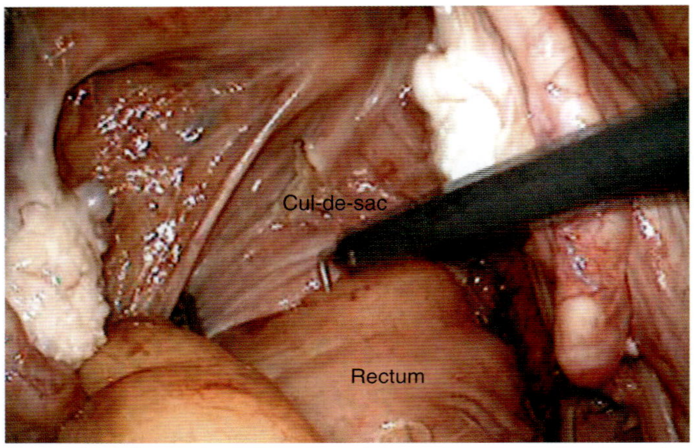

Figure 16-9

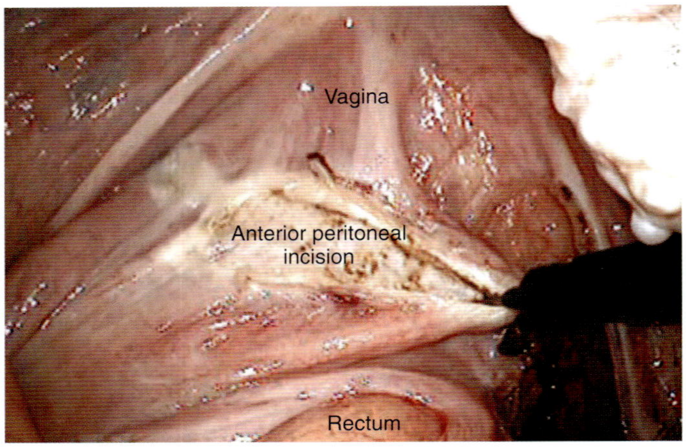

Figure 16-10

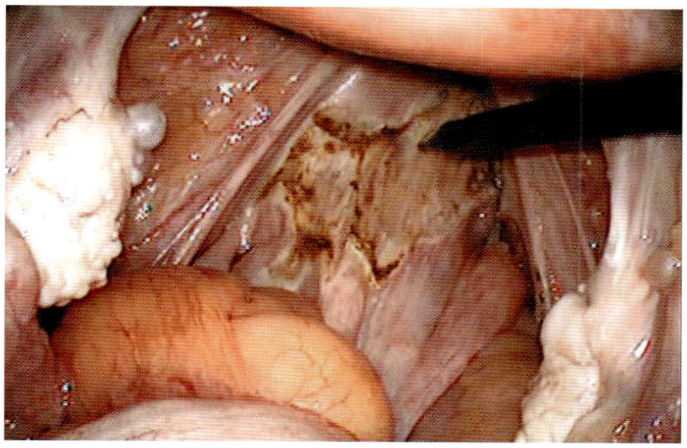

Figure 16-11

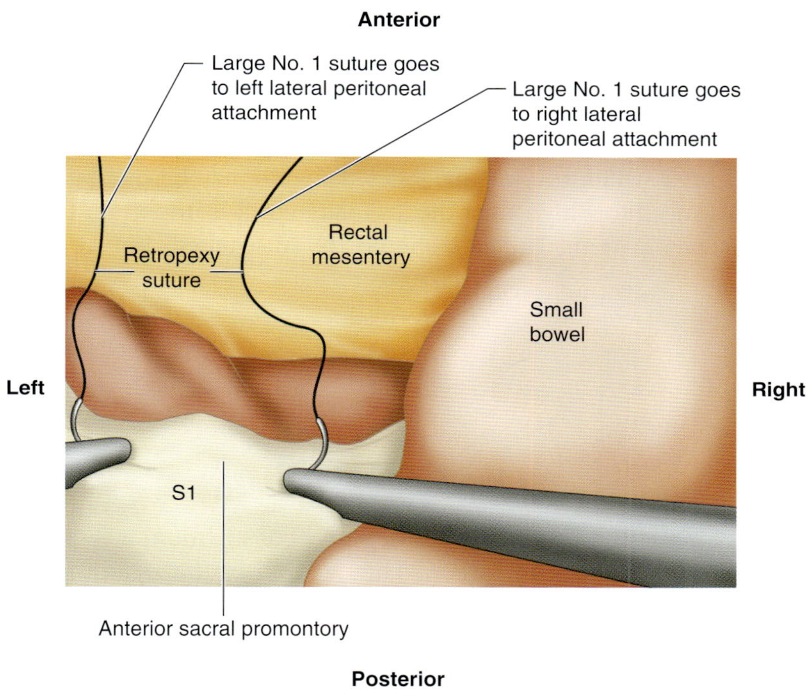

Figure 16-12

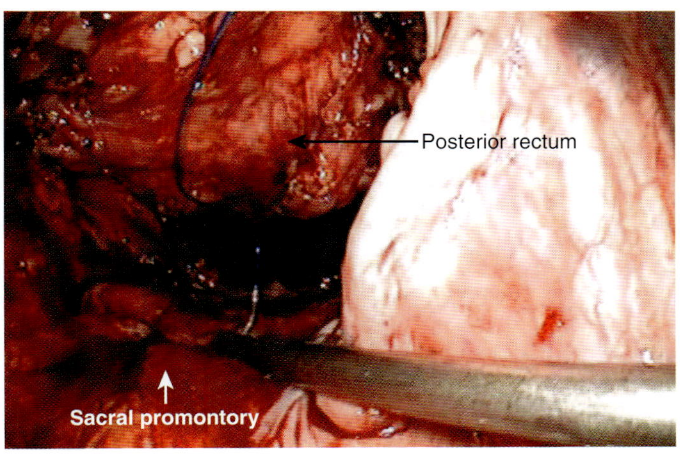

Figure 16-13

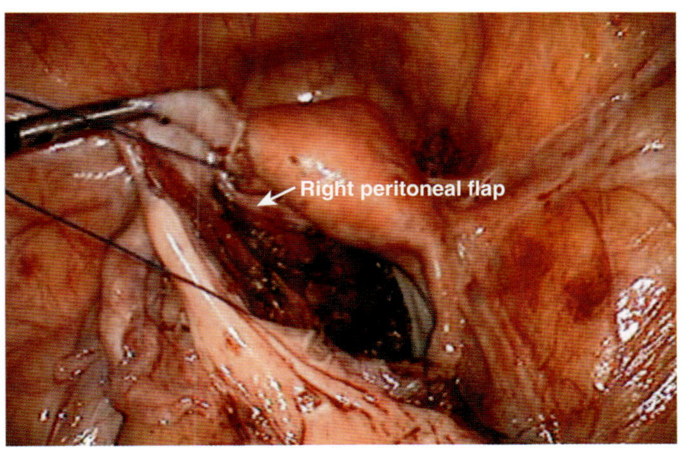

Figure 16-14

- With the right-sided and left-sided stitches in place, the rectum is pulled out of the pelvis so that the anterior rectal wall is taut. The suture is passed back through the peritoneum of the anterior lateral mesorectum (Figure 16-15). The sigmoid colon is returned to its position (Figure 16-16). A closed suction drain is placed posteriorly into the pelvis to drain fluid and blood (Figure 16-17).

Step 4: Postoperative Care

Patients are ambulated early. Intravenous fluid replacement is given to maintain a urine output of greater than 30 mL/hr. Nasogastric decompression is not required unless the patient becomes nauseated. Most patients tolerate clear liquids within 24 to 48 hours, and the diet can be advanced as tolerated. Patients should be given antibiotics for 24 hours, incentive spirometry, and deep vein thrombosis prophylaxis and encouraged to ambulate as much as possible during the early postoperative period. Postoperative analgesia is usually managed with patient-controlled analgesia followed by a switch to oral analgesics. Patients may be discharged home on a low-residue diet and advanced to a high-fiber diet as tolerated. It is important to prevent the patient from developing constipation. Patients should be instructed not to strain with bowel movements.

Step 5: Pearls and Pitfalls

In patients with a long redundant sigmoid colon and constipation, a resection rectopexy may be more appropriate than simple rectopexy. The overfold of the sigmoid after rectopexy may cause partial colonic obstruction and exacerbate constipation.

Stretching the rectum too tight results in recurrence as the sutures have a tendency to pull through the peritoneal flaps. The use of mesh provides more security but markedly increases the risk of fistula formation or obstruction at the mesh band.

Selected Readings

Byrne CM, Smith SR, Solomon MJ, et al. Long-term functional outcomes after laparoscopic and open rectopexy for the treatment of rectal prolapse. Dis Colon Rectum 2008;51:1597–1604.

Kariv Y, Delaney CP, Casillas S, et al. Long-term outcome after laparoscopic and open surgery for rectal prolapse: a case-control study. Surg Endosc 2006;20:35–42.

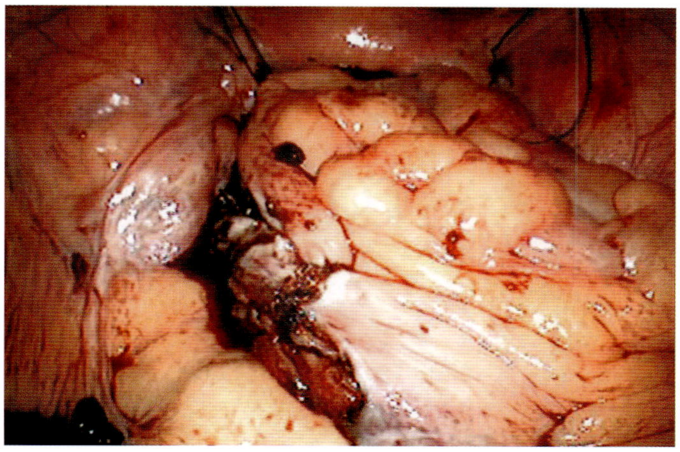

Figure 16-15

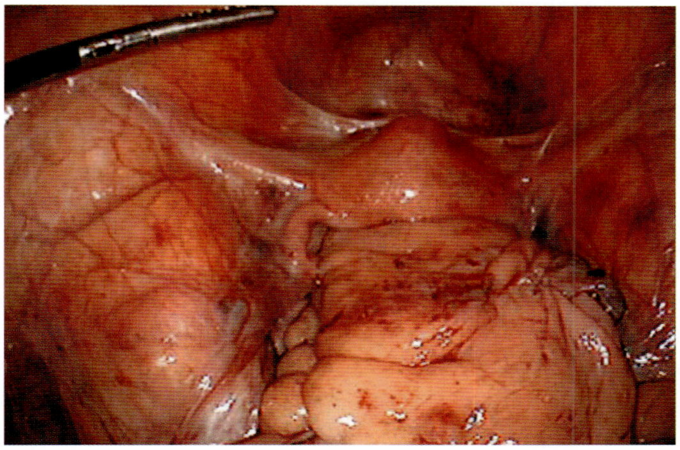

Figure 16-16

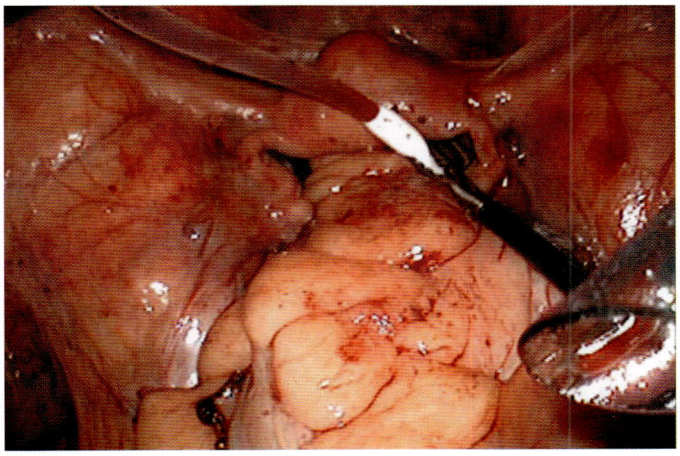

Figure 16-17

CHAPTER 17

Completion Proctectomy for Crohn's Disease

Anne Y. Lin

Step 1: Clinical Anatomy

The external anal sphincter is a cylindrical sheet of striated, voluntary muscle extending from the puborectalis and levator ani muscles in the pelvic floor down to the perineal skin at the anal verge. The circular formation allows closure of the anal canal with contraction of the muscular tube. The internal sphincter is the thickened continuation of the circular muscle fibers of the rectal wall. The dentate line marks the fusion of the rectal mucosa and the anoderm. The skin of the anal canal proper has no hair follicles. The anal verge is palpated at the distal end of the internal and external sphincter where there is a palpable groove known as the intersphincteric groove (Figure 17-1*A*). Within the intersphincteric groove, the longitudinal fibers of the rectal wall travel to the perineal skin as the corrugator cutanei ani muscles (Figure 17-1*B*). The upper extent of the external anal sphincter is the levator ani thickening called the puborectalis. In females, the anterior sphincter has attachments to the transverse perineal muscle and the posterior vagina.

Step 2: Preoperative Considerations

The technique of completion proctectomy for benign disease involves an intersphincteric dissection because this results in a smaller defect, which facilitates closure. The preparation for completion proctectomy, which usually follows an initial total abdominal colectomy and ileostomy, includes preoperative antibiotics and deep vein thrombosis prophylaxis with sequential compression devices.

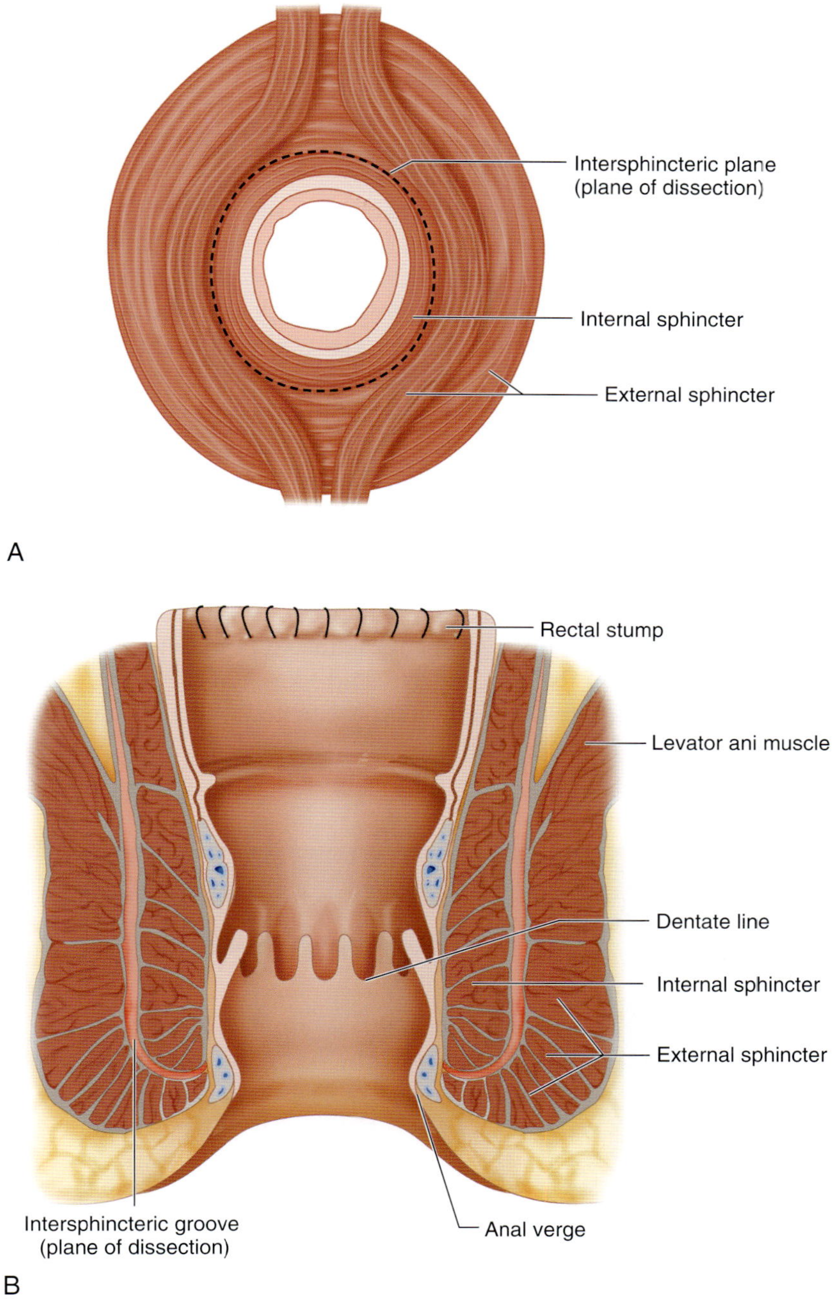

Figure 17-1A-B

Step 3: Operative Steps

See Chapter 10 for the details of the abdominal portion of the procedure, specifically mobilization of the rectum down to the level of the levators. A totally perineal dissection is possible if the rectum is divided at a level below the midportion of the sacrum during the initial colectomy.

- The patient is placed in the prone-flexed position. The anal orifice is sutured closed using a 0-silk purse-string suture to minimize spillage.
- The perineum is prepared and draped in standard sterile fashion.
- The perineum is exposed with the use of a Lone Star Retractor (Lone Star Medical Products, Inc., Stafford, Tex.). An incision is outlined to include all the fistula tracts (Figure 17-2).
- Using electrocautery, the intersphincteric groove is marked at the anal verge, and dissection is performed along the internal sphincter and rectal wall with care taken to preserve the outer external sphincter muscle cuff (Figure 17-3).
- The dissection proceeds along the rectal wall posteriorly and laterally up to the level of the abdominal rectal dissection at the levators and puborectalis (Figure 17-4). Care is taken to avoid injury to the vagina (or urethra and prostate) during anterior dissection with frequent digital examination of the posterior vaginal wall or palpation of the bladder catheter. The rectal remnant is completely divided by transecting the levators close to the rectal wall (Figure 17-5).
- A suction drain is placed into the pelvis to exit anteriorly through the closure (Figure 17-6).
- The muscle layers of the pelvic floor are reapproximated in individual layers—levators, external sphincter (Figure 17-7), ischiorectal fat, and skin (Figure 17-8)—using 2-0 and 3-0 absorbable sutures. The skin may be left unapproximated if there is great concern for wound infection and the wound is packed with gauze.

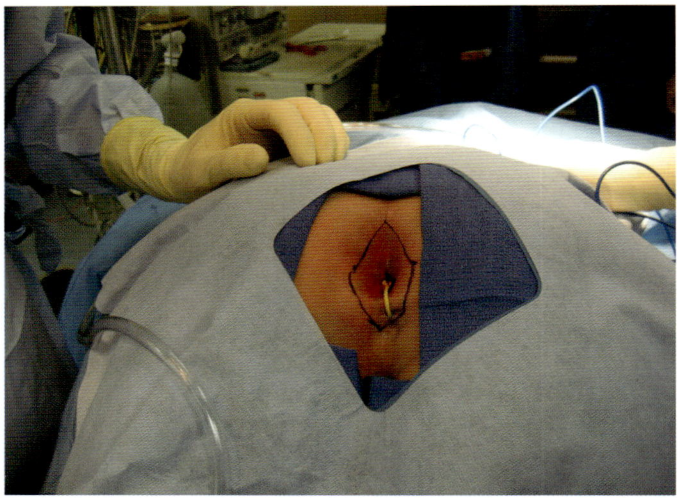

Figure 17-2

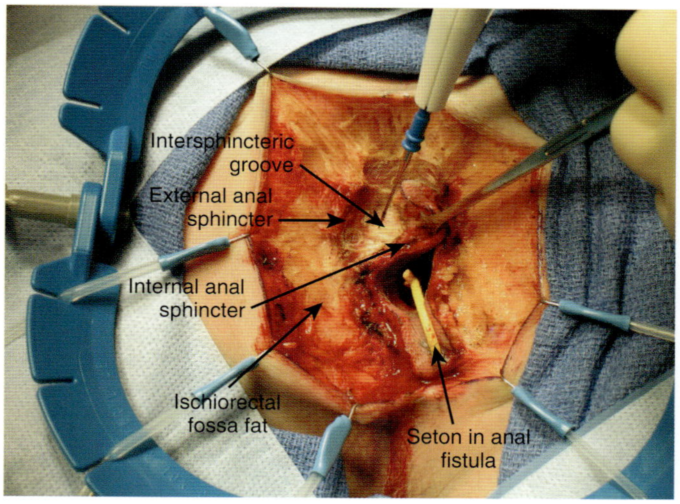

Figure 17-3

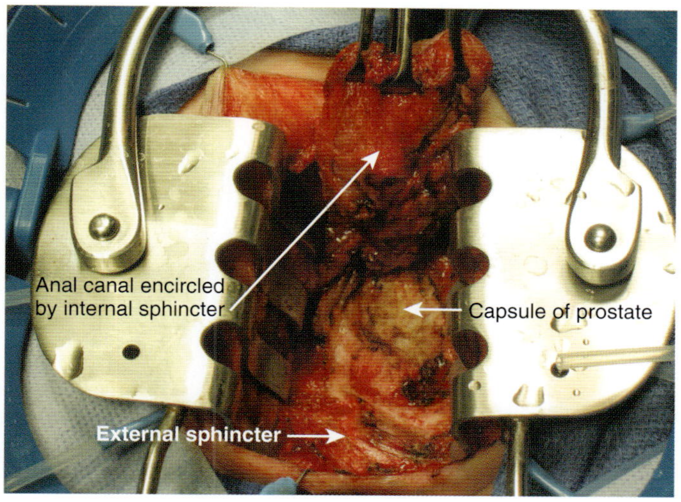

Figure 17-4

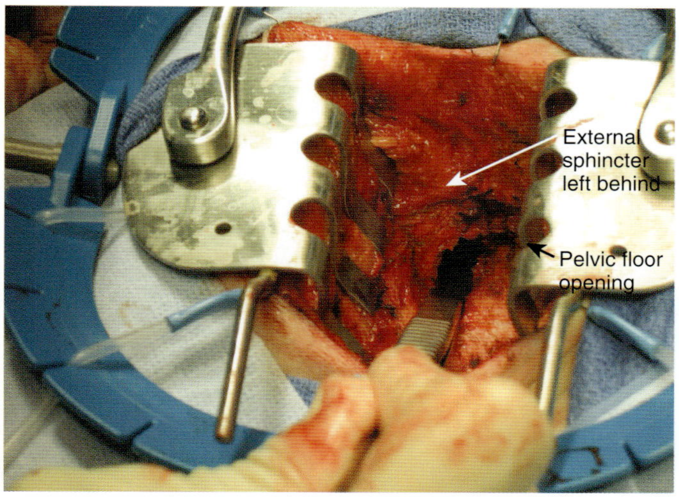

Figure 17-5

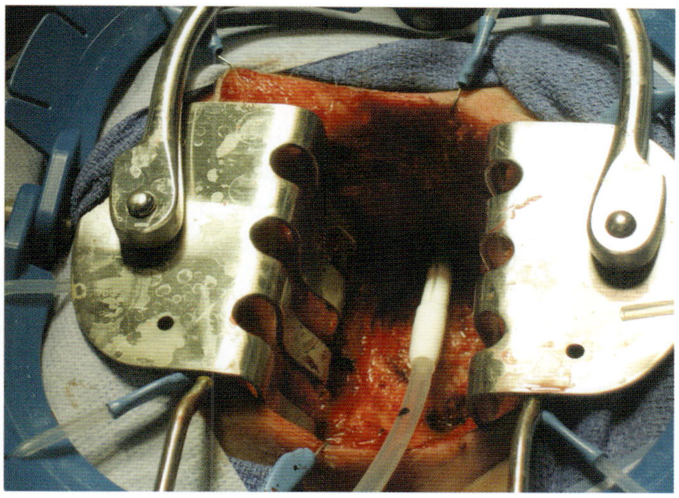
Figure 17-6

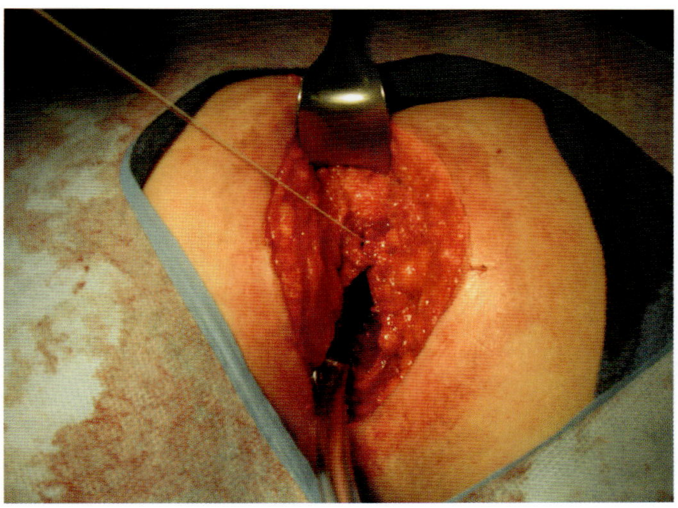
Figure 17-7

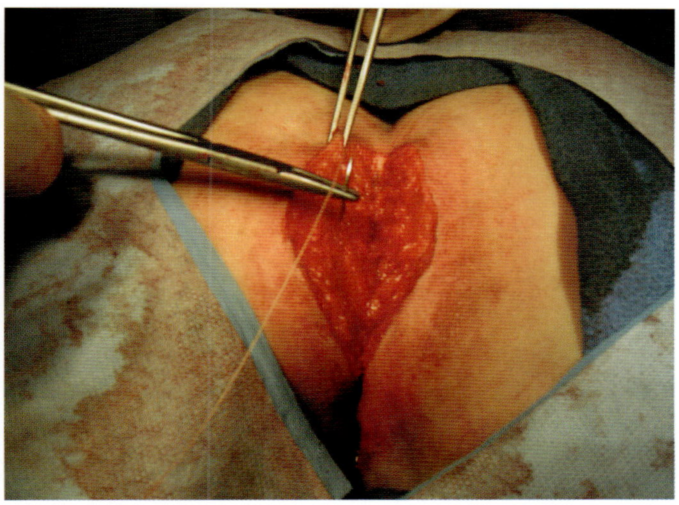
Figure 17-8

Step 4: Postoperative Care

Pain is managed with patient-controlled analgesia. The drain may be removed when minimal output is noted. The patient is asked not to sit, scoot, or drive for 2 weeks.

Step 5: Pearls and Pitfalls

Major risks are abscess formation or breakdown of the perineal wound. Consideration should be given to leaving the skin open if the perineal skin is excoriated from Crohn's disease. Maintenance of the intact external sphincter provides well-vascularized tissue to close the midline defect. Care must be taken to remove all fistula tracts or other aspects of active Crohn's disease to prevent recurrent purulent disease.

Selected Readings

Cattan P, Bonhomme N, Panis Y, et al. Fate of the rectum in patients undergoing total colectomy for Crohn's disease. Br J Surg 2002;89:454–9.

Yamamoto T, Keighley MR. Fate of the rectum and ileal recurrence rates after total colectomy for Crohn's disease. World J Surg 2000;24:125–9.

CHAPTER 18

Transanal Excision of Rectal Lesions

Steven R. Hunt and James W. Fleshman, Jr.

Step 1: Clinical Anatomy

For transanal excision, the relevant anatomy involves the anus and distal rectum; tumors above 8 to 10 cm from the anal verge are difficult to remove by conventional means. Important anatomic landmarks include the anal verge, which is the distal end of the anal canal with the buttocks effaced. The dentate line is a visible, irregular line that separates the columnar epithelium of the rectum and the stratified epithelium of the anal canal. Its location within the anal canal varies from patient to patient. The surgical anal canal refers to the area from the anal verge to the top of the anal sphincter complex. The upper edge of the anal canal is defined by the anorectal ring. Above the anorectal ring, the rectum becomes much more distensible and capacious. The anal canal is of varying length depending on the habitus of the patient and can range in length from 2 to 5 cm. The muscularis propria of the rectum consists of inner circular smooth muscle fibers and an outer layer of longitudinal smooth muscle fibers. Posteriorly and laterally, the mesorectal fat surrounds the rectum. In females, the vagina is immediately anterior to the muscularis propria above the anal canal. In males, the prostate gland and seminal vesicles are encountered anteriorly above the anal verge. The anterior peritoneal reflection varies between males and females and can vary according to the habitus of the patient. Generally, the anterior peritoneal reflection lies somewhere between 8 and 10 cm above the anal verge anteriorly and anterolaterally to the rectum.

Step 2: Preoperative Considerations

Before embarking on a transanal excision, the tumor must be evaluated carefully to confirm that it is amenable to transanal excision. Examination in the office should consist of a careful digital rectal examination to determine the level of the tumor and its mobility. A transrectal ultrasound scan should be performed to rule out invasion. Although it is often difficult to differentiate between an adenoma and a superficial T1 tumor, it is important to rule out deeper invasion by transrectal ultrasound. The office examination should also include rigid proctoscopy to determine the distance of the tumor from the anal verge and to localize the tumor. The laterality and anterior-posterior localization of the tumor is important in the positioning of the patient for the procedure. All biopsy results of any tumors that are considered for local excision should be carefully reviewed. If transanal excision is to be performed for cancer, a staging workup consisting of a computed tomography scan, carcinoembryonic antigen, chest radiography, and complete colonoscopy should be done.

We prepare each patient with two Fleet enemas before surgery. Preoperative antibiotics and deep vein thrombosis prophylaxis are generally unnecessary. We do not routinely place a bladder catheter.

Step 3: Operative Steps

- Patient positioning depends on the location of the lesion. Anterior and lateral lesions are best approached with patients in the prone jackknife position. The patient's buttocks should be pulled laterally with tape to efface the anus partially (Figure 18-1). Patients with posterior lesions should be placed in the dorsal lithotomy position with the buttocks taped apart.
- The choice of anesthesia depends on surgeon preference. It is possible to perform a local excision under monitored anesthesia care/local, spinal, or general anesthesia. The anus is effaced with a Lone Star Retractor (Lone Star Medical Products, Inc., Stafford, Tex.). (Figure 18-2). Visualization is best accomplished with a lighted anoscope. It may be necessary to place stay sutures at the lateral margins of higher tumors to provide traction and pull the tumor into view. The tumor itself should not be handled with instruments. The default procedure should be a full-thickness excision, unless the tumor is definitely benign, in which case, a submucosal excision is acceptable.
- A 1-cm margin is scored around the tumor with the cautery (Figure 18-3). In scoring the margin, it is necessary to create a char rather than mere blanching of the mucosa because visualization of this margin in the latter portions of the procedure can become difficult owing to blood. After the margins have been scored circumferentially, the full-thickness excision should begin. It is easiest to start the excision at the distal margin of the tumor. During this incision, the operator should take note of each layer as it is crossed—submucosa, muscularis layer, and exposure of the perirectal fat (Figure 18-4). For lower tumors, there may be a paucity of perirectal fat, and the levator muscles may become immediately visible on full incision of the muscularis propria. Anteriorly, there is also scant mesorectal fat, and the vagina or Denonvilliers' fascia of the prostate may be encountered immediately after incising through the rectal wall.
- After a full-thickness incision has been made, the incision should be extended laterally around the tumor. Placing an Allis-Adair clamp on the margins of the specimen facilitates visualization (Figure 18-5). Dissection in the mesorectal fat should begin underneath the tumor to leave a wide margin of mesorectal fat on the specimen. Finally, the remaining superior rectal wall is divided (Figure 18-6). Although we use the electrocautery for most of the dissection, vessel sealing devices can also prove helpful to obtain hemostasis during the dissection.

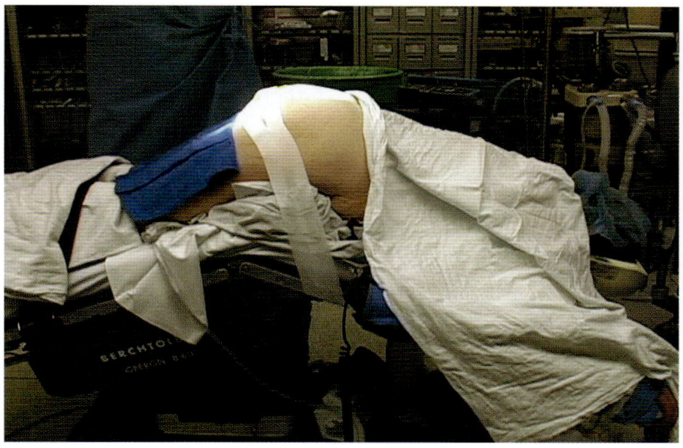

Figure 18-1

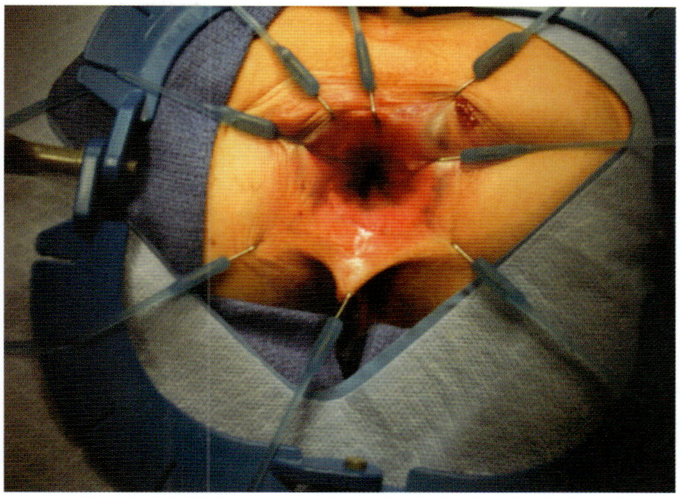

Figure 18-2

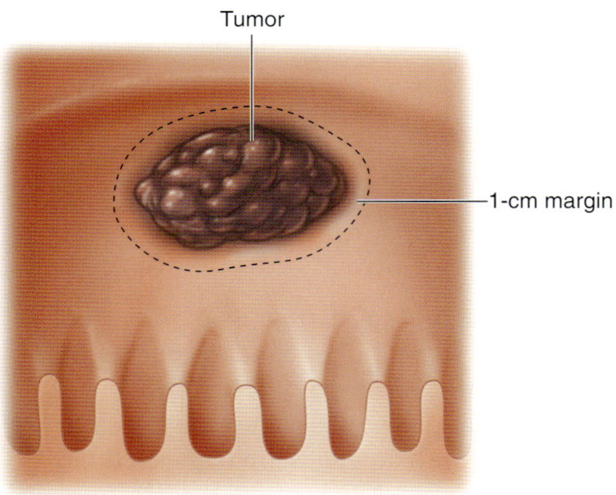

Figure 18-3

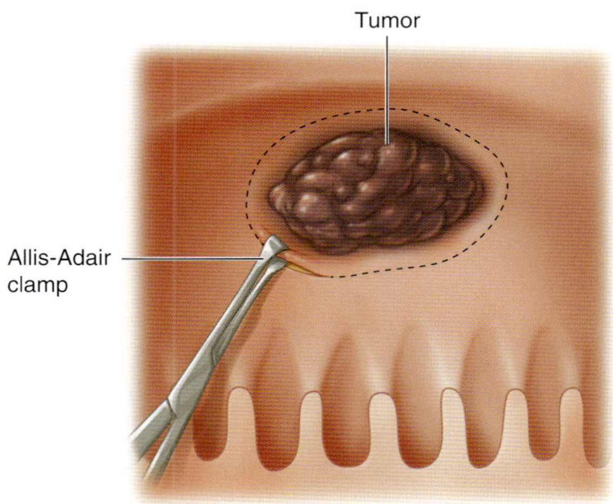

Figure 18-4

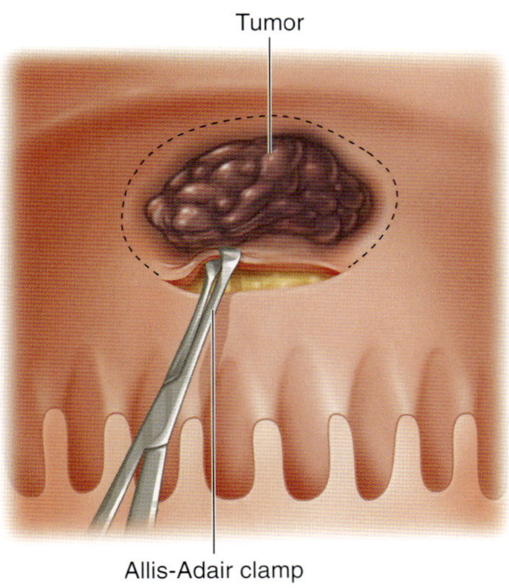

Figure 18-5

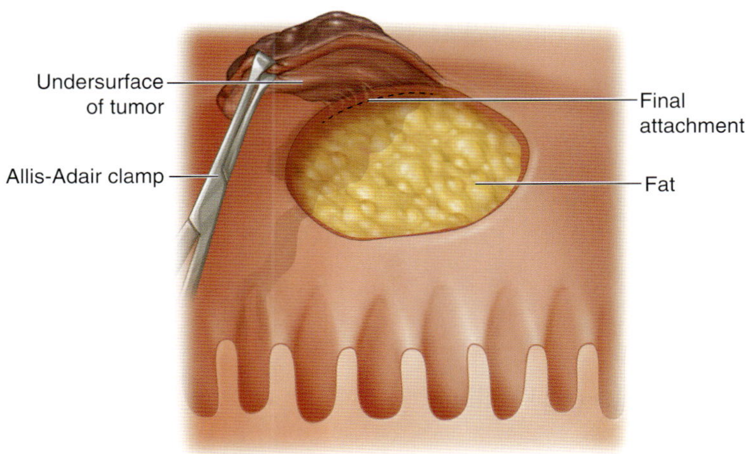

Figure 18-6

- When the tumor has been excised, it should be removed and oriented for the pathologist by pinning to a corkboard. The defect should be inspected and irrigated with saline, and meticulous hemostasis should be obtained with electrocautery.
- The defect is closed transversely with running absorbable sutures (Figure 18-7). For large defects, it is helpful to orient the transverse closure by starting with a single suture in the center to approximate the two edges and orient the line of closure (Figure 18-7).
- After closure, the suture line should be inspected and interrogated for any defects. The rectal lumen above the line of closure should also be inspected to confirm that the rectal lumen has not been obliterated by the closure (Figure 18-8). If closure of the mucosal/rectal wall defect is not possible, it may be left open to granulate and close secondarily.

Step 4: Postoperative Care

Most patients can be treated in the outpatient setting. Because urinary retention is a common postoperative complication, patients should be able to void before discharge. In our practice, patients who have an open wound are discharged with a 7-day regimen of oral antibiotics. Patients should be given an ample supply of pain medications and stool softeners. Sitz baths may provide some relief for patients with low lesions that extend down into the anal canal.

Step 5: Pearls and Pitfalls

In many cases, closure of the wound is difficult or results in significant narrowing of the rectal lumen. In these cases, it is safe to leave these wounds open to heal by secondary intention; however, in our experience, these patients have significantly more pain postoperatively.

In the rare cases of a pedunculated or extremely mobile rectal polyp, it is sometimes possible to evert the polyp through the anal canal and excise the lesion with an endoscopic linear cutter stapler. Although more proximal rectal polyps often must be excised by transanal endoscopic microsurgery or low anterior resection, it is possible to excise lesions using an operating proctoscope and a transanal snare. Because this is not a full-thickness excision, it should be reserved for benign tumors. When attempting to remove a lesion with the snare, great care must be taken with anterior and anterolateral tumors to avoid entering the peritoneal cavity. Larger lesions should be excised in a piecemeal fashion because an en bloc snare excision can often result in a full-thickness injury to the rectal wall.

Complications with transanal excisions are similar to complications of other anorectal procedures and include urinary retention and bleeding. Although pelvic sepsis is rare, it should be considered in patients who develop fever, worsening pain, or delayed urinary retention. If sepsis is suspected, the patient should be taken to the operating room expeditiously for an examination under anesthesia. Rectal or anal stenosis after a transanal excision is a rare complication that is usually corrected with simple dilation.

Selected Readings

Nascimbeni R, Burgart LJ, Nivatvongs S, et al. Risk of lymph node metastasis in T1 carcinoma of the colon and rectum. Dis Colon Rectum 2002;45:200–6.

Touzios J, Ludwig KA. Local management of rectal neoplasia. Clin Colon Rectal Surg 2008;21:291–9.

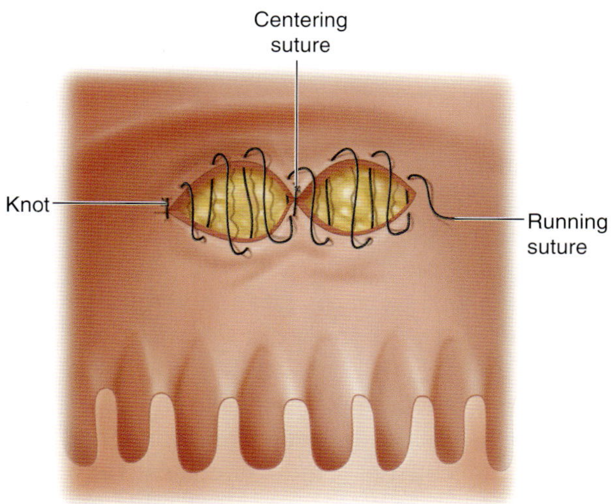

Figure 18-7

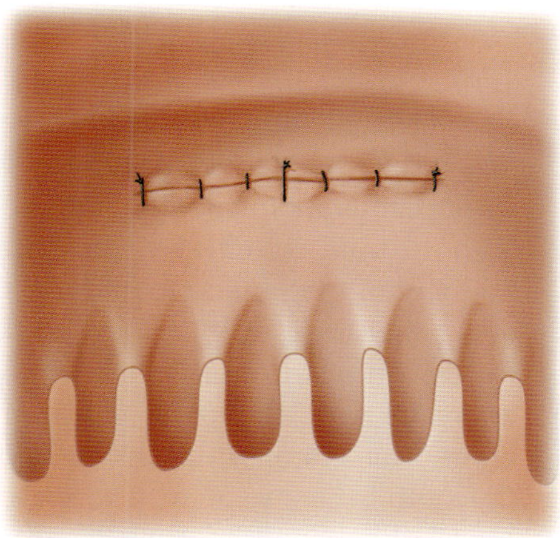

Figure 18-8

CHAPTER 19

Transanal Endoscopic Microsurgery

Steven R. Hunt

Step 1: Clinical Anatomy

In transanal endoscopic microsurgery (TEM), the relevant anatomy consists of the rectum within 15 cm of the anal verge; tumors higher than this level are very difficult to remove by TEM. Important anatomic landmarks include the anal verge, which is the distal end of the anal canal with the buttocks effaced. The dentate line is a visible, irregular line that separates the columnar epithelium of the rectum and the stratified epithelium of the anal canal. Its location within the anal canal varies from patient to patient. The anal canal refers to the area from the anal verge to the top of the anal sphincter complex. The upper edge of the anal canal is defined by the anorectal ring. Above the anorectal ring, the rectum becomes much more distensible and capacious. The length of the anal canal varies depending on the habitus of the patient and can range in length from 2 to 5 cm. The muscularis propria of the rectum consists of inner circular smooth muscle fibers and an outer layer of longitudinal smooth muscle fibers. The internal sphincter thickens at the distal end and is palpable under the skin at the anal verge. The longitudinal outer muscles splay out to insert into the skin and create a gap palpable outside the internal sphincter, known as the intersphincteric groove, at the anal verge. Posteriorly and laterally, the mesorectal fat surrounds the rectum above the anal canal. In females, the vagina is immediately anterior to the muscularis propria above the anal canal. In males, the prostate gland and seminal vesicles are encountered anteriorly above the anal verge. The anterior peritoneal reflection, which indicates the start of the exposed anterior rectum, inside the pelvis, varies in its position between males and females and according to the habitus of the patient. Generally, the anterior peritoneal reflection lies somewhere between 8 and 10 cm above the anal verge anteriorly and anterolaterally to the rectum.

Step 2: Preoperative Considerations

Before embarking on a TEM procedure, the tumor must be evaluated carefully to confirm that it is amenable to TEM. Examination in the office should consist of a careful digital rectal examination to determine the level of the tumor and its mobility. A transrectal ultrasound scan should be performed to rule out invasion. Although it is often difficult to differentiate between an adenoma and a superficial T1 tumor, it is important to rule out deeper invasion by transrectal ultrasound. The office examination should also include rigid proctoscopy to determine the distance of the tumor from the anal verge and to localize the tumor. The lateral and anterior-posterior localization of the tumor is extremely important in the positioning of the patient for the TEM procedure. All biopsy results of tumors that are considered for TEM should be carefully reviewed. If TEM is to be performed for cancer, a staging workup consisting of a computed tomography scan, carcinoembryonic antigen, chest radiography, and complete colonoscopy should be done.

We prepare each patient with a complete mechanical bowel preparation; this allows for a clear field of view and clears the colon should it become necessary to create a diverting loop ileostomy in the case of a complicated procedure. Patients should be given preoperative antibiotics. Deep vein thrombosis prophylaxis should be routine; we use sequential compression devices. A Foley catheter should be placed before beginning the procedure.

Step 3: Operative Steps

- The positioning of the patient is critical to the successful completion of a TEM procedure. Because of the angulation of the scope and camera, the tumor must be positioned in a downward direction. The operator must be able to move the scope in a free range of motion. The handle of the TEM scope points downward, and the patient's legs and the operating table must not interfere with movement of the scope. For anterior tumors, we position patients in a prone-kneeling position with the hips flexed at 90 degrees (Figure 19-1). An alternative for anterior lesions is to abduct the patient's legs on leg-spreader bars to allow the operator to stand between the patient's legs (Figure 19-2). For lateral tumors, patients are positioned in the lateral decubitus position with the hips flexed at 90 degrees. This position can be achieved with arm boards or with leg-spreader bars bent out at 90 degrees from the end of the table (Figure 19-3). The patient's buttocks should be at the end of the operating table. For posterior tumors, patients should be positioned in the lithotomy position with the buttocks at the edge of the table (Figure 19-4).
- After the patient is positioned, the TEM scope fixation apparatus should be affixed to the side of the bed. The anus should be gently dilated with two fingers and a generous amount of lubricant. The TEM scope is gently inserted so that it passes easily into the anal canal with gentle rotation on the scope. The scope should be fixed, and the faceplate should be attached (Figure 19-5). The rectum is insufflated with carbon dioxide to a pressure of 12 mm Hg. The lesion should be visualized and centered within the visualized field.

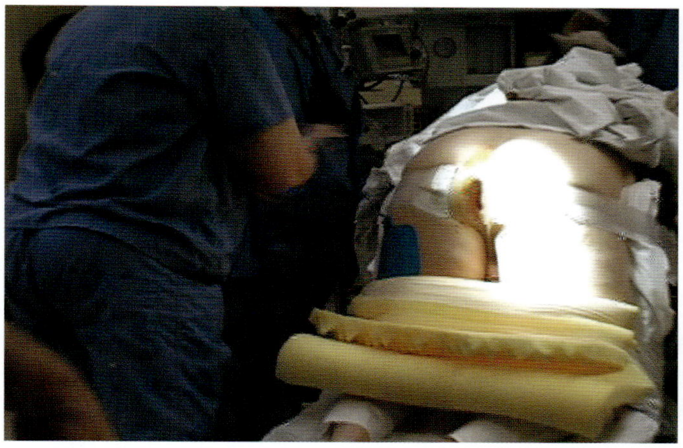
Figure 19-1

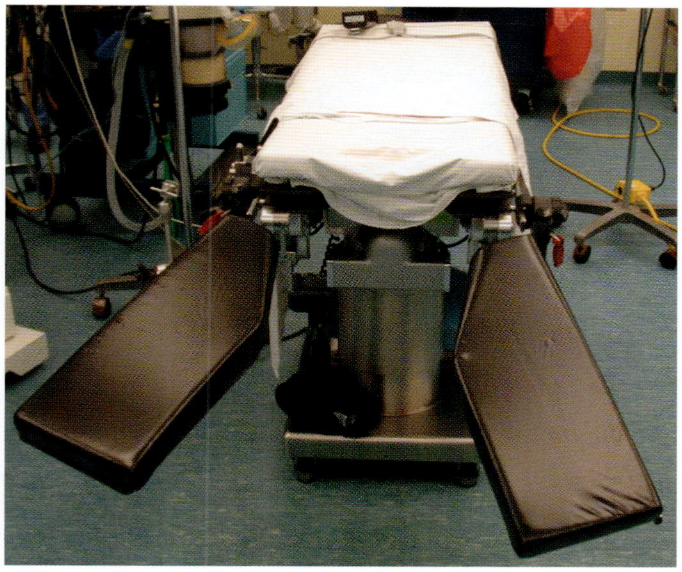
Figure 19-2

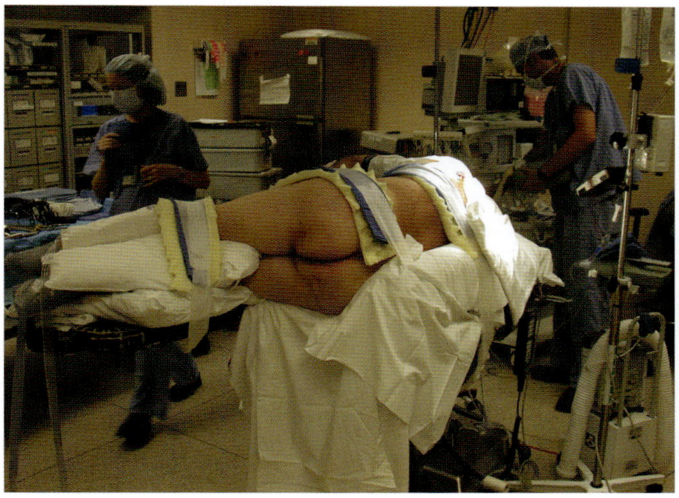
Figure 19-3

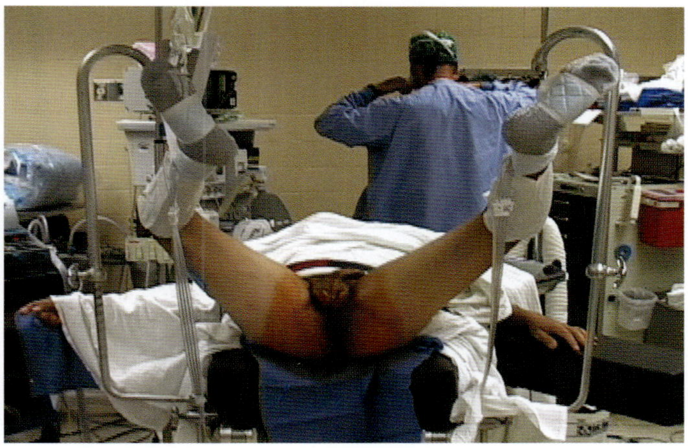
Figure 19-4

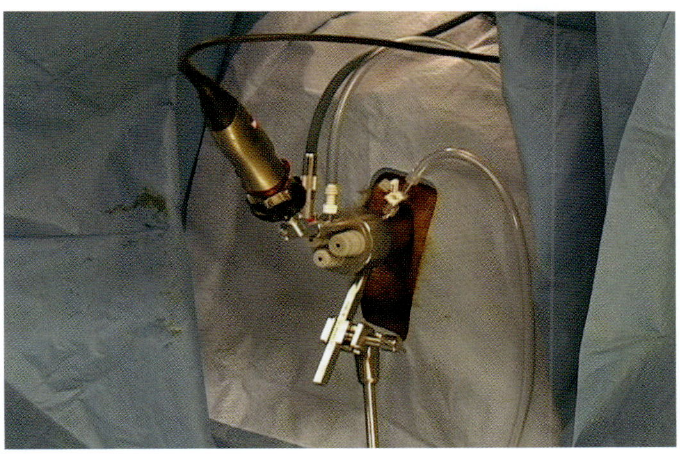
Figure 19-5

- A 1-cm margin should be scored around the tumor with the needle tip cautery (Figure 19-6). To judge the 1-cm margin appropriately, a clamp should be measured in the open position and used as a reference point. In scoring the 1-cm margin, it is necessary to create a char during the score rather than mere blanching of the mucosa because visualization of this margin in the latter portions of the procedure can become difficult owing to blood. After the margins have been scored circumferentially, the full-thickness excision should begin. It is easiest to start this full-thickness excision between the 3 o'clock and 6 o'clock positions relative to the tumor (Figure 19-7). During this incision, the operator should take note of each layer as it is crossed—submucosa (Figure 19-8), muscularis layer, and perirectal fat (Figure 19-9). For lower tumors, there may be a paucity of perirectal fat, and the levator muscles may become immediately visible on full incision of the muscularis propria. Anteriorly, there is also scant mesorectal fat, and the vagina or Denonvilliers' fascia of the prostate may be encountered immediately after incising through the rectal wall. In the upper rectum, for anterior tumors, incision through the full thickness of the rectal wall may gain entrance into the peritoneal cavity. Great care should be taken to avoid injury to the small bowel if entrance into the peritoneal cavity is anticipated. It is often helpful to place patients in Trendelenburg position to evacuate the small bowel from the pelvis.
- After a full-thickness incision has been made, the incision should be extended between the 3 o'clock and 9 o'clock positions around the inferior border of the tumor. Dissection in the mesorectal fat should begin underneath the tumor to leave a wide margin of mesorectal fat on the specimen. Although we use the electrocautery for most of the dissection, vessel sealing devices can also prove helpful to obtain hemostasis during the dissection (Figure 19-10).

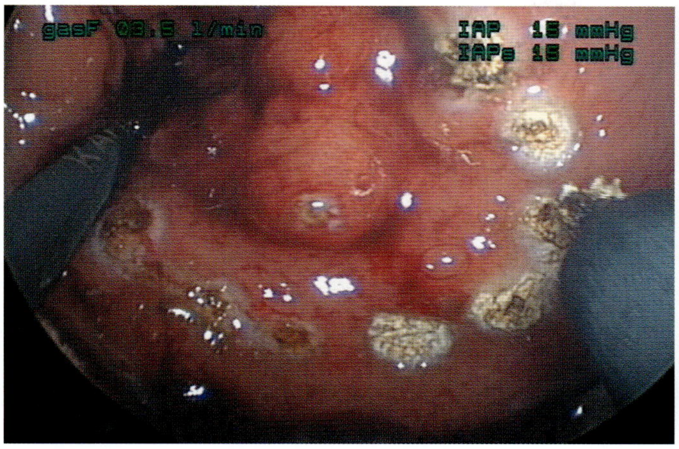

Figure 19-6

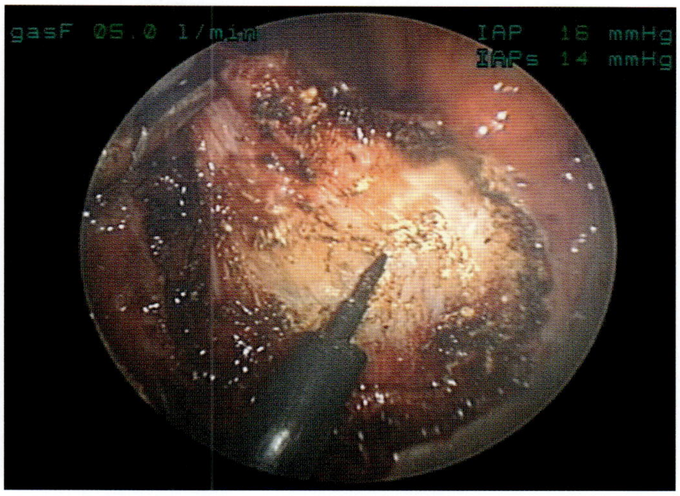

Figure 19-7

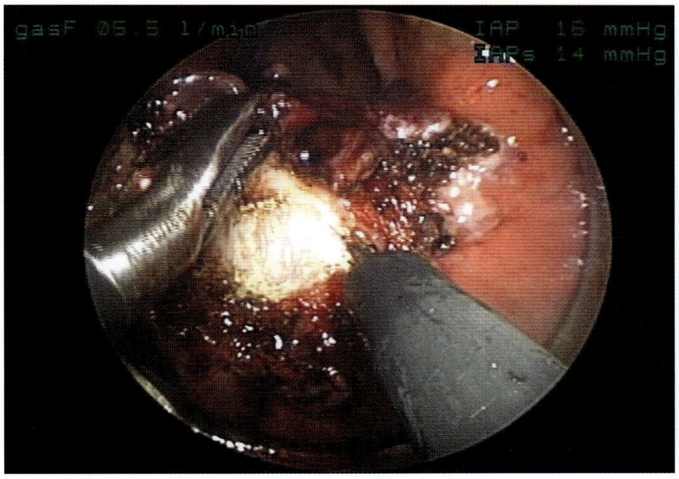

Figure 19-8

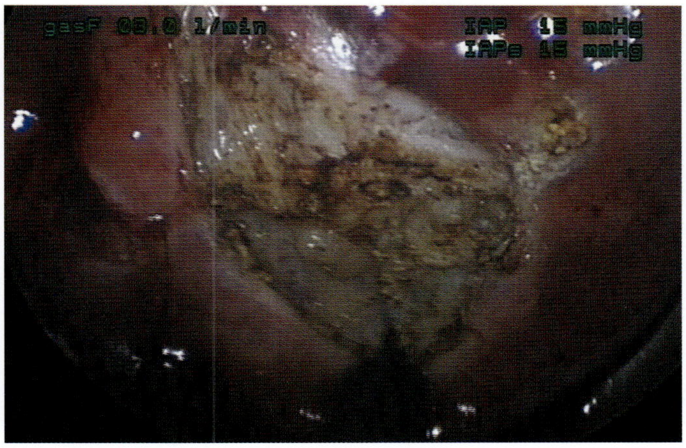

Figure 19-9

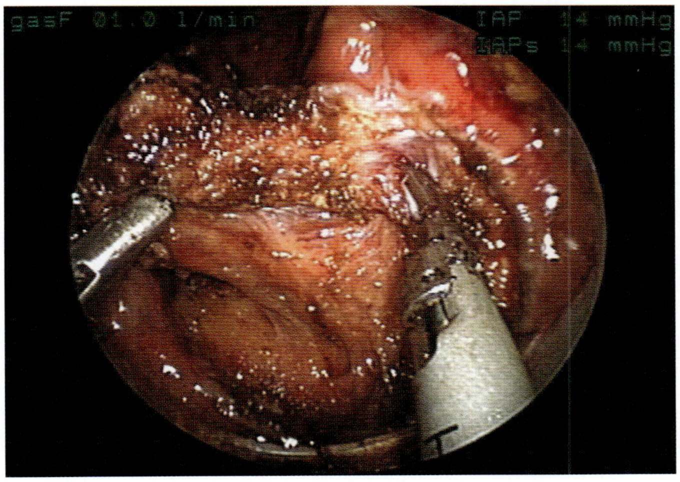

Figure 19-10

- After the lower border of the rectal wall has been incised, dissection should continue around the lateral and superior edges of the tumor using countertraction with the left hand to achieve appropriate exposure. The upper margins of the excision frequently can prove to be the most difficult, and it is often helpful to use a hook cautery to complete the excision of the upper portions of the rectal wall.
- When the tumor has been excised, it should be removed and oriented for the pathologist. Rectal insufflation is obtained again. The defect should be inspected and irrigated with saline (Figure 19-11). Meticulous hemostasis should be obtained with electrocautery.
- The defect is closed transversely with absorbable monofilament sutures. The ends of the suture can be secured with either a silver clip or a Lapra-Ty clip (Figure 19-12). Closure is achieved most easily by proceeding from the right side of the monitor to the left (Figure 19-13). For large defects, it is helpful to orient the transverse closure by starting with a single suture in the center to approximate the two edges.
- After closure, the suture line should be inspected and interrogated for any defects. The rectal lumen above the line of closure should also be inspected to confirm that the rectal lumen has not been obliterated by the closure.

Step 4: Postoperative Care

Most patients are admitted overnight for 23-hour observation. Because of the high rate of urinary retention postoperatively, the Foley catheter is left in overnight and removed early in the morning of postoperative day 1. Patients are started on a clear liquid diet on arrival to the floor, and their diet is advanced as tolerated. No postoperative antibiotics are indicated if the wound is completely closed. Patients can generally be discharged on postoperative day 1.

Step 5: Pearls and Pitfalls

For very large intraluminal polyps, it is often difficult to complete the dissection on the superior edge of the polyp because the view of the upper margins can be obscured by the large mobile polyp. In these cases, it is often helpful to use a transanal snare through the TEM scope to débride the intramucosal portion of the polyp down to a relatively flat polyp base. If such débridement is undertaken, the débrided portion of the polyp should be sent as a separate pathologic specimen from the base to assess the true margin accurately. After the polyp has been débrided, it is often easy to excise the base of the polyp in full thickness as described previously.

Polyps that extend down into the anal canal can prove to be very challenging for TEM excision. The anal canal does not distend with rectal insufflation. The field of view and working space can be extremely limited. It is often better to excise these polyps using a conventional transanal approach. TEM can prove helpful if the polyp extends for several centimeters above the anal canal, in which case it would be very difficult to perform the upper dissection transanally.

In a very small subset of patients, a submucosal excision of the polyp is acceptable; this includes polyps that are quite high in the rectum, in which case the operator is unsure that he or she would be able to achieve closure of the wound should the peritoneal cavity be entered. Such an approach should be used only for polyps that are almost definitely benign or with the understanding that cancer in the specimen would be an indication for rectal resection.

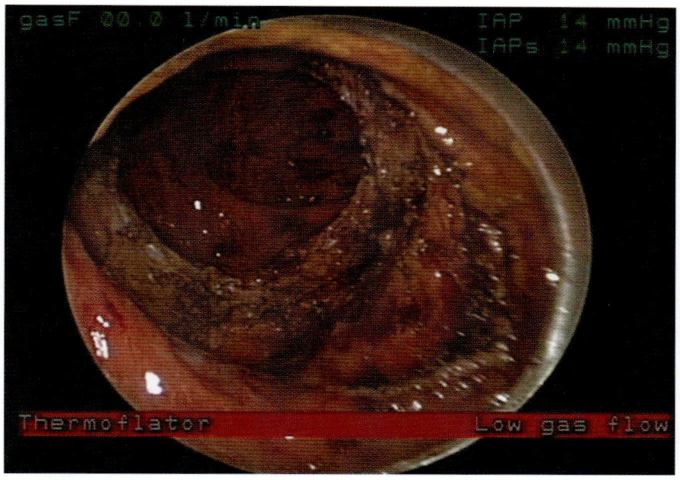

Figure 19-11

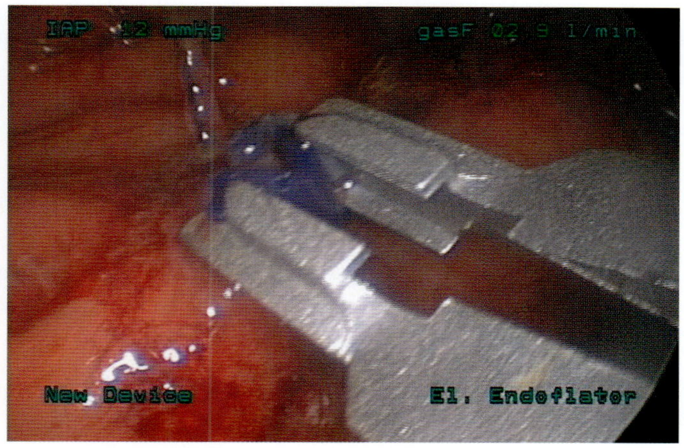

Figure 19-12

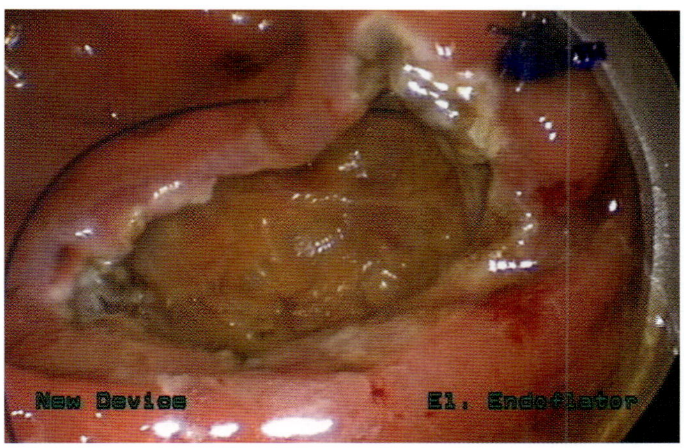

Figure 19-13

One of the most challenging aspects of performing a TEM dissection is the parallel position of the working instruments because they are functioning in a long cylinder. For this reason, many of the TEM instruments have 30-degree bends at the effector end to allow the instruments to approach the tumor more perpendicularly and to work at right angles to the opposite instrument. Torquing of these bent instruments is often necessary to achieve appropriate lines of dissection.

In many cases, closure of the wound is difficult or results in significant narrowing of the rectal lumen. In these cases, provided that there is no concern about entry into the peritoneal cavity, it is safe to leave these wounds open to heal by secondary intention. In our practice, patients who have an open wound are discharged with a 7-day regimen of oral antibiotics.

Selected Readings

Jeong WK, Park JW, Choi HS, et al. Transanal endoscopic microsurgery for rectal tumors: experience at Korea's National Cancer Center. Surg Endosc 2009;23:2575–9.

Moore JS, Cataldo PA, Osler T, et al. Transanal endoscopic microsurgery is more effective than traditional transanal excision for resection of rectal masses. Dis Colon Rectum 2008;51:1026–30.

CHAPTER 20

Anal Strictureplasty and Skin Flaps

Ira J. Kodner

Step 1: Clinical Anatomy

The external anal sphincter is a cylindrical sheet of striated, voluntary muscle extending from the puborectalis and levator ani muscles in the pelvic floor down to the perineal skin at the anal verge. The circular formation allows closure of the anal canal with contraction of the muscular tube. The internal sphincter is the thickened continuation of the circular muscle fibers of the rectal wall. The dentate line marks the fusion of the rectal mucosa and the anoderm. The skin of the anal canal proper has no hair follicles. The anal verge is palpated at the distal end of the internal and external sphincter where there is a palpable groove known as the intersphincteric groove. Within the intersphincteric groove, the longitudinal fibers of the rectal wall travel to the perineal skin. The upper extent of the external anal sphincter is the levator ani thickening called the puborectalis. In females, the anterior sphincter has attachments to the transverse perineal muscle and the posterior vagina.

Step 2: Preoperative Considerations

Skin flaps to increase the skin within the anal canal have been used to treat anal stricture and correct anal ectropion. The mobilization of inner buttock skin into the anal canal can be accomplished based on the principles of plastic surgery flap construction. The base of the flap should be broad enough to maintain an adequate blood supply. The dissection should be performed with as little cautery as possible, and the mobility of the flap toward the anal canal should be maximized by releasing the tethering attachments under the donor site rather than under the flap skin itself.

The patient should undergo a complete bowel preparation and receive preoperative antibiotics. The patient should be informed that a period of low activity without sitting, driving, or climbing steps is required for 2 weeks after surgery. The decision whether to do a single flap versus a simultaneous second flap should be made preoperatively and based on the amount of skin available within the anal canal.

Consideration should be given to the etiology of the stricture before recommending skin flap advancement. Crohn's disease has very limited indications because the healing process is impaired. Radiation-induced strictures most likely involve damage to the perianal skin and may have some skin impairment. The most common cause for anal strictures is an overzealous hemorrhoidectomy with removal of more viable anoderm than is adequate to dilate the anal canal. Replacement of this anoderm with skin from the inner buttock is the ideal indication for skin flap advancement for treatment of strictureplasty.

An inappropriately performed Whitehead hemorrhoidectomy with circumferential excision of the anoderm of the anal canal will result in an ectropion of rectal mucosa and stricture formation at the neo-mucocutaneous junction in most patients. The ectropion can be reduced into the anal canal and the stricture treated at the same procedure using a broad-based house-shaped skin flap. Patients who have no ectropion but have normal external anoderm and normal rectal mucosa and simply have lost dermis at the level of the dentate line benefit most from a diamond-shaped skin advancement flap.

Step 3: Operative Steps

V-Shaped, U-Shaped, or House-Shaped Flap

- The patient should be placed in the prone-jackknife position with the buttocks taped apart. The perineum is prepared and draped sterilely. The patient is sedated to relax the muscle and facilitate the injection of local anesthetic. Epinephrine should not be used because of its vasoconstrictive features. The flap should be drawn on the inner aspect of the buttock with a broad base encompassing approximately the entire side of the anal canal in the case of strictures. The length of the flap is determined by the base and should be two to three times the length of the base.
- The flap lines are drawn with indelible marker (Figure 20-1). The flap is incised along the lines of the drawing and carried into the anal canal on either side of the ectropion down to normal mucosa. The edges of the flap are protected. The tethering attachments to the flap are released by undermining under the edges of the donor site rather than the flap itself. The pedicle is released at the apex of the tip of the flap on the buttock to allow the redundant skin to move toward the anal canal with very little tension (Figure 20-2).
- The advanced skin is secured at the new inner site. If the ectropion is moved inward into the anal canal, the redundant mucosa is banded with internal elastic ligation as if treating internal hemorrhoids. The edges of the flap are secured at its new position with interrupted 3-0 polypropylene (Prolene) horizontal mattress sutures incorporating the subcuticular layer of the flap and the full thickness of the adjacent donor skin to avoid piercing the flap and to protect the blood supply. The opening of the donor site is closed in a linear fashion with interrupted vertical mattress sutures to close the donor site behind the skin flap (Figures 20-3 and 20-4). A dressing of antibiotic ointment and fluff gauze is applied.

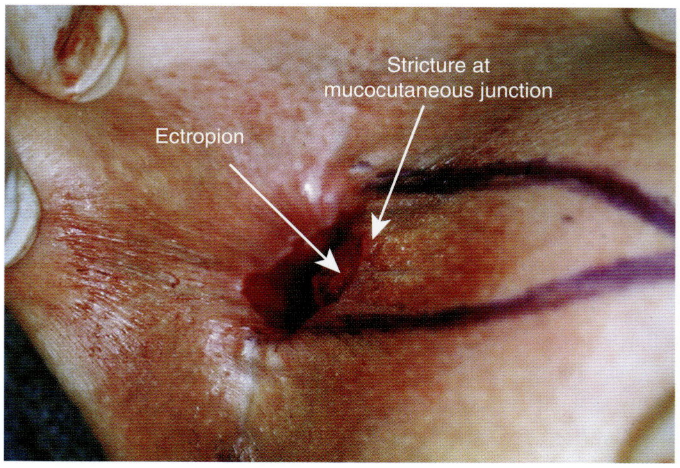

Figure 20-1

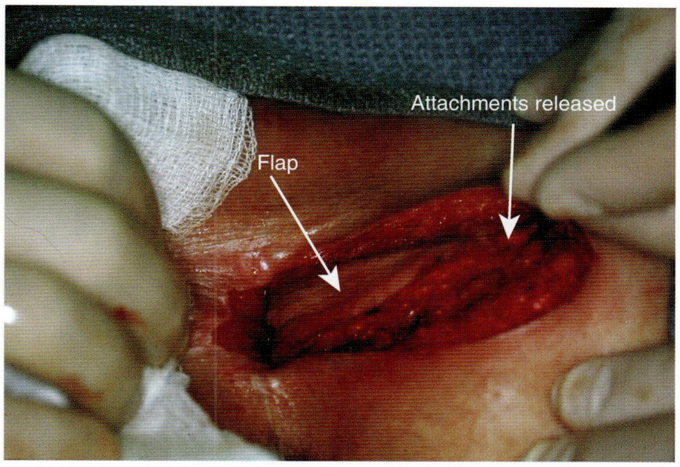

Figure 20-2

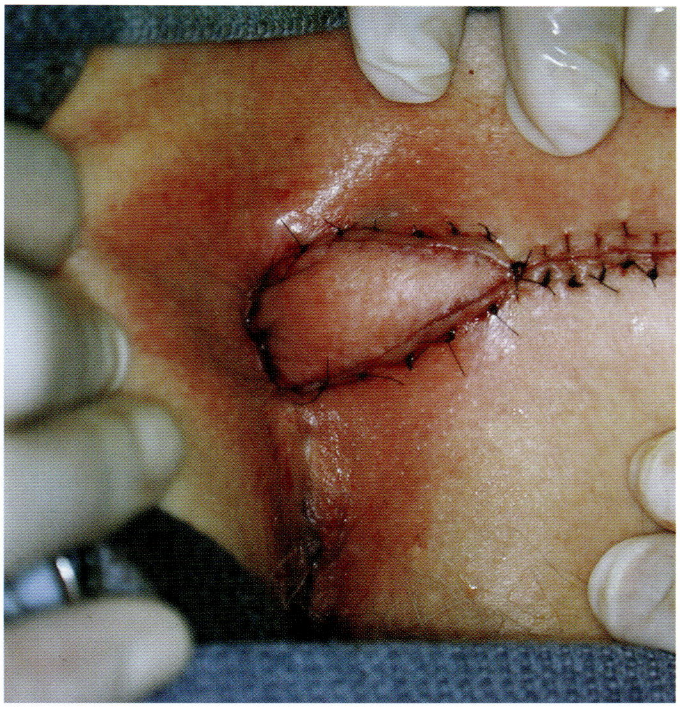

Figure 20-3

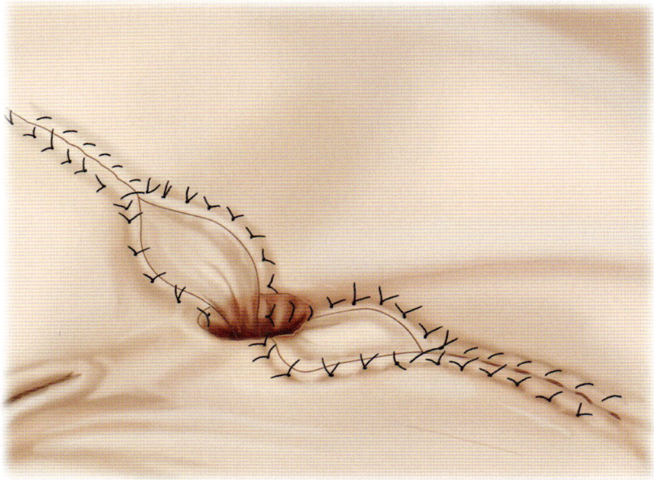

Figure 20-4

Diamond-Shaped Flap

- The diamond-shaped skin flap, designed to expand the available tissue in the anal canal, is begun with the patient in the prone-jackknife position with the buttocks taped apart and the perineum partially draped sterilely. Proctoscopy can be performed to empty the rectum, and the rectum can be irrigated with povidone-iodine. During dilation of the anal canal, it is typical for fissures to occur in the lateral positions of the anal canal, and these fissures become the basis for the receptive site for the skin to be introduced. The flaps are drawn on the skin with the inner tip of the diamond at the edge of the fissures in the anal canal stricture. The stricture is incised at these fissure sites, and the scar is divided. The underlying internal sphincter and external sphincter are protected, and the incision sites are enlarged to accommodate the postage stamp–sized diamond flap (Figure 20-5).
- The diamond-shaped flaps are incised on the skin maintaining broad-based pedicles of fat under the flaps by undermining the attachments under the donor skin to allow the broad base of the diamond flap to slide into the anal canal. The blood supply is protected. The skin is handled very gently, and the skin is pushed into the defect in the stricture (Figure 20-6).
- The donor sites are closed behind the diamond flap, and the edges of the diamond flap are secured in the donor site with horizontal mattress sutures of 3-0 absorbable suture between full-thickness outer skin and subcuticular layer of the flap skin. The apex of the diamond within the anal canal is secured with a full-thickness 3-0 absorbable suture to fix the tip flap within the anal canal at the apex of the fissure defect, and the edges are sewn in around the shape of the diamond. The donor site is closed in a linear fashion to keep the flap from pulling out (Figure 20-4). Antibiotic ointment and a fluff gauze are applied.

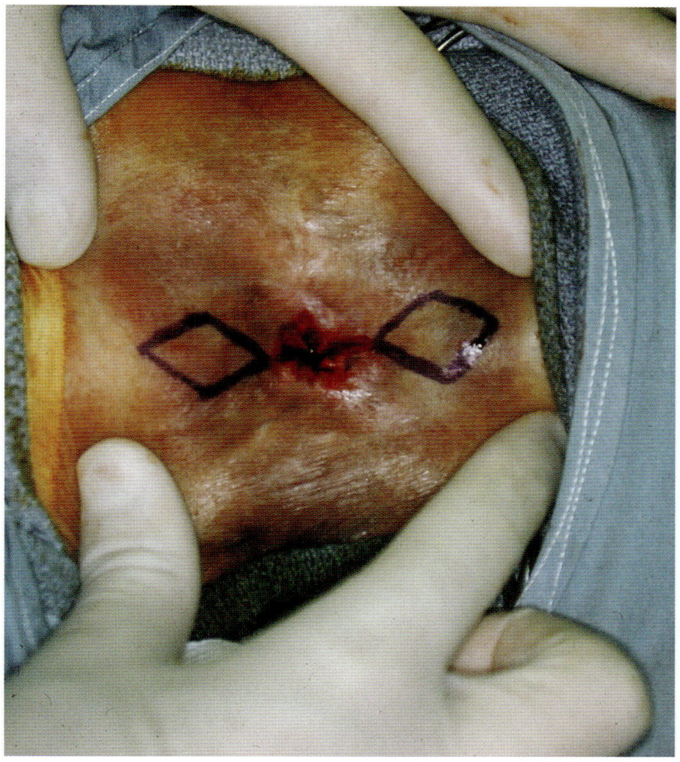

Figure 20-5

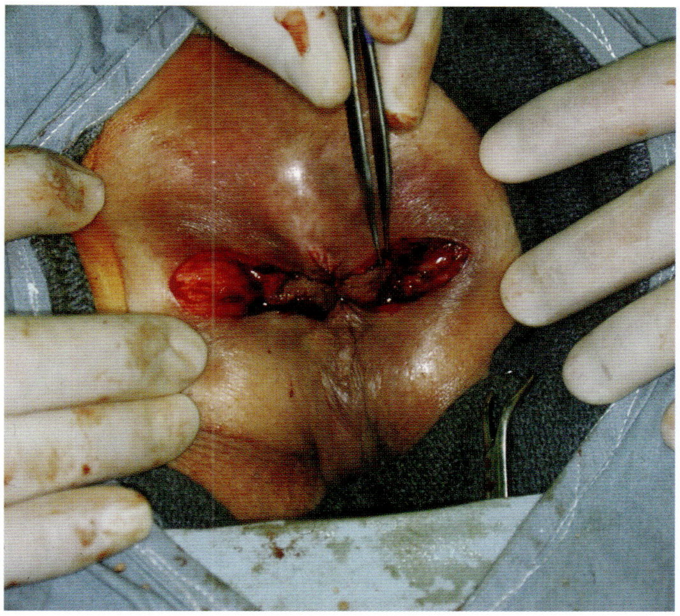

Figure 20-6

Step 4: Postoperative Care

Patients with either of these flaps are managed similarly. The patient receives antibiotics in the hospital on bowel rest without sitting or climbing stairs for 3 days. On postoperative day 3, the patient is begun on a liquid diet, stool softeners, and laxatives. On postoperative day 4, the patient is allowed to resume a regular diet and warned against constipation. The patient is allowed to leave the hospital but is instructed not to sit, climb stairs, drive, or do strenuous exercise for 2 weeks. At the end of the 2-week period, if healing has progressed and the sutures can be removed, the patient is allowed to increase activity.

Step 5: Pearls and Pitfalls

Because this is a very unsterile area, the likelihood of infection is high; however, the flaps can be saved in the event of infection. Examination under anesthesia and débridement is an appropriate first maneuver. Long-term antibiotics can also reduce the likelihood of poor outcome.

It is usually unnecessary to perform repeated dilations after a flap procedure. A single anoscopy after 2 weeks of healing reveals an adequate anal canal, and the patient can be reassured that the stenosis is resolved.

Flap viability is an issue when patients are obese, have known cardiovascular disease, and smoke. Patients should be instructed to avoid cigarettes for 2 weeks before the procedure and 4 weeks afterward.

Selected Readings

Duieb Z, Appu S, Hung K, et al. Anal stenosis: use of an algorithm to provide a tension-free anoplasty. Aust N Z J Surg 2010;80:337–40.

Pearl RK, Hooks VH 3rd, Abcarian H, et al. Island flap anoplasty for the treatment of anal stricture and mucosal ectropion. Dis Colon Rectum 1990;33:581–3.

CHAPTER 21

Excisional Hemorrhoidectomy

Elisa H. Birnbaum

Step 1: Clinical Anatomy

Venous drainage of the anal canal begins with the hemorrhoidal plexus. The external hemorrhoidal plexus is situated subcutaneously around the anal canal below the dentate line. When dilated, these vessels constitute the external hemorrhoids. The internal hemorrhoidal plexus is situated above the dentate line and located submucosally. The internal hemorrhoids originate from the internal hemorrhoidal plexus in the upper anal canal. There are three anorectal arterial venous plexi, located in the (1) left lateral position, (2) right anterior position, and (3) right posterior position. These plexi drain into the paired inferior and middle hemorrhoidal veins, which drain into the internal iliac vein and a single superior hemorrhoidal vein that drains into the inferior mesenteric vein. Each of these venous complexes is associated with an arterial supply within the connective tissue cushion surrounding the veins.

Step 2: Preoperative Considerations

Excisional hemorrhoidectomy is indicated for patients with large symptomatic third-degree (prolapsing, bleeding, reducible) and fourth-degree (nonreducible) internal hemorrhoids that cannot be treated with ligation and patients with symptomatic combined internal and external hemorrhoids (mixed) who have failed or are not candidates for nonoperative treatments. Preoperative counseling is important regarding dietary and medical bowel control for constipation, expected postoperative anal discomfort, and urinary retention that can be common after an excisional hemorrhoidectomy. A mechanical bowel preparation is unnecessary, but a Fleet enema is given several hours before surgery. Prophylactic antibiotics are not indicated for a hemorrhoidectomy in most patients.

Step 3: Operative Steps

- Intravenous sedation is given to the patient with plans for local anesthesia; however, spinal anesthesia or general anesthesia can be used if chosen by the anesthesiologist and patient.
- The patient is placed in the prone-jackknife position. Retraction tape placed on the buttocks is used to help expose the perianal region, and the skin is prepped. An anal field block is established using approximately 20 mL of 0.25% bupivacaine injected starting at the lateral midpoint of the anal verge in a fan shape deep and superficial in the ischiorectal fossa on each side of the anal canal to a total of 40 to 60 mL. Care must be taken to cross the midline anteriorly and posteriorly during the injections. The pudendal nerve and vessels should be included in the deep posterior injection on both sides of the anal canal. The largest hemorrhoid is approached first (Figures 21-1 and 21-2). A curved Hill-Ferguson retractor is placed within the anal canal identifying the hemorrhoidal complex. The hemorrhoid is grasped on the external and internal components with curved clamps (Figure 21-3), and a deep apical suture of absorbable suture is placed encompassing all of the vascular pedicle 3 to 4 cm above the dentate line and is tied (Figure 21-4). An elliptical or diamond-shaped incision is made around the hemorrhoidal complex with a scalpel or cautery (Figure 21-5). The perianal skin is placed on traction, and the hemorrhoid is dissected off of the internal sphincter using cautery or sharp dissection of the submucosal plane (Figure 21-6).

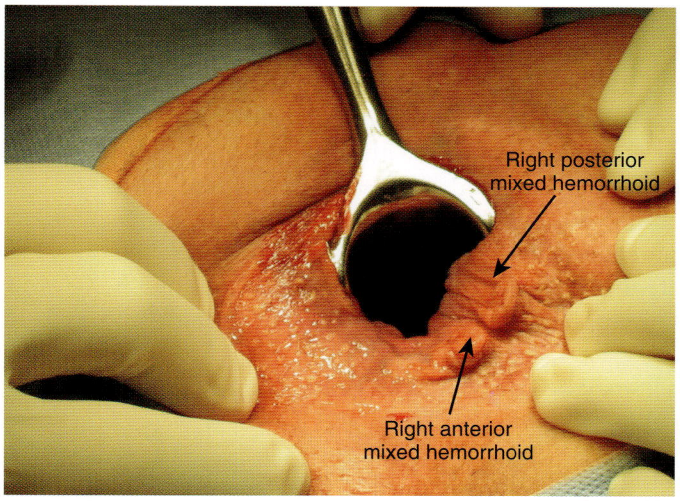

Figure 21-1

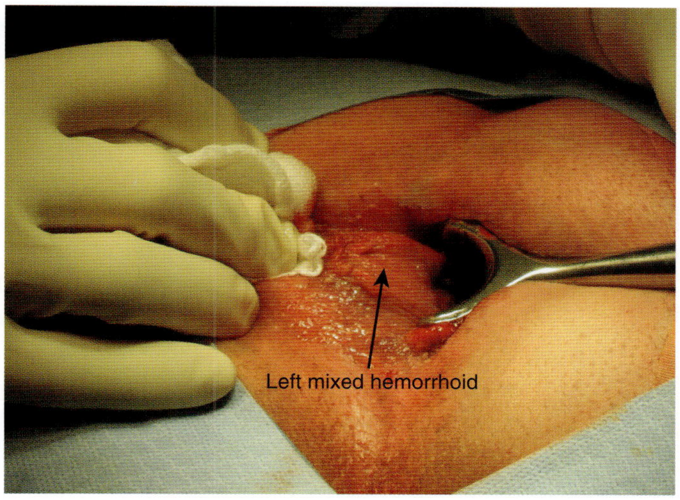

Figure 21-2

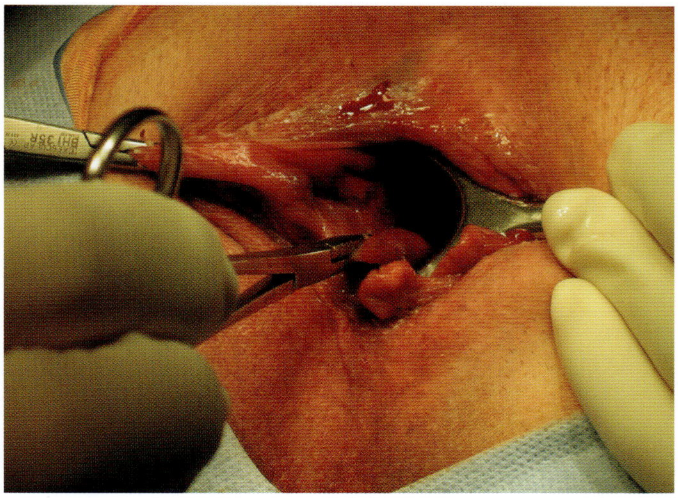

Figure 21-3

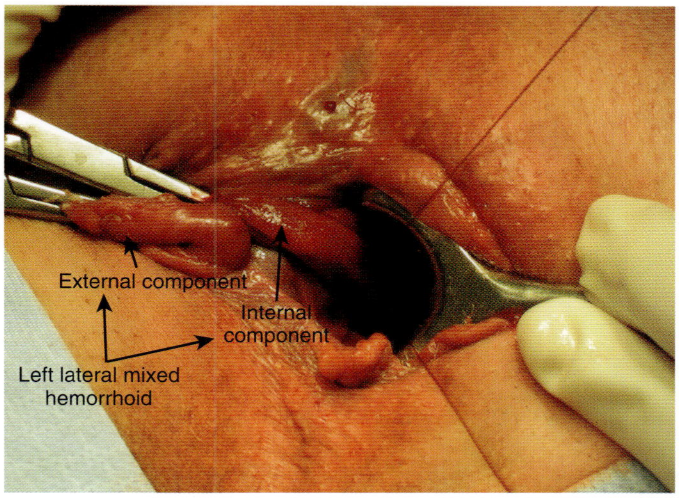

Figure 21-4

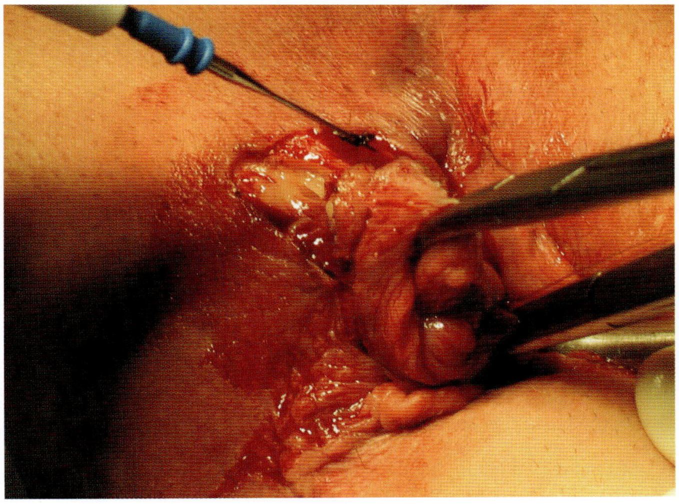

Figure 21-5

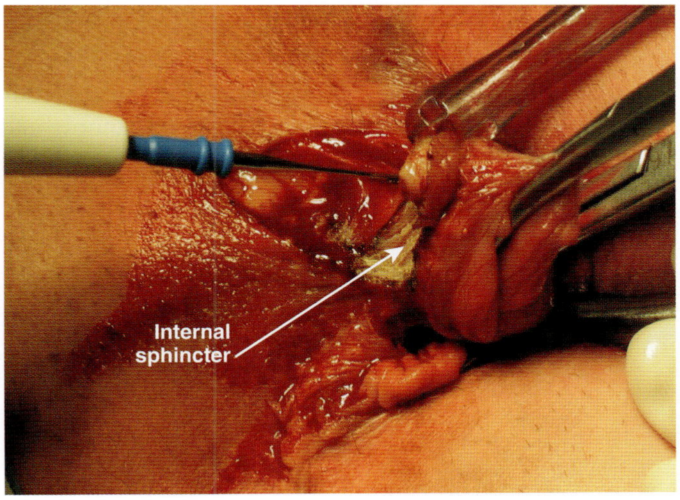

Figure 21-6

- On reaching the apical suture, the hemorrhoid is excised, and the wound is irrigated (Figure 21-7). Hemostasis is obtained using the cautery. The apical suture is used to reinforce control of the vascular pedicle before starting the closure (Figure 21-8). The apical suture is extended outward along the defect to close the mucosa edges and obliterate the potential space beneath the mucosa by catching small portions of the internal sphincter with each passage of the needle (Figure 21-9). The entire elliptical defect is closed, and hemostasis is ensured with additional sutures as needed (Figure 21-10).
- The next largest hemorrhoidal complex is approached in a similar fashion followed by the third complex if necessary (Figure 21-11). Care must be taken to avoid removal of too much of the anoderm around the level of the dentate line and outer anal canal, which results in stricture formation.
- A double elastic ligation of the vascular pedicle may be considered to guarantee hemostasis and remove any more proximal redundant mucosa (Figure 21-12).

Step 4: Postoperative Care

Narcotics are often required to control postoperative pain, and intravenous narcotics can be given initially if the patient is admitted for 23-hour observation. Patients can be discharged when their pain is under control; they should be instructed to maintain pain control with oral analgesics. Urinary retention can occur in one third of patients. This problem can be minimized by limiting intravenous fluids that are given by the anesthesia team in the perioperative period. Constipation owing to pain and narcotic use is common, and patients should be instructed on the use of stool softeners and laxatives for several weeks in the postoperative period.

Step 5: Pearls and Pitfalls

Fecal incontinence is uncommon. Care in dissecting the hemorrhoidal complex off the internal sphincter prevents injury of the internal sphincter. Infections are rare and can be minimized by loosely approximating the mucosa and using a dissolvable suture. Strictures are more common after a Whitehead hemorrhoidectomy (circumferential lifting of the anoderm at the dentate line); however, they also can occur with an overzealous excisional hemorrhoidectomy that removes the bridges of anoderm between the hemorrhoidal complexes. A conscious effort to retain anoderm between suture lines helps to prevent this complication.

The complexity and difficulty of excisional hemorrhoidectomy are sometimes underestimated. The deep anal canal of an obese man is the most challenging. Long, fine instruments and adequate retraction (lighted Hill-Ferguson retractor) with experienced assistance are key to a stress-free, bloodless excisional hemorrhoidectomy.

Selected Readings

Giordano P, Gravante G, Sorge R, et al. Long-term outcomes of stapled hemorrhoidopexy vs conventional hemorrhoidectomy: a meta-analysis of randomized controlled trials. Arch Surg 2009;144:266–72.

Tan EK, Cornish J, Darzi AW, et al. Meta-analysis of short-term outcomes of randomized controlled trials of LigaSure vs conventional hemorrhoidectomy. Arch Surg 2007;142:1209–18.

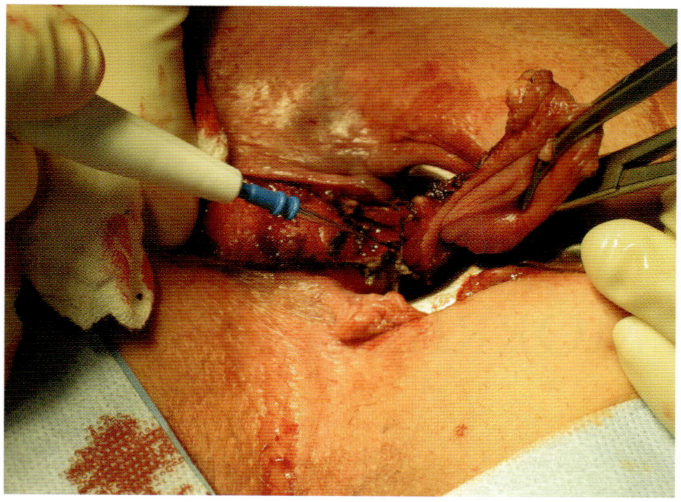

Figure 21-7

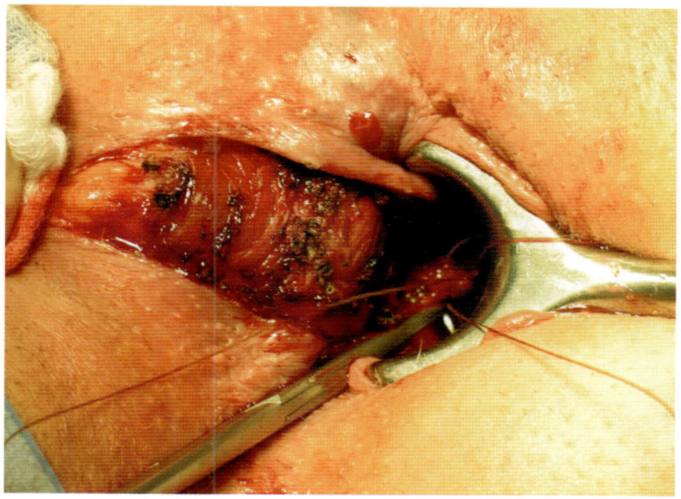

Figure 21-8

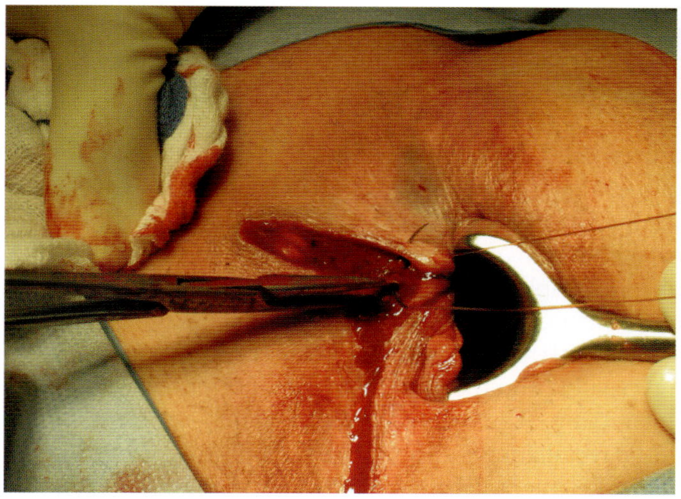

Figure 21-9

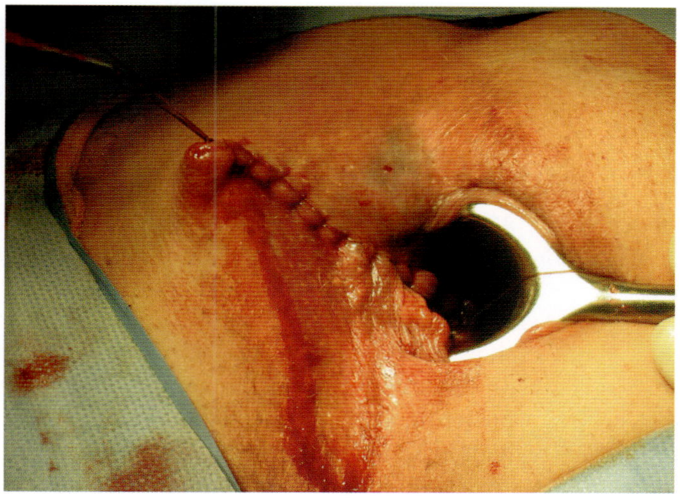

Figure 21-10

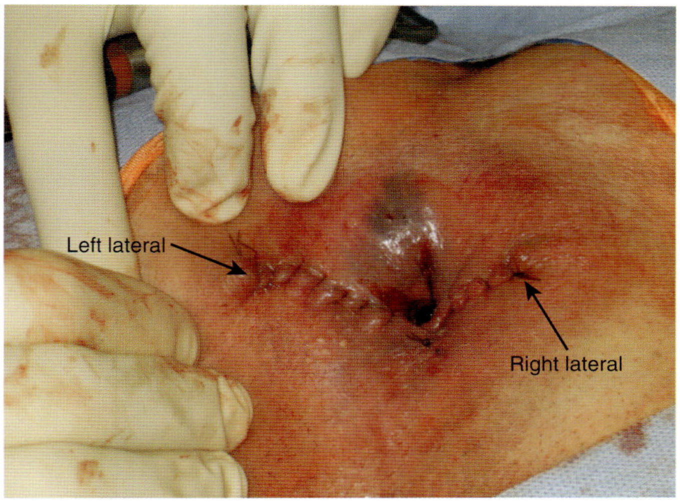

Figure 21-11

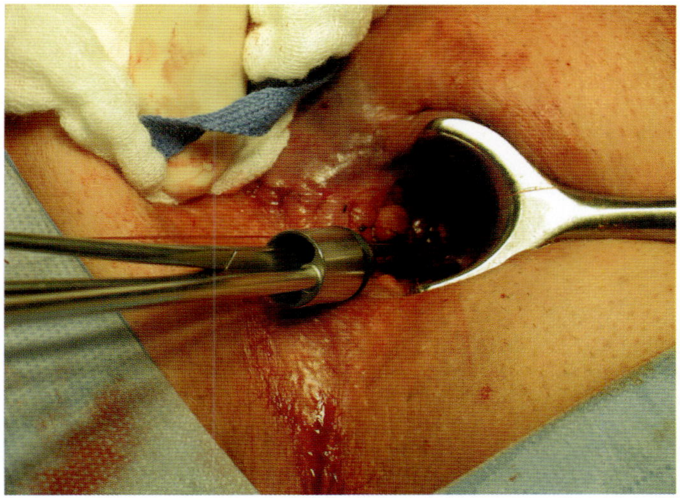

Figure 21-12

CHAPTER 22

Stapled Hemorrhoidectomy

Matthew G. Mutch

Step 1: Clinical Anatomy

The main anatomic points of interest for stapled hemorrhoidectomy are the anal verge, dentate line, and anorectal ring. The anal verge is found in the perineal skin at the intersphincteric groove where the internal anal sphincter ends distally. The dentate line is the junction of columnar epithelium from the rectum and the squamous epithelium of the perineal skin. The anorectal ring is the top or proximal extent of the anal sphincter complex; it is palpable as the puborectalis muscle circles behind the rectum. There are two main hemorrhoidal complexes: internal hemorrhoids, which are located above the dentate line, and external hemorrhoids, which are located on the anal verge. The internal hemorrhoids are typically prominent in the right anterior, right posterior, and left lateral quadrants of the distal rectum. The arterial blood supplies to the hemorrhoidal "cushions" are the superior and middle rectal arteries. The venous drainage occurs via the superior rectal vein to the portal system for the internal hemorrhoids and the inferior pudendal vein to the inferior vena cava for the external hemorrhoids. The sensory innervation for the epithelium distal to the dentate line, which conveys sensations of heat, cold, and pain, is provided by the inferior rectal nerves. The most intensely innervated area of the anal canal is the anal transition zone, which is the 2 cm of cuboidal epithelium within the dentate line crypts up to 1 cm above the Morgagni columns. The parasympathetic fibers are responsible for conveying sensation for the epithelium proximal to the dentate line. As a result, there is very little or only poorly defined sensation above this point.

Step 2: Preoperative Considerations

The patient must be thoroughly examined and appropriately selected for a stapled hemorrhoidectomy. Anal stenosis, cancer, proctitis, and radiation damage are contraindications. This procedure is most effective for larger circumferential grade III hemorrhoids that cannot be treated by ligation owing to volume of tissue, and it is ineffective for grade IV hemorrhoids. Patients should receive two enemas to cleanse the rectum and sigmoid colon. Perioperative antibiotics and deep vein thrombosis prophylaxis are unnecessary for this short operation. The procedure can be performed under a general anesthetic or with a regional anesthetic with intravenous sedation and a perianal block with a local anesthetic. Patients should be informed that there will be a severe rectal pressure for at least 24 hours after the procedure.

Step 3: Operative Steps

- The patient can be placed in the prone-jackknife or lithotomy position based on the surgeon's preference.
- After adequate general or local anesthesia has been induced, the anal canal and distal rectum must be examined to confirm the diagnosis and the appropriateness of the anatomy for the procedure.

- The external hemorrhoids are grasped with atraumatic clamps to evert the anal canal. The anal dilator and obturator unit is inserted (Figure 22-1). The obturator is removed, leaving the clear anal dilator in place. It can be secured to the perineal skin with sutures or by an assistant.
- The dentate line is identified through the clear sides of the operating dilator (Figure 22-2). The operating anoscope is inserted, and a line is drawn on the anoscope at 5 cm above the dentate line to mark the line for the purse-string suture (Figure 22-3). The purse-string suture is placed 4 cm above the dentate line with eight stitches placed no deeper than the submucosa, starting posteriorly and ending posteriorly.
- When the purse-string suture is in place, the index finger is placed through the purse-string, and the suture is pulled to ensure there are no gaps in the purse-string (Figure 22-4).
- The stapler anvil is passed above the purse-string suture, taking time to ensure the anvil is above all of the purse-string (Figure 22-5), and the purse-string is tied securely but loosely around the post of the stapler (Figure 22-6).

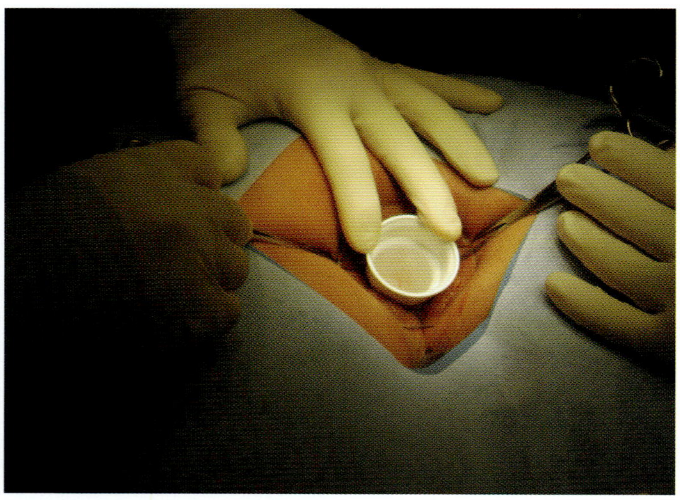

Figure 22-1

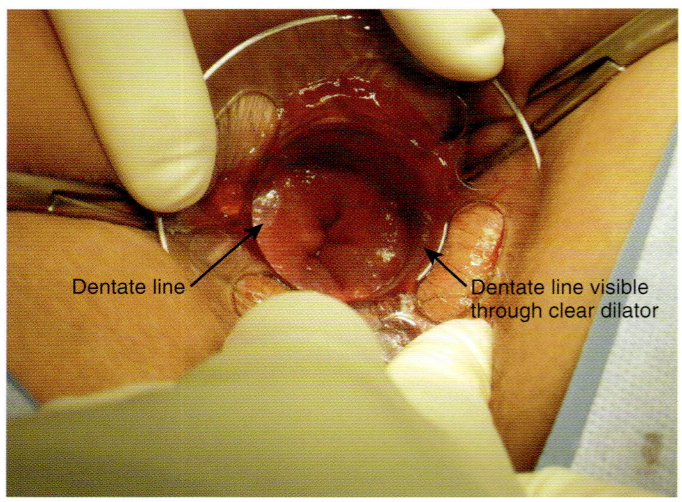

Figure 22-2

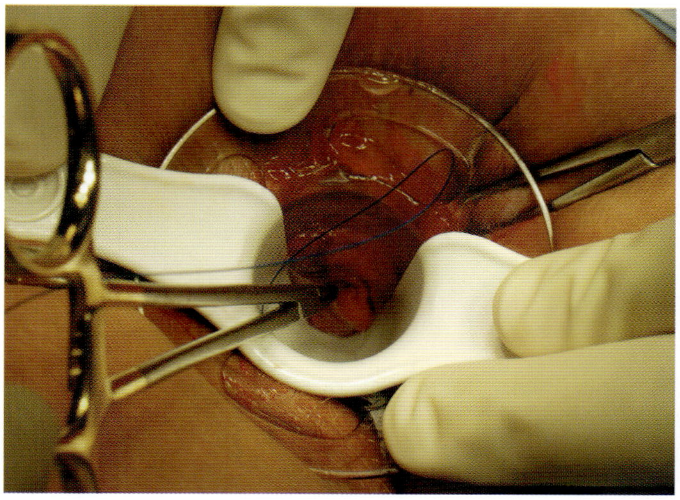

Figure 22-3

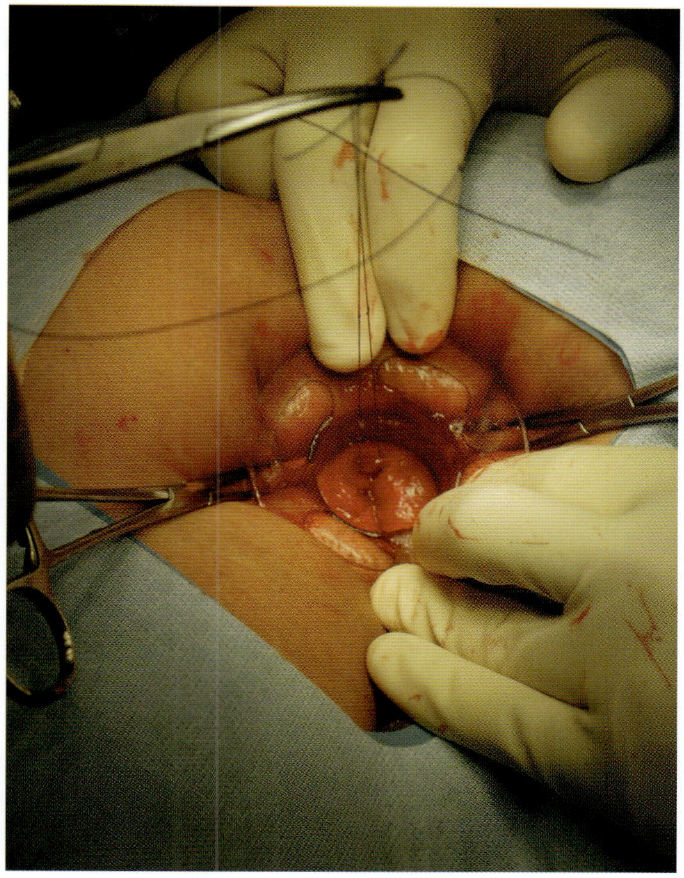

Figure 22-4

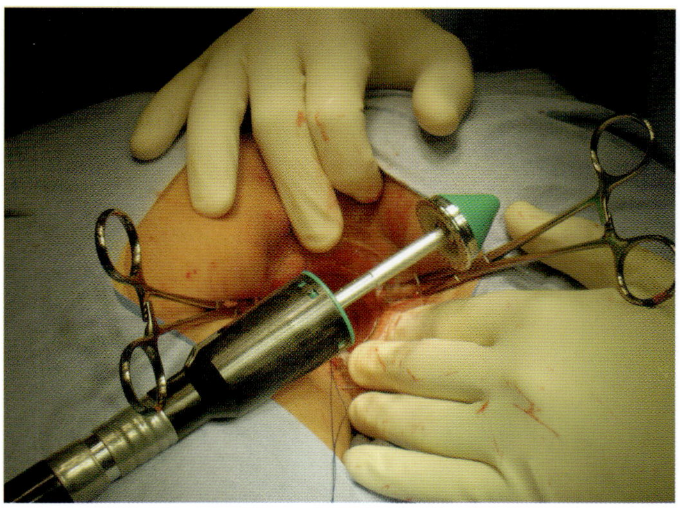

Figure 22-5

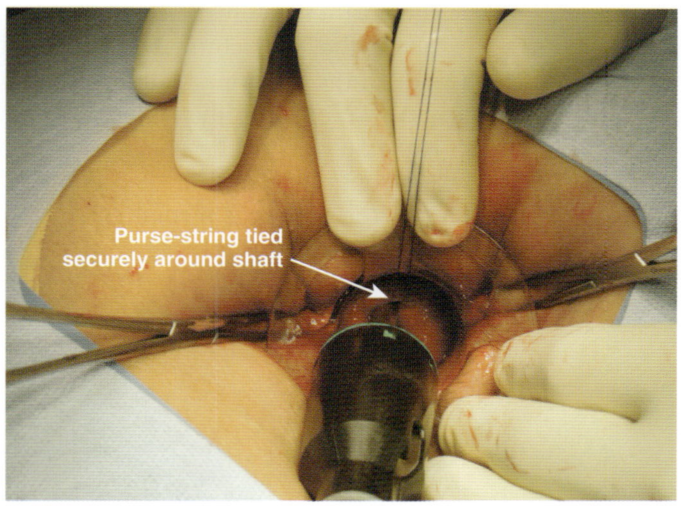

Figure 22-6

- The ends of the suture are brought through the side ports of the stapler to help create traction on the redundant mucosa captured by the purse-string suture (Figures 22-7 and 22-8). The stapler is tightened as it is pushed up to the level of the purse-string, all the while pulling down on the suture (Figure 22-9). The closed stapler is inspected, a finger is placed in the vagina if the patient is female, and the trigger is fired. The stapler is held closed for 2 minutes for hemostasis.
- The hemorrhoidal doughnut is inspected (Figure 22-10) for completeness.
- After the stapler is fired, the staple line is closely inspected, and any bleeding is ligated with suture. The staple line is reinforced at the three hemorrhoidal pedicles with a figure-eight suture, which crosses the staple line to prevent and manage bleeding (Figure 22-11). Figure 22-12 is a diagram of the final position of the staple line, ideally 4 cm above the dentate line.

Step 4: Postoperative Care

The patient may be discharged the day of surgery if he or she is able to void. Patients should be provided with adequate pain control and placed on a high-fiber diet. Appropriate stool softeners are prescribed to prevent constipation.

Step 5: Pearls and Pitfalls

The placement of the suture line and subsequent staple line is paramount for success. A staple line placed too low can result in substantial anal pain, and a staple line placed too high does not effectively treat the symptomatic hemorrhoids. The low rectal mucosa should be resuspended in its normal anatomic position as an "anopexy." Delayed postoperative bleeding requires an examination under anesthesia because exposed submucosal vessels can lead to significant blood loss. These can be suture ligated. Persistent pain, fever, or urinary retention may be signs of perineal sepsis. Partial inclusion of the purse-string suture would result in only partial hemorrhoidectomy. Partial capture of the rectal wall results in creation of a mucosal bridge across the low rectum. Acute angulation of the stapler during closure can result in capture of the side of the rectum and almost total occlusion of the rectum as the purse-string is pulled to the side. Removal of the stapler without complete transection of the mucosa has been the cause of massive hemorrhage and rectal perforation. This is a simple procedure; however, there are severe consequences if the procedure is performed improperly. A learning curve of 10 cases with a proctor present is recommended.

Selected Readings

Jayaraman S, Colquhoun PH, Malthaner RA. Stapled hemorrhoidopexy is associated with a higher long-term recurrence rate of internal hemorrhoids compared with conventional excisional hemorrhoid surgery. Dis Colon Rectum 2007;50:1297–305.

Senagore AJ, Singer M, Abcarian H, et al. A prospective, randomized, controlled multicenter trial comparing stapled hemorrhoidopexy and Ferguson hemorrhoidectomy: perioperative and one-year results. Dis Colon Rectum 2004;47:1824–36.

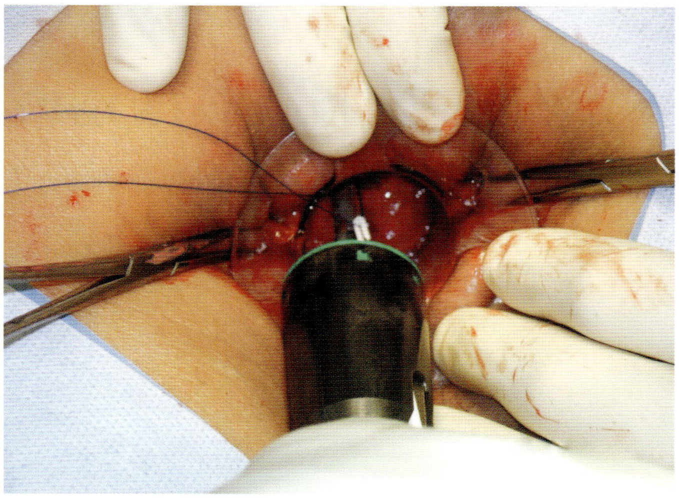

Figure 22-7

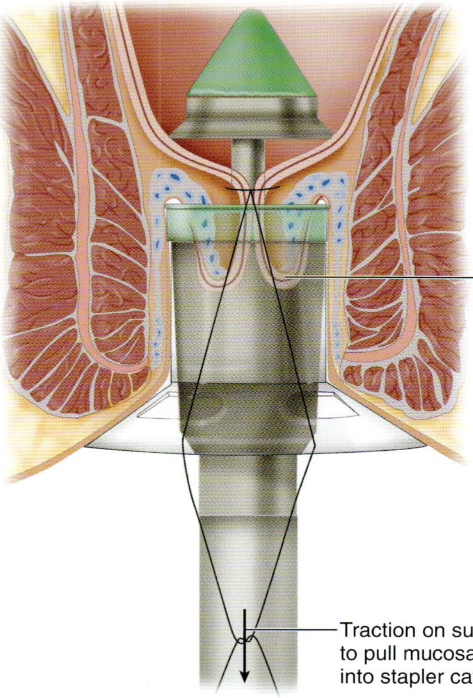

Figure 22-8

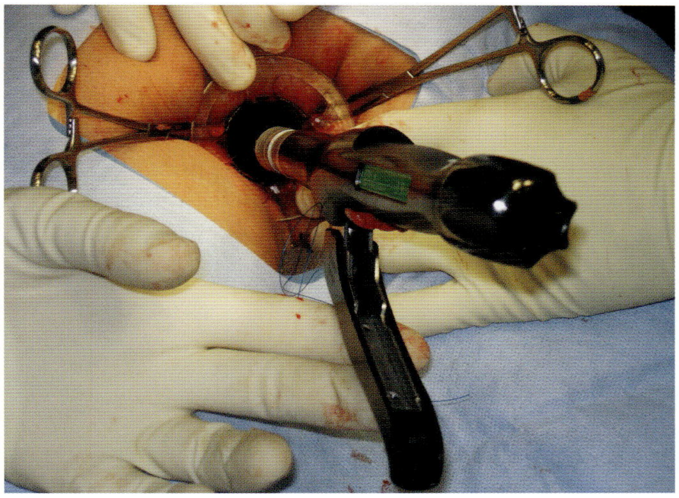

Figure 22-9

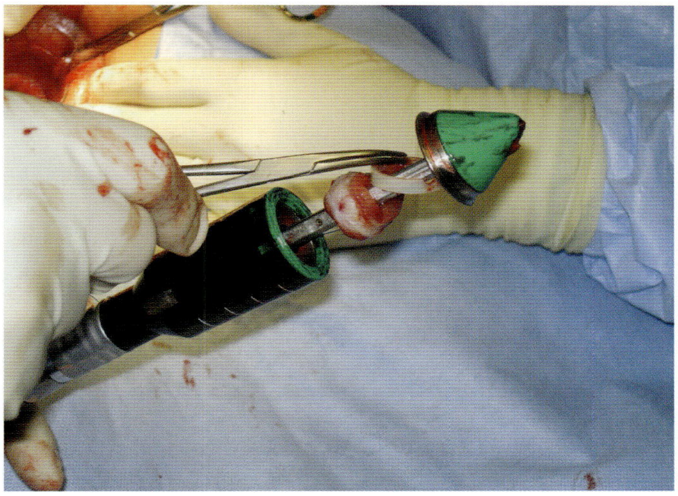

Figure 22-10

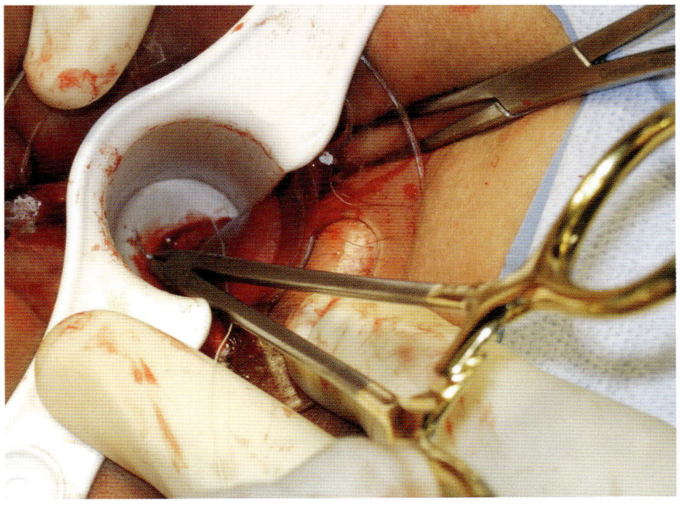

Figure 22-11

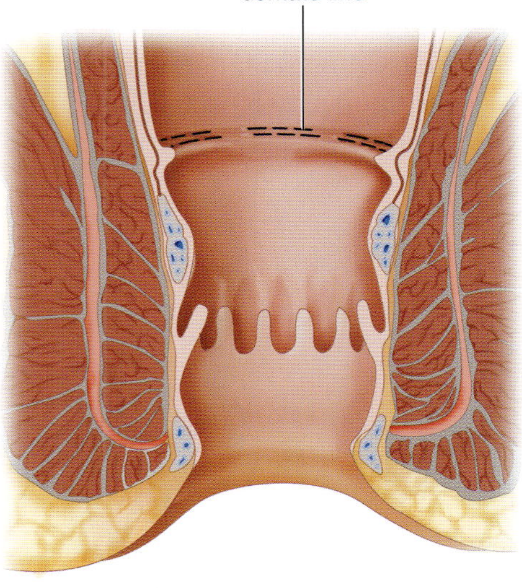

Figure 22-12

CHAPTER 23

Open Lateral Internal Sphincterotomy

Bashar Safar and Ira J. Kodner

Step 1: Clinical Anatomy

The anal canal is enveloped by two muscles, the internal sphincter, which is innervated by the autonomic nervous system, and the external sphincter, which has somatic innervation. The external sphincter extends slightly beyond the internal sphincter at the anal verge, which allows clear identification of the intersphincteric groove. The intersphincteric groove is a bloodless plane that runs between the two sphincter muscles and extends up to the levator ani muscle. Anal fissures occur in the anterior and posterior midline and result most commonly from a combination of internal sphincter spasm and ischemia. Dividing the internal sphincter in a lateral position allows the fissure to heal, although this is associated with a small risk of incontinence.

Step 2: Preoperative Considerations

Anal fissures produce a distinctive set of symptoms. Good history taking and a thorough examination in the office are sufficient tools in most cases to establish a diagnosis. Most fissures are idiopathic and are located posteriorly (80%) or anteriorly (20%), distal to the dentate line. An unusual presentation and location should alert the treating physician to the possibility of other pathology, such as Crohn's disease, cancer, or sexually transmitted diseases, which would not respond to therapies employed for chronic fissures.

When the diagnosis of anal fissure is established, the patient should be started on medical management including agents that induce chemical relaxation of the internal sphincter, fiber supplementation, sitz baths, and steroid suppositories. Medical management should be continued for at least 1 month, at which time more than two thirds of patients will have improved. Surgical management may be recommended in patients who fail medical management with persistent symptoms and fissure on examination. Most acute anal fissures respond to medical management; however, a few persist and become chronic.

Lateral internal sphincterotomy is a procedure commonly employed in the management of chronic anal fissure. Chronicity can be defined by appearance and timing. A chronic fissure is defined by symptoms lasting longer than 3 months and an examination that reveals exposed internal sphincter at the base of the ulcer, a sentinel pile, edema, and fibrosis. Lateral internal sphincterotomy for chronic anal fissure is associated with a very high success rate with a small, but significant, risk of incontinence, especially in women.

Step 3: Operative Steps

- These procedures can be performed under conscious sedation with local anesthesia, spinal anesthesia, or general anesthesia.
- The patient is placed in the prone-jackknife position with the pressure points protected, and the buttocks are taped apart to efface the anus using 3-inch silk tape. Sedation is administered by the anesthesia staff, and an anal block is performed with local infiltration of the canal, ischiorectal fossa, and pudendal nerves using long-acting local anesthetic (Figure 23-1).
- The anal canal is examined using a curved Hill-Ferguson anoscope to confirm the diagnosis and exclude other causes of anal pain. The hypertrophied band of the internal anal sphincter is usually the length of the anal fissure ulcer split (Figure 23-2).
- With the anoscope facing the left lateral or right lateral wall, the surgeon slides the index finger across the anal canal from the dentate line to the anal verge to find the intersphincteric groove.
- A radial incision is made over the groove (Figure 23-3), and a clamp is inserted between the two sphincters (Figure 23-4). The clamp is spread gently, and the tip of the clamp is elevated through the incision to expose the hypertrophied fibers of the internal sphincter.

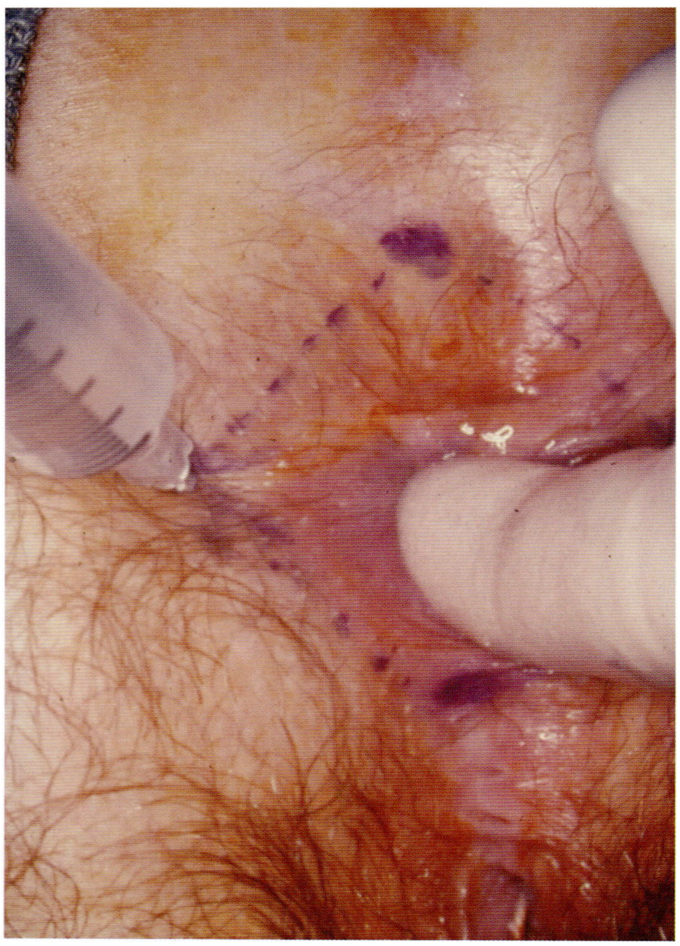

Figure 23-1

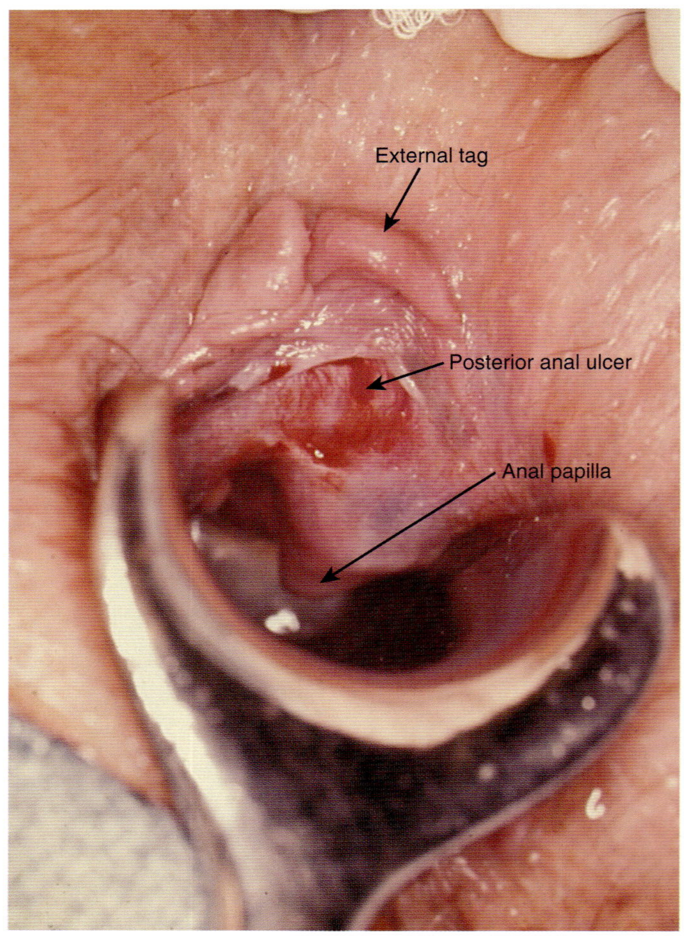

Figure 23-2

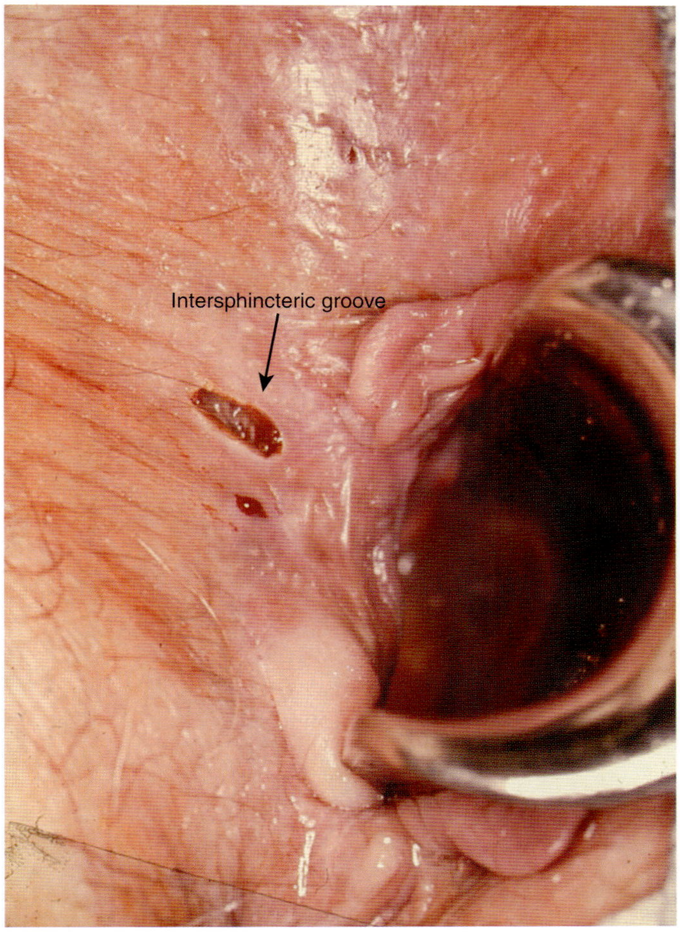

Figure 23-3

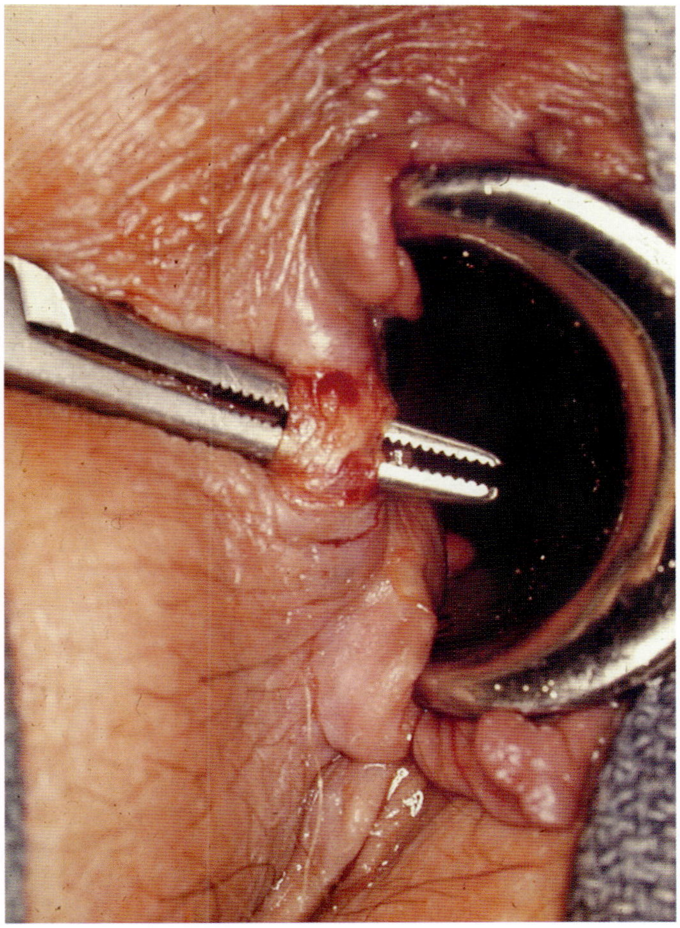

Figure 23-4

- The sphincter is divided under direct vision to the level of the dentate line or enough to remove the hypertrophied band (Figures 23-5 and 23-6*A*-*C*).
- Hemostasis is accomplished with electrocautery or pressure.
- The incision is reapproximated with 3-0 absorbable suture. An antibiotic ointment and gauze dressing is applied.
- A closed sphincterotomy can be performed through the radial incision in the midlateral position. A No. 11 blade is guided into the intersphincteric groove with a finger in the anal canal. The knife is turned toward the lumen, and a sawing motion is used to divide the internal sphincter hypertrophied fibers without damaging the overlying mucosa (Figure 23-7*A* and *B*).

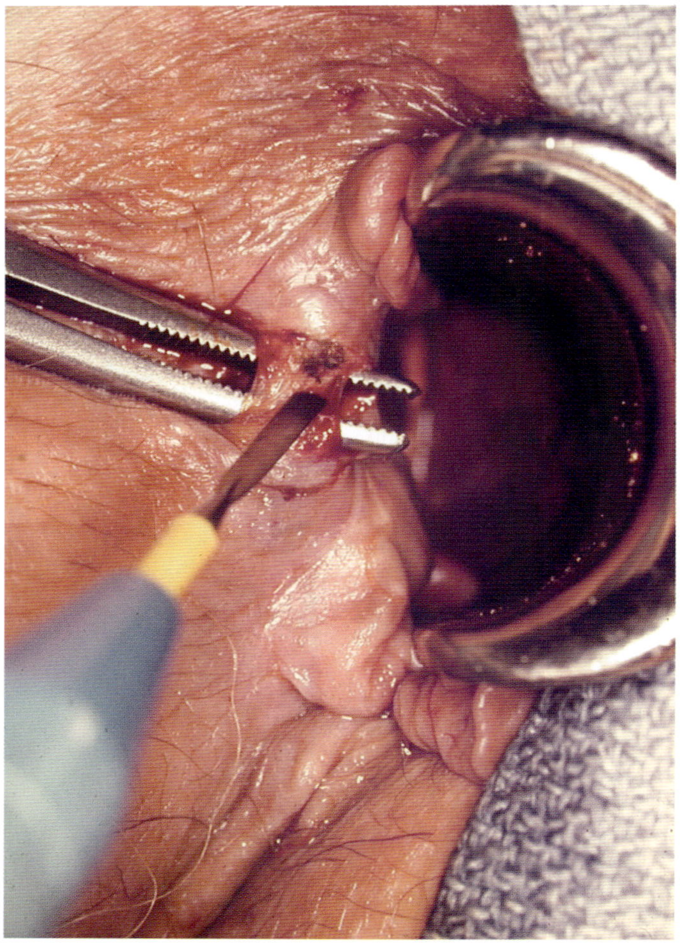

Figure 23-5

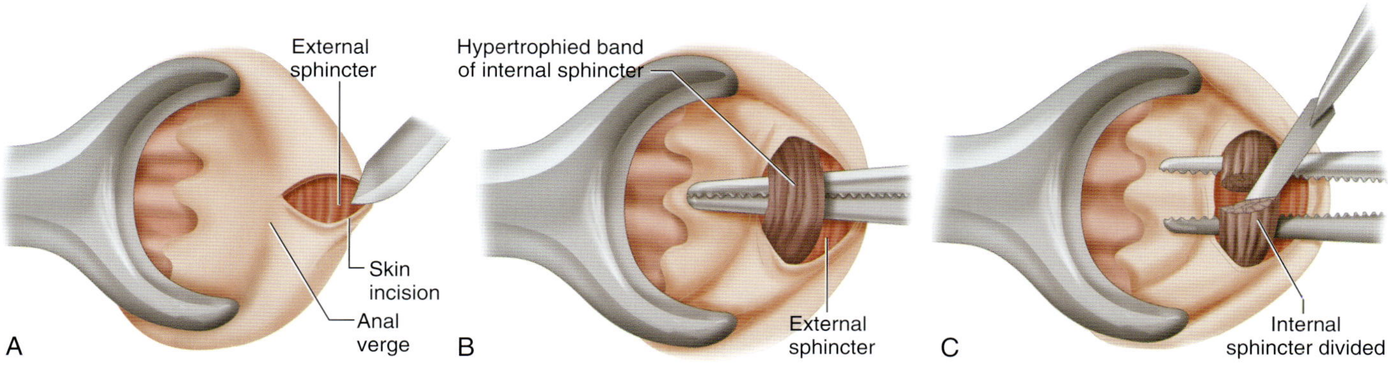

Figure 23-6A-C

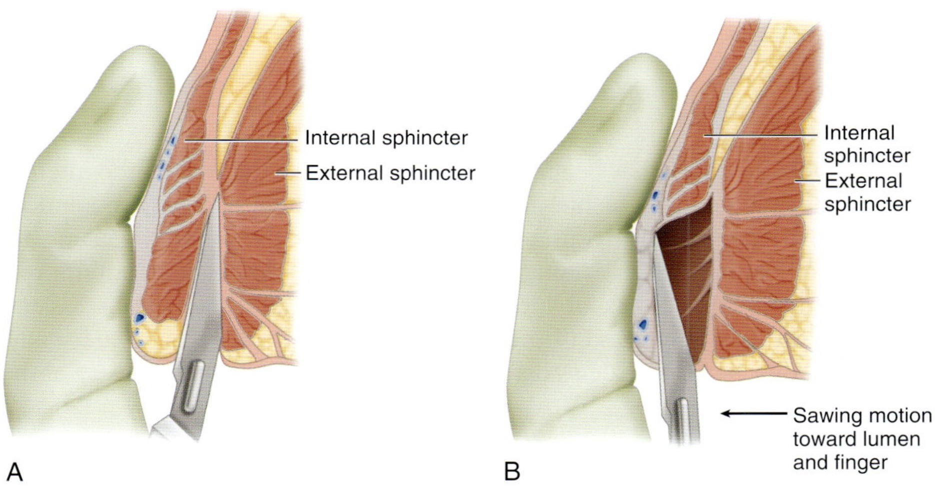

Figure 23-7A-B

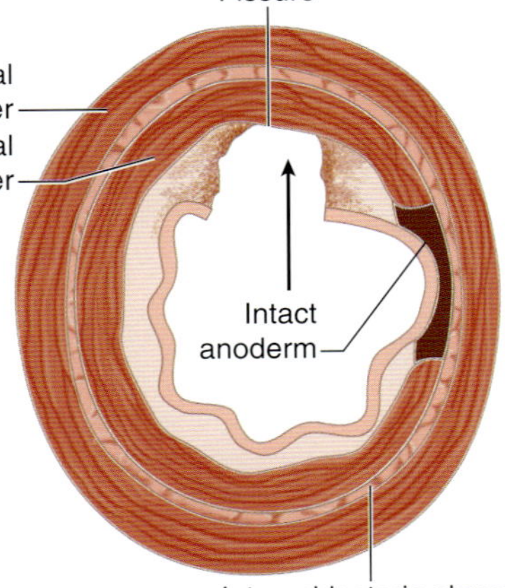

Figure 23-8

Step 4: Postoperative Care

The patient is continued on fiber supplement with stool softeners, tub soaks three times per day, and nifedipine ointment to the perianal skin to relieve spasm. The patient is seen in the office 2 to 4 weeks postoperatively to check the wound.

Step 5: Pearls and Pitfalls

The extent of sphincterotomy has been debated in the literature. Dividing the internal sphincter to the level of the dentate line to achieve adequate relaxation has been recommended. However, most experts now recommend dividing the sphincter up to the proximal extent of the fissure and the thickened band of muscle. Longer sphincterotomies do not result in improved healing and may result in increased risk of incontinence (Figure 23-8). If an abscess forms in the sphincterotomy site, simple release of the purulence through the incision is usually adequate. If a fistula forms, this is usually due to damage of the rectal wall during delivery of the sphincter through the incision.

Selected Readings

Brown CJ, Dubreuil D, Santoro L, et al. Lateral internal sphincterotomy is superior to topical nitroglycerin for healing chronic anal fissure and does not compromise long-term fecal continence: six-year follow-up of a multicenter, randomized, controlled trial. Dis Colon Rectum 2007;50:442–8.

Elsebae MM. A study of fecal incontinence in patients with chronic anal fissure: prospective, randomized, controlled trial of the extent of internal anal sphincter division during lateral sphincterotomy. World J Surg 2007;31:2052–7.

CHAPTER 24

Sliding Flap Repair of Rectovaginal Fistula

Bashar Safar and Ira J. Kodner

Step 1: Clinical Anatomy

The upper anal canal begins at the puborectalis sling or the anorectal ring, which sits at the level of the pelvic floor and can be palpated through the anal canal as a bulge posteriorly. The longitudinal muscles of the rectum continue into the anus as the intersphincteric plane demarcating the line between autonomic internal sphincter and somatic external sphincter fibers all the way down to the level of the anal canal skin where the intersphincteric groove is palpable. The ischiorectal fossa fat is found outside the circular fibers of the external sphincter that encircle the rectum.

The rectovaginal and rectoprostatic septum descends all the way to the level of the perineum anteriorly. The transverse perinei muscle separates the anterior and posterior perineum. The terminal fibers of the longitudinal muscle of the rectum insert into the skin of the anal canal just outside the anal verge as the corrugator cutanei ani and cause the ridges that are noticed around the anal canal. The internal sphincter is the hypertrophied circular muscle of the wall of the rectum. The lowest portion of the internal sphincter can be palpated as a groove where the longitudinal fibers insert on the skin.

Within the anal canal, the dentate line is the junction between the cuboidal epithelium of the anal transition zone, which is the terminal mucosal layer of the rectum, and the stratified epidermal cells of the anal canal skin. Gland openings (or crypts) are found in the dentate line at the base of the Morgagni columns, which are interdigitating lines of squamous epithelium into the cuboidal and columnar epithelium of the distal rectum. The anal transition zone is the most highly innervated section of the rectum and anal canal and contains nerve endings sensing temperature, vibration, electrical stimulation, pressure, liquid, solid, and gas. The dentate line lies approximately halfway along the surgical anal canal, which extends from the palpable anal verge all the way up to the anorectal ring palpated at the puborectalis sling posteriorly. The anoderm within the anal canal, cephalad to the anal verge, has no hair follicles.

Step 2: Preoperative Considerations

The most common cause of rectovaginal fistula is obstetric trauma. The combination of Crohn's disease and obstetric injury may increase the risk. Cryptoglandular disease rarely causes a rectovaginal fistula in the isolated setting of a normal anal canal and a perirectal abscess. However, the combination of a previous obstetric injury with scarring of the anterior anal sphincter complex and an anterior perirectal cryptoglandular abscess may result in a late rectovaginal fistula remote from the time of the obstetric injury.

The level of the fistula determines in some way the extent of the procedure needed to correct the fistula. A very low rectovaginal fistula between the dentate line and the introitus can be managed with a simple, short sliding flap repair with advancement of normal mucosa over the rectal internal opening to prevent egress of material through the rectovaginal septum into the vagina. A high rectovaginal fistula caused by cancer, radiation, iatrogenic trauma, or sexual trauma may require a more complicated flap procedure with placement of intervening muscle and vascularized tissue to achieve final healing. A high colovaginal or rectovaginal fistula from diverticulitis almost always requires a bowel resection to close the upper vaginal opening. Sliding flap repair for a mid to low rectovaginal fistula is described for fistula induced by obstetric injury or fistula induced by cryptoglandular disease or Crohn's disease.

Before the operation, a complete bowel preparation is recommended. Enemas and clear liquids may be used to empty the left side of the colon. The patient can be constipated to prevent bowel movement in the early postoperative period. Intravenous antibiotics are normally given prophylactically at the beginning of the procedure. Deep vein thrombosis prophylaxis is required in the form of sequential compression devices because the patient is most commonly placed in the prone-jackknife position for more than 30 minutes for the operation. A bladder catheter should be placed to help identify the urethra in complicated cases and to decompress the bladder for several days postoperatively to avoid the need for sitting on the toilet.

Step 3: Operative Steps

- The patient is placed in the prone-jackknife position with the buttocks taped apart and the perineum prepared and draped sterilely with antiseptic material. The vagina and perineum are prepared. Rigid proctoscopy should be performed to wash the rectum completely clear of its contents followed by irrigation with povidone-iodine (Betadine) to reduce bacterial load. The operation is normally best performed with a general anesthetic if the fistula is large; however, regional anesthesia is possible for a fistula that requires only a short sliding flap. A Lone Star retractor (CooperSurgical, Stafford, Texas) is placed to expose the anal canal, and a lighted Hill-Ferguson retractor can be used to expose the anterior anal canal (Figure 24-1).
- The anterior anal mucosal flap is created by incising around the anterior half of the anal canal at the dentate line and extending the incision to include the internal opening of the fistula. If this is on the anoderm, a portion of the anoderm should be removed. If the fistula tract is on the mucosa only, a portion of the mucosa and the dentate line only should be removed (Figure 24-2).

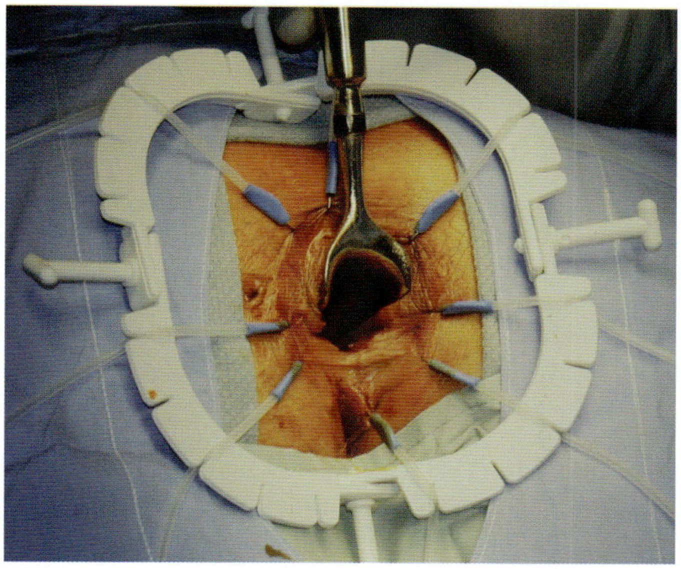

Figure 24-1

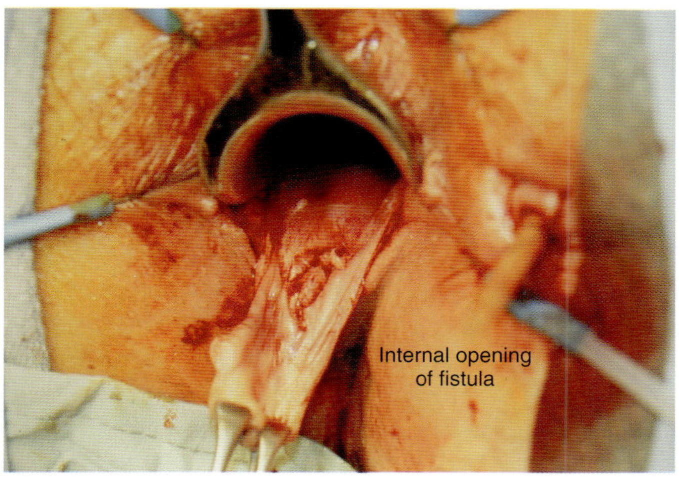

Figure 24-2

- The flap is extended to the top of the anal canal muscular ring to provide adequate mucosal extension and advancement. A portion of the internal muscle is sometimes removed with the flap to make it thicker. If the fistula tract opening is much higher in the anal canal, the full-thickness flap should be carried through the rectal wall in the rectovaginal septum to allow full-thickness rectum to be pulled down to the anal canal. This maneuver must be done very carefully, and the surgeon must keep in mind the need to close the redundant opening in the lateral aspects of the flap harvest site that occur when the anterior rectal wall is brought down to the anal canal. The internal sphincter is preserved. The internal portion of the fistula tract is closed with a figure-eight suture of absorbable suture at the level of the muscle (Figure 24-3).
- The tissue in the anterior anal canal is reefed toward the midline with a series of figure-eight sutures of absorbable suture to approximate the internal sphincter across the midline and to increase the amount of tissue between the rectum and the vagina. This reefing generally incorporates most of the internal sphincter but may also capture the scar and some of the external sphincter muscle from the previous obstetric injury to bolster the anterior muscle. A dilator should be used within the anal canal to calibrate the closure of the anal canal and prevent stricturing. The mucosal flap is pulled down over the muscle repair to guarantee adequate mobility of the flap (Figure 24-4).
- The flap is advanced to the level of the perineal skin to cover the defect. The skin and mucosa are reapproximated with interrupted absorbable sutures around the anterior anal canal. The redundant anal canal skin may be closed in a vertical manner toward the posterior aspect of the vagina to create a T-shaped closure. The reapproximated sphincter may decrease the circumference of the anal canal and leave a redundant portion of skin opening. An open mushroom catheter drain should be placed through the external opening of the fistula tract to counter drain any remaining cavity or tract, or a closed Blake suction drain can be placed in the space between the mucosa and the muscular repair to remove any chance of hematoma or abscess formation (Figures 24-5 and 24-6).

Step 4: Postoperative Care

Postoperative care for sliding flap repair requires a period of bowel rest or at least soft, easy stools to prevent tearing the advanced flap from the mucocutaneous junction. The patient is given intravenous antibiotics for 24 hours postoperatively and maintained on NPO status ("nothing per mouth") or at least on liquids for 2 to 3 days, and the bladder catheter is removed only when the anal canal is adequately sealed. The mushroom catheter or Blake drain may be removed when drainage has stopped. Routine daily tub soaks and tub soaks after bowel movements are recommended to keep the perineum clean.

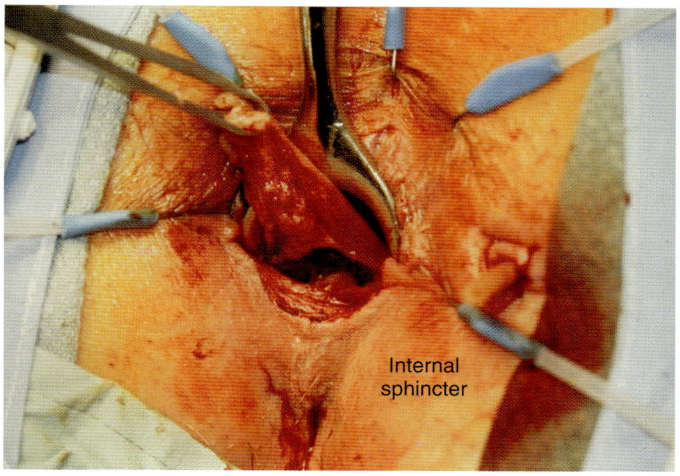

Figure 24-3

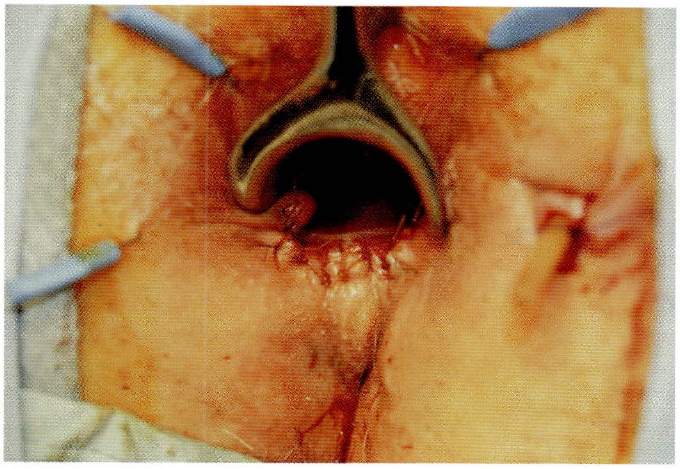

Figure 24-5

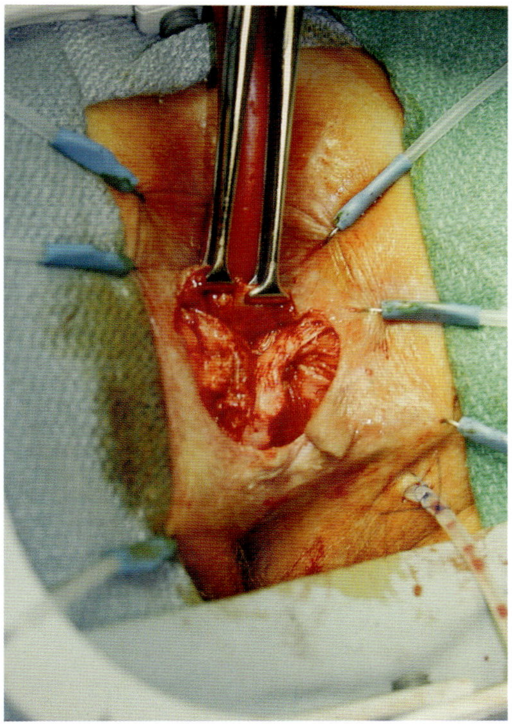

Figure 24-4

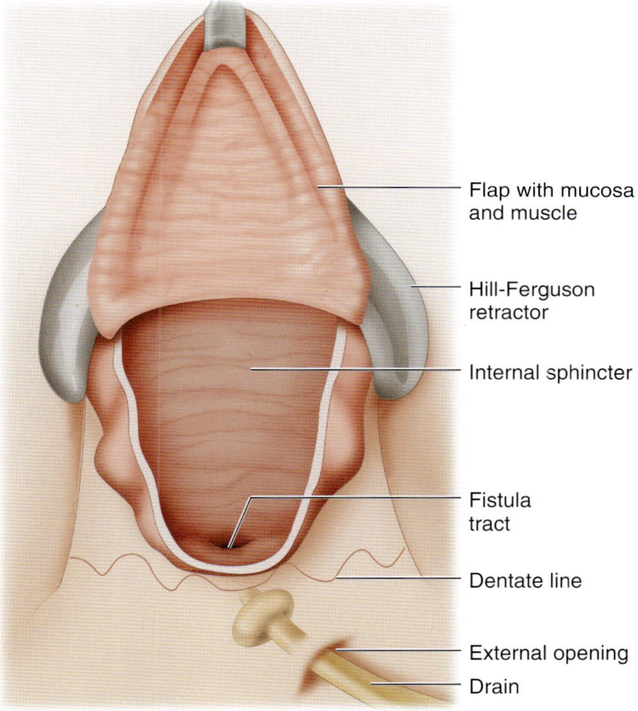

Figure 24-6

Step 5: Pearls and Pitfalls

The mobility of the flap that is advanced must be tempered with the adequacy of blood supply. The broader the base of the flap, the better the blood supply. As the flap needs to be more mobile, the proximal dissection within the rectovaginal septum becomes essential. Placement of an intervening portion of muscle from a gracilis muscle transfer or placement of biologic mesh between the two edges of the fistula may be beneficial.

Use of an external drain is not always necessary but may prevent recurrence of an abscess in the external portion of the fistula. The recurrence of the abscess does not mean a failed fistula repair, and the drainage procedure should be performed under anesthesia to look at the sliding flap repair.

In the circumstance where the flap separates because of ischemia or a hard bowel movement, the flap can be examined under anesthesia, freshened, and resutured or left open to granulate with the patient on an elemental diet. A diverting stoma would be recommended only in the rarest circumstances in the case of a large, high rectovaginal fistula or in the case of a failed fistula after multiple previous attempts.

Selected Readings

Pinto RA, Peterson TV, Shawki S, et al. Are there predictors of outcome following rectovaginal fistula repair? Dis Colon Rectum 2010;53:1240–7.

Soltani A, Kaiser AM. Endorectal advancement flap for cryptoglandular or Crohn's fistula-in-ano. Dis Colon Rectum 2010;53:486–95.

CHAPTER 25

Excision of Anal Bowen's or Paget's Disease with a V-Y Advancement Flap

Bashar Safar and Ira J. Kodner

Step 1: Clinical Anatomy

The upper anal canal begins at the puborectalis sling or the anorectal ring, which sits at the level of the pelvic floor and can be palpated through the anal canal as a bulge posteriorly. The longitudinal muscles of the rectum continue into the anus as the intersphincteric plane demarcating the line between autonomic internal sphincter and somatic external sphincter fibers all the way down to the level of the anal canal skin where the intersphincteric groove is palpable. The ischiorectal fossa fat is found outside the circular fibers of the external sphincter that encircle the rectum.

The rectovaginal and rectoprostatic septum descends all the way to the level of the perineum anteriorly. The transverse perinei muscle separates the anterior and posterior perineum. The terminal fibers of the longitudinal muscle of the rectum insert into the skin of the anal canal just outside the anal verge as the corrugator cutanei ani and cause the ridges that are noticed around the anal canal. The internal sphincter is the hypertrophied circular muscle of the wall of the rectum. The lowest portion of the internal sphincter can be palpated as a groove where the longitudinal fibers insert on the skin.

Within the anal canal, the dentate line is the junction between the cuboidal epithelium of the anal transition zone, which is the terminal mucosal layer of the rectum, and the stratified epidermal cells of the anal canal skin. Gland openings (or crypts) are found in the dentate line at the base of the Morgagni columns, which are interdigitating lines of squamous epithelium into the cuboidal and columnar epithelium of the distal rectum. The anal transition zone is the most highly innervated section of the rectum and anal canal and contains nerve fibers sensing temperature, vibration, electrical stimulation, pressure, liquid, solid, and gas. The dentate line lies approximately halfway along the surgical anal canal, which extends from the palpable anal verge all the way up to the anorectal ring palpated at the puborectalis sling posteriorly. The anoderm within the anal canal, cephalad to the anal verge, has no hair follicles.

Step 2: Preoperative Considerations

Extramammary Paget's disease or adenocarcinoma of the perianal skin and extensive anal Bowen's disease have been considered indications for excision of perianal skin and replacement with V-Y advancement flaps of inner buttock skin. Anal Bowen's disease is due to regional human papillomavirus, and performance of this procedure does not relieve the physician from long-term screening of the intra-anal mucosa for the development of dysplasia or cancer in the future. If the patient is extremely symptomatic from itching and raised lesions, the excision of the anal canal disease and advancement of inner buttock skin is an option. The existence of intradermal adenocarcinoma or extramammary Paget's disease should automatically result in excision and screening of the rest of the colon for the existence of other areas of adenocarcinoma. If extramammary Paget's disease progresses to invasive cancer, the only option is an abdominal perineal resection. As a result, early excision of Paget's disease is required.

To guarantee that all of the disease is removed at the time of excision, some surgeons still recommend mapping of the area at a separate operation using punch biopsies in concentric rings around the anal canal with careful documentation of the position of the removed areas according to a drawn map, which is correlated to the pathologic findings.

Wide local excision of a perianal lesion requires 1 cm of clear margin to guarantee a low risk of local recurrence. Adequate skin must be available to replace the removed tissue. The use of house-shaped or V-Y advancement flaps is appropriate. If a larger portion of skin is needed, an S-shaped advancement flap may be preferred to roll more of the buttock skin into the anal canal.

The operation is performed with the patient in the prone-jackknife position under a general anesthetic because of the need to harvest tissue wide out onto the buttock. Epinephrine should be avoided in any additional local anesthetic that is applied to reduce the risk of flap necrosis.

Patients must be warned that they will be restricted from sitting, driving, or climbing stairs for at least 2 weeks and may spend a portion of their time in the hospital not lying on their back, depending on the size of the donor sites. It is possible to treat half of the lesion at one setting and return for a second procedure on the opposite side of the anal canal if there is a question of ability to restrict mobility.

Step 3: Operative Steps

- The patient is placed in the prone-jackknife position, and the lesion is mapped and distinguished from normal tissue (Figures 25-1*A* and 25-2). The patient should undergo complete bowel preparation for clearance of the anal canal, and the rectum should be irrigated with povidone-iodine (Betadine) after clearing all solid material. Postoperative constipation may be appropriate depending on the size of the lesions removed. The patient is given prophylactic antibiotics intravenously within 1 hour before the incision is made. A bladder catheter is placed to reduce the need for mobility. Deep vein thrombosis prophylaxis with sequential compression devices or chemical prophylaxis is appropriate depending on the length of the operation with the patient in the prone-jackknife position. Positioning is accomplished with a roll under the hips, the table flexed, and chest rolls applied because the patient requires intubation for general anesthetic.
- The disease is completely excised, and a V-shaped flap corresponding to the width of the excised disease is made out onto the perianal skin or inner aspect of the buttock. The flap is raised by incising through the dermis and undermining the lateral edges of the donor skin rather than the flap itself to prevent encroachment on the blood supply to the flap. The lateral attachments of the flap are incised over the inner aspect of the buttock, and this allows the skin to move toward the midline and fill the defect of the excised area (Figure 25-1*B*).

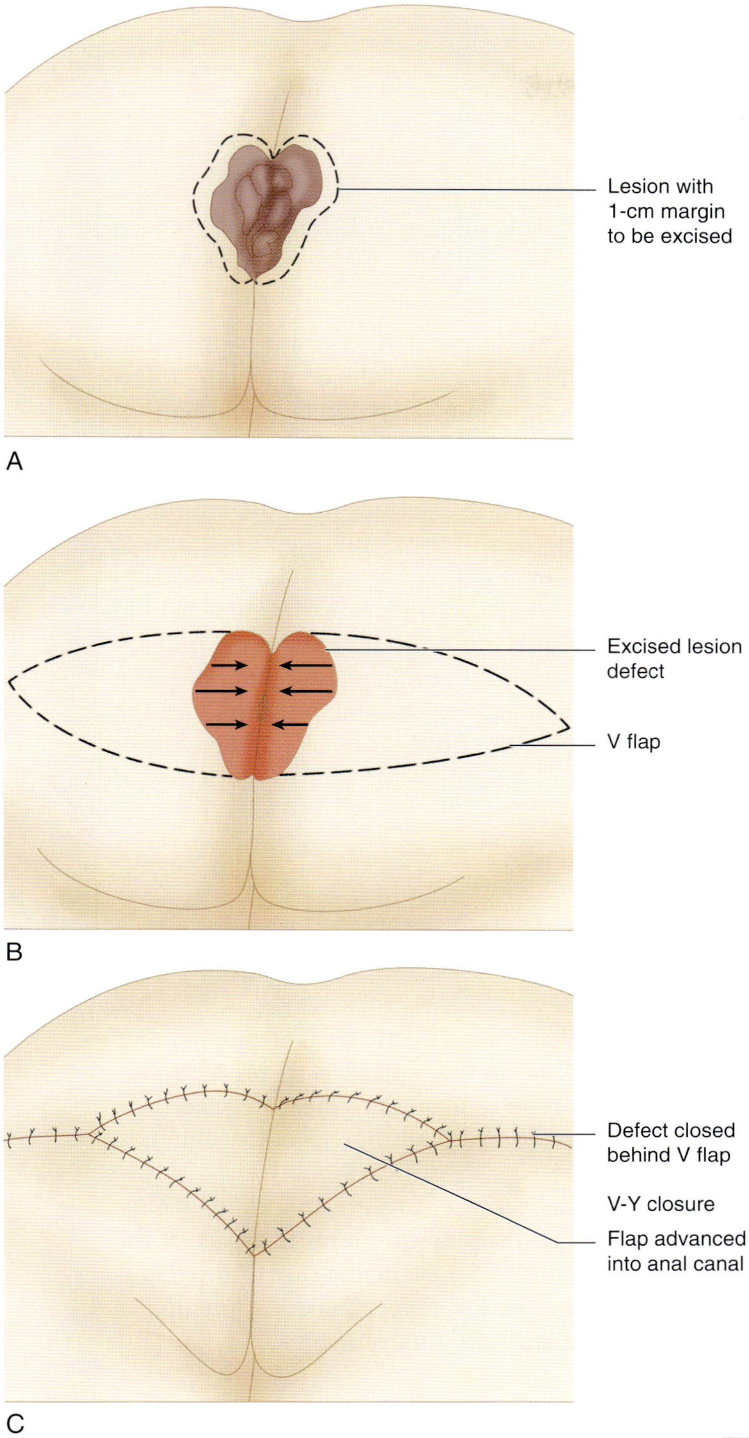

Figure 25-1A-C

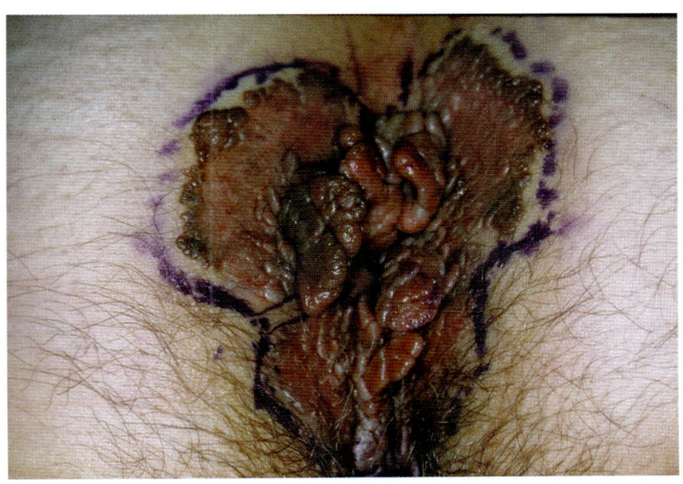

Figure 25-2

- The inner aspect of the "V," which is the clear margin of the excision, is reapproximated to the inner margin of the lesion in the anal canal—either the mucosa or the dentate line. Interrupted absorbable sutures are used. The flap should be approximated loosely without tension and should cover all of the exposed fat or muscle. In the anterior and posterior midline, the contralateral flap may be sewn to the flap to replace anterior and posterior skin. The sides of the "V" are secured by placing interrupted horizontal mattress sutures from the full thickness of the donor skin to the subcuticular layer of the flap to avoid full-thickness capture of the donated skin and reduce the risk of ischemia (Figure 25-3).
- The donor site of the flap is reapproximated to close the defect in a linear fashion behind the apex of the "V" so that a linear closure is accomplished out onto the apex of the buttock on each side of the anal canal resulting in a "Y" shape to the closed flap and donor site. The area is covered with antibiotic ointment and fluff gauze pads to prevent pressure, and the patient is returned to a cushioned bed to avoid any pressure on the flap or the donor sites (Figures 25-1C and 25-4).

Step 4: Postoperative Care

Antibiotics are continued for 24 hours postoperatively. The bladder catheter is maintained for several days until the flaps have begun to heal before allowing the patient to sit on the toilet. The patient is maintained either on his or her side or prone to avoid any pressure placed on the flaps. When ambulation is resumed, the patient should avoid sitting, scooting, climbing stairs, or driving for 2 weeks.

Resumption of diet is left to the discretion and judgment of the surgeon. In a difficult procedure with possible tension on flaps or questionable blood supply to the inner aspect of the flap, the patient should be maintained on bowel rest or at least an elemental diet. If the flap is healing rapidly and there is little likelihood of disruption of the mucocutaneous junction, a regular diet may be resumed with precautions to avoid hard bowel movements.

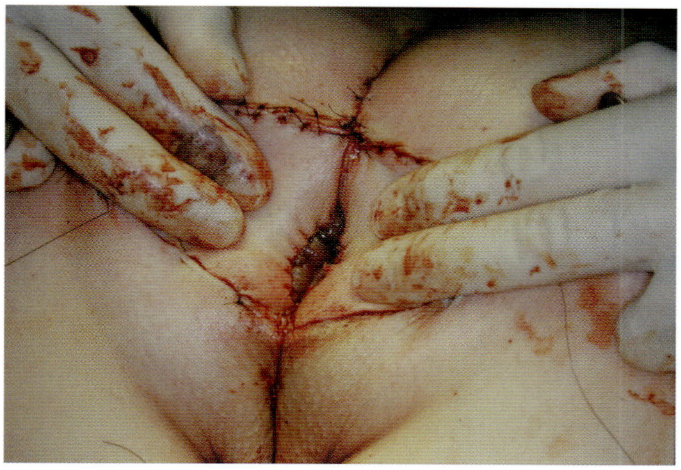

Figure 25-3

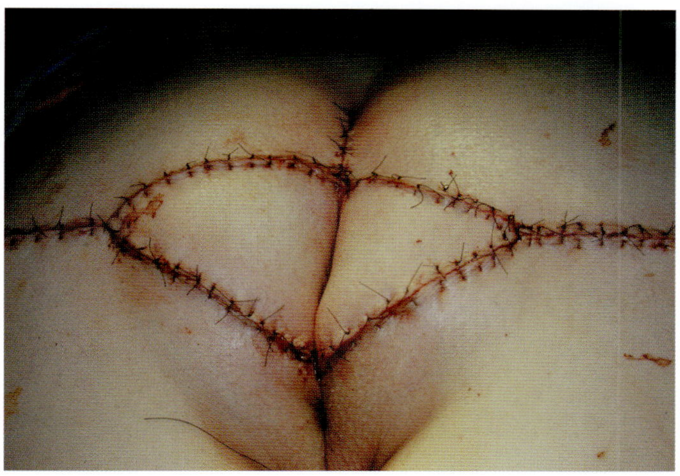

Figure 25-4

Step 5: Pearls and Pitfalls

As in all plastic surgery procedures, the breadth of the flap should be considered in determining the length of the flap with a 2:1 ratio of length to breadth. The donor site should be free of any scars or areas of questionable blood supply, such as a previous decubitus ulcer. The management of a disrupted or infected flap requires rapid return to the operating room for examination under anesthesia, decompression of any fluctuance or abscess, and local care with intensive cleaning to preserve the mucocutaneous junction and the flap. It is usually unnecessary to place drains in the donor site unless there is ongoing oozing.

Selected Readings

Margenthaler JA, Dietz DW, Mutch MG, et al. Outcomes, risk of other malignancies, and need for formal mapping procedures in patients with perianal Bowen's disease. Dis Colon Rectum 2004;47:1655–60.

Pineda CE, Welton ML. Management of anal squamous intraepithelial lesions. Clin Colon Rectal Surg 2009;22:94–101.

CHAPTER 26

Hanley Procedure for Fistula and Abscess

Bashar Safar and Ira J. Kodner

Step 1: Clinical Anatomy

The anus and rectum are surrounded by many potential spaces that could potentially harbor abscesses and give rise to fistulae. The perianal space surrounds the anal canal at the anal margin. It is bounded by the subcutaneous fat laterally, anal canal medially, intersphincteric space superiorly, and skin inferiorly. The superficial postanal space connects the two perianal spaces below the anococcygeal ligament.

The intersphincteric plane is the space between the autonomic circular fibers of the internal sphincter and the somatic circular external sphincter and extends upward between the internal and external sphincters. It contains the terminal fibers of the longitudinal fibers of the rectal wall and the glands of the anal canal at the level of the dentate line.

The ischiorectal space is bounded by the levator ani muscle and external sphincter medially, obturator internus and ischium laterally, perianal skin inferiorly, and levator ani and obturator fascia superiorly. The right and left ischiorectal spaces communicate posteriorly above the anococcygeal ligament giving rise to the deep postanal space, also known as the retrosphincteric space of Courtney.

A horseshoe abscess results from a postanal space abscess extending laterally to the ischiorectal fossa on both sides of the anal canal. The offending gland is in the posterior midline at the dentate line. Abscesses may necessitate to the skin in the anterior ischiorectal fossa near the perineal body.

Step 2: Preoperative Considerations

The Hanley procedure provides drainage of a perianal abscess or fistula that communicates through the deep postanal space. Superficial postanal space extensions can be treated by dividing the internal sphincter muscle for the length of the abscess. A significant amount of external sphincter may have to be divided to obtain adequate drainage of the posterior anal space. The basis of the Hanley procedure is a midline incision through the internal and external sphincter to unroof the postanal space, destroy the internal opening at the dentate line and infected anal gland, and open the skin over the postanal space. Lateral (or off midline) deviation damages the circle of the external sphincter. Inquiry regarding preoperative sphincter function may be appropriate to document sphincter dysfunction.

Step 3: Operative Steps

- Either spinal or general anesthesia can be used. The patient is placed in the prone-jackknife position with the buttocks taped apart. Anoscopy is performed to confirm the posterior midline internal opening. A probe is placed through the internal opening into the posterior space (Figure 26-1*A*). An incision is made through most of the sphincter mechanism making sure to unroof the entire sinus tract (Figure 26-1*B*). Care must be taken not to divide the puborectalis muscle or deviate from the midline.

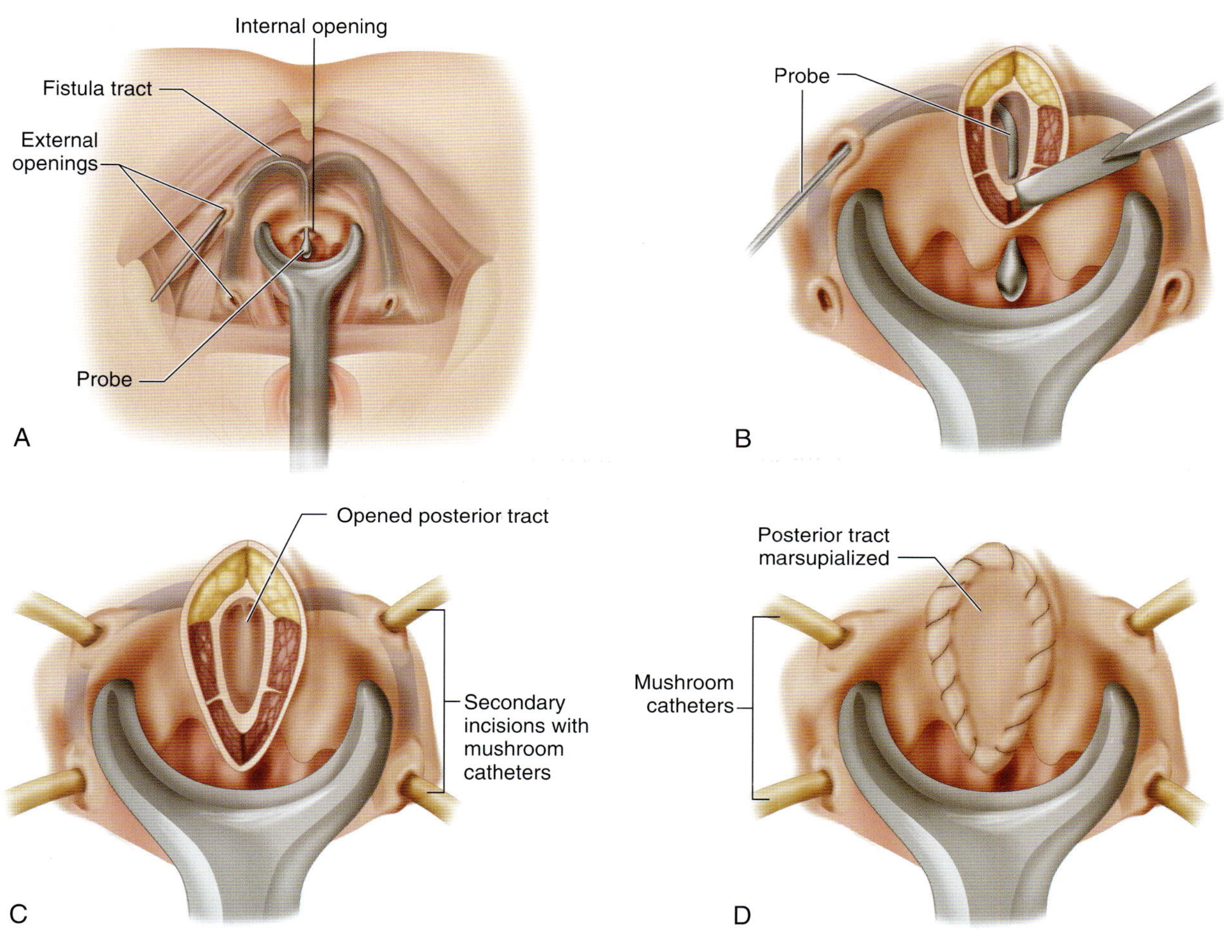

Figure 26-1A-D

- The anterior extension of the abscess in the ischiorectal fossa is drained separately on both sides of the anal canal (Figure 26-2). After draining is accomplished, povidone-iodine (Betadine) is irrigated through the right and left external ischiorectal drainage sites. Both ischiorectal fossa tracts should communicate to the posterior incision. The tracts that connect the anterior openings with the posterior space should be drained by passing a small Penrose drain through the posterior incision to the anterior drainage site (Figure 26-3). If this is not possible, a second incision can be made in the posterior skin over the tract lateral to the anal canal, and the Penrose drain can be used to encircle the skin bridge and drain the ischiorectal fossa completely. Deep extensions of the ischiorectal fossa can be drained through a separate incision with placement of a mushroom catheter and fixed in place with a permanent suture (Figure 26-1*C*).
- Marsupialization of the posterior space is accomplished with running suture of 3-0 chromic catgut (Figure 26-1*D*). Hemostasis is verified. Continuity of the puborectalis is verified by placing a finger in the anal canal to confirm the presence of the posterior muscular sling at the level of the pelvic floor. Polysporin ointment and a wound dressing are applied.

Step 4: Postoperative Care

The patient is discharged home on the same day with pain relief medications and stool softeners with instructions to perform sitz baths three times a day and after every bowel movement. The drain and setons are inspected in the office 2 weeks postoperatively. The mushroom catheter is removed if the abscess cavity is completely granulated. The Penrose setons are removed when the drainage has stopped and no active infection is identified. The posterior incision is examined with a finger to separate any cross-healing of the skin over the postanal space and clear any debris that may have accumulated.

Step 5: Pearls and Pitfalls

In the acute setting, the abscess is best drained through a posterior incision with division of the internal and external sphincter. Counterincisions are made on the left and right sides, and a Penrose seton is placed. The decussating fibers of the external sphincter reapproximate and scar together to restore a concentric functioning sphincter. Unless the entire tract is opened, the patient may develop a recurrent abscess or fistula or both. This situation would require repeat division of the external sphincter posteriorly. Chronic inflammation and scarring may prevent healing of the circular sphincter and cause incontinence. The incision of the internal sphincter in the midline almost always causes a keyhole deformity, which results in leakage of mucus, soft stool, and gas. This deformity is difficult to repair even when an operative internal sphincter repair is used.

Selected Readings

Hyman N, O'Brien S, Osler T. Outcomes after fistulotomy: results of a prospective, multicenter regional study. Dis Colon Rectum 2009;52:2022–7.

Rosa G, Lolli P, Piccinelli D, et al. Fistula in ano: anatomoclinical aspects, surgical therapy and results in 844 patients. Tech Coloproctol 2006;10:215–21.

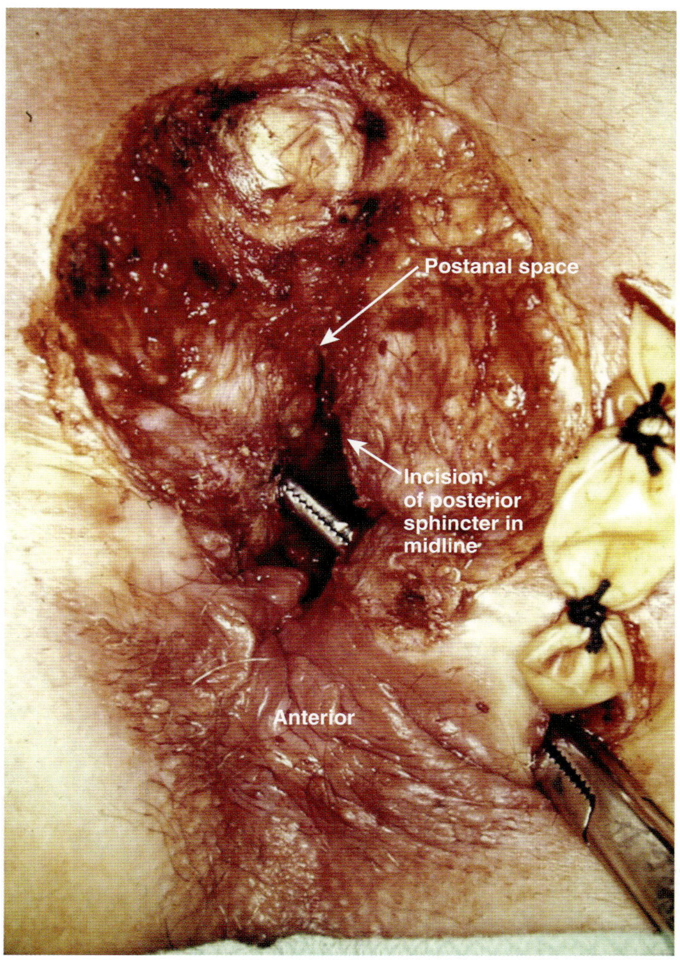

Figure 26-2

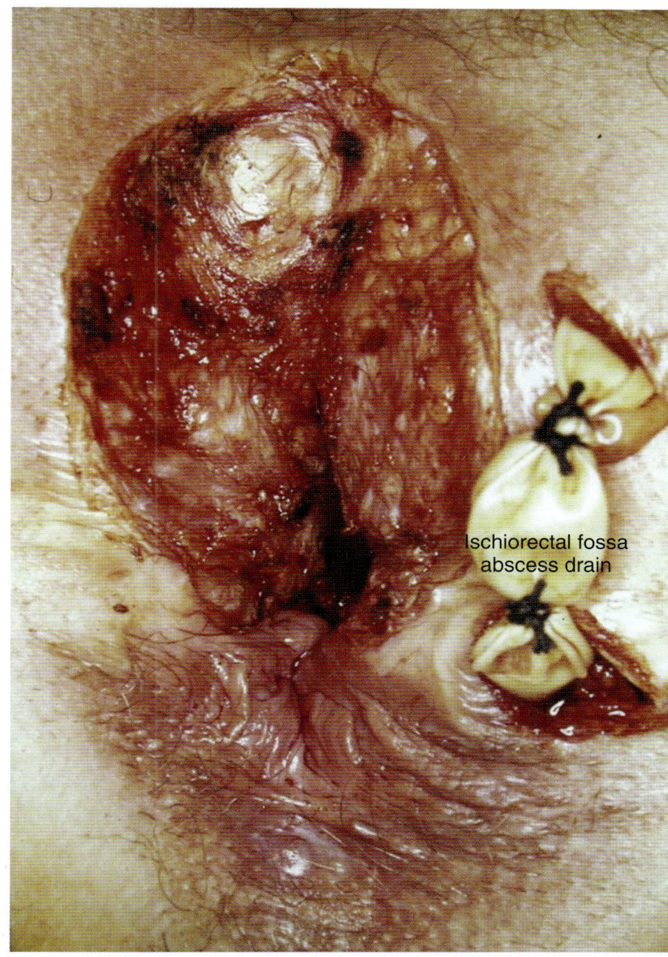

Figure 26-3

CHAPTER 27

Anal Sphincter Reconstruction

Bashar Safar and Ira J. Kodner

Step 1: Clinical Anatomy

The upper anal canal begins at the puborectalis sling or the anorectal ring, which sits at the level of the pelvic floor and can be palpated through the anal canal as a bulge posteriorly. The longitudinal muscles of the rectum continue into the anus as the intersphincteric plane demarcating the line between autonomic internal sphincter and somatic external sphincter fibers all the way down to the level of the anal canal skin where the intersphincteric groove is palpable. The ischiorectal fossa fat is found outside the circular fibers of the external sphincter that encircle the rectum. The pudendal nerve and vessels traverse the ischiorectal fat diagonally posterior to anterior from each ischial spine through Alcock's canal to the posterolateral aspect of the anal canal. During the perineal portion of a procedure, the pudendal nerves and vessels must be controlled.

The rectovaginal and rectoprostatic septum descends all the way to the level of the perineum anteriorly. The transverse perinei muscle separates the anterior and posterior perineum. The terminal fibers of the longitudinal muscle of the rectum insert into the skin of the anal canal just outside the anal verge as the corrugator cutanei ani and cause the ridges that are noticed around the anal canal. The internal sphincter is the hypertrophied circular muscle of the wall of the rectum. The lowest portion of the internal sphincter can be palpated as a groove where the longitudinal fibers insert on the skin (Figure 27-1).

Within the anal canal, the dentate line is the junction between the cuboidal epithelium of the anal transition zone, which is the terminal mucosal layer of the rectum, and the stratified epidermal cells of the anal canal skin. Gland openings (or crypts) are found in the dentate line at the base of the Morgagni columns, which are interdigitating lines of squamous epithelium into the cuboidal and columnar epithelium of the distal rectum. The anal transition zone is the most highly innervated section of the rectum and anal canal and contains nerve fibers sensing temperature, vibration, electrical stimulation, pressure, liquid, solid, and gas. The dentate line lies approximately halfway along the surgical anal canal, which extends from the palpable anal verge all the way up to the anorectal ring palpated at the puborectalis sling posteriorly. The anoderm within the anal canal, cephalad to the anal verge, has no hair follicles.

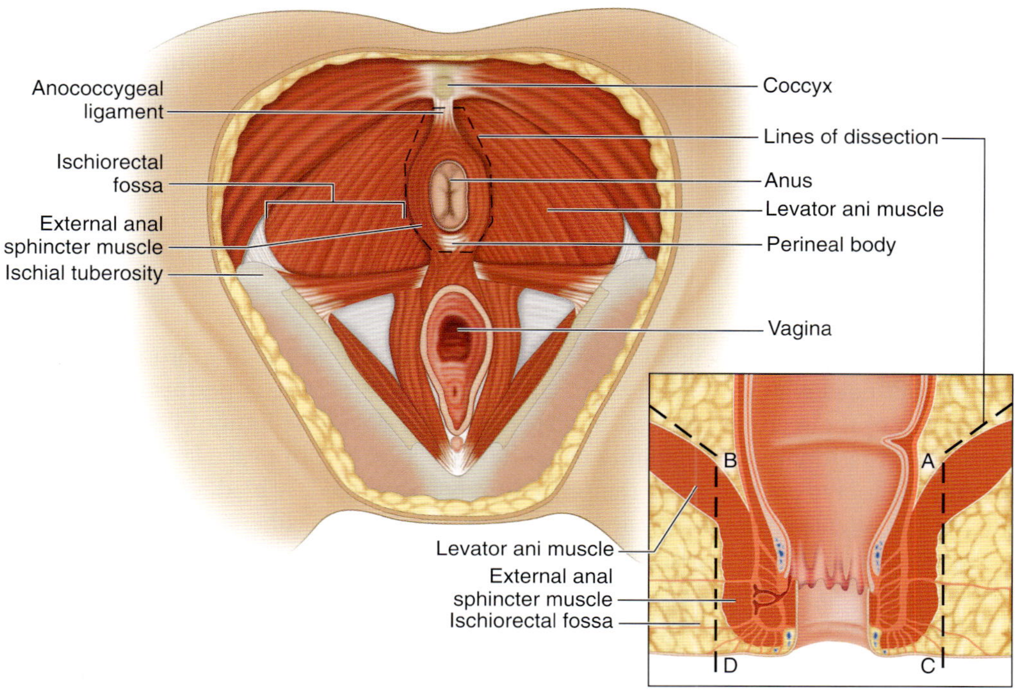
Anococcygeal ligament
Ischiorectal fossa
External anal sphincter muscle
Ischial tuberosity
Coccyx
Lines of dissection
Anus
Levator ani muscle
Perineal body
Vagina
B
A
Levator ani muscle
External anal sphincter muscle
Ischiorectal fossa
D
C

Figure 27-1

Step 2: Preoperative Considerations

Anal sphincter reconstruction is performed for patients with a demonstrable external sphincter defect and significant incontinence to stool. Anal manometry and transrectal ultrasound are helpful to document dysfunction and the site of the sphincter defect if this is not obvious on physical examination.

Most of these procedures are performed for anterior sphincter defects that result from obstetric injuries. At the time of the sphincter injury during delivery, a simple reapproximation of the torn or cut ends of the muscle should be attempted without further dissection; this preserves the planes for a future repair and allows for scar tissue to form, which is useful during a future repair.

Full mechanical bowel preparation is used. A constipating agent can be started on the night before the operation. Intravenous antibiotics are administered within 1 hour of the incision and continued until the patient is discharged home.

Step 3: Operative Steps

- After adequate spinal or general anesthesia, the patient is placed in a prone flexed position, and the buttocks are taped apart with silk tape. Sigmoidoscopy is performed with complete evacuation of the rectum followed by irrigation with povidone-iodine (Betadine) solution. If there is any residual stool, copious irrigation is performed to evacuate the stool. If a large amount of stool is encountered, the procedure is abandoned. A bladder catheter is placed to gravity. The intended site for incision is injected with local anesthetic mixed with epinephrine for hemostasis. A self-retaining retractor is applied, and an anterior circumanal incision is made (Figures 27-2*A* and 27-3).
- A flap of rectal wall including partial thickness of the internal sphincter muscle is created, and the plane is developed superiorly until the entire sphincter is exposed (Figures 27-2*B* and 27-4).
- Attention is turned to identifying the external sphincter laterally. The perineal skin is dissected and reflected inferiorly until the ischiorectal fat is encountered; this allows identification of the external surface of the external sphincter muscle on each side (Figure 27-5). The muscle is mobilized laterally no further than the horizontal midline to preserve the pudendal nerves and medially to the anteroposterior midline and released from the vagina (Figure 27-6). The anterior scar is transected. The upper attachments of the muscles are released to provide mobility of the muscle flaps (Figure 27-2*C*). The internal and external sphincter muscles are mobilized as a unit and released from the mucosa of the rectum to the level of the pelvic floor and laterally to the point of ischiorectal fossa release.

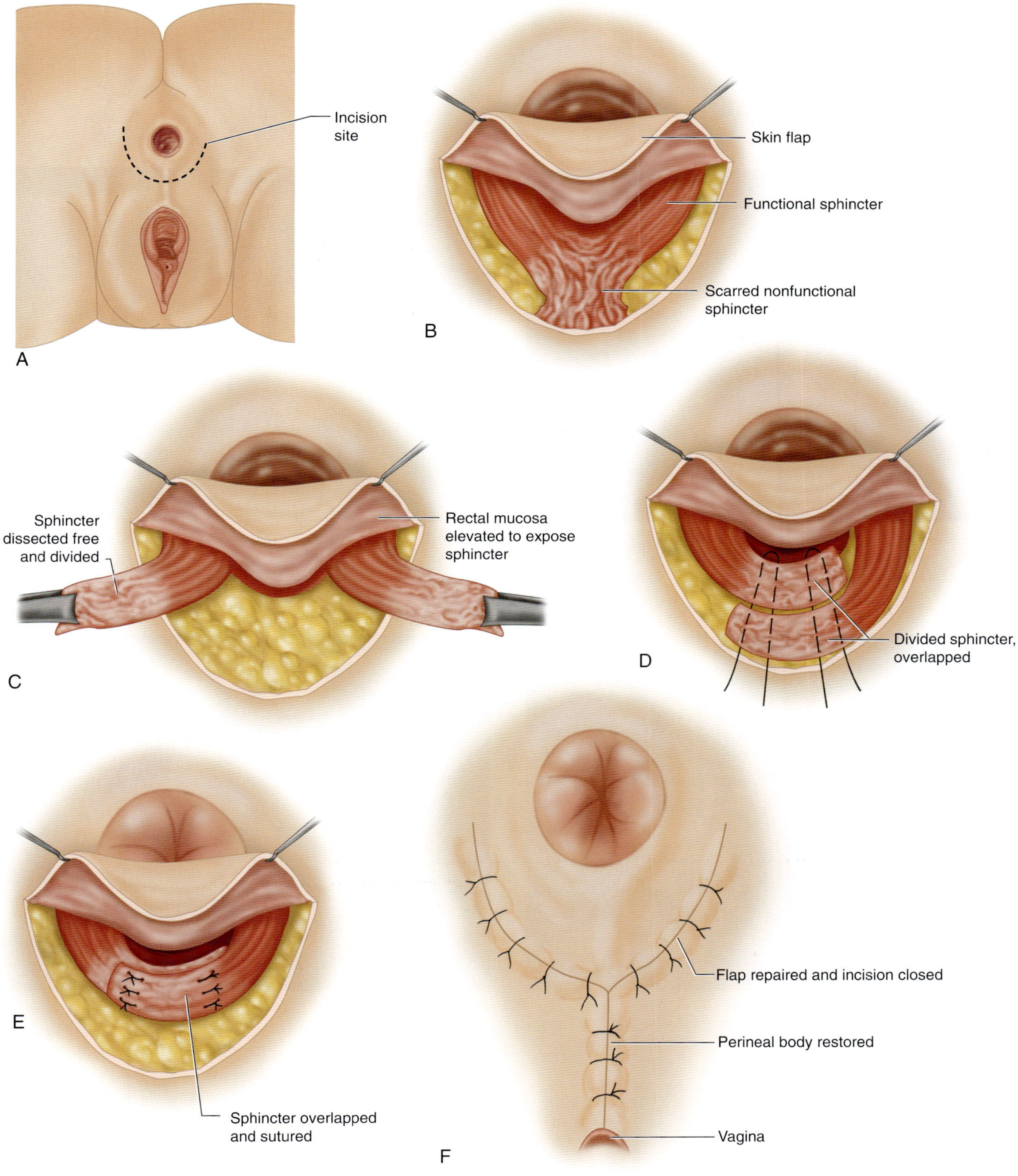

Figure 27-2A-F

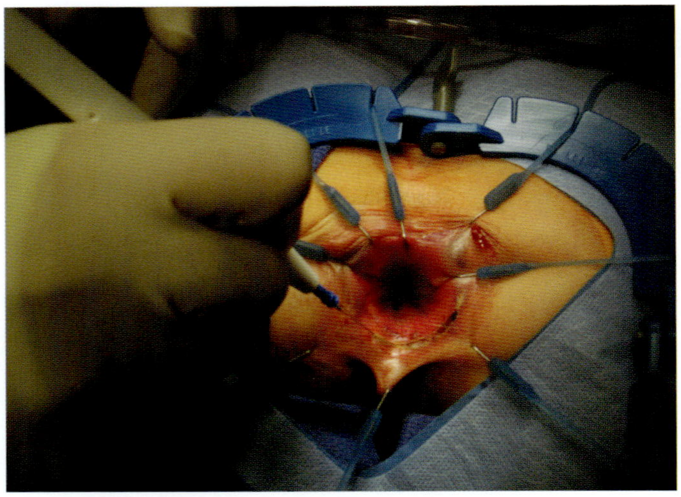

Figure 27-3

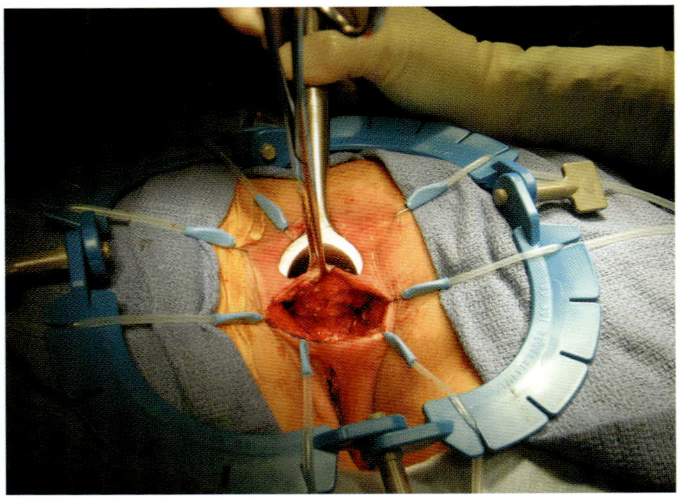

Figure 27-4

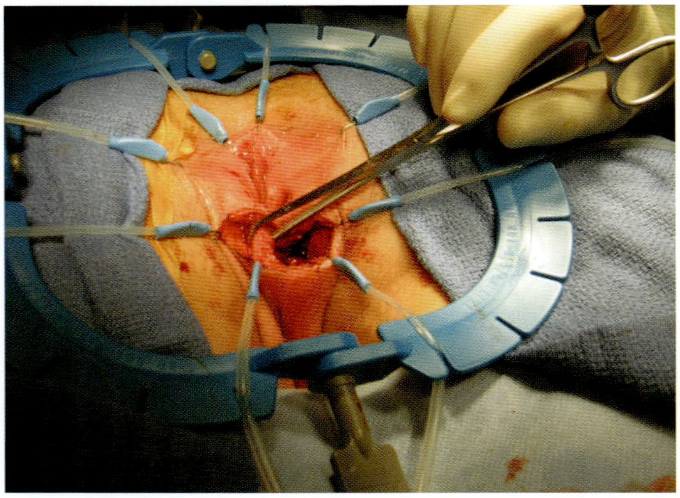

Figure 27-5

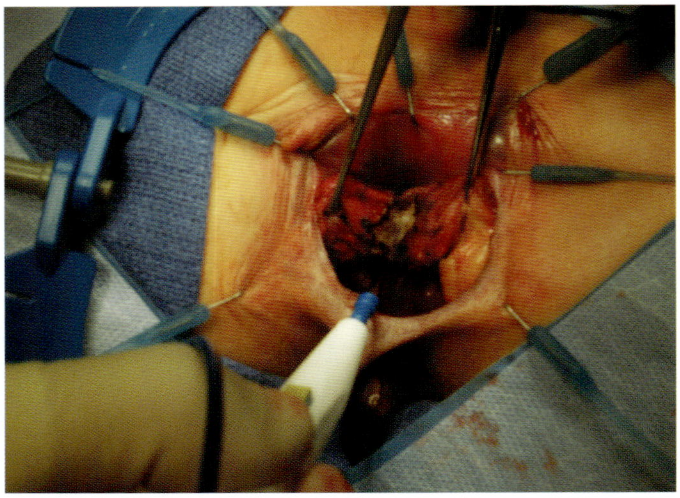

Figure 27-6

Overlapping Reconstruction

- The muscle is reconstructed after adequate hemostasis. The muscle flaps are pulled across the midline to overlap the pedicles of the muscle (Figure 27-7). It does not matter which side is pulled over or under. Horizontal mattress sutures of 0 polypropylene are placed in two rows of three on either side of the midline (Figure 27-8). This technique fixes the tip of the flap of each muscle to the base of the opposite pedicle (Figures 27-2*D* and *E* and 27-9). A small stab incision is made in the lateral aspect of the perineum, and a No. 10 round Jackson-Pratt drain is inserted deep to the repair and held in place with 3-0 Prolene suture (Figure 27-10). The flap is resutured to the perineal skin with interrupted 3-0 absorbable sutures, and the resulting Y-shaped closure restores the skin of the perineal body to provide distance between the anus and the vagina (Figure 27-2*F*).

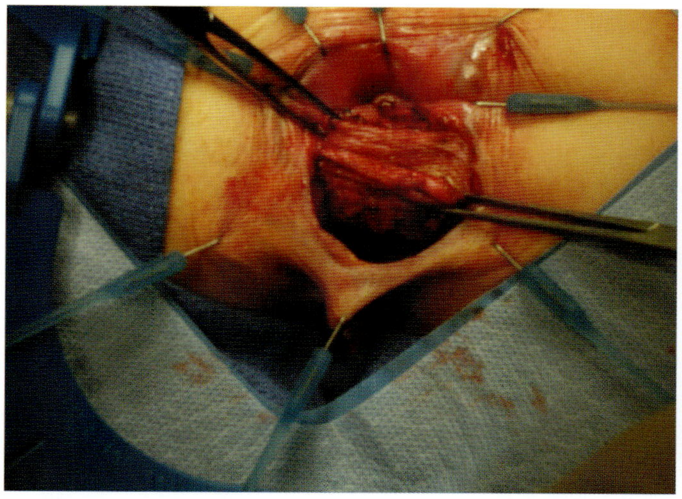

Figure 27-7

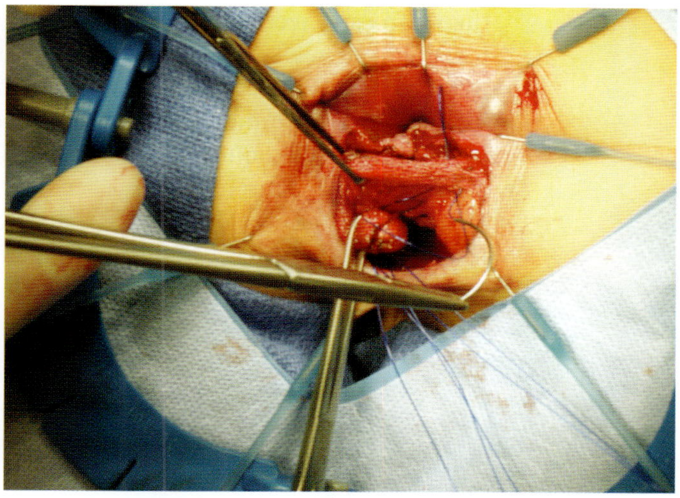

Figure 27-8

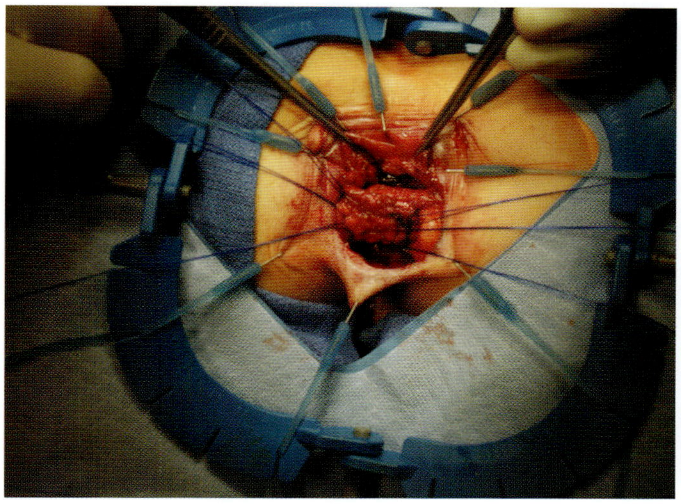

Figure 27-9

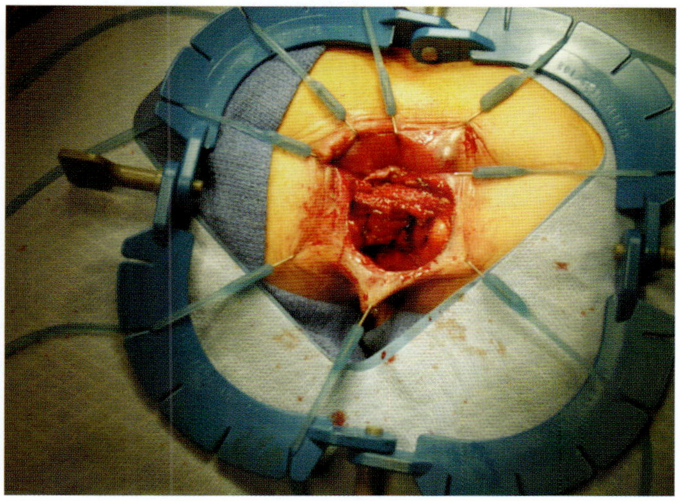

Figure 27-10

Reefing Reconstruction

- The same process is followed as for overlapping repair until muscle mobilization. Reefing repair of the anal sphincter requires less mobilization of the rectal mucosa from the sphincter and less lateral mobilization of the external sphincter from the ischiorectal fossa fat. The rectal mucosal flap is freed in the midline to release the scar of the anterior mechanism of the sphincter. The two ends of the scar and the muscle are pulled to the midline (Figure 27-11). A single row of three horizontal mattress sutures of 0 polypropylene are used to reef the muscle in the midline with the scar folded anteriorly toward the posterior vagina (Figures 27-12 and 27-13*A*). This redundant tissue serves to fill the perineal body space and separates the vagina and rectum (Figures 27-13*B* and 14). If the scar is divided and the muscles pulled together and reefed (Figure 27-13*C*), extra tissue can be brought to the midline from the ischiorectal fossa to restore the perineal body.
- The skin of the perineum is approximated loosely with absorbable interrupted vertical mattress sutures in an anterior to posterior direction to the perineal body behind the vagina.
- The mucocutaneous junction is reconstructed with simple sutures of absorbable material. Hemostasis is again verified. The drain deep to the repair is irrigated with antibiotic solution to ensure patency and a watertight repair (Figure 27-2*F*).

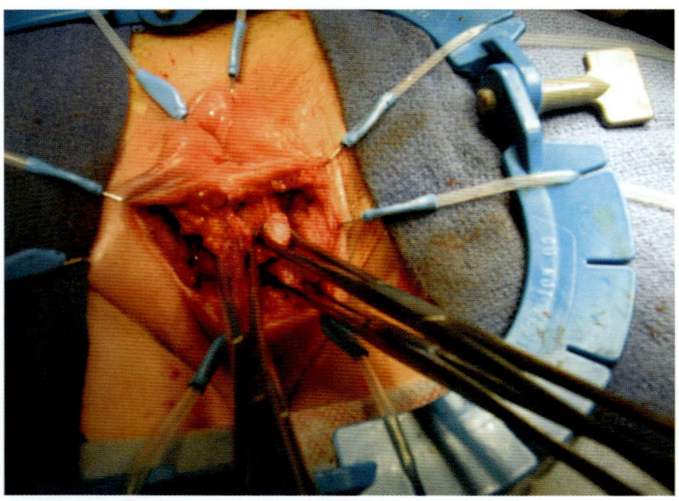

Figure 27-11

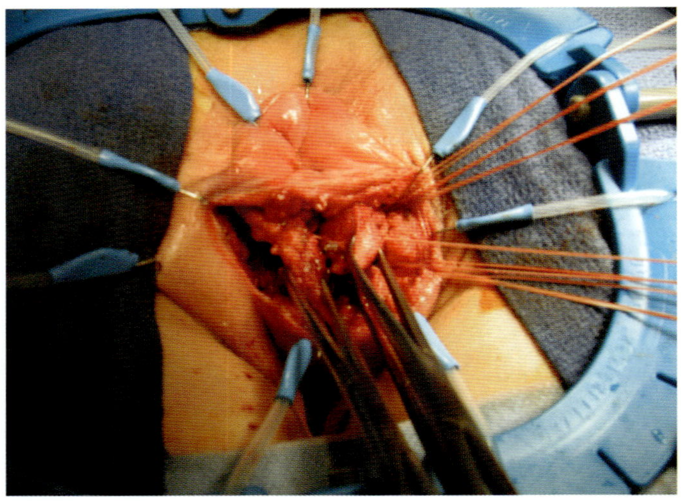

Figure 27-12

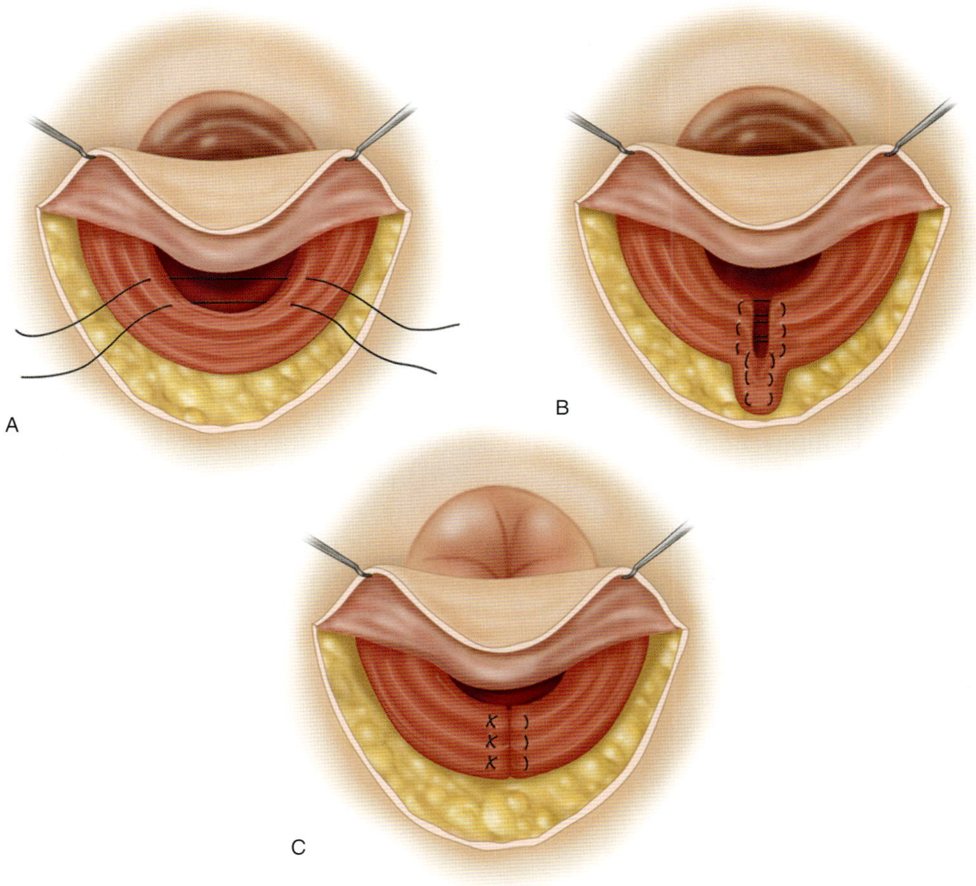

Figure 27-13A-C

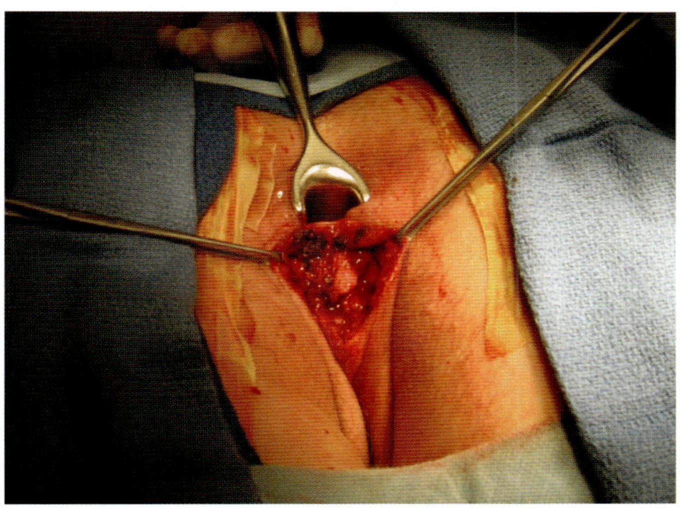

Figure 27-14

Step 4: Postoperative Care

The patient is admitted for bowel rest with a constipating agent for 2 days. The bladder catheter is removed when the patient is able to ambulate freely. On postoperative day 3, the constipating agent is stopped, and the diet is advanced. The patient is discharged with stool softeners after passage of stool. Intravenous antibiotics are continued while the patient is in the hospital and then converted to broad-spectrum agents orally for another week.

The Jackson-Pratt bulb is cut on discharge, leaving the drain in place for another few days to be removed in the office. Sutures are removed in the office, if still undissolved, after the incision has healed without signs of infection. Early function is not perfect, but function should improve over 6 months. Patients should not drive, lift, climb stairs, or engage in sexual intercourse until seen 1 month after discharge to ensure healing.

Step 5: Pearls and Pitfalls

Minimal use of electrocautery is encouraged to minimize tissue trauma and collateral tissue damage. Electrocautery is reserved for hemostasis and avoided during the dissection. Placing a 1- to 2-cm sizer in the anal canal at the time of suture placement in the muscle prevents any likelihood of obliterating the anal canal and of performing a very tight repair that is likely to break down.

A large hematoma between the vagina and the rectum may result from drain malfunction or occlusion. A return to the operating room with drainage through the perineal body closure and hemostasis should preserve the repair and prevent later infection. The perineal wound can be left open and packed if infection is suspected.

Constipation and stool impaction must be avoided in the early postoperative period. Worsening anal pain and pressure sensation in the pelvis indicates fecal impaction or hematoma. Passage of a large hard stool may threaten the repair. Digital disimpaction under sedation may prevent repair breakdown during the critical period of healing.

Selected Readings

Fleshman JW, Peters WR, Shemesh EI, et al. Anal sphincter reconstruction: anterior overlapping muscle repair. Dis Colon Rectum 1991;34:739–43.

Malouf AJ, Norton CS, Engel AF, et al. Long-term results of overlapping anterior anal-sphincter repair for obstetric trauma. Lancet 2000;355:260–5.

Maslekar S, Gardiner AB, Duthie GS. Anterior anal sphincter repair for fecal incontinence: good long-term results are possible. J Am Coll Surg 2007;204:40–6.

Young CJ, Mathur MN, Eyers AA, et al. Successful overlapping anal sphincter repair: relationship to patient age, neuropathy, and colostomy formation. Dis Colon Rectum 1998;41:344–9.

CHAPTER 28

End Ileostomy and Loop Ileostomy

Anne Y. Lin

Step 1: Preoperative Considerations

The most common reason for making an end ileostomy is inflammatory bowel disease after a total proctocolectomy. A well-functioning stoma can restore quality of life to a patient with severe colitis. Placing a stoma in the correct site is crucial for minimizing appliance application difficulties. Using the stoma appliance, a site should be marked on the skin within the right lower quadrant rectus muscle outline on the infraumbilical fat roll. The patient should be observed in a sitting position, which allows full apposition of the faceplate, specifically away from the costal margin, anterior superior iliac spine, umbilicus, and any scars or creases on the abdominal surface.

The most common reason for loop ileostomy is to protect a distal anastomosis (low colorectal or high-risk ileocolic anastomosis). No bowel preparation is needed for an emergent operation.

Step 2: Operative Steps

End Ileostomy

- A 3-cm-diameter circle of skin is excised at the stoma site. The fascia is grasped at the medial edge of the incision opposite the stoma site and retracted medially. A folded laparotomy sponge is placed in the abdomen and held in place below the peritoneum. A longitudinal incision is made through the anterior rectus fascia to match the vertical diameter of the skin opening. The rectus muscle fiber is separated to expose the posterior rectus fascia and peritoneum. This layer is incised longitudinally to provide an opening to pass two fingers. The opening is dilated with two fingers (Figure 28-1).
- The cut end of the ileum is pulled out through the opening using a Babcock clamp with gentle pushing intra-abdominally and external traction. Care is taken to ensure that the ileostomy is correctly oriented and that the mesentery is not twisted (Figure 28-2). The ileostomy can be fashioned with the mesentery position cephalad. The mesentery can be secured to the anterior abdominal wall to prevent rotation or herniation (Figure 28-3). The cut end of the ileum is brought out a distance of 5 cm beyond the skin (Figure 28-4).

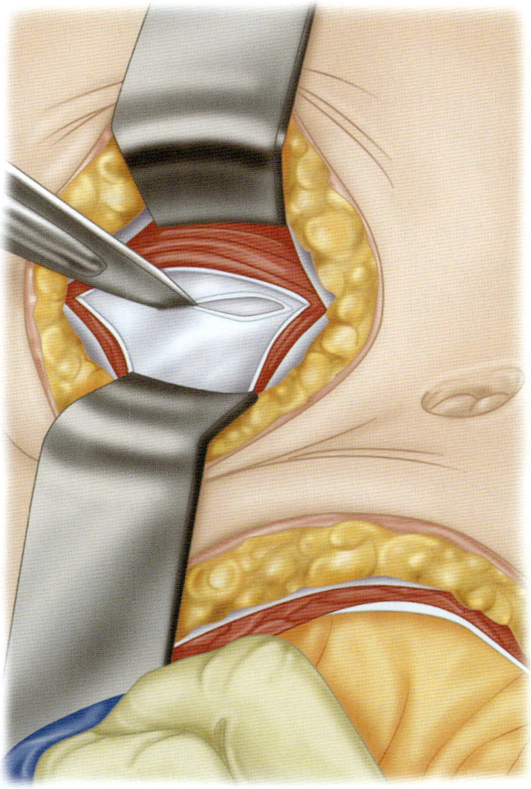

Figure 28-1

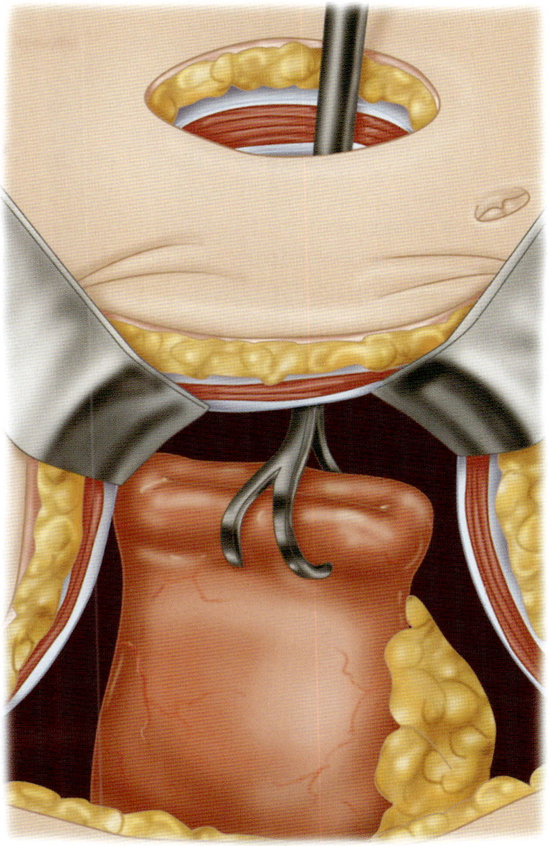

Figure 28-2

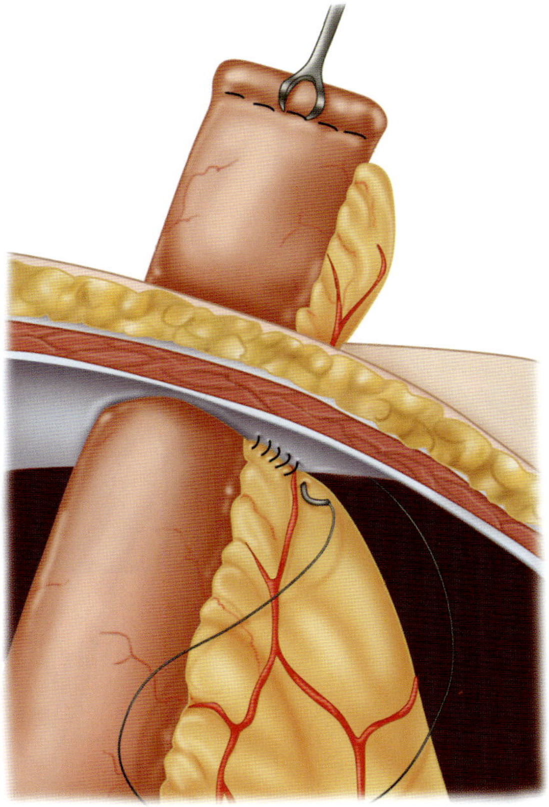

Figure 28-3

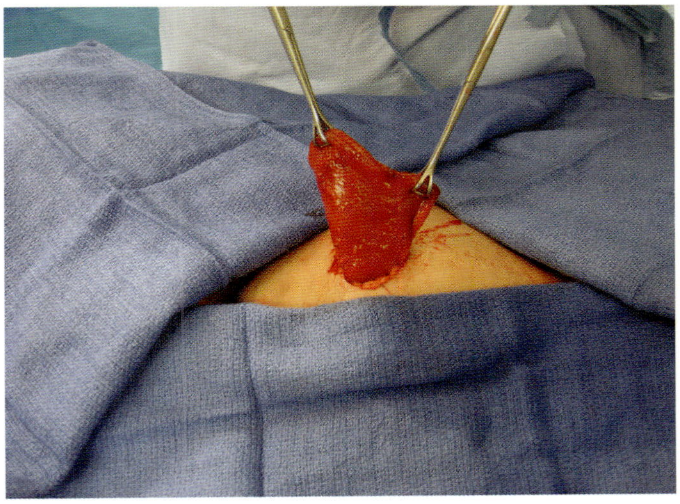

Figure 28-4

- The first suture is placed on the mesenteric edge of the bowel (full thickness) and then to the subcuticular layer at the cephalad apex of the stoma opening (Figure 28-5).
- Placement of 3-0 absorbable sutures is done to create a Brooke stoma (spigot) using a full-thickness suture through the cut edge of the terminal ileum (Figure 28-6), followed by a seromuscular bite of the ileum a distance of 5 cm from the edge (Figure 28-7), followed by a subcuticular bite (Figures 28-8 and 28-9). Hemostats are used to hold the sutures until sutures have been placed in all four quadrants and the intervening spaces (Figure 28-10).

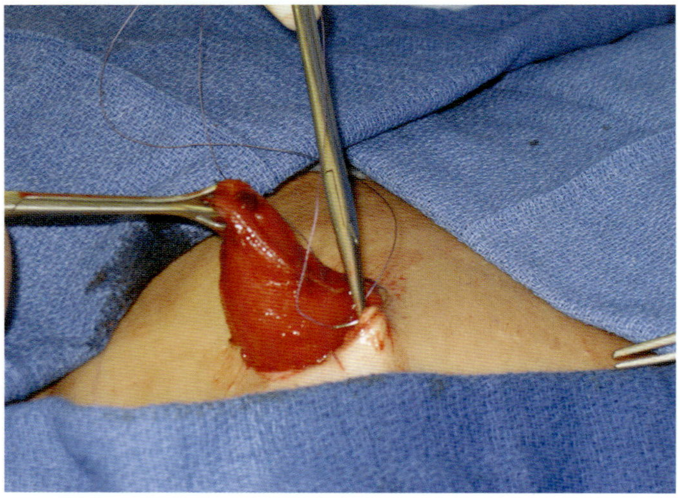

Figure 28-5

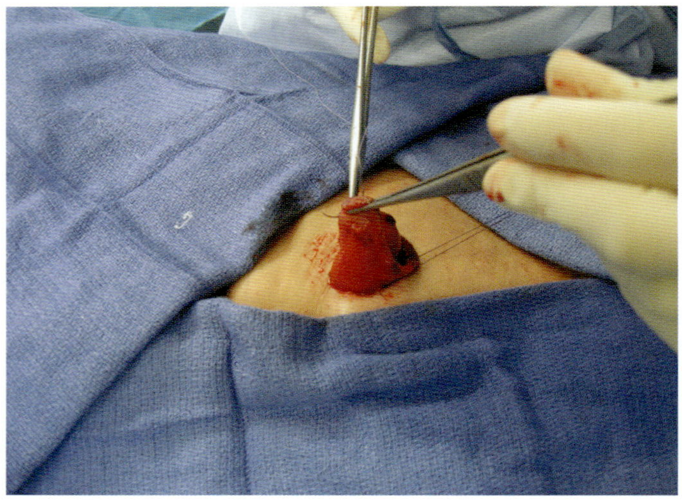

Figure 28-6

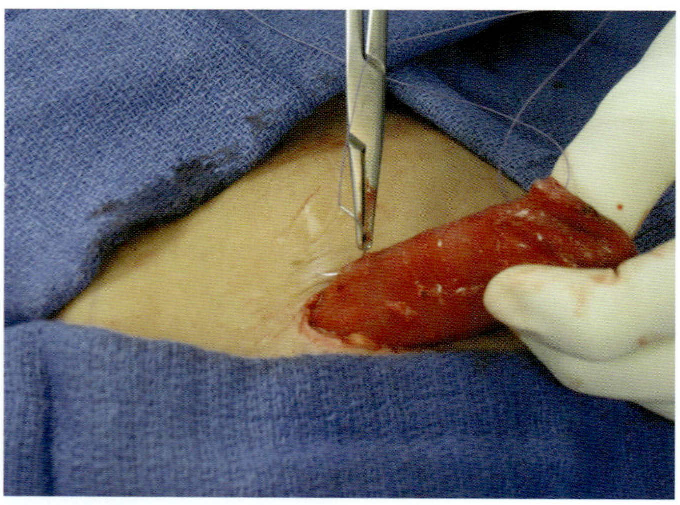

Figure 28-7

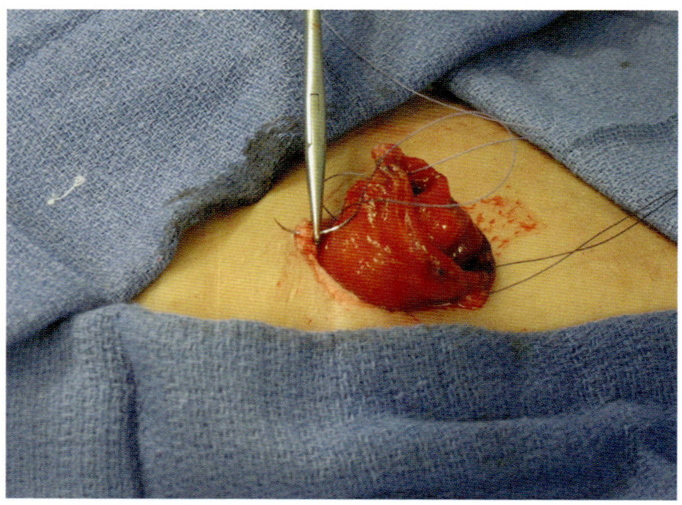

Figure 28-8

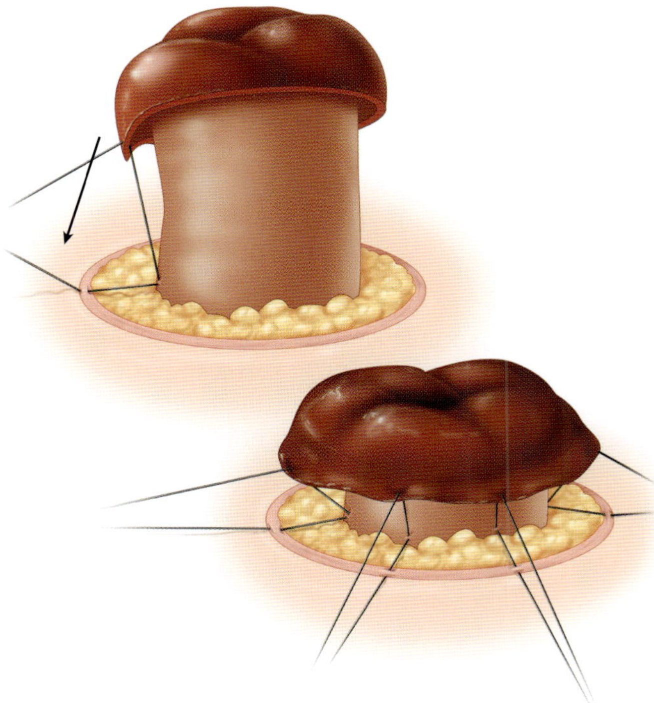

Figure 28-9

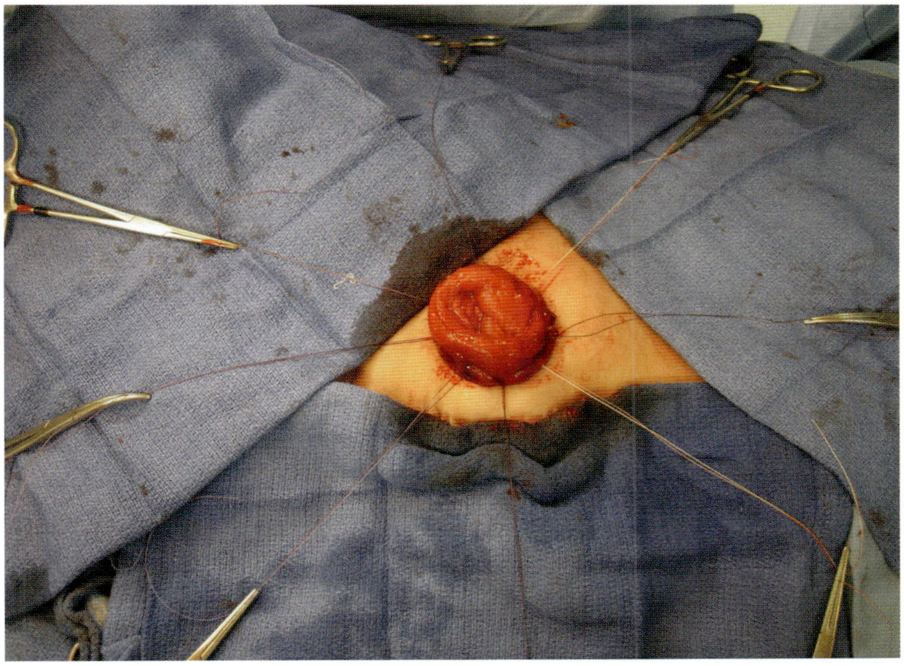

Figure 28-10

- The ileum is everted, and the sutures are tied.
- The ostomy appliance is applied (Figure 28-11). The size of the appliance opening is usually 1 inch or $1\frac{1}{8}$ inches in diameter using the cutting guides on the appliance. The appliance should touch the stoma on all sides but should not cut the mucosa.

Loop Ileostomy

- The chosen loop of ileum is pulled out through the prepared abdominal wall opening using a Babcock clamp with gentle pushing intra-abdominally and external traction. Care is taken to ensure that the ileostomy is correctly oriented and that the mesentery is not twisted. The ileostomy is pulled out with the proximal limb oriented cephalad (Figure 28-12). If a rod is needed for support in patients with a thick abdominal wall, a small opening is made in the mesentery, and an ileostomy rod is passed beneath the bridge of bowel close to the distal limb. A suture can be placed through the eyes of the rod to create a loop of suture to allow retrieval if the rod slips.

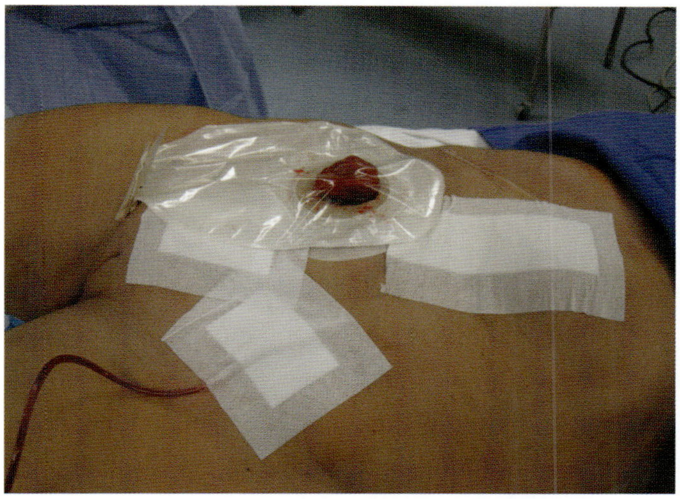

Figure 28-11

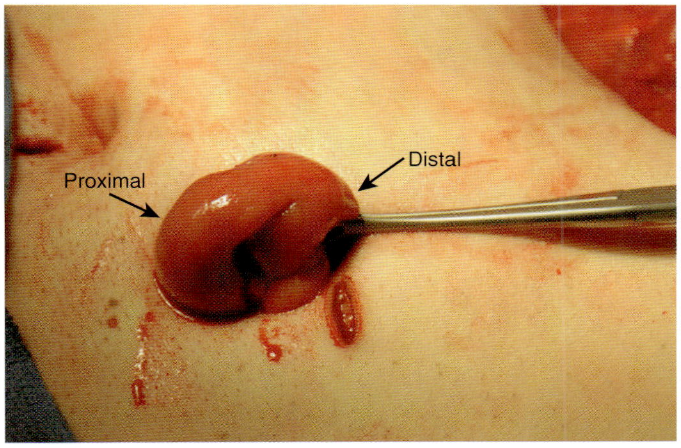

Figure 28-12

- The bowel is incised 80% around the circumference at the level of the skin on the inferiorly placed distal (bypassed) limb (Figures 28-13*A* and 28-14). Simple full-thickness sutures are placed through the distal ileal limb and subcuticular skin to secure the distal limb flush to the skin (Figure 28-15). The proximal ileal limb is everted in a Brooke fashion using a full-thickness suture through the terminal ileum, followed by a seromuscular bite of the ileum a distance of 5 cm from the edge, followed by a subcuticular skin suture (Figure 28-16). This process is repeated around the upper limb four times equidistant around the bowel to evert the proximal limb (Figures 28-13*B* and 28-17). The bridge of bowel wall between proximal and distal limb is secured to the lower portion of the skin opening to keep the midportion of the bowel from retracting and to close the distal limb partially when the rod is not needed (Figures 28-13*C* and 28-18).
- The sutures are tied to evert the spigot of the stoma (Figure 28-19), and an appliance is applied (Figure 28-20).

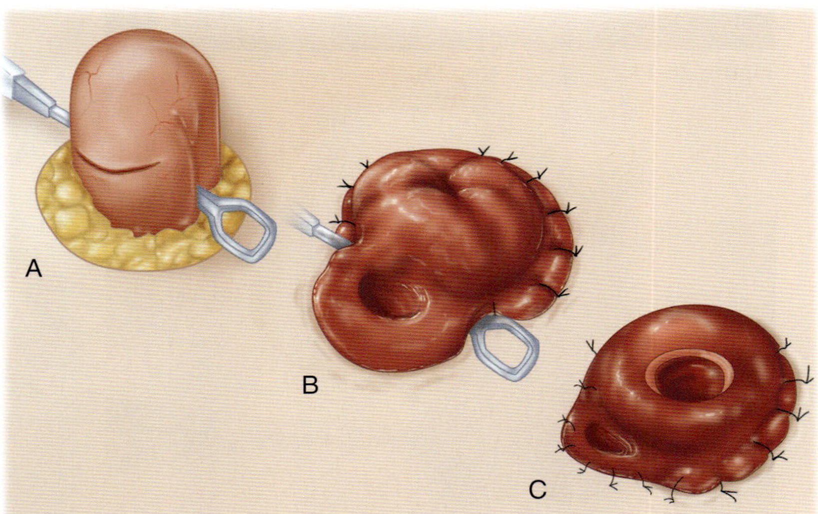

Figure 28-13A-C

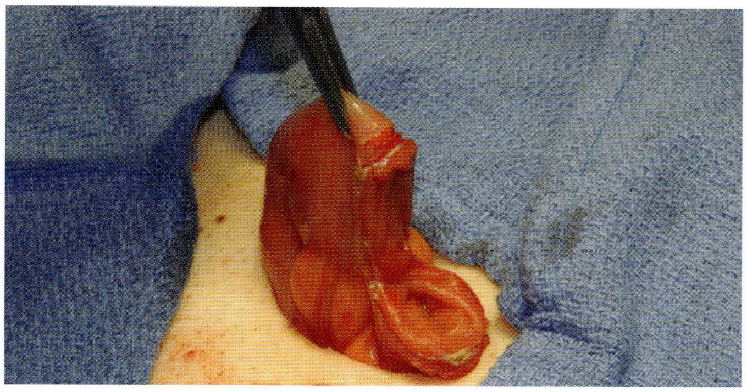

Figure 28-14

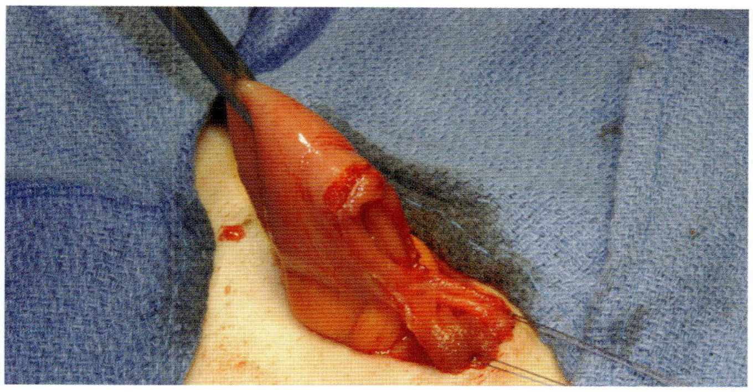

Figure 28-15

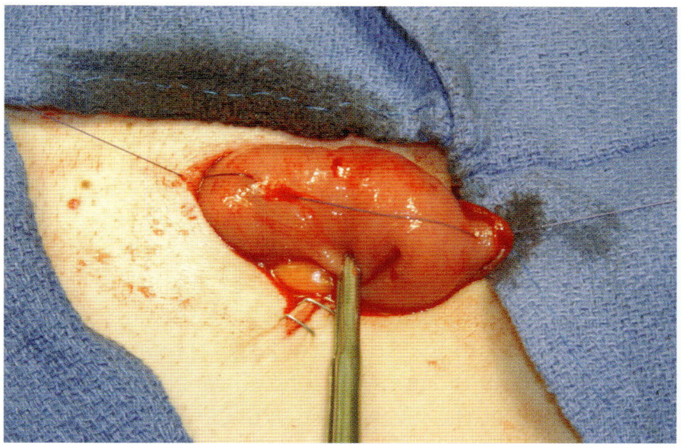

Figure 28-16

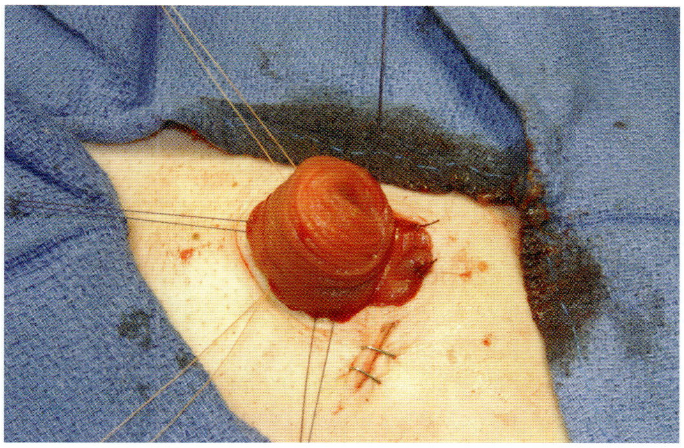

Figure 28-17

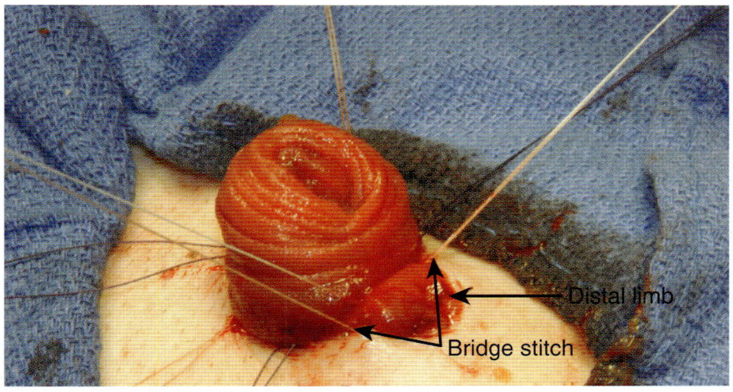

Figure 28-18

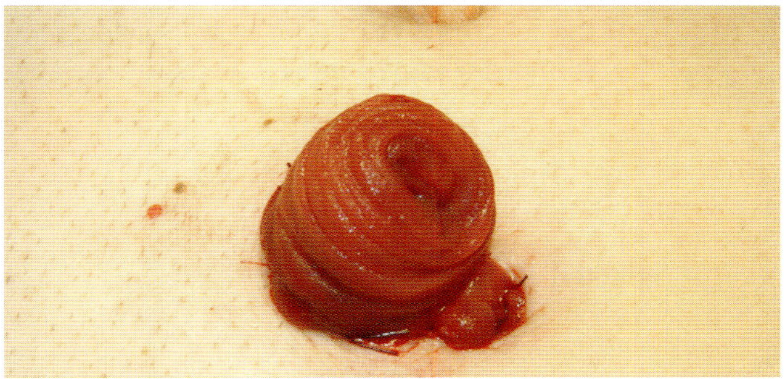

Figure 28-19

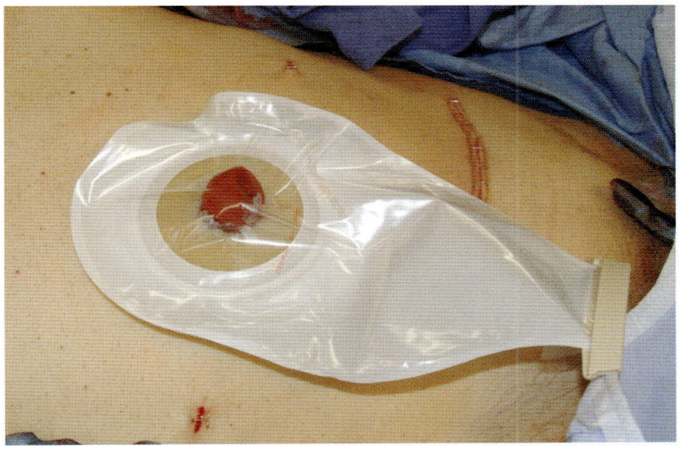

Figure 28-20

Step 3: Postoperative Care

Diet may be advanced when bowel function returns. An enterostomal therapist should be involved in the postoperative care and training of the patient. The ileostomy rod should be removed at postoperative day 5.

Step 4: Pearls and Pitfalls

The fascial opening should be widened sufficiently to allow the ileum to be pulled out an adequate length without compromising the mesenteric blood supply. An overly large opening can lead to stomal prolapse or hernia formation. Poor placement of sutures can result in stomal retraction. Sutures placed too deep into the wall of the ileum at the level of the skin can cause a fistula.

The ileostomy rod is needed only in patients with a thick abdominal wall when there is obvious tension on the loop brought through the opening. The thickened mesentery may require a larger abdominal wall opening to facilitate passage. A more proximally placed stoma along the length of the ileum may provide more mobility. Finally, if it is absolutely necessary, the stoma site can be moved to the upper abdomen where the subcutaneous fat is thinner.

Selected Readings

Güenaga KF, Lustosa SA, Saad SS, et al. Ileostomy or colostomy for temporary decompression of colorectal anastomosis. Cochrane Database Syst Rev 2007;(1):CD004647.

Rondelli F, Reboldi P, Rulli A, et al. Loop ileostomy versus loop colostomy for fecal diversion after colorectal or coloanal anastomosis: a meta-analysis. Int J Colorectal Dis 2009;24:479–88.

CHAPTER 29

Colostomy: End and Divided Loop

Anne Y. Lin and Elisa H. Birnbaum

Step 1: Clinical Anatomy

The left colon lies along the left side of the abdomen suspended from the splenic flexure to the pelvic brim by lateral peritoneal attachments. The mesentery of the left colon arises from the midline of the abdomen along the aorta. The sigmoid colon has no lateral peritoneal attachments other than some congenital adhesions that fix the apex of the sigmoid to the pelvic brim and the iliac fossa. The sigmoid colon is attached to the retroperitoneum through a midline mesentery arising from the inferior mesenteric artery (IMA) and extending down into the pelvis to the mesorectum. The splenic flexure is attached to the undersurface of the tip of the spleen, the lower edge of the tail of the pancreas, and the anterior surface of the left kidney by various levels of suspensory ligaments and peritoneal extensions. The blood supply to the left colon is based on the IMA, which arises from the anterior surface of the aorta just above the bifurcation of the common iliac arteries. The IMA extends anteriorly and bifurcates to produce the superior rectal artery feeding the sigmoid colon and the rectum. The left colic artery extends cephalad to provide the left colon and distal splenic flexure with blood supply through the arcade at the mesenteric edge known as the marginal artery of Drummond. The retroperitoneum behind the left colon contains the left ureter and the gonadal vessels lying over the psoas muscle. The ureter crosses the iliac vessels at the bifurcation of the iliac vessels into the external and internal iliac branches.

Step 2: Preoperative Considerations

End colostomies are constructed typically when an abdominal perineal resection is performed for rectal carcinoma or when a Hartmann procedure is performed for treatment of diverticulitis or obstructing carcinoma. Typically, the descending colon is used as the end stoma. The sigmoid colon is usually removed because it has been irradiated during neoadjuvant treatment of rectal carcinoma or involved with the disease process in the case of diverticulitis. A divided loop stoma can be performed as an end loop colostomy. These stomas provide complete diversion of stool and decompression of the distal end. The stomas also provide an advantage, in that laparotomy is not required for takedown. An end loop stoma can also be used to overcome lack of reach for a loop colostomy in an obese patient with a thick abdominal wall.

Ideally, the stoma site should be marked in the left lower quadrant within the rectus outline on the infraumbilical fat fold by an enterostomal therapist or an individual well versed in creation of stomas. Care should be taken to avoid skin folds, scars, and bony protuberances, which would dislodge the ostomy appliance. The patient's preference on waistline should be taken into account when placing an ostomy. A bowel preparation is unnecessary if a patient is undergoing an operation that will not result in an anastomosis. Prophylactic antibiotics are given within 1 hour of the incision.

Step 3: Operative Steps

- The patient is typically placed in the lithotomy position, and the site is marked on the skin with parallel scratch marks so that the site can be identified at the end of the procedure (Figure 29-1*A*). The sigmoid and left colon are mobilized by incising the lateral peritoneal reflection as for a left colectomy, and the colon and its mesentery are mobilized away from the retroperitoneum toward the central vessels. After selecting the most distal colonic segment, the bowel is mobilized until the segment reaches the abdominal wall. This maneuver may require mobilization of the colon to the splenic flexure and occasionally mobilization of the splenic flexure to get adequate length.

End Colostomy

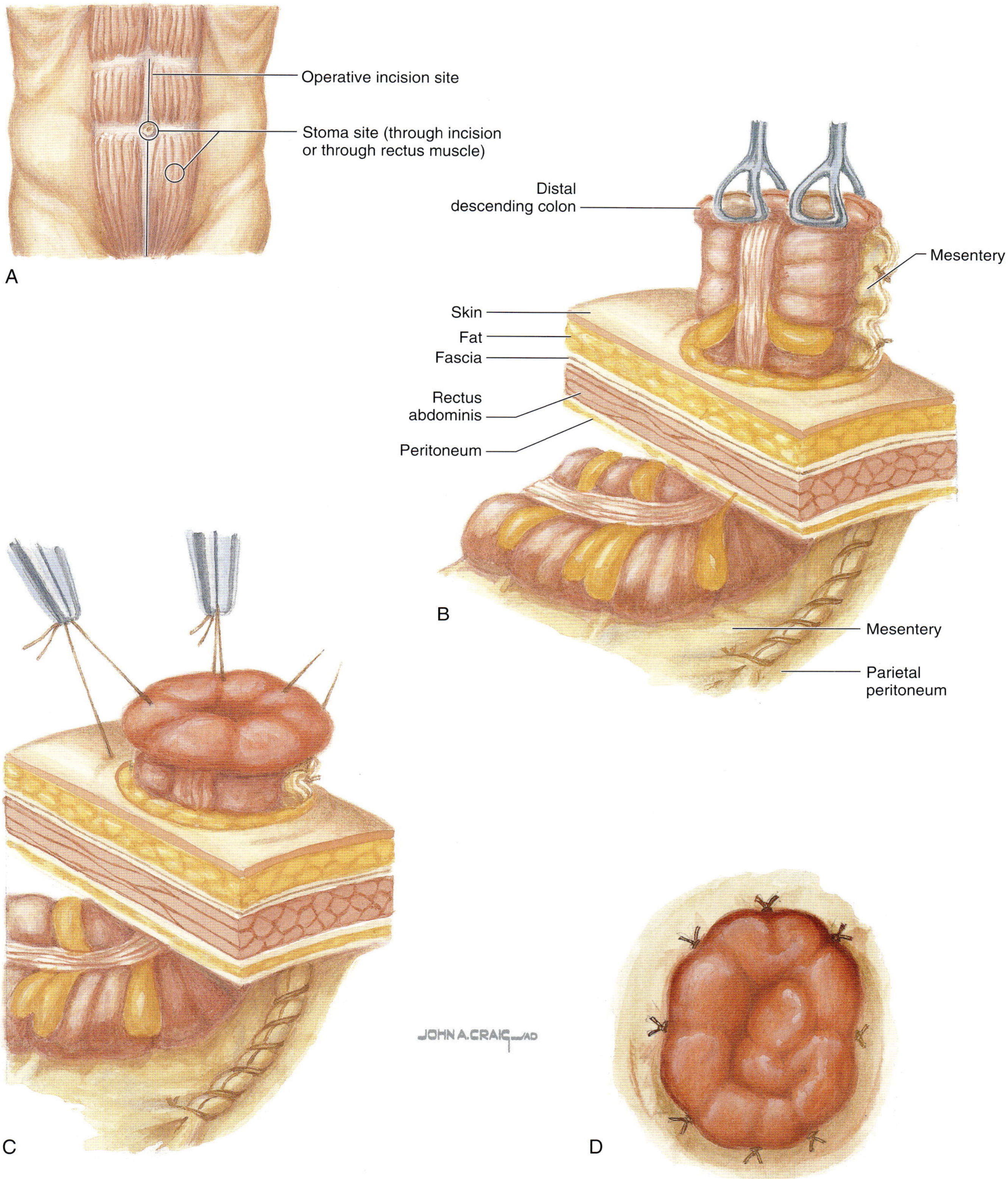

Figure 29-1A-D *Netter illustration from www.netterimages.com.*

End Colostomy

- After resection of the vascular supply to the distal bowel and division of the mesentery up to the chosen site for the stoma (Figure 29-2), the bowel is divided with a GIA stapler (Covidien, Mansfield, Mass.), and the specimen is removed from the operative field (Figure 29-3). The mesenteric vessels may be preserved at the aorta in most cases, but occasionally the IMA must be sacrificed to reach through a thick abdominal wall.
- A Kocher clamp is applied to the fascial edge just across from the stoma site, and a second Kocher clamp is placed on the subcuticular layer. A folded laparotomy pad is placed beneath the abdominal wall under the planned stoma site, and the Kocher clamps are used to line up the abdominal wall layers (Figure 29-4). A 3- to 4-cm-diameter circular skin incision is made at the marked site using the cautery for the skin and subcutaneous tissues. In an obese patient, a core of subcutaneous fat can be removed. In thin patients, the skin disk is removed. The dissection is carried to the fascial layer, and the fascia is exposed using Army-Navy retractors. The fascia is divided vertically over a distance of 3 cm, and a small "T" incision is made in the midportion of this incision. The abdominal wall is tented up with the laparotomy sponge, and a clamp or curved scissor is used to split the rectus muscle in the direction of its fibers down to and through the posterior peritoneum.
- The peritoneum and posterior rectus fascia are incised vertically for a distance adequate to place two to three fingers through this new stoma opening (Figure 29-5).
- A Babcock clamp is placed from the skin aperture through the stoma site into the abdominal cavity, and the bowel end is grasped (Figures 29-1*B* and 29-6). If the fascial opening is too tight, it should be opened further, and the colon should be drawn through the abdominal wall by gently pushing the colon into the opening from the abdomen with traction on the Babcock clamp. The midline abdominal wall opening is closed.
- The GIA staple line is excised, and the stoma is sewn to the skin with 3-0 absorbable suture through the full-thickness bowel edge and through the skin (Figure 29-1*C*). These sutures are placed at the top, bottom, left, and right quadrants, and a second series of sutures is placed equidistant between each of these quadrant sutures (Figures 29-1*D* and 29-7).

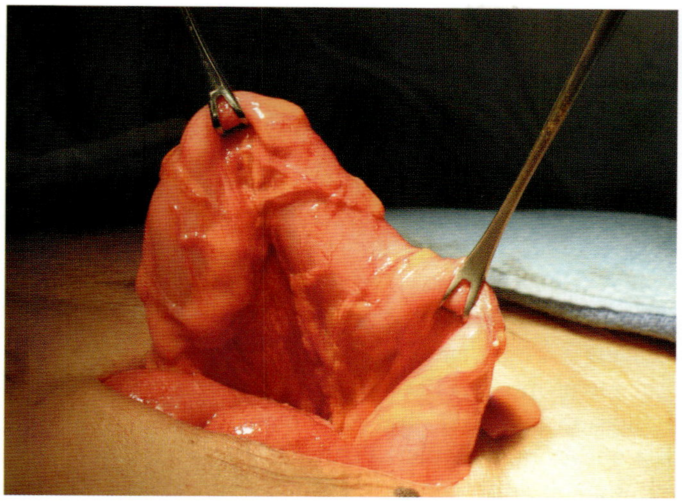

Figure 29-2

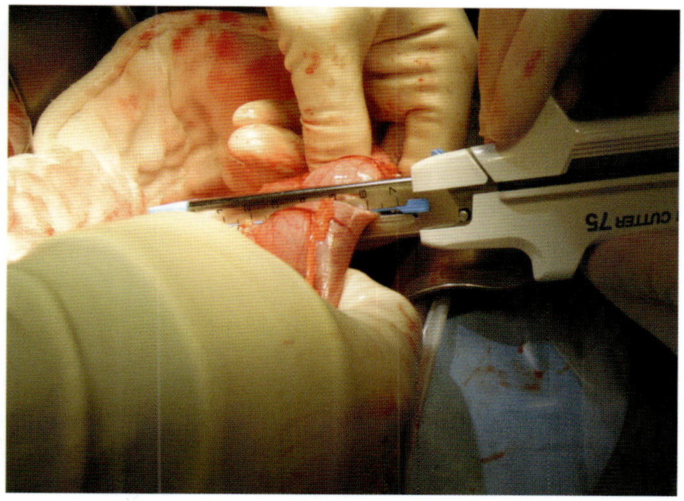

Figure 29-3

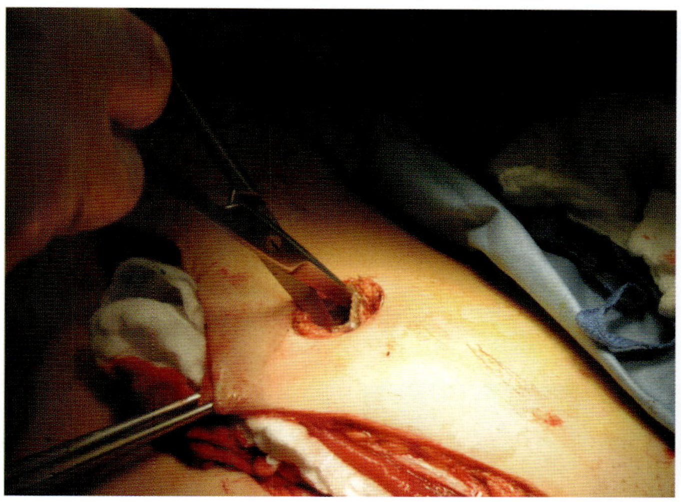

Figure 29-4

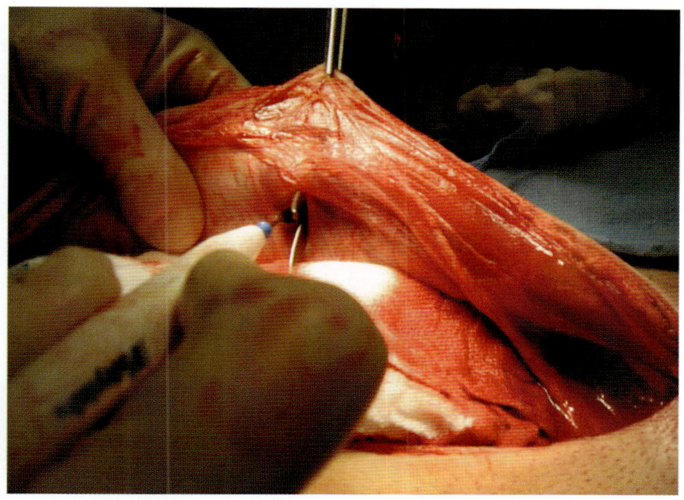

Figure 29-5

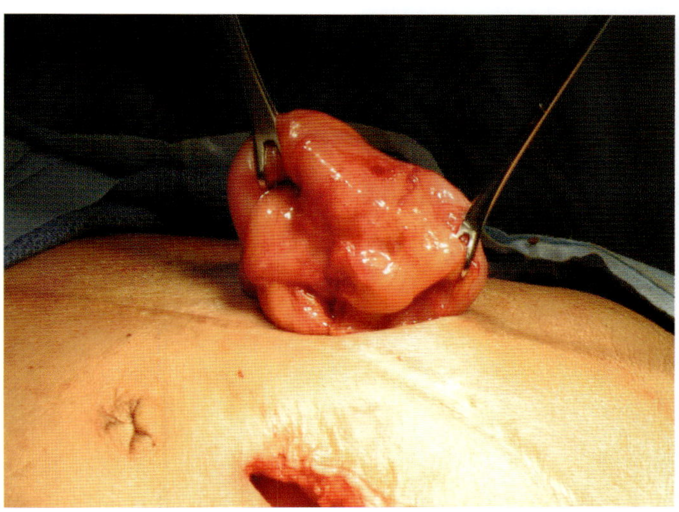

Figure 29-6

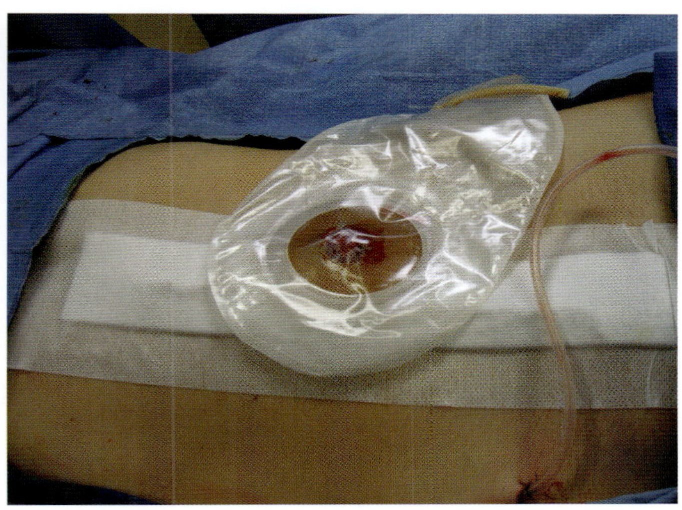

Figure 29-7

Divided Loop Colostomy

- After laparoscopic or open mobilization of the colon, as described in previous chapters, the abdominal wall stoma opening is created by excising a 3-cm-diameter disk of skin and fat to deliver two fingers through the midportion of the rectus muscle. The loop of colon is brought out through the colostomy site, the midline incision is closed, and the colon is divided antimesenteric to mesenteric in direction with a linear cutter stapler (Figure 29-8).
- The full circumference of the proximal bowel and the antimesenteric corner of the distal bowel is brought out through the stoma opening (Figure 29-9*A*).
- The antimesenteric corner of the transverse staple line of the distal bowel is cut off to create no more than a 1-cm-diameter opening in the colon to provide a vent to an obstructing distal lesion (Figure 29-9*B*). The distal bowel is matured to the stoma site dermis with several full-thickness 3-0 absorbable sutures placed at 6 o'clock on the stoma site (Figure 29-10). Alternatively, if complete diversion is needed, the staple line is left intact, and the corner of the staple line is sutured to the skin with two sutures at 6 o'clock on the stoma opening.
- The functioning limb of the stoma is matured by excising the staple line on the proximal bowel (Figure 29-9*C*). For a divided loop colostomy, the bowel is sutured to the skin in the top, right, and left positions and sutured to the distal limb with a single 3-0 chromic suture to create a small bridge. Intervening sutures are placed as needed around the open bowel. For the end loop colostomy, the proximal functioning end is matured at skin level with full-thickness sutures around the circumference, which cover the corner of the still-stapled-closed distal bowel in the lower part of the stoma (not shown).

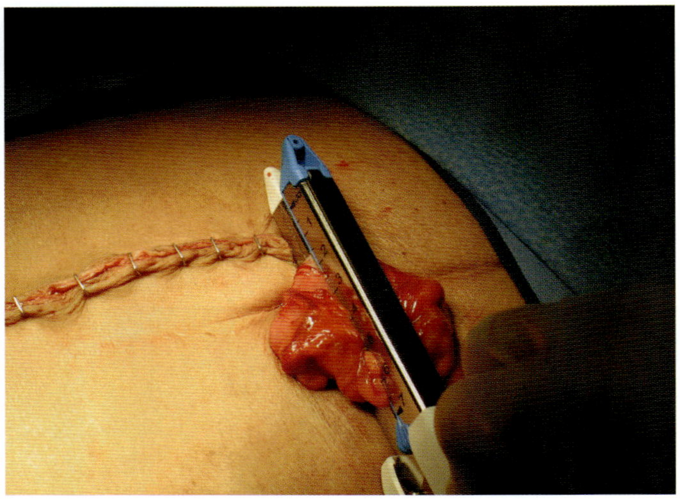

Figure 29-8

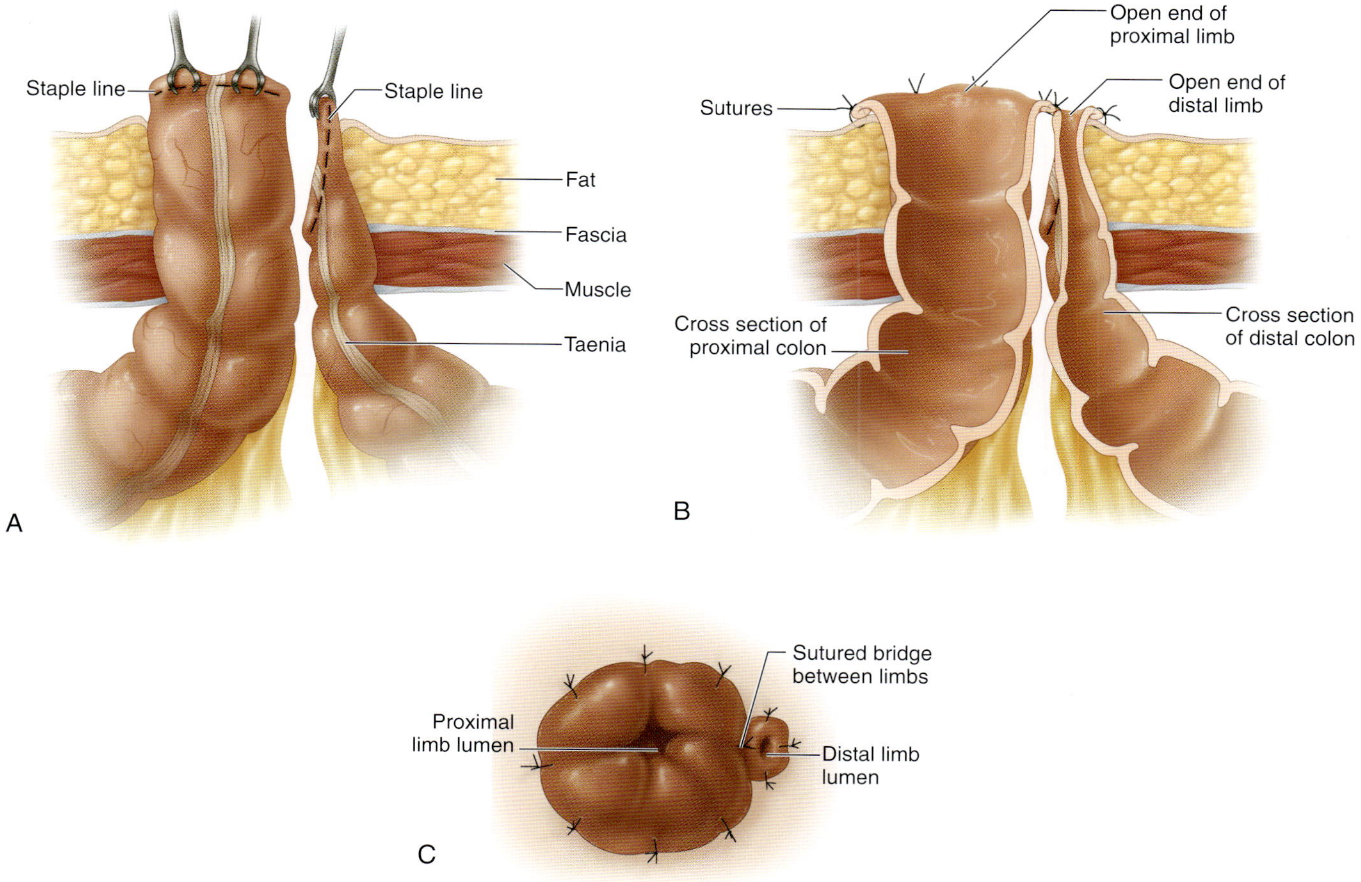

Figure 29-9A-C

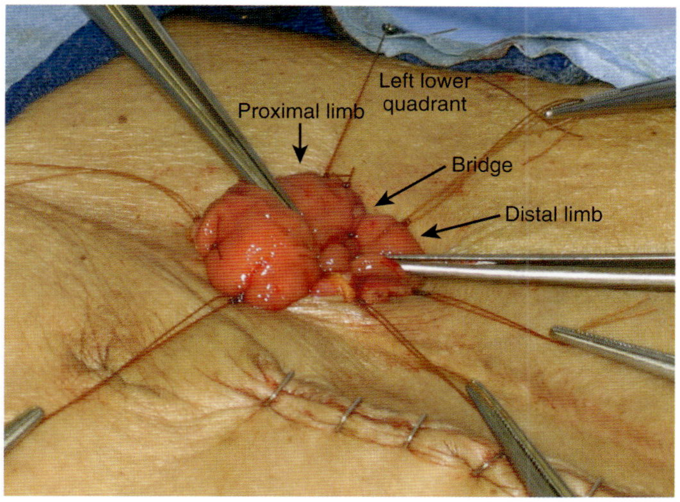

Figure 29-10

Step 4. Pearls and Pitfalls

Occasionally, the bowel cannot reach the skin, and further colonic mobilization is required. Incising the left colon mesentery in the central avascular window allows the colon to stretch up to the next vascular arcade. The mesentery or bowel may be too edematous or too fat to fit through a stoma opening two to three fingerbreadths wide, and the abdominal wall opening should be enlarged and the high probability of a hernia forming accepted as a reasonable risk.

When forming a temporary stoma after an open operation, the use of an adhesion barrier around the limbs of the colostomy should be considered. This barrier reduces the need for adhesiolysis at the time of takedown. The open mucus fistula is essential for impending or complete obstruction in a distal lesion. However, the mucus fistula continues to make mucus, and the appliance must accommodate this output or peristomal irritation will occur.

Selected Readings

Güenaga KF, Lustosa SA, Saad SS, et al. Ileostomy or colostomy for temporary decompression of colorectal anastomosis. Cochrane Database Syst Rev 2007;(1):CD004647.

Rondelli F, Reboldi P, Rulli A, et al. Loop ileostomy versus loop colostomy for fecal diversion after colorectal or coloanal anastomosis: a meta-analysis. Int J Colorectal Dis 2009;24:479–88.

CHAPTER 30

Local Parastomal Hernia Repair

Matthew G. Mutch

Step 1: Clinical Anatomy

The stoma aperture is created within the rectus muscle. Herniation can occur via two mechanisms. First, the limb of bowel leading to the stoma can protrude through a normal opening in the abdominal wall and become adherent to subcutaneous tissues. Second, an enlarged fascial opening at the stoma aperture can lead to herniation of adjacent bowel. Attention should be paid to the presence of another hernia associated with the midline incision. Stomas created lateral to the rectus muscle have been shown to herniate more frequently and have a less appropriate surface to maintain an appliance.

Step 2: Preoperative Considerations

The anatomy of the hernia should be thoroughly evaluated. A good physical examination is necessary, and a computed tomography scan is often helpful. The current site of the stoma must be assessed to ensure that a local repair of the hernia would result in good pouching and improved quality of life. Otherwise, the stoma may need to be moved to a new site. An enterostomal therapist can assist with site marking and patient education and postoperative care. If the stoma is a colostomy, mechanical bowel preparation is needed. Preoperative antibiotic prophylaxis that continues for 24 hours postoperatively is preferred. Deep vein thrombosis prophylaxis with sequential compression devices is required and may be supplemented with subcutaneous heparin.

Step 3: Operative Steps

- The patient is placed supine on the operating table. The abdomen is prepared and draped in the usual sterile fashion. If a lateral approach is used, the stoma is covered with an adhesive drape to exclude it from the operating field.
- The hernia can be accessed by detaching the stoma from the mucocutaneous junction (Figure 30-1) or through an incision that is made lateral to the stoma. A self-retaining ring retractor is helpful to expose the subcutaneous space after the mucocutaneous junction is incised.
- In the subcutaneous space, the stoma is mobilized circumferentially into the peritoneal cavity (Figure 30-2). The stoma can be closed to prevent spillage of enteric contents by placing a staple line across the opening of the bowel or applying Allis clamps across the bowel.
- The hernia is reduced (Figure 30-3). The fascial defect is repaired with interrupted, permanent sutures (Figure 30-4). The repair is reinforced with biologic mesh. A cruciform hole is made in the center of the mesh (Figure 30-5). The stoma is brought through the defect in the mesh and seated on top of the fascia (Figure 30-6). The mesh is fastened to the fascia

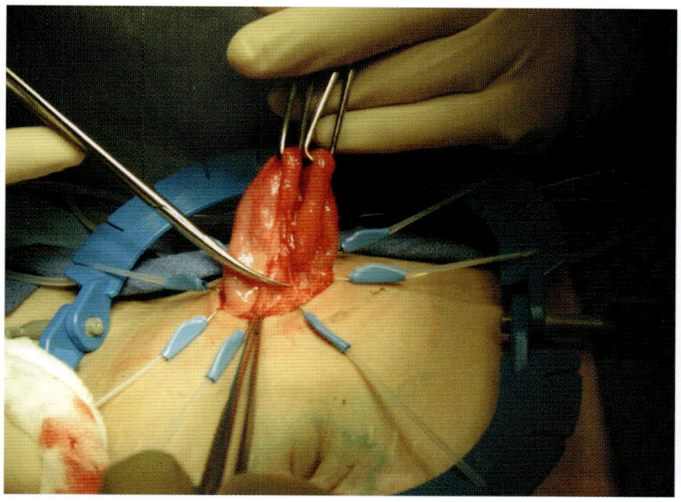

Figure 30-1

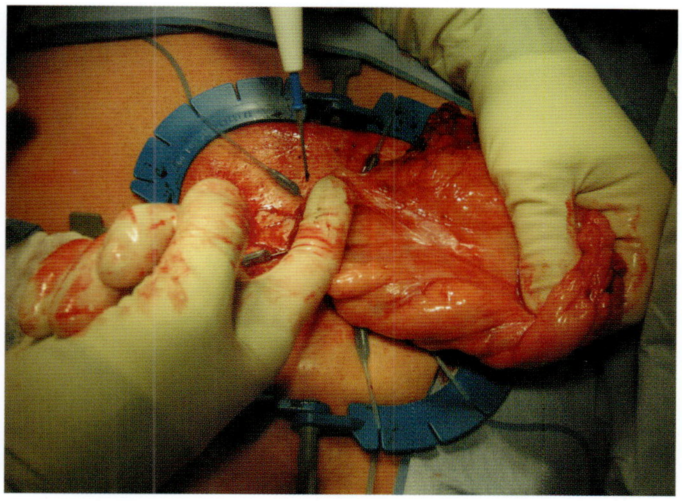

Figure 30-2

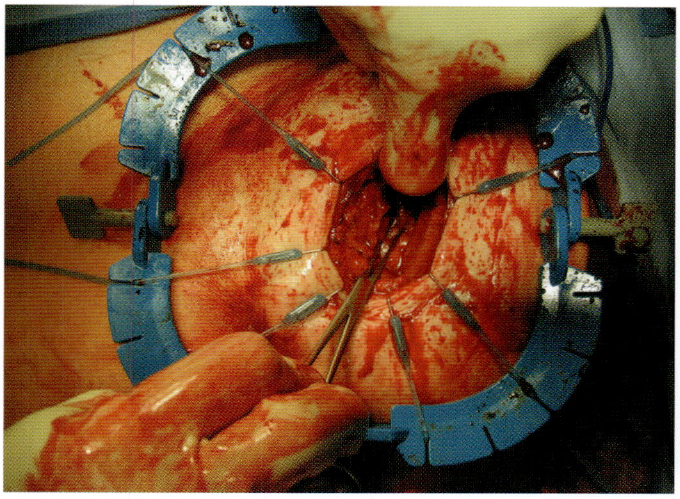

Figure 30-3

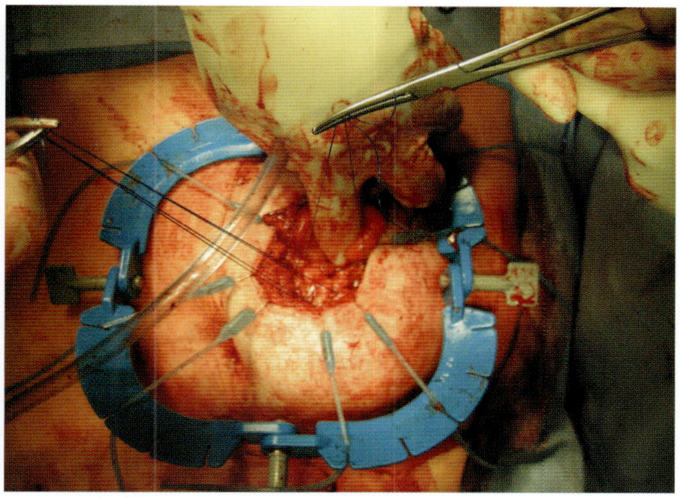

Figure 30-4

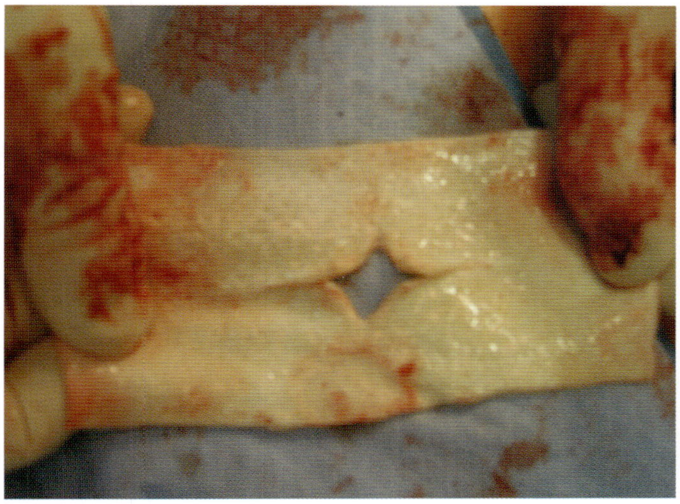

Figure 30-5

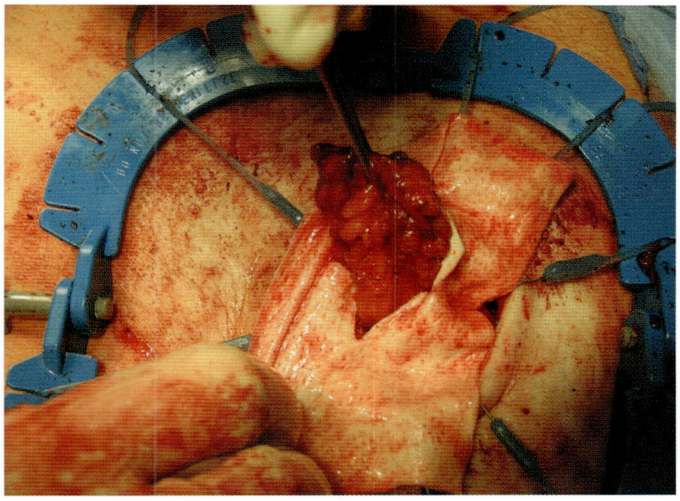

Figure 30-6

either with a fascial stapler (Figures 30-7 and 30-8) or with permanent suture (Figure 30-9*A*). The stoma is matured to the skin (Figure 30-10) with a drain in the hernia space under the fat.

- Submuscular repair can be accomplished by creating a pocket behind the rectus muscle but anterior to the posterior rectus fascia and sliding the mesh along the bowel to lie in the pocket flat on the posterior fascia (Figure 30-9*B*). There is no need for sutures or staples to fix the mesh in place because the rectus muscle falls back on top of the mesh in the pocket.

Step 4: Postoperative Care

The patient can be started on a clear liquid diet the day of surgery. When adequate stoma function is confirmed, the patient is tolerating solid food, and the patient's pain is under control, the patient may be discharged to home. Patients should be restricted to lifting no more than 10 lb for at least 8 weeks. The drain, which is draining the subcutaneous pocket and old hernia sac, is removed when output is less than 15 mL/day.

Step 5: Pearls and Pitfalls

A local repair is more likely to result in recurrent hernia but should be considered as first-line treatment because moving the stoma to a new site may eventually become necessary. After removal of the sac, drainage of the subcutaneous hernia space usually prevents a parastomal abscess. The tightness of the abdominal wall opening after completion of the repair is critical to avoid recurrent hernia and prevent ischemia of the ostomy. Measurement of the opening in the mesh and the fascia with two large fingers is usually enough of a precaution. The size of the ostomy opening in the skin should be reduced to less than $1\frac{1}{2}$ inches in diameter to facilitate ostomy appliance adherence. A radial suture line in the inferior portion of the large skin opening, resulting in a racquet-shaped "incision," can bring the stoma back to size.

Selected Readings

Saclarides TJ, Hsu A, Quiros R. In situ mesh repair of parastomal hernias. Am Surg 2004;70:701–5.

Wijeyekoon SP, Gurusamy K, El-Gendy K, et al. Prevention of parastomal herniation with biologic/composite prosthetic mesh: a systematic review and meta-analysis of randomized controlled trials. J Am Coll Surg 2010;211:637–45.

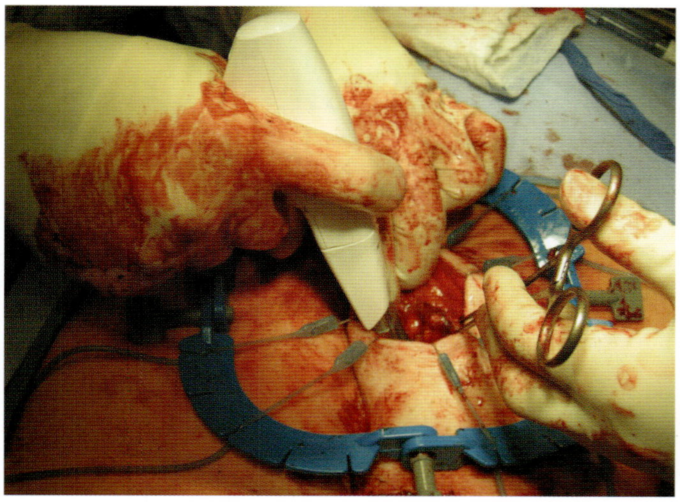

Figure 30-7

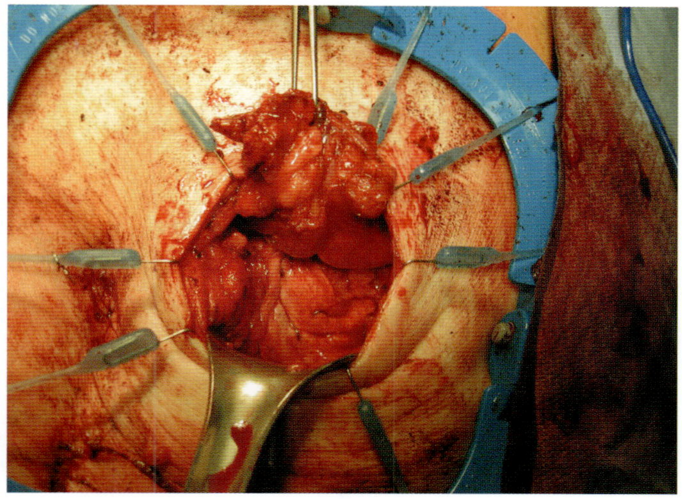

Figure 30-8

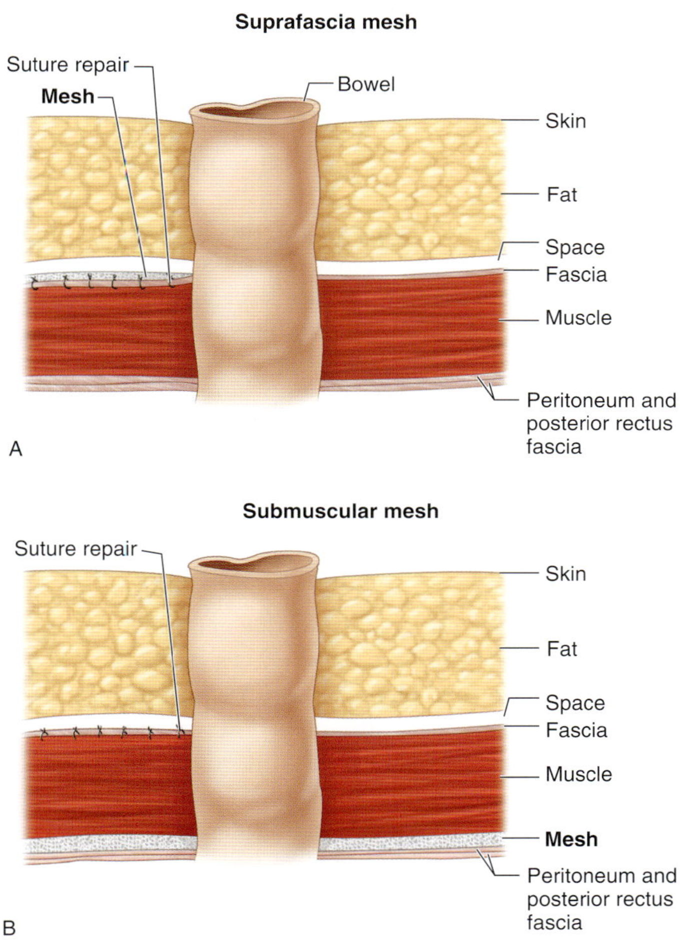

Figure 30-9A-B

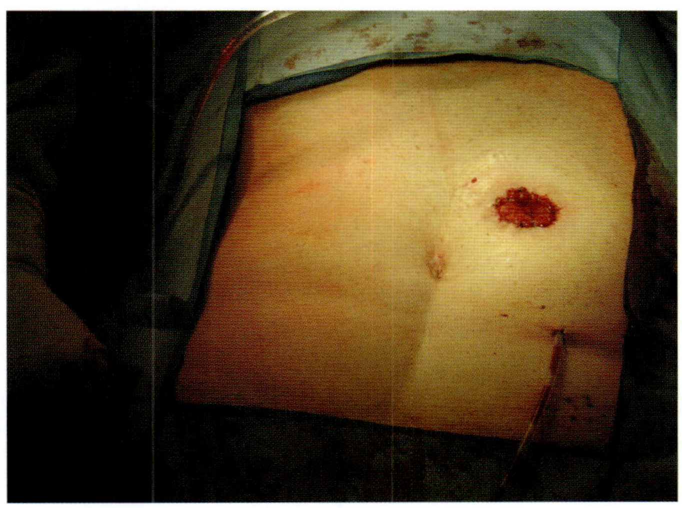

Figure 30-10

CHAPTER 31

Small Bowel Strictureplasty

Steven R. Hunt

Step 1: Clinical Anatomy

The anatomy relating to a strictureplasty is straightforward. Most strictureplasties are performed in the small intestine. There is no clear transition point between the jejunum and ileum, and treatment is not differentiated based on this designation. Generally, the ileum has more fat in the mesentery and more complex arterial arcades with less distinct terminal vasa recta in the mesentery.

A noteworthy structure is the ligament of Treitz, which is the point where the jejunum emerges from the transverse colon mesentery. Generally, measurement of small bowel length is begun at the ligament of Treitz. A second important landmark is the fold of Treves (or ligament of Treves). On the terminal ileum at the ileocecal junction, this antimesenteric fat fold is the only nonmesenteric fat over the course of the entire small bowel.

Step 2: Preoperative Considerations

Strictureplasty was developed for the treatment of strictures of the small intestine related to Crohn's disease. The technique allows small bowel length to be preserved and allows patients to avoid short bowel syndrome. A strictureplasty may be performed alone, in series with multiple other strictureplasties, or in combination with resection.

Laparoscopy is not an option for patients who are identified preoperatively to need a strictureplasty. Generally, the thickened and shortened mesentery of diseased small bowel does not lend itself to delivery through a small incision. Additionally, strictureplasty techniques require a significant amount of palpation, and performing a strictureplasty with straight laparoscopy is not recommended.

Preoperative imaging studies include computed tomography, magnetic resonance enterography, small bowel follow-through studies, or a barium enema. These studies should be done as needed to delineate the relevant anatomy and to rule out active inflammation.

Strictureplasty is best performed on chronic fibrotic strictures. If a phlegmon or abscess is present, the patient should be given ample time to allow for the inflammation to resolve, or resection should be planned.

Strictureplasty for Crohn's disease should be considered in patients with multiple strictures and patients who have had multiple previous small bowel resections in whom repeat resection could lead to short bowel syndrome. It is best to avoid strictureplasty in the following situations:

- ▲ Localized perforation or phlegmon
- ▲ Fistula
- ▲ Multiple strictures over a short segment of small bowel
- ▲ A stricture near the site of a planned resection
- ▲ Radiation strictures
- ▲ Colonic strictures
- ▲ Malnutrition

As with other small bowel procedures, there is no need for a bowel preparation. Broad-spectrum antibiotics and deep vein thrombosis prophylaxis should be administered preoperatively. Provided that there is no colonic disease and no need for access to the rectum, these procedures can be done in the supine position.

Step 3: Operative Steps

- ◆ The length of the stricture determines the appropriate type of strictureplasty. For shorter strictures (<10 cm), a Heineke-Mikulicz strictureplasty should be performed. For strictures longer than 10 cm, a Finney or Jaboulay strictureplasty should be performed. In the unusual case where a stricture is longer than 20 to 25 cm, a divided side-to-side isoperistaltic strictureplasty can be performed. Each of these procedures is described separately.

Heineke-Mikulicz Strictureplasty

- After a stricture has been identified as appropriate for a Heineke-Mikulicz strictureplasty, two stay sutures should be placed on each side of the antimesenteric edge of the small bowel at the midpoint of the stricture. A longitudinal incision should be created on the antimesenteric side of the small bowel (Figure 31-1). The incision is made with the electrocautery. The incision should begin 2 cm proximal to the stricture. The incision is initially made through normal small bowel proximal to the stricture. A tonsil clamp can be used to guide the remainder of the longitudinal enterotomy over the entire length of the stricture and 2 cm out onto normal bowel at the distal end of the stricture.
- Tension is placed on the stay sutures at the midpoint of the longitudinal incision (Figure 31-2). A central suture is placed across the central portion of this transverse closure at each point of the apices of the initial incision. The suture is tightened down to show that the transverse closure of this strictureplasty is possible. If this central suture can be tied down without significant tension, it is appropriate to proceed with closure.
- The incision is closed transversely with an absorbable suture (Figure 31-3), starting at each stay suture and proceeding to the middle of the transverse opening (Figure 31-4). The choice of simple interrupted sutures, as opposed to a running inverted baseball stitch suture line, is left to the discretion of the surgeon. There are no data to support one technique over the other. A single-layer closure is usually adequate (Figure 31-4). Oversewing the thickened bowel with Lembert sutures can be quite difficult and can result in further narrowing of the strictureplasty, defeating the purpose of the procedure.
- As an alternative to single-layer closure, the transverse closure can be bolstered with wide bites of simple interrupted absorbable sutures across this transverse closure suture line.
- An endoscopic biopsy forceps should be used to capture a portion of the mesenteric surface (usually an ulcer is present) at the center of the stricture to screen for cancer, or a shave biopsy can be obtained from the antimesenteric cut surface.

Finney (Jaboulay) Strictureplasty

- The Finney strictureplasty is appropriate for strictures 10 to 20 cm long. These strictures generally are not suitable for Heineke-Mikulicz closure because it is difficult to bring the midpoint of the transverse closure of such a strictureplasty into approximation.
- To begin this strictureplasty, the bowel should be folded into a "U" configuration with either end of the stricture as the apex of the "U" (Figure 31-5). A single stay suture should be placed at the apex of the "U" and at the top of the arms of the "U" on normal bowel to maintain the bowel in this "U" configuration.
- An antimesenteric incision should be made 2 cm out onto normal bowel, beyond the stricture and the same length on the normal limb of the "U."
- An absorbable suture is used in a running fashion to complete the strictureplasty. The initial suture is started at the folded edge of the back walls of the strictureplasty. The simple suture line is sewn down to and around the corner bringing the two limbs together. A second running suture should be started on the antimesenteric surface at the apex of the "U" and sewn in a running fashion along the anterior wall to meet the other suture and complete the closure of the newly enlarged lumen (Figure 31-6).

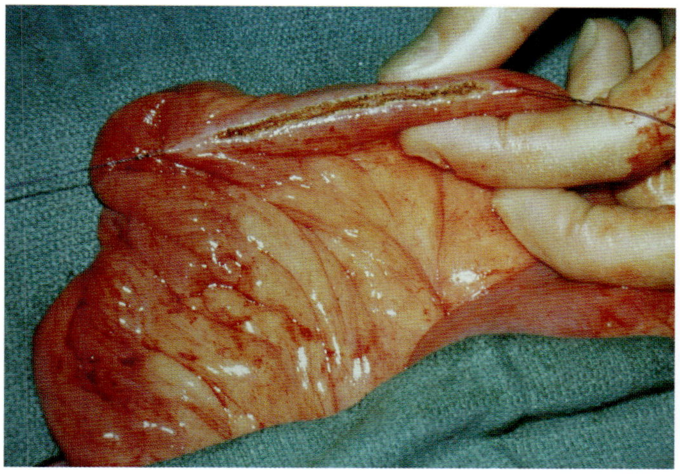

Figure 31-1

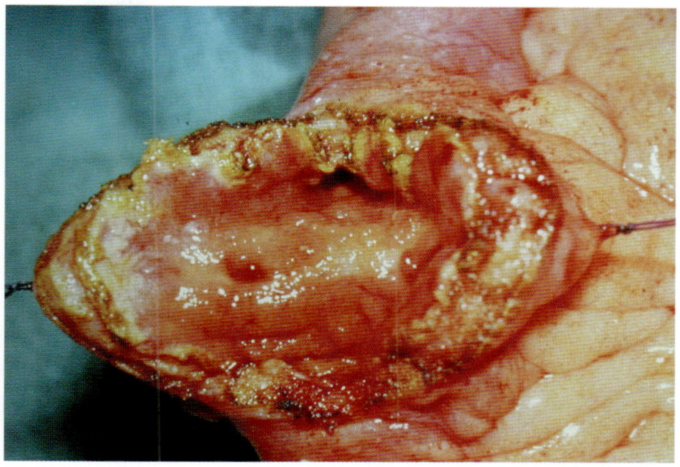

Figure 31-2

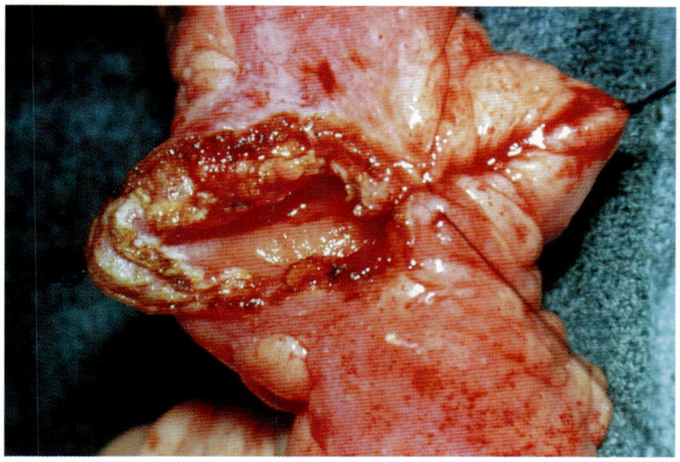

Figure 31-3

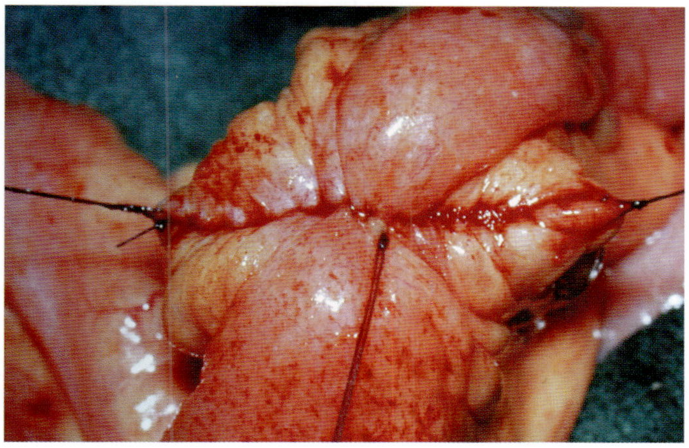

Figure 31-4

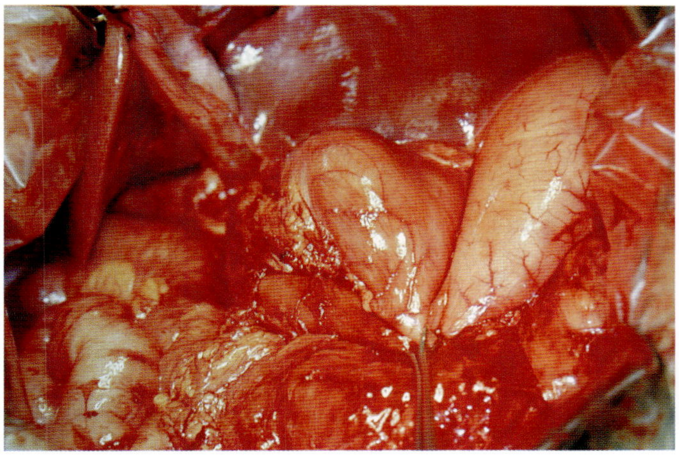

Figure 31-5

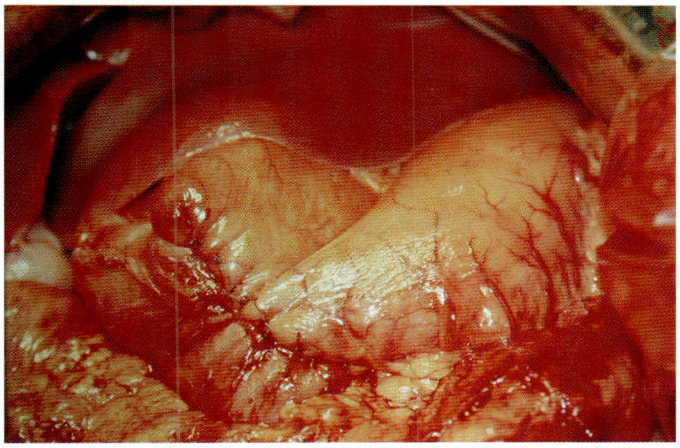

Figure 31-6

Side-to-Side Isoperistaltic Strictureplasty

- For strictures longer than 20 to 25 cm, the entire length of the stricture should be elevated into the wound to display the mesentery. The bowel at the midpoint of the stricture should be divided transversely with the electrocautery. The mesentery to this bowel should be divided in a perpendicular fashion to preserve blood flow to both ends of the bowel.
- After the mesentery is divided, the proximal limb of the diseased bowel is overlapped with the distal limb of bowel. On each end, the diseased bowel should overlap the normal bowel by at least 2 cm. These two limbs of bowel are laid side by side.
- An outer row of simple interrupted Lembert stay sutures is placed along the mesenteric edge to approximate and hold the two limbs. After this suture line is placed, each limb of the bowel is opened longitudinally on the antimesenteric border. The incision should extend out onto the normal small bowel, proximally and distally, to accommodate for the overlapping diseased segment. The ends of each limb are spatulated to facilitate the closure in the corners. The inner layer of the back row is completed with two running, simple, absorbable sutures, each starting at the midpoint of the back row. The sutures are continued around each corner and across the anterior closure until they meet and are tied to each other. A second layer of simple interrupted sutures is placed to reinforce the anterior closure line.
- Small titanium vascular clips should be placed at the mesenteric border of the middle of each strictureplasty site to act at the ends of the stricture as a marker to identify each site (by the number or pattern of clips at each site).

Step 4: Postoperative Care

Patients should be maintained on intravenous fluids until they can resume adequate oral intake. Patients who require multiple strictures at a single operation should be decompressed with a nasogastric tube until resolution of ileus is documented. Otherwise, patients are begun on a liquid diet on postoperative day 1, and the diet is advanced as tolerated. Patients are discharged only when they show adequate bowel function and can tolerate a regular diet. Prophylactic antibiotics are continued for a total coverage period of 24 hours. Deep vein thrombosis prophylaxis is continued until discharge with either pneumatic compression boots or subcutaneous heparin. Patients are ambulated on postoperative day 1, and the Foley catheter is removed as soon as the patient is ambulatory.

Step 5: Pearls and Pitfalls

Hemorrhage is a common complication after a strictureplasty. It usually manifests as gastrointestinal bleeding and results from hypervascularity of the cut edge of the bowel involved in the strictureplasty. The hemorrhage usually can be treated with supportive care including correction of coagulopathy, serial hemoglobin determinations, and transfusion as appropriate. In refractory cases, hemorrhage may be treated angiographically. The titanium clips placed at the time of the initial strictureplasty can facilitate the identification of the bleeding sites. If embolization fails, patients may need to return to the operating room. An enteric leak may occur at the site of the strictureplasty. If the leak is contained, it is best treated with radiographically guided drainage. If there is free leakage of enteric contents in the peritoneal cavity, re-exploration is necessary.

It is often difficult to determine whether a stricture is symptomatic based on its external appearance. Generally, bowel that permits the passage of a Foley balloon filled with 3 mL of saline should not be symptomatic. The presence of "occult" strictures of the small intestine can be identified using a Foley catheter. At a point where there is a known stricture, after the enterotomy has been made, a Foley catheter with the balloon inflated to 3 cm with saline may be inserted proximally and distally. The balloon can be withdrawn through the bowel to identify other points of stricture.

In circumstances where short bowel syndrome is a possibility, it is necessary to measure the small bowel; this is generally done starting at the ligament of Treitz. A 75-cm umbilical tape is marched along the bowel to determine the actual length of the bowel. This measurement should be recorded in the operative note for reference in the future.

Although the incidence is quite low, adenocarcinoma can develop in the small bowel in cases of chronic active Crohn's disease. During strictureplasty, biopsy specimens of any suspicious areas of the small bowel mucosa and the area of ulceration on the mesenteric aspect of the stricture should be obtained and sent for frozen-section analysis to rule out the presence of an adenocarcinoma.

Titanium hemoclips should be used to mark the proximal and distal extent of each strictureplasty to allow for radiographic identification in the future. These clips can be useful in cases where there is postoperative bleeding, cases with a diagnosis of cancer in the biopsy specimen of the stricture, or when patients develop subsequent strictures to identify the site of the previous strictureplasty.

More recent studies have shown that it is safe to perform strictureplasties across an ileocolic anastomosis. Depending on the configuration of the stricture and the anastomosis, either a Heineke-Mikulicz strictureplasty or a Finney strictureplasty may be used.

Selected Readings

Dietz DW, Fazio VW, Laureti S, et al. Strictureplasty in diffuse Crohn's jejunoileitis: safe and durable. Dis Colon Rectum 2002;45:764–70.

Shatari T, Clark MA, Yamamoto T, et al. Long strictureplasty is as safe and effective as short strictureplasty in small-bowel Crohn's disease. Colorectal Dis 2004;6:438–41.

Yamamoto T, Fazio VW, Tekkis PP. Safety and efficacy of strictureplasty for Crohn's disease: a systematic review and meta-analysis. Dis Colon Rectum 2007;50:1968–86.

CHAPTER 32

Resection of Rectorectal Tumor with Sacrectomy

Anne Y. Lin and James W. Fleshman, Jr.

Step 1: Clinical Anatomy

Pelvic Anatomy

The pelvic anatomy is complex with interrelationships between the rectum, vagina, uterus, ovaries, bladder, and prostate. The anatomy is important for pelvic dissection because of the various structures that are at risk, such as the splanchnic nerves (innervation of the bladder and sexual organs), the ureters, and the organs themselves. The common iliac artery and vein on each side of the sacral promontory course along the posterior aspect of the pelvic brim. The hypogastric plexus of parasympathetic and sympathetic nerves is found between the bifurcation of the aorta and common iliac vessels. This plexus coalesces to the right and left to become the splanchnic pelvic nerves, which run along the inner aspect of the pelvic side wall to the level of the obturator fossa and the anterolateral ligaments carrying the middle hemorrhoidal vessels. Nerve fibers course from the splanchnic nerve to the rectum through the anterolateral ligaments along the middle hemorrhoidal vessels. These nerves continue to either the vagina or the prostate as the nervi erigentes. A clear understanding of this nerve anatomy is critical because it is easily damaged during dissection and results in both sexual dysfunction and urinary bladder dysfunction (Figure 32-1*A*).

At the level of the sacral promontory, an areolar tissue plane begins behind the superior hemorrhoidal artery. The superior hemorrhoidal artery descends from the bifurcation of the inferior mesenteric artery and splits at approximately S1-2 to give two major trunks down the posterior aspect of the rectum. The mesorectal envelope encases the fat, lymphatic, and vascular structures to the rectum. The areolar tissue plane outside the mesorectal envelope is known as the "holy plane" and guides the dissection in the pelvis. A cross-sectional diagram of the pelvis shows the visceral peritoneum encasing the mesorectum with the areolar tissue plane between the visceral peritoneum and the parietal peritoneum posteriorly. The parietal peritoneum covers a nerve and venous plexus over the sacrum and the musculature of the side wall of the pelvis. Maintaining dissection within the areolar tissue plane between the parietal peritoneum and the visceral peritoneum protects all of the crucial structures in the pelvis (Figure 32-1*B*).

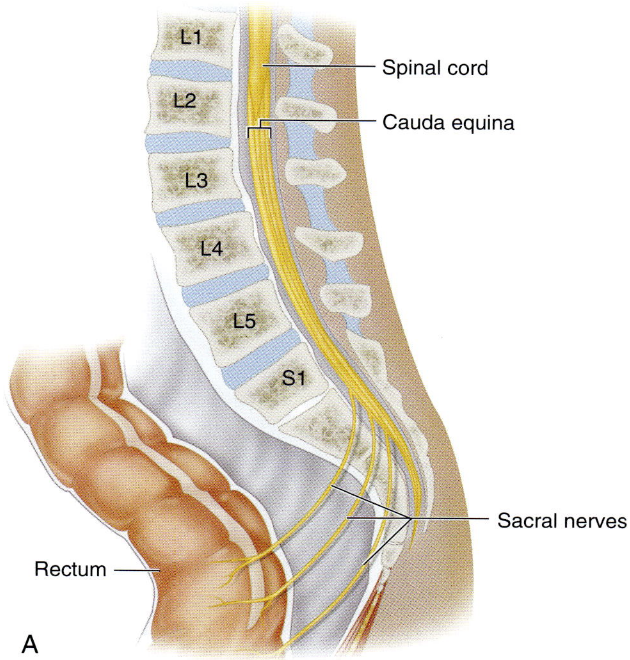

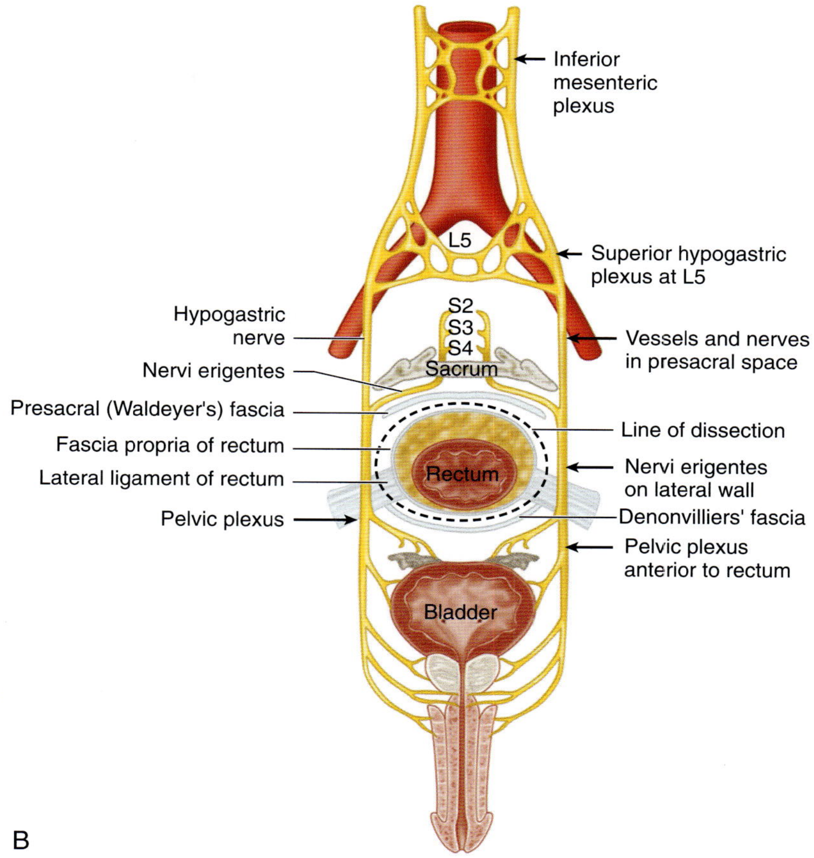

Figure 32-1

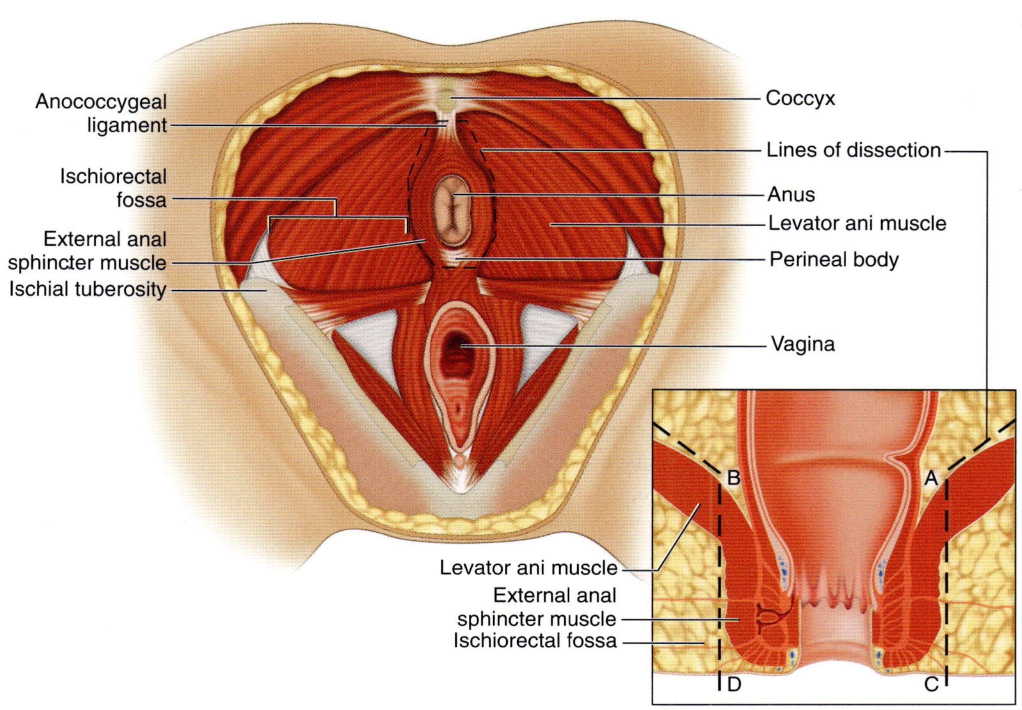

Figure 32-2

The rectum descends through the middle of the pelvis following the curve of the sacrum and at the level of the coccyx makes a right angle to exit through the pelvic floor via the anal canal. The levator ani muscles on either side of the pelvic floor form the support diaphragm of the pelvis and extend up onto the side wall of the pelvis to insert in the ischiospinous ligament attachments covering the nerves and vessels of the deep pelvic floor. The tip of the coccyx attaches to the pubococcygeal ligament, which supports the puborectalis muscle as a semicircular sling from the pubis around the back of the rectum. This muscle closes the top of the anal canal anterior to posterior (Figure 32-2).

The anterior pelvic structures including the bladder, prostate, and vagina are separated from the rectum by the rectoprostatic or rectovaginal septum. A visceral peritoneal layer known as Denonvilliers' fascia is the posterior boundary of the anterior structures. This fascia protects the seminal vesicles and prostate during dissection. The areolar tissue plane surrounding the fat of the mesorectum continues around the entire rectum to the anterior surface of the rectum below the cul-de-sac of the pelvis. The plane is found behind or posterior to Denonvilliers' fascia. The anterolateral ligaments of the rectum carry the middle hemorrhoidal vessels into the mesorectal envelope through the visceral fascia from an anterolateral direction. Dissection and transection of these middle hemorrhoidal vessels reveals the anterior areolar tissue plane behind Denonvilliers' fascia, which can be followed all the way down to the anal canal.

The ureters, which have been described as running into the pelvic area over the pelvic brim crossing the common iliac artery and vein on either side of the pelvis, continue into the pelvis along the side wall of the pelvis toward the posterior aspect of the bladder. In a nonoperated, pristine pelvis, the ureters are higher up along the side wall of the pelvis aiming toward the posterior aspect of the trigone of the bladder. In females, the ureters run between the arterial blood supply of the uterus along the anterolateral side wall of the pelvis. In males, ureters are not exposed during the distal pelvic dissection. The ureters may be drawn posteriorly after a previous operation but are normally fairly well protected anteriorly and laterally. In a previously operated pelvis, it is always wise to place ureteral stents at the beginning of the procedure to aid in identification of the aberrantly placed ureters.

Anal Anatomy

The upper anal canal begins at the puborectalis sling or the anorectal ring, which sits at the level of the pelvic floor and can be palpated through the anal canal as a bulge posteriorly (Figure 32-2). The longitudinal muscles of the rectum continue into the anus as the intersphincteric plane demarcating the line between autonomic internal sphincter and somatic external sphincter fibers all the way down to the level of the anal canal skin where the intersphincteric groove is palpable. The ischiorectal fossa fat is found outside the circular fibers of the external sphincter that encircle the rectum. The pudendal nerve and vessels traverse the ischiorectal fat from each ischial spine through Alcock's canal to the posterolateral aspect of the anal canal. During the perineal portion of a procedure, the pudendal nerves and vessels must be controlled.

The rectovaginal and rectoprostatic septum descends all the way to the level of the perineum anteriorly. The transverse perinei muscle separates the anterior and posterior perineum. The terminal fibers of the longitudinal muscle of the rectum insert into the skin of the anal canal just outside the anal verge as the corrugator cutanei ani and cause the ridges that are noticed around the anal canal. The internal sphincter is the hypertrophied circular muscle of the wall of the rectum. The lowest portion of the internal sphincter can be palpated as a groove where the longitudinal fibers insert on the skin.

Within the anal canal, the dentate line is the junction between the cuboidal epithelium of the anal transition zone, which is the terminal mucosal layer of the rectum, and the squamous epidermal cells of the anal canal skin. Gland openings (or crypts) are found in the dentate line at the base of the Morgagni columns, which are interdigitating lines of squamous epithelium into the cuboidal and columnar epithelium of the distal rectum. The anal transition zone is the most highly innervated section of the rectum and anal canal and contains nerve fibers sensing temperature, vibration, electrical stimulation, pressure, liquid, solid, and gas. The dentate line lies approximately halfway along the surgical anal canal, which extends from the palpable anal verge all the way up to the anorectal ring palpated at the puborectalis sling posteriorly. The anoderm within the anal canal, cephalad to the anal verge, has no hair follicles.

Step 2: Preoperative Considerations

The most common indication for sacrectomy and pelvic floor resection are retrorectal tumors arising in the distal third of the sacrum, including chordomas, costochondral sarcomas, or invasive cancers, usually adenocarcinoma, from duplication cysts of the low rectum. Many other rare tumors may manifest in this area and require excision with sacrectomy. In the case of recurrence of adenocarcinoma in the low pelvis, a sacrectomy is indicated only if there is no other systemic disease present and the tumor can be removed completely with sacrectomy. The risk of local recurrence in this situation is extremely high, and the morbidity of the procedure is also high, which makes the benefit-to-risk ratio unacceptable in all but the rarest circumstance. Anal canal cancer recurs frequently in the anal canal after chemoradiation or abdominal perineal resection and can be resected locally if there is no evidence of systemic disease and salvage chemoradiation is not an option.

Preoperative imaging is critical to plan the operation and determine resectability. Combined computed tomography scan and magnetic resonance imaging provides clear evidence of level of sacrum involvement. Tumors below the level of the body of S2 usually are considered resectable. However, local ingrowth into the table of S2 may be resectable if a nerve-sparing procedure can be done in conjunction with neurosurgery or orthopedic surgery. The key to deciding whether a higher resection level is possible is the ability to restore stability to the sacrum after resection of the bone. Nerve preservation should be considered for nerve roots S1 and S2, but S3 and S4 can usually be sacrificed without marked debility. S1 and S2 greatly influence ambulation, and S3 and S4 affect pelvic floor, bladder, and sexual function. In circumstances where the bladder and rectum are both sacrificed, the effects of S3 and S4 are usually not noticeable (Figure 32-3).

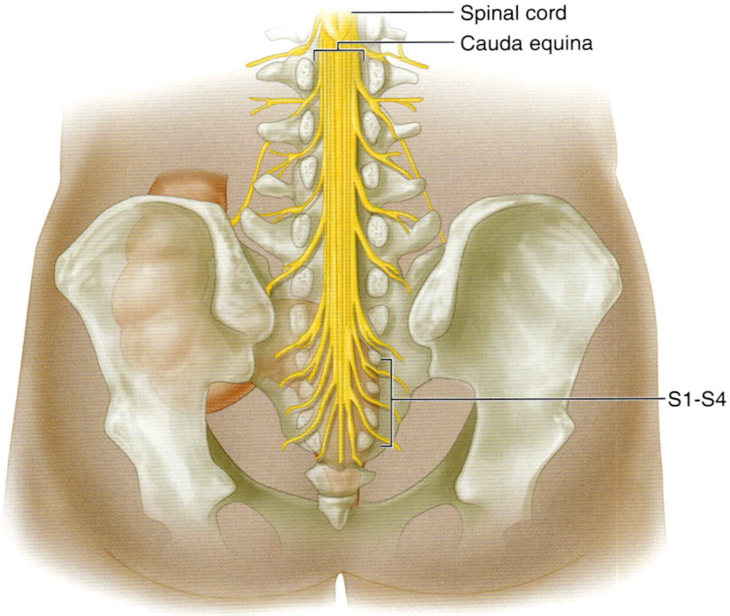

Figure 32-3

The spinal cord and cauda equina end at the level of L2 and L3. The nerves run within the spinal cord sac in the cauda equina to the level of the distal sacrum. In the areas of the sacrum, the nerves that are at risk are still only S2, S3, and S4 if the resection is at the S2-3 junction. Any resection higher than the level of S3-4 requires ligation of the dural sac and either ligation of the selected nerves or preservation of the important nerve roots S1-2.

Almost all patients require a colostomy after a major sacrectomy. In cases where a retrorectal tumor is being resected, an abdominal approach to the pelvis may be adequate to free the rectum from the anterior aspect of the tumor without risk of local recurrence. In these circumstances, the function of the pelvic floor and rectum should be considered based on the involvement of the nerve roots. If possible, the rectum and the pelvic floor should be spared, and the sacrectomy should be focused toward removing the tumor alone. When considering a permanent stoma, preoperative marking by an enterostomal therapist is helpful.

In patients with recurrent disease after a previous operation, ureteral stent placement is helpful to avoid damage to the ureters and the pelvis. The abdominal approach to releasing any abdominal contents from the pelvis before performing the sacrectomy should be considered.

A multidisciplinary team approach involving an orthopedist, neurosurgeon, urologist, and plastic surgeon is important, with the roles of all team members established before the operation to avoid confusion at the time of the procedure. Muscle flaps, skin flaps, cystectomy, ureteral reimplantation, nerve root identification, and dural ligation all are components of the procedure that may require other services. A bowel preparation is not essential but should be considered. Preoperative antibiotics and deep vein thrombosis (mechanical and chemical) prophylaxis should be considered. In patients who have had previous deep vein thromboses, a filter should be considered because of the high risk of pelvic venous thrombosis during the procedure. The pelvic portion of the procedure should be performed with the patient in the prone-jackknife position under general anesthesia with a roll under the hip, rolls under the chest, and the airways secured.

Step 3: Operative Steps for Sacrectomy below S1

- The patient is prepared and draped with the outline of the excision drawn on the buttock, gluteal cleft, and sacrum. The posterior ischial tuberosities and level of the lumbar sacral junction are marked (Figure 32-4).
- An elliptic incision is created to excise the area of tumor or to expose the sacrum adequately. A bear claw St. Mark's retractor is used to separate the edges of the incision, and the skin edges of the specimen are held together with Kocher clamps to provide traction. The sacrum is exposed at the upper limits of the sacrum to begin the dissection (Figure 32-5).
- The sacrum is completely exposed down to the tip of the coccyx. The anal canal or gluteal cleft skin is left attached to the specimen as the dissection is begun. Self-retaining retractors are placed to hold the edges of the wound apart and provide exposure. The sacrum is exposed all the way up to the level of S1 for proximal exposure (Figure 32-6).
- Rongeur bone cutters are used to open the S1-2 joint to expose the dural sac and the nerve roots as dictated by the tumor recurrence from anal cancer (Figure 32-7).

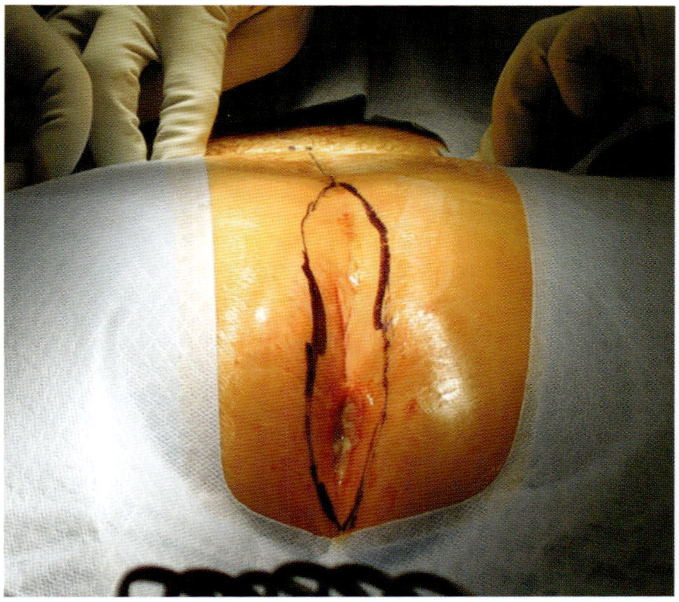

Figure 32-4

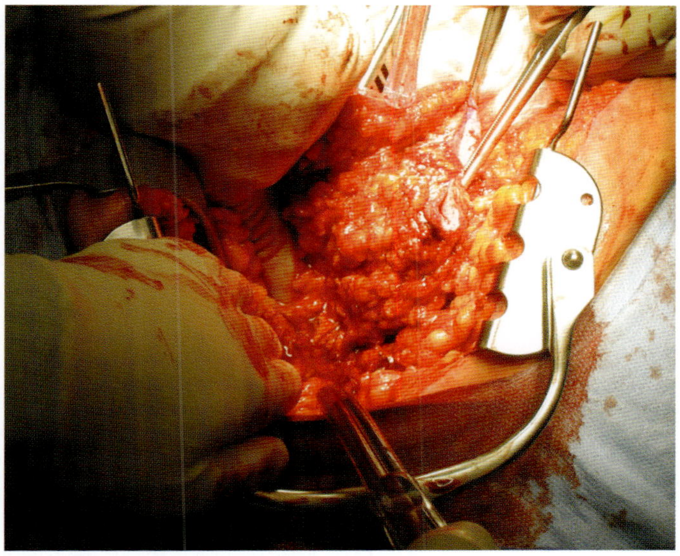

Figure 32-5

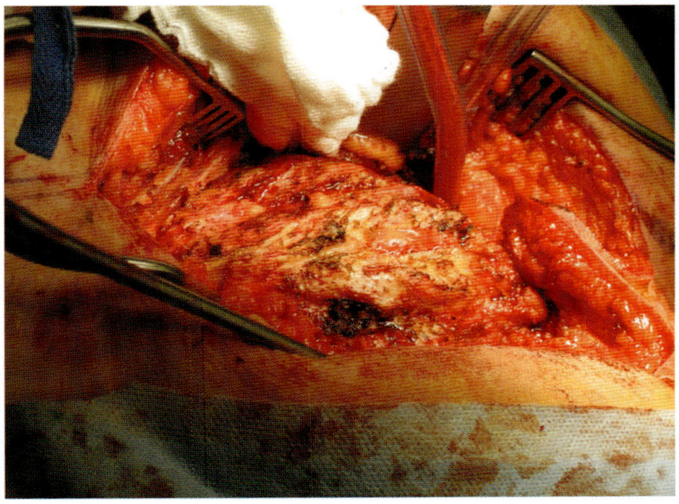

Figure 32-6

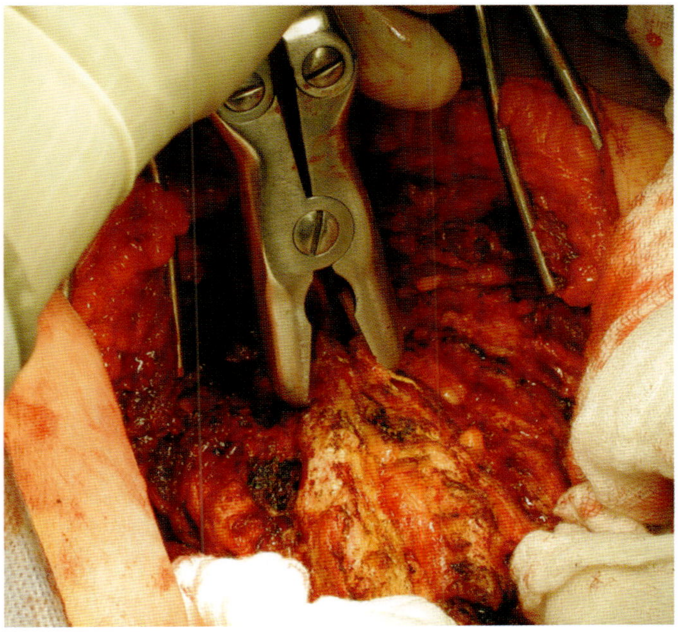

Figure 32-7

- The dura is exposed, and the dissection is carried down the cauda equina with good hemostasis and careful management of the dura (Figure 32-8). The medially placed S1-2 nerves are protected, and the laterally placed S3-4 nerves are isolated and divided (Figure 32-9*A*). The nerve roots are individually ligated, and the dural sac is ligated separate from the nerve roots, and S1 and S2 nerve roots are spared (Figure 32-9*B*).
- Using an osteotome, the anterior table of the sacrum between S1 and S2 is transected to enter the pelvis. Alternatively, a rotary saw can be used carefully. During the abdominal portion of the procedure, it is important to place a laparotomy sponge anterior to the sacrum to protect any of the abdominal contents from contact with the sharp orthopedic instruments (Figure 32-10).
- The cut surface of the S1 vertebral body is covered with bone wax, and the parietal peritoneum and the vessels of the presacrum are incised and controlled with either electrocautery or with individual ligation leaving the distal sacrum free and attached to the specimen (Figure 32-11).

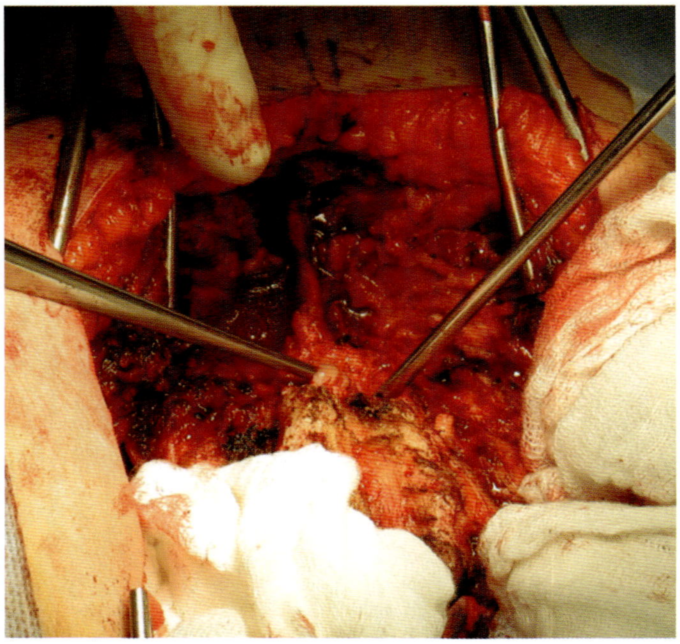

Figure 32-8

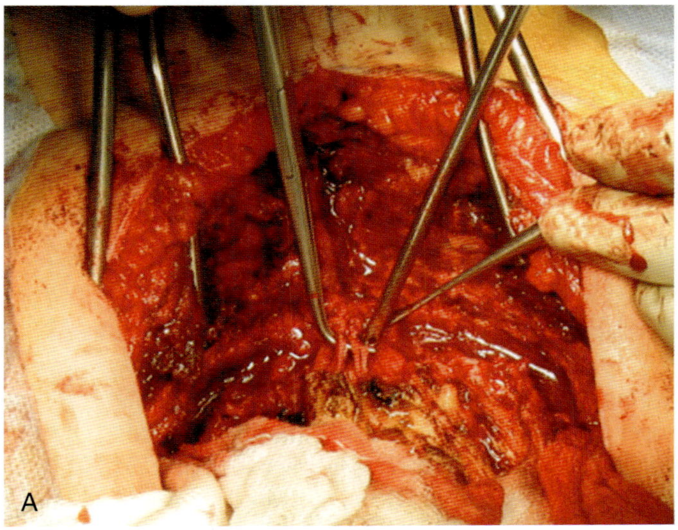

Figure 32-9A

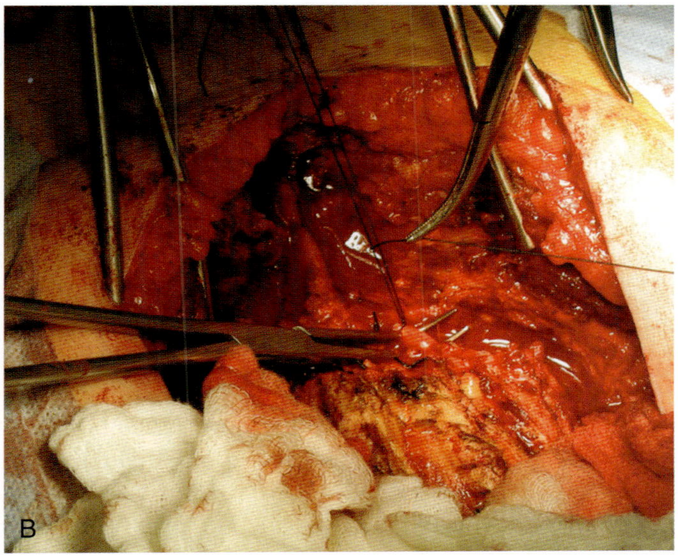

Figure 32-9B

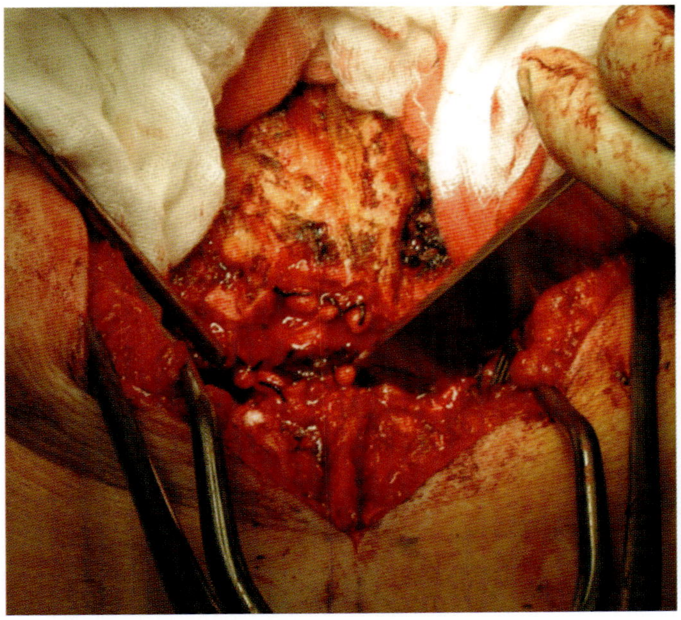

Figure 32-10

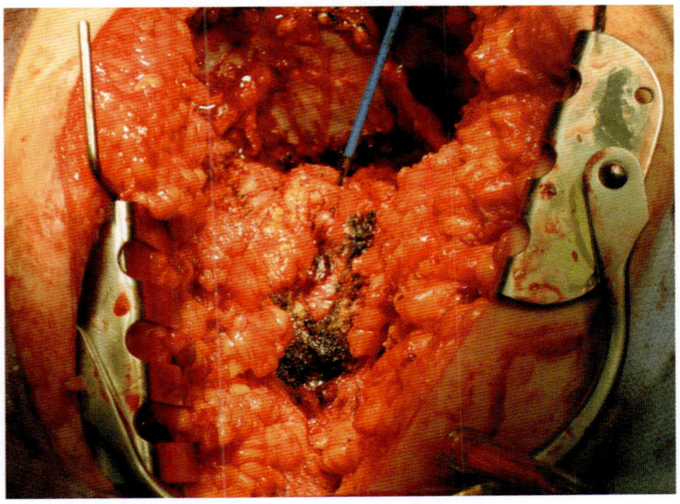

Figure 32-11

- With the sacrum freed from the upper levels of the vertebral column, the lateral muscular attachments of the sacrum to the pelvic floor are incised over guidance with a finger or with a large clamp (Figure 32-12). When both sides of the sacrum have been freed with incision of the pelvic muscles, the specimen can be removed en bloc to expose the anterior pelvis, the base of the upper sacrum, and the nerve roots that have been spared (Figure 32-13).
- The posterior pelvic drains should be placed in the abdomen and brought out through the gluteal flaps. The muscles are released to meet in the midline as far as possible and reapproximated with running nonabsorbable suture (Figure 32-14).
- The remaining defect is closed with biologic mesh if necessary. In extremely wide resections, it may be appropriate to begin with the mesh closure rather than trying to raise flaps. The pelvic drains are placed, and the mesh is secured to the cuff of the lateral pelvic floor muscles in a running horizontal mattress closure with permanent suture (Figures 32-15 and 32-16); this places the mesh within the pelvis overlaying the underlying muscles and provides a stronger repair than if the mesh was sewn to the outside of the muscle (Figure 32-17). The mesh should be placed in the defect and stretched as tightly as possible to provide a matrix for the muscles of the pelvic floor to grow across and prevent the development of herniation.
- The skin is mobilized with the underlying fat from the gluteal muscles to meet in the midline. The deep fat layer is approximated with interrupted figure-eight sutures of 2-0 or 3-0 absorbable suture, and the skin is closed with interrupted vertical mattress sutures to maintain closure. A large suction drain can be placed external to the biologic mesh to remove any accumulated fluid and reduce the risk of infection. Antibiotics are maintained for the length of time the drains are in place during the hospital stay.

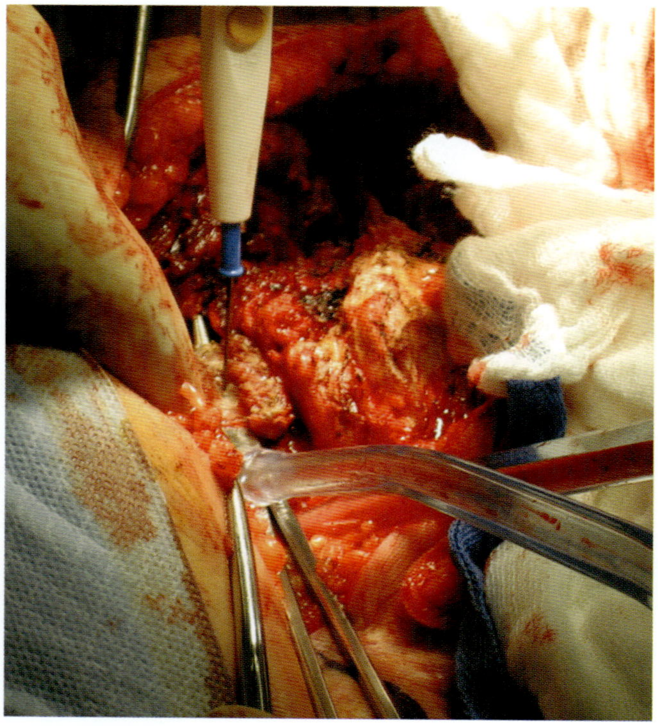

Figure 32-12

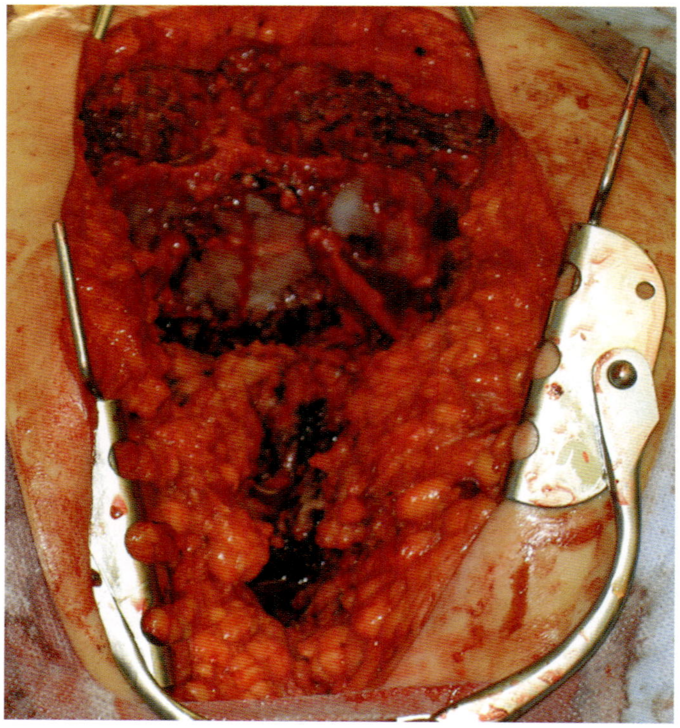

Figure 32-13

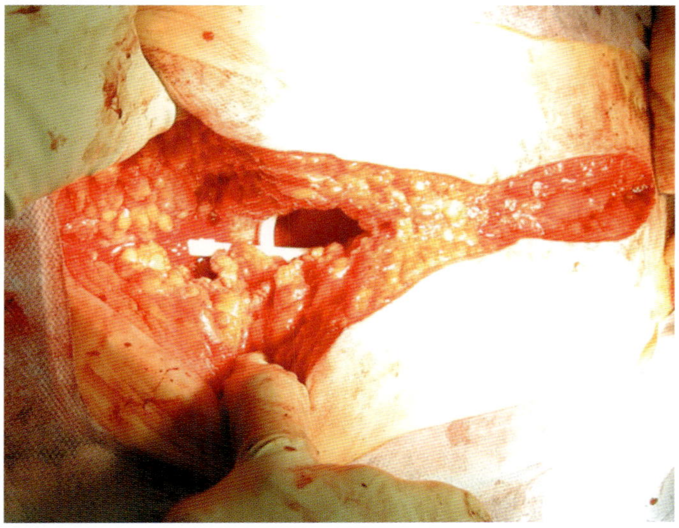

Figure 32-14

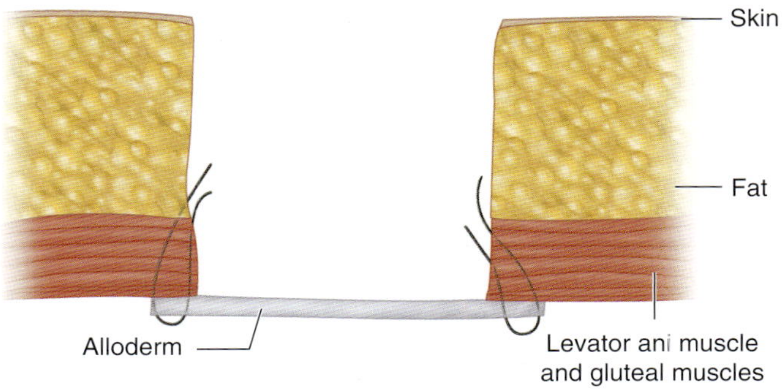

Figure 32-15

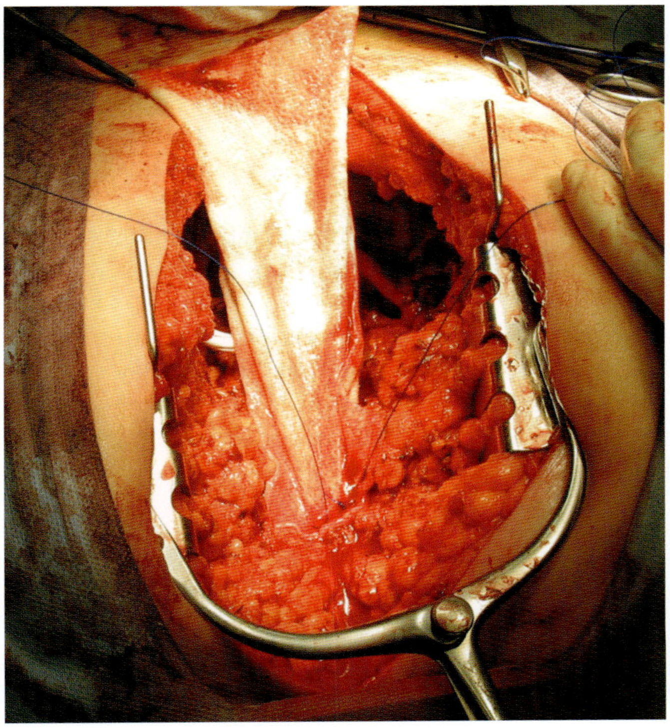

Figure 32-16

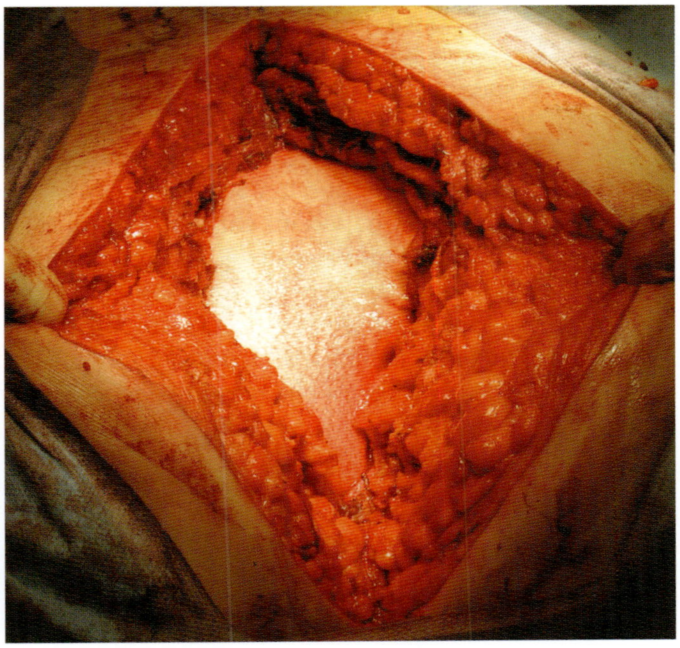

Figure 32-17

Step 4: Postoperative Care

This extensive procedure demands a longer in-hospital observation period in most circumstances. The patient is asked to avoid lying on the back for at least 5 days. In cases where most of the sacrum is removed and only S1 is left behind, there is risk of instability, and the patient is supported with physical therapy and ambulatory assistance at all times. Patients in whom only S3 to the coccyx is removed are allowed early mobility without restriction.

In the case of postoperative wound infection of the perineal wound, examination under anesthesia is required, and washout and decompression of any collection is required. If a pelvic collection develops during the postoperative period, it is advisable to perform an interventional radiology drainage procedure to avoid opening the wound if possible. The use of antibiotics as indicated is necessary to avoid severe infection and sepsis. The patient is requested not to sit, scoot, drive, or climb stairs for at least 2 weeks after surgery.

Step 5: Pearls and Pitfalls

As mentioned previously, this procedure requires a multidisciplinary team. The planning of the surgery requires input from an orthopedist or neurosurgeon; urologist; and colon and rectal surgeon, general surgeon, or oncologic surgeon. The decision to save or resect levels of sacrum should be made in conjunction with a radiologist experienced in identifying invasion of bone by pelvic tumors to determine the adequacy of the resection level.

The patient should be warned about the deficits that may occur after sacrectomy. With this communication, the patient develops appropriate expectations and is able to participate in the physical therapy recovery that is required.

Advance notice to the pathologist is key to receiving a comprehensive report on tumor resection. It is important to invite the pathologist to come to the operating room at the time of specimen removal to orient the pathologist to the specimen and enable him or her to provide information regarding the adequacy of margins.

Familiarity with available biologic mesh is critical in deciding on the closure technique. If the tumor is large and it is known early that flaps or transfer of muscle is required, a plastic surgeon may be an important part of the team early on.

The age of the patient is a major factor in the recovery of the patient. Young patients with severe disease may have an excellent outcome. Elderly patients with less significant disease may have a much worse outcome simply because the reserve of the patient is inadequate to overcome the debilitation that results from such a major resection as S2 through coccyx sacrectomy. Getting to know the patient is extremely important in the selection process.

Selected Readings

Dozois EJ, Jacofsky DJ, Billings BJ, et al. Surgical approach and oncologic outcomes following multidisciplinary management of retrorectal sarcomas. Ann Surg Oncol 2011;18:983–8.

Glasgow SC, Birnbaum EH, Lowney JK, et al. Retrorectal tumors: a diagnostic and therapeutic challenge. Dis Colon Rectum 2005;48:1581–7.

CHAPTER 33

Debulking and Peritoneal Stripping with Placement of Intraperitoneal Catheters for Carcinomatosis

James W. Fleshman, Jr.

Step 1: Clinical Anatomy

The right colon lies on the patient's right side suspended by peritoneal attachments to the right side of the abdominal wall, the undersurface of the liver, and the posterior diaphragm and by its mesentery from the medial aspect through which the ileocolic artery and vein and the right colic vessels, if present, run. The colon is adherent to the retroperitoneum on the right side of the abdomen and covers the right gonadal vessels and right ureter. The inferior vena cava is the next most medial structure on the right side. The hepatic flexure or the fold at the junction between the right colon and transverse colon is adherent to the anterior surface of the kidney by avascular attachments over the outside of Gerota's fascia. First and second portions of the duodenum are adherent to the undersurface of the mesentery of the right colon and the proximal aspect of the transverse colon. The gallbladder is sometimes adherent to the cephalad surface of the transverse colon at the hepatic flexure. The space behind the right colon is triangle-shaped with the flat horizontal surface at the hepatic flexure running from the abdominal side wall toward the midline along the line of the greater curve of the stomach. The vertical axis is found along the right gutter at the peritoneal attachment to the lateral side wall of the abdomen, and the hypotenuse runs from the fusion plane of the cecum at the pelvic brim over the top of the right iliac artery and vein at about the point where the ureter passes over the iliac vessels toward the midline over the aorta up to the base of the pancreas along the third portion of the duodenum. This triangular retroperitoneal area is an avascular space and allows the right colon to be lifted completely from the retroperitoneum during dissection; this allows the right colon to be made into a midline structure. The ileocolic artery and vein arise from the superior mesenteric artery and vein in the midportion of the superior mesenteric artery below the point of exit above the duodenum. The right colic artery is a variable structure and may not exist. The right branch of the middle colic artery exits through the pancreatic tissue from its origin on the superior mesenteric artery as a portion of the middle colic trunk at the base of the transverse mesocolon.

The left branch of the middle colic artery and vein arise adjacent to the right branch of the middle colic trunk and are found at the third portion of the duodenum over the pancreas. The inferior mesenteric vein travels along the window of the base of the mesentery of the left colon and enters the portal vein adjacent to the ligament of Treitz at the base of the splenic flexure mesentery. This area of the vasculature to the colon is extremely complex and should be studied carefully before mobilization of the transverse colon. The mesentery of the transverse colon itself is sometimes attached to filmy attachments of the posterior aspect of the stomach. The omentum falls from the gastroepiploic artery along the greater curve of the stomach over the transverse colon where it attaches tangentially to the antimesenteric surface of the transverse colon and continues to the lower aspect of the abdomen free-floating over the surface of the small bowel.

The splenic flexure of the colon sits in the left upper quadrant with a surface adherent to the undersurface of the tip of the spleen, the anterior surface of the left kidney, and the anterior surface of the tail of the pancreas. A portion of the base of the mesentery of the transverse colon is attached to the undersurface of the tail of the pancreas starting at the level of the inferior mesenteric vein and extending laterally toward the left side of the abdomen. These attachments can be released by developing avascular planes given knowledge of the peritoneal windows, areolar tissue planes, and structural relationships. The left colon itself is adherent to the retroperitoneum in the left gutter via an avascular filmy tissue plane that attaches the mesentery and left colon to the posterior abdominal wall where the ureter and gonadal vessels are found. The peritoneal attachments along the left gutter of the abdomen suspend the left colon from the left side of the abdomen from the pelvic brim all the way up to the splenic flexure. The splenic flexure is a fold of the colon with its apex attached to the tip of the spleen by omental congenital adhesions.

The splenic flexure is usually covered by the omentum as it falls over the top of the transverse colon along the left gutter, and numerous embryologic attachments can occur between the antimesenteric surface of the proximal left colon and the omentum at the splenic flexure. The left colon descends along the left gutter to the level of the pelvic brim where the colon becomes free from the pelvic side wall and falls into an S-shaped structure known as the sigmoid colon. The sigmoid colon lies free in the pelvis, attached only posteriorly to its vascular attachments at the midline over the sacral promontory.

The inferior mesenteric artery arises from the anterior surface of the aorta, proximal to the bifurcation at the common iliac vessels. The inferior mesenteric artery branches to give the superior hemorrhoidal artery descending to become the posterior mesorectal vessels and the ascending left colic vessel, which sweeps up toward the splenic flexure. The inferior mesenteric vein runs across the base of the mesentery of the left colon, crossing the superior hemorrhoidal and left colic vessels on its way to the duodenum. There is a clear peritoneal window between the aorta and the inferior mesenteric vein that can be used to enter the avascular plane behind the left colon mesentery and the retroperitoneum.

Pelvic Anatomy

The pelvic anatomy is complex with interrelationships between the rectum, vagina, uterus, ovaries, bladder, and prostate. The anatomy is important for pelvic dissection because of the various structures that are at risk, such as the splanchnic nerves (innervation of the bladder and sexual organs), the ureters, and the organs themselves. The common iliac artery and vein on each side of the sacral promontory course along the posterior aspect of the pelvic brim. The hypogastric plexus of parasympathetic and sympathetic nerves is found between the bifurcation of the aorta and common iliac vessels. This plexus coalesces to the right and left to become the splanchnic pelvic nerves, which run along the inner aspect of the pelvic side wall to the level of the obturator fossa and the anterolateral ligaments carrying the middle hemorrhoidal vessels.

Nerve fibers course from the splanchnic nerve to the rectum through the anterolateral ligaments along the middle hemorrhoidal vessels. These nerves continue to either the vagina or the prostate as the nervi erigentes. A clear understanding of this nerve anatomy is critical because it is easily damaged during dissection and results in both sexual dysfunction and urinary bladder dysfunction.

At the level of the sacral promontory, an areolar tissue plane begins behind the superior hemorrhoidal artery. The superior hemorrhoidal artery descends from the bifurcation of the inferior mesenteric artery and splits at approximately S1-2 to give two major trunks down the posterior aspect of the rectum. The mesorectal envelope encases the fat, lymphatic, and vascular structures to the rectum. The areolar tissue plane outside the mesorectal envelope is known as the "holy plane" and guides the dissection in the pelvis. A cross-sectional diagram of the pelvis shows the visceral peritoneum encasing the mesorectum with the areolar tissue plane between the visceral peritoneum and the parietal peritoneum posteriorly. The parietal peritoneum covers a nerve and venous plexus over the sacrum and the musculature of the side wall of the pelvis. Maintaining dissection within the areolar tissue plane between the parietal peritoneum and the visceral peritoneum protects all of the crucial structures in the pelvis.

The rectum descends through the middle of the pelvis following the curve of the sacrum and at the level of the coccyx makes a right angle posteriorly to exit through the pelvic floor via the anal canal. The levator ani muscles on either side of the pelvic floor form the support diaphragm of the pelvis and extend up onto the side wall of the pelvis to insert in the ischiospinous ligament attachments covering the nerves and vessels of the deep pelvic floor. The tip of the coccyx attaches to the pubococcygeal ligament, which supports the puborectalis muscle as a semicircular sling from the pubis around the back of the rectum. This muscle closes the top of the anal canal anterior to posterior.

The anterior pelvic structures including the bladder, prostate, and vagina are separated from the rectum by the rectoprostatic or rectovaginal septum. A visceral peritoneal layer known as Denonvilliers' fascia is the posterior boundary of the anterior structures. This fascia protects the seminal vesicles and prostate during dissection. The areolar tissue plane surrounding the fat of the mesorectum continues around the entire rectum to the anterior surface of the rectum below the cul-de-sac of the pelvis. The plane is found behind or posterior to Denonvilliers' fascia. The anterolateral ligaments of the rectum carry the middle hemorrhoidal vessels into the mesorectal envelope through the visceral fascia from an anterolateral direction. Dissection and transection of these middle hemorrhoidal vessels reveals the anterior areolar tissue plane behind Denonvilliers' fascia, which can be followed all the way down to the anal canal.

The ureters, which have been described as running into the pelvic area over the pelvic brim crossing the common iliac artery and vein on either side of the pelvis, continue into the pelvis along the side wall of the pelvis toward the posterior aspect of the bladder. In a nonoperated, pristine pelvis, the ureters are higher up along the side wall of the pelvis aiming toward the posterior aspect of the trigone of the bladder. In females, the ureters run between the arterial blood supply of the uterus along the anterolateral side wall of the pelvis. In males, ureters are not exposed during the distal pelvic dissection. The ureters may be drawn posteriorly after a previous operation but are normally well protected anteriorly and laterally. In a previously operated pelvis, it is always wise to place ureteral stents at the beginning of the procedure to aid in identification of the aberrantly placed ureters.

Step 2: Preoperative Considerations

The existence of abdominal carcinomatosis secondary to colon cancer that is confined to the abdominal cavity is a rare circumstance. However, these patients may benefit from a debulking of the tumor and application of intraperitoneal chemotherapy to provide some palliation or chance for cure. Carcinomatosis secondary to appendiceal adenocarcinoma and low-grade appendiceal mucin-producing neoplasm (pseudomyxoma peritonei), as it is now called, are also indications for debulking, peritoneal stripping, and placement of peritoneal dialysis catheters for intraperitoneal chemotherapy. It is imperative to rule out other disease outside of the abdominal cavity or within the liver. The poor prognosis associated with these diagnoses far outweighs the benefits of performing this extensive debilitating operation. The use of hyperthermic intraperitoneal early chemotherapy (HIPEC) has been associated with a very high incidence of complications. The use of delayed intraperitoneal chemotherapy with peritoneal dialysis catheters placed at the time of debulking has alleviated some of these complications and allowed patients to receive a full dose of intraperitoneal chemotherapy. Early results suggested outcomes equivalent to HIPEC.

Patients should be counseled regarding the potential for a wide excision of the colon and rectum and portions of the small intestine, stomach, spleen, tail of pancreas, and diaphragms. The debulking procedure works only if the final result is a complete removal of all disease. A complete debulking (CC-O = Completeness of Cytoreduction to <2 mm maximum size of residual tumor) results in a better outcome and the longer disease-free survival for the patient.

The patient should undergo a complete bowel preparation and receive appropriate prophylactic antibiotics. An enterostomal therapist should mark the potential stoma site, and an intensive care unit (ICU) bed should be reserved for the patient postoperatively because of the massive fluid shifts that occur. Chemical and mechanical deep vein thrombosis prophylaxis is recommended because of the high likelihood of thromboembolic disease in the setting of cancer and in long operations. The average time for this procedure is 4 hours.

Step 3: Operative Procedure

- The patient is placed in the supine position with sequential compression devices in place and a bladder catheter in place, and the abdomen is prepared and draped sterilely. A midline incision is used to enter the abdomen from xiphoid to pubis; a Bookwalter retractor is very helpful for exposure. The operation is begun by debulking the mesenteric and serosal surface implants, removing any portions of small bowel, spleen, and stomach that can be removed (Figure 33-1). The dissection of the mesenteric implants can be performed in such a way that the underlying vessels of the mesentery are preserved. Only the peritoneal surface and a very thin layer of the fat is removed, and the serosal implants are plucked from the surface of the bowel if there is no invasion (Figure 33-2). Invasive cancer has to be removed with resection of the bowel. It is important to minimize the length of bowel removed by consolidating the number of implants in the resected specimens.
- The omentum is removed from the greater curve of the stomach using either ties to control the short gastric vessels and gastroepiploic arcade or a sealing source that employs radiofrequency ablation or ultrasound. The procedure is generally speeded up when sealing instrumentation is available. The entire omentum along the greater curve adjacent to the spleen all the way to the first portion of the duodenum is removed because of the high likelihood of cancer cells being present within the omentum (Figure 33-3).
- The abdominal wall peritoneal surface is removed along the midline incision initially. The posterior fascia of the rectus is removed with the peritoneum from the upper to the lower portion of the rectus (Figures 33-4 and 33-5). The posterior rectus fascia tends to adhere densely to the lateral edge of the rectus muscle, and this must be incised to enter the more lateral space to begin the lateral peritoneal dissection (Figure 33-6).

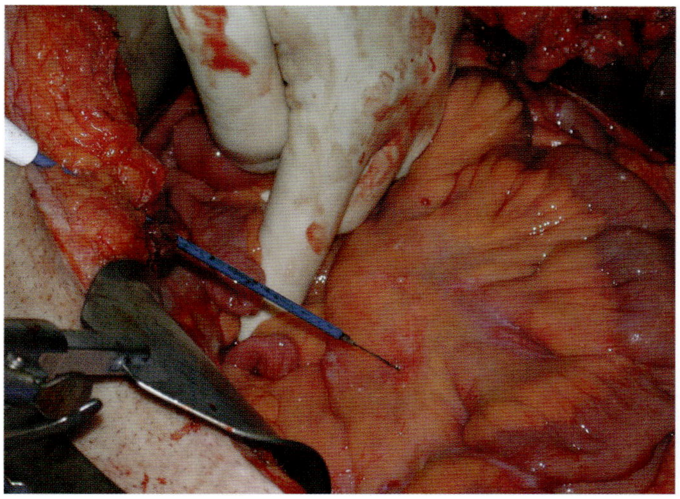

Figure 33-1

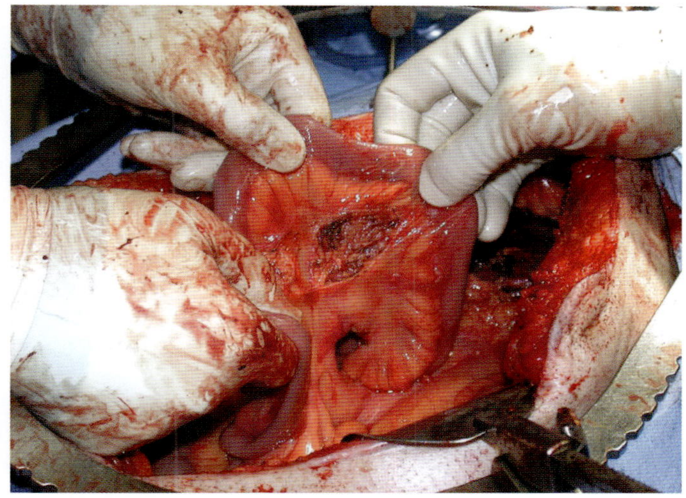

Figure 33-2

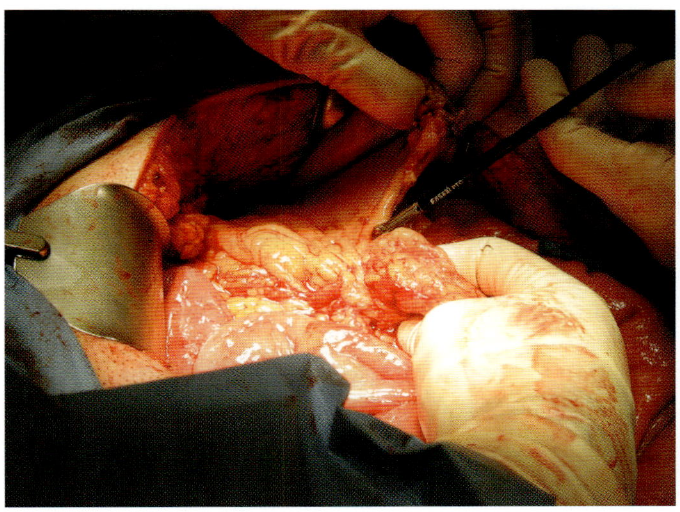

Figure 33-3

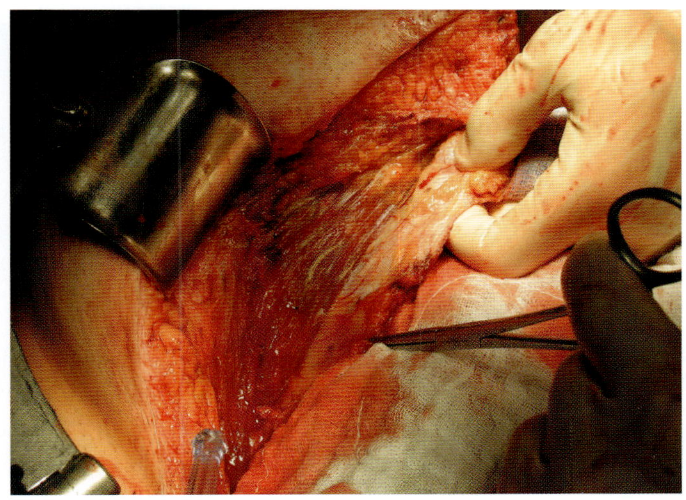

Figure 33-4

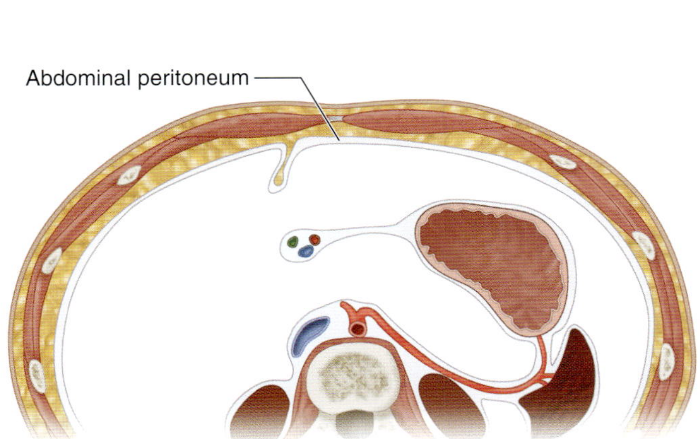

Figure 33-5

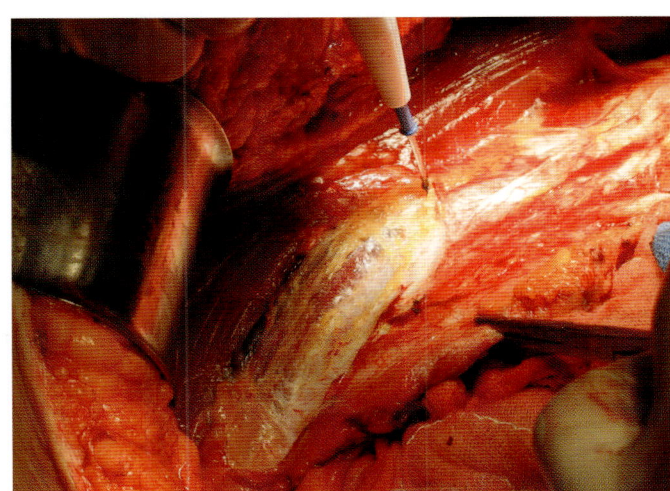

Figure 33-6

- The transition between the posterior rectus fascia and into the lateral retromuscular space requires a very detailed dissection to avoid making holes in the peritoneum outside the rectus sheath. There is no posterior fascia of the transversalis muscle, but the fat in this area provides a plane for cautery dissection as tension is applied to the peritoneum toward the midline and lateral traction is provided on the muscle with the Bookwalter retractor (Figure 33-7).
- The right gutter and the right retroperitoneum become visible at the lateral extent of the abdominal wall. The avascular plane becomes usable behind the colon, and this can be followed all the way to the midline over the inferior vena cava on the right and up to the aorta on the left. The muscle should be released from the fold in the peritoneal reflection, and the peritoneum should be peeled out of the retroperitoneum toward the midline (Figure 33-8).
- Next, the peritoneal covering of the side wall of the abdomen can be lifted up as a whole (Figure 33-9). The entire dissection has progressed from the right upper quadrant to the pelvis. Removing the undersurface of the diaphragm is more difficult, and this should be done in a separate effort beginning at the anterior midline and extending toward the dome of the diaphragm on the right and left in separate dissections. The cardia of the diaphragm is very difficult to dissect, and this portion of the diaphragm may be left unremoved; this can be excised only with use of a mesh replacement. The muscles of the diaphragm are attached to the peritoneal surface and can, with some difficulty, be released from the peritoneum.
- The iliac fossa on the right is uncovered all the way to the edge of the bladder and over the iliac vessels protecting the ureter, gonadal vessels, and hypogastric and lateral femoral cutaneous nerves, if possible. Any or all of these structures may be involved with overlying tumor invasion and can be sacrificed as needed. The iliac fossa peels toward the midline in the same avascular plane behind the colon up onto the back of the bladder (Figure 33-10).
- The left side of the abdomen can be released in the same way as the right beginning at the midline and extending to the lateral edge of the rectus removing the posterior rectus fascia and entering the avascular plane behind the left colon along the left gutter (Figure 33-11).
- The left iliac fossa with the inguinal ring, gonadal vessels, and ureter is freed toward the midline into the pelvis with the overlying peritoneal flap intact (Figure 33-12).

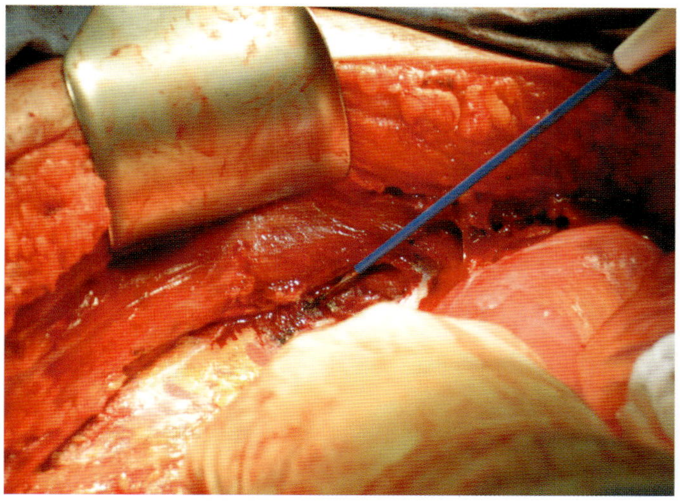

Figure 33-7

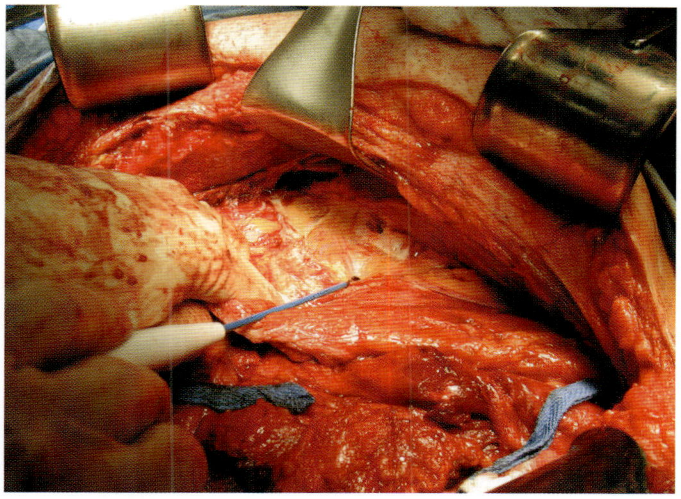

Figure 33-8

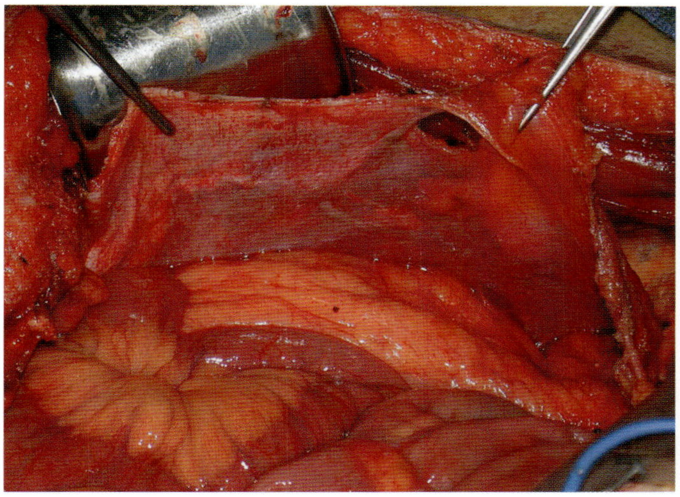

Figure 33-9

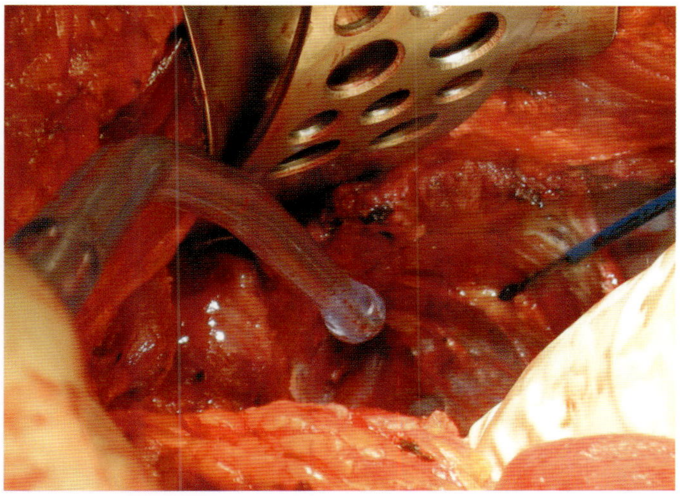

Figure 33-10

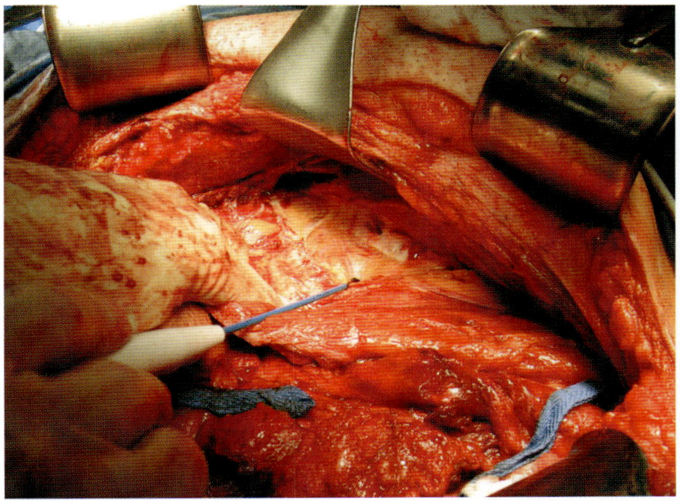

Figure 33-11

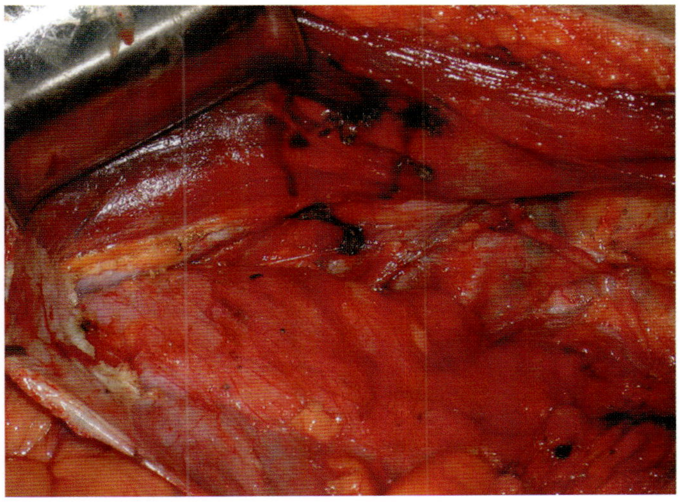

Figure 33-12

- The small bowel is packed from the pelvis using a flexible sponge-covered retractor (Figure 33-13), and the dissection begins in the pelvis using the same avascular plane at the pelvic brim on both sides to dissect behind the rectum down to the pelvis, around the pelvic side walls, and up onto the back of the bladder (Figure 33-14).
- After the peritoneum has been dissected from the posterior aspect of the bladder, the rectum is divided below the cul-de-sac in an area where there is no tumor. The bladder is freed from the pubis and the posterior peritoneum to ensure that all of the tissue in the anterior pelvis has been removed (Figure 33-15).

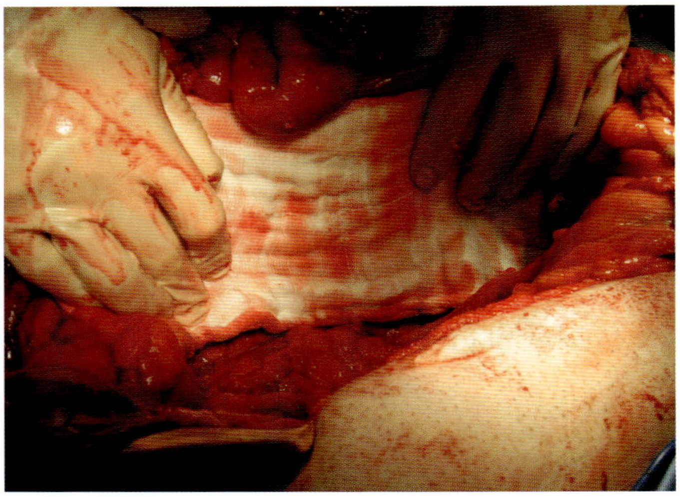

Figure 33-13

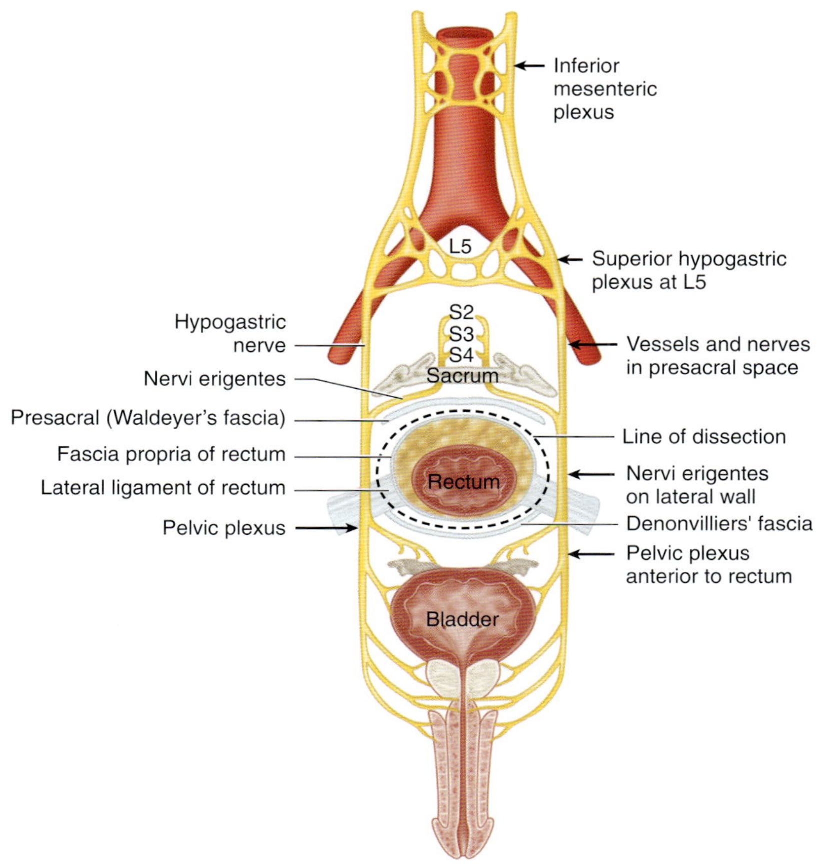

Figure 33-14

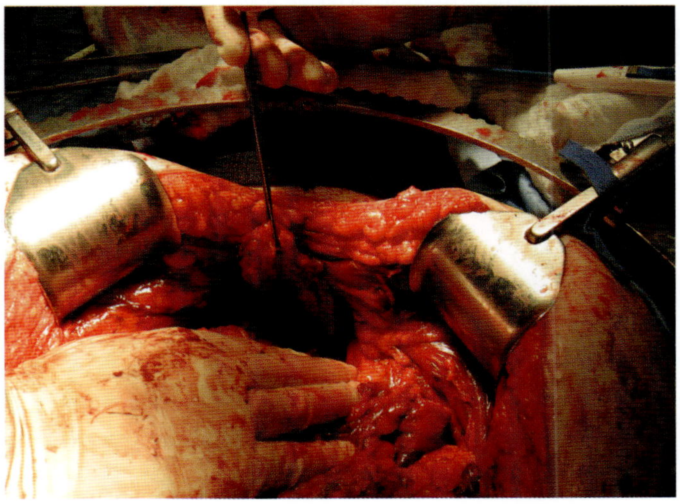

Figure 33-15

- The specimen can be removed after the colon with implants has been freed from the posterior vascular pedicles along the left side at the inferior mesenteric artery and vein, in the middle at the transverse colon at the middle colic vessels, and along the right side removing the ileocolic vessels and dividing the terminal ileum at a site where there is no disease. The resulting specimen en bloc is very large. The rectum, posterior bladder, and cul-de-sac are a closed envelope without tumor present on the surface (Figure 33-16).
- After the colon, peritoneal omentum, rectum, and portion of small bowel have been removed, the abdomen is relatively empty with the retroperitoneal structures preserved and all bulk disease removed (Figure 33-17). A patient who has had a total proctocolectomy is given a permanent end ileostomy unless there is enough small bowel and distal rectum left to perform an ileal pouch–anal anastomosis in the future, after 1 year of recovery without recurrence of disease.
- Placement of the peritoneal dialysis catheters requires a creation of a pocket in the subcutaneous tissue over the lower rib cage on the left and right. A site for tunneling the peritoneal dialysis catheter is made in the upper portion of the rectus muscle in a line inferior to the access pocket site (Figure 33-18).
- The peritoneal dialysis catheter is tunneled from the access pocket site to the abdominal insertion site over the rectus muscle and into the abdominal cavity. This tunneling is performed on both sides of the abdomen (Figure 33-19).
- The peritoneal dialysis catheter is trimmed and hooked to the access port. The port is inserted into the pocket and secured with 3-0 permanent sutures in two positions. The skin is closed over the pocket and the tunneling site with staples (Figure 33-20).
- Once both ports have been placed and the peritoneal dialysis catheters are within the abdominal cavity, 12 full sheets of an adhesion barrier are placed throughout the abdominal cavity to cover all raw surfaces and to provide adequate diffusion space for intraperitoneal chemotherapy (Figure 33-21).

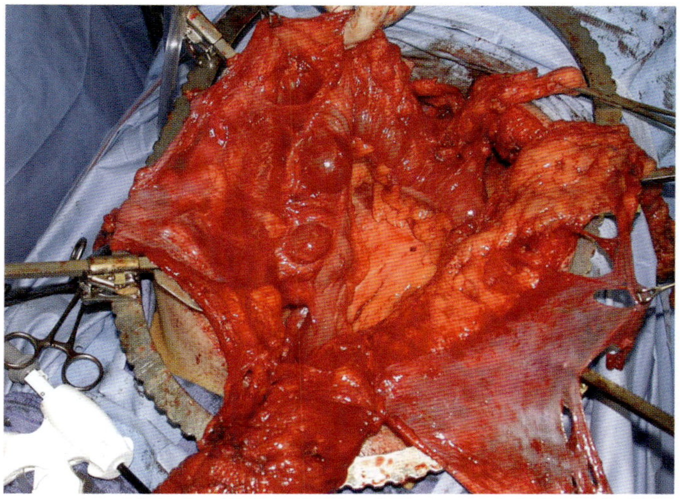
Figure 33-16

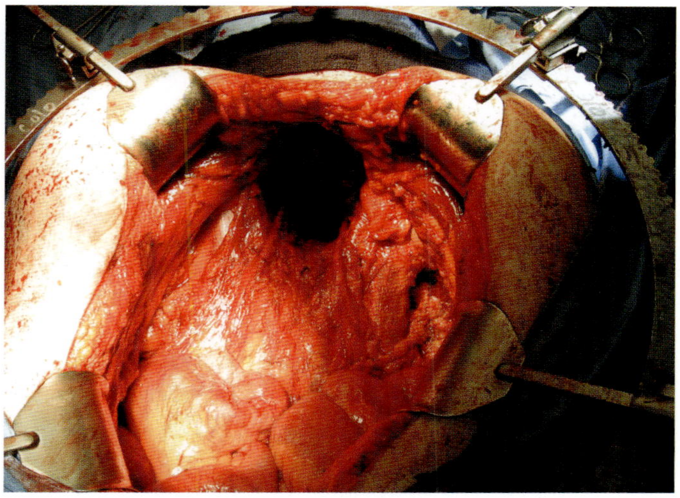
Figure 33-17

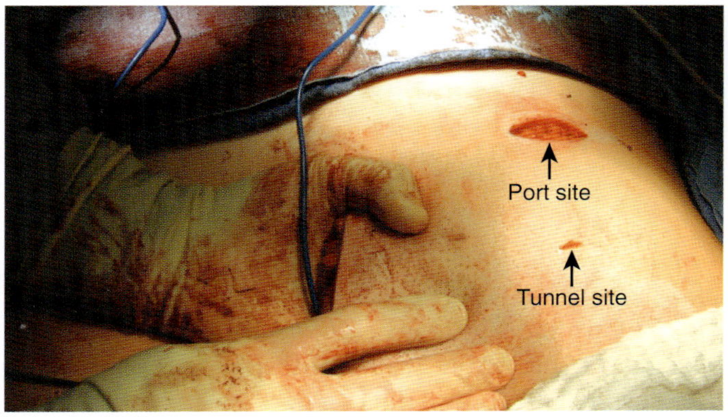

Figure 33-18

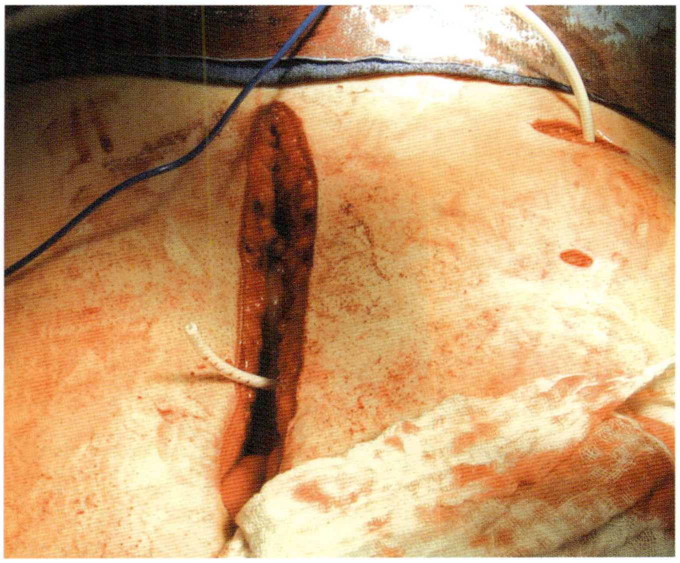
Figure 33-19

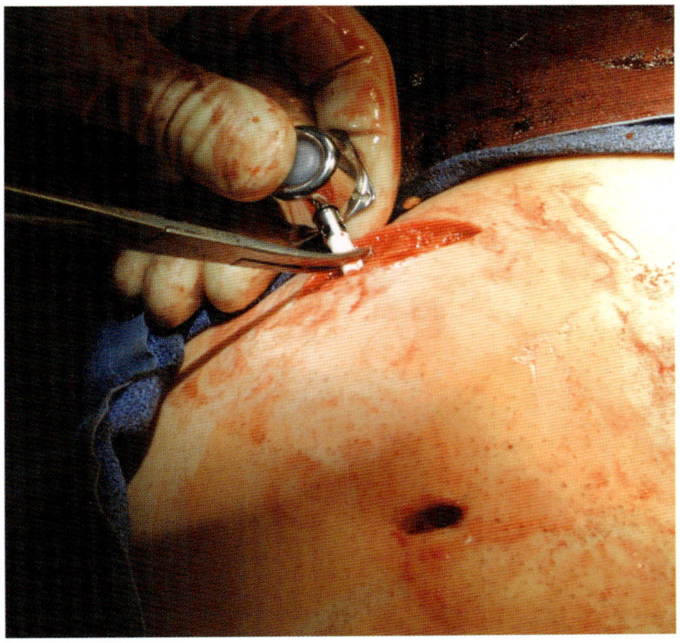
Figure 33-20

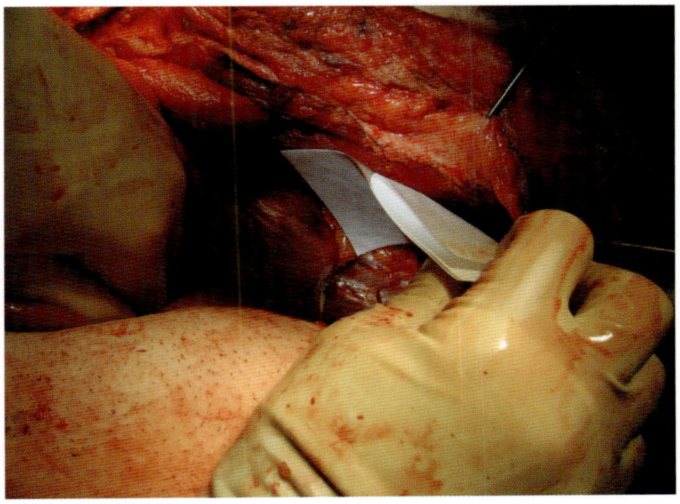
Figure 33-21

- The adhesion barrier is wrapped around the peritoneal dialysis catheter within the abdominal cavity to protect the catheter from any adhesion formation. The surfaces of the small bowel are also covered. The pelvis and the surfaces under the diaphragm are also protected (Figure 33-22).
- The ileostomy is brought out through the appropriate site at the previously marked stoma site. An adhesive barrier is placed around the stoma and over the peritoneal dialysis catheter lateral to the ileostomy site to provide adequate diffusion space lateral to the stoma (Figure 33-23). The abdominal wall is closed with a running No. 1 absorbable suture. The subcutaneous skin is irrigated and closed with skin staples. The wound is protected, and the ileostomy is matured by placing three-point sutures of 3-0 absorbable material around the circumference to create a 2.5-cm spigot. The ostomy appliance is applied taking care to avoid any contamination to the access port sites. The patient is returned to the surgical ICU for close monitoring, fluid replacement, and blood product replacement as needed.

Step 4: Postoperative Care

The usual course of a patient undergoing this massive operation is 2 weeks in the hospital with 1 week spent in an ICU setting or at least an observation unit setting. The peritoneal dialysis catheters should not be used for at least 1 month after the procedure. Before infusion of chemotherapy, a technetium-99m scan should be performed with injection of both ports to ensure that there is space for infusion of chemotherapy. If one port does not function properly, the other port may function adequately to provide benefit to the patient.

The return of ileostomy function signals the bowel is ready for alimentation. Patients are advanced in their diet and learn stoma care from the enterostomal therapy nurse. Patients are maintained on antibiotics throughout the course of the hospital stay because the catheters are placed in a potentially contaminated setting. Chemical and mechanical deep vein thrombosis prophylaxis is continued. Ambulation is possible early after the operation. Follow-up is usually within 2 weeks after discharge.

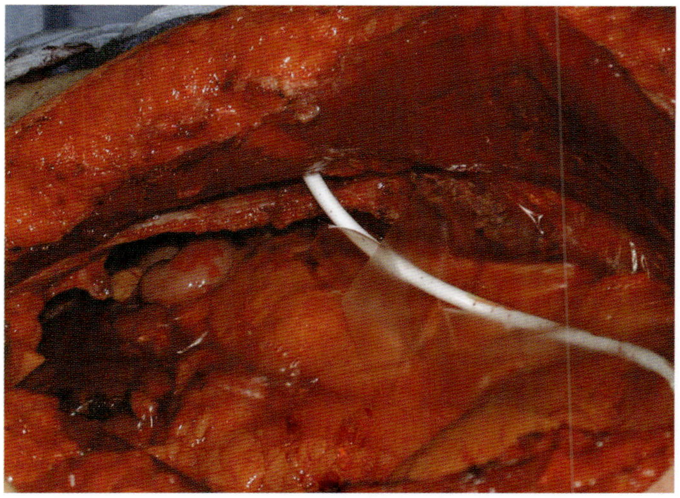

Figure 33-22

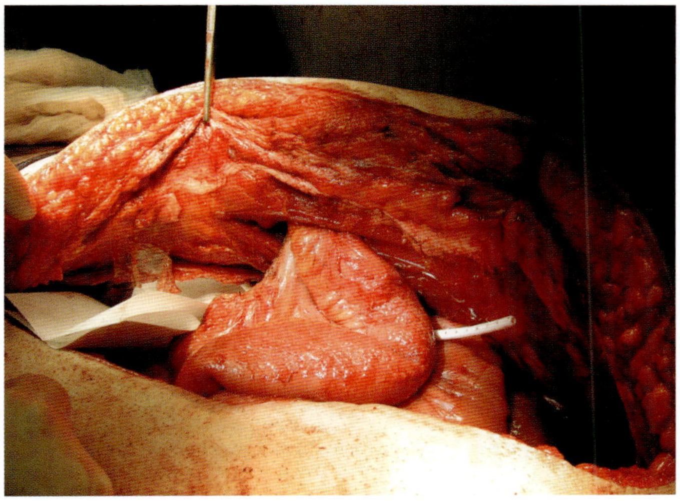

Figure 33-23

Step 5: Pearls and Pitfalls

Total proctocolectomy is not always necessary for complete debulking. The minimization of anastomoses within the abdominal cavity is important. However, complete debulking of the tumor should be the goal, as opposed to preservation of bowel or organs.

The dialysis catheters may not function properly at the early injection of technetium-99m during the planning of intraperitoneal chemotherapy. If the patient returns 2 to 4 weeks later and repeats the infusion, the adhesive process may have softened enough to allow diffusion through one or the other of the catheters.

Infection of the catheter or access port requires removal, as does erosion of the catheter or port through the skin. Care must be taken to avoid superficial placement of the peritoneal dialysis catheter during the tunneling process. The goal should be that this is always behind Scarpa's fascia.

The decision to proceed with a massive debulking and creation of a short bowel syndrome should be discussed with the patient before the operation. If this outcome is a possibility, abortion of the procedure is the usual approach rather than forcing the patient to accept a lifetime of total parenteral nutrition and high stoma output. The use of octreotide, codeine, opium drops, and maximalization of loperamide (Imodium) and diphenoxylate (Lomotil) can sometimes reverse the short bowel syndrome. However, if the patient is an accepting candidate for operation and postoperative chemotherapy, a procedure resulting in maximum debulking is appropriate. The indications for this procedure are rare. Embarking on this course of treatment for an unknowing, unsuspecting patient can bring suffering to the patient and the physician. A complete, well-informed consent is necessary before recommending such an invasive operation.

Selected Readings

Vaira M, Cioppa T, D'Amico S, et al. Treatment of peritoneal carcinomatosis from colonic cancer by cytoreduction, peritonectomy and hyperthermic intraperitoneal chemotherapy (HIPEC): experience of ten years. In Vivo 2010;24:79–84.

Verwaal VJ, Bruin S, Boot H, et al. 8-year follow-up of randomized trial: cytoreduction and hyperthermic intraperitoneal chemotherapy versus systemic chemotherapy in patients with peritoneal carcinomatosis of colorectal cancer. Ann Surg Oncol 2008;15:2426–32.

Index

Page numbers followed by f indicate figures.